Textbook of
Advanced Cardiac Life Support

Editor

Richard O. Cummins, MD, MPH, MSc

Subcommittee on Advanced Cardiac Life Support, 1991-1994

Richard O. Cummins, MD, MPH, MSc, Chair
Joseph P. Ornato, MD, Immediate Past Chair
Norman S. Abramson, MD
Lance Becker, MD
John E. Billi, MD
Charles G. Brown, MD
Nisha Chibber Chandra, MD

Roy V. Ditchey, MD
Jay L. Falk, MD
Nora F. Goldschlager, MD
Edgar R. Gonzalez, PharmD
Jerris R. Hedges, MD, MS
Karl B. Kern, MD
Katherine A. Littrell, MSN, RN

Mary E. Mancini, MSN, RN
Arthur J. Moss, MD
Paul E. Pepe, MD
Linda Quan, MD
Arthur B. Sanders, MD
Corey Slovis, MD

Committee on Emergency Cardiac Care, 1991-1994

Joseph P. Ornato, MD, Chair
Richard E. Kerber, MD, Immediate Past Chair
Richard O. Cummins, MD, Vice-Chair
Richard K. Albert, MD

Donald D. Brown, MD
Nisha Chibber Chandra, MD
Mary Fran Hazinski, MSN, RN
Richard J. Melker, MD, PhD

Linda Quan, MD
W. Douglas Weaver, MD

© 1994, American Heart Association

ISBN 0-87493-626-8

Contributors and Consultants

Harold P. Adams, Jr., MD
Wendy Adams, RN
Richard V. Aghababian, MD
James M. Atkins, MD
Thomas P. Aufderheide, MD
John Auricchio, PharmD
William H. Barth, Jr., MD
Dean Brooke, REMT-P
Frederick M. Burkle, Jr., MD
Leon Chameides, MD
James Christenson, MD
Timothy J. Crimmins, MD
Paula Derr, RN
Steven Dronen, MD
Mickey S. Eisenberg, MD, PhD

Gordon A. Ewy, MD
Phil B. Fontanarosa, MD
Mads Gilbert, MD
Judith Reid Graves, RN, EMT-P
Allan S. Jaffe, MD
William Kaye, MD
Walter G. J. Kloeck, MD, BCh
Kristian Lexow, MD
Bernard Lo, MD
L. Murray Lorance
Kevin M. McIntyre, MD, JD
Terry Mengert, MD
George E. Membrino, PhD
Steven G. Miller, MD
William H. Montgomery, MD

Lawrence D. Newell, EdD, EMT-D
Norman A. Paradis, MD
John A. Paraskos, MD
Ronald W. Quinsey, NREMT-P
Peter Safar, MD
Richard Swanson, MD
Scott Syverud, MD
William H. Thies, PhD
Andrew D. Weinberg, MD
Roger D. White, MD
Nancy Wood, RN
Brian S. Zachariah, MD
Arno Zaritsky, MD

Reviewers

Jeanette Abundis, MN, RN
John W. Becher, DO
Ron Benoit, EMT-P
Nancy Bernard, RN
Susan Callaghan-Montella, RN

David M. Cline, MD
David Connor, MD
Nabil El Sanadi, MD
David L. Freedman, MD
Donald J. Gordon, MD

Joel Harrison, DMD
Thomas Herrin, MD
Mitchell L. Mutter, MD
Henry Perez, MD
Amelia Selph, RN

Special Acknowledgments

Many AHA staff members have worked diligently to make the *Textbook of Advanced Cardiac Life Support* possible. Their contribution to this edition of the textbook is reflected in its high quality, and for this we thank them. In particular, we thank F. G. Stoddard, AHA copy editor, who has devoted long hours to shaping this work in all dimensions — style, literacy, accuracy, and organization. He is highly competent, hardworking, and blessed with a sparkling wit and good humor. The final quality of this textbook is due in large part to his labors. The editor and contributors extend to F. G. our deepest gratitude.

Contents

Preface

Ask any healthcare worker, "Do you remember your first ACLS course?" You will be greeted with a wry smile and a nodding head. Most people recall vividly that information-packed, intense weekend course where instructors first introduced them to "the ACLS approach." The American Heart Association, with its support of emergency cardiac care training, has achieved an enormous educational success. Almost every medical institution and Emergency Medical Services System in the United States conducts BLS and ACLS training year round. Almost every doctor, nurse, medical student, respiratory therapist, emergency technician, and paramedic can be glimpsed, at some point in their career, clutching this ACLS textbook in their hand and cramming for an ACLS course.

ACLS "clicked" with many of these participants. They caught the resuscitation bug. Over the years they continued to devote a major part of their professional life to learning more about cardiac emergencies. They became ACLS instructors, imparting their lessons to the next generations of ACLS providers. Most of the contributors to this textbook will see themselves in these words. Some of you reading this book for the first time will join the ranks of seasoned instructors and mature researchers.

ACLS challenges people with its "high density" of information. We must, however, avoid viewing ACLS as simply algorithms, protocols, and drug doses to stuff into our memories and regurgitate for some unsmiling instructor. The ACLS concept embodies much more than a collection of cognitive and psychomotor skills. At its core, ACLS presents a way of thinking, a systematic approach to dealing with people experiencing a cardiopulmonary emergency or even sudden death. ACLS presents a way for resuscitation providers to treat a desperately ill patient in a coordinated way, regardless of whether the response team consists of one person, two people, or a swirling group of 15. ACLS-trained providers will use the same guidelines, the same approaches, inside the hospital as outside the hospital, nationally as well as internationally.

Of necessity, ACLS also deals with death. ACLS starts with those people experiencing severe cardiopulmonary compromise. Their hearts have either stopped to function or are about to stop. Some hearts are too good to die — some are too sick to live. Part of your job is to determine which one you are treating. ACLS helps distinguish between those people who, through your quick and diligent efforts, return to continue their life and those people who plainly have reached the end of their life. They may need a hand to hold rather than a hand to pump their chest.

You are not going to save everyone with your ACLS techniques. In fact, most of your ACLS efforts for people in cardiac arrest will fail. The majority of resuscitation attempts end with death, not life. Life continues, however, in the victim's friends, relatives, and loved ones and in your colleagues who helped in the resuscitation attempt. Remember, the moment resuscitative efforts stop, you acquire a new set of patients — the family, the survivors, your team members, and yourself.

Sometimes ACLS leaves us with a tragedy — the tragedy of people whose hearts we get back but not their minds. These are the victims whose thoughts, creativity, and emotions diminish, perhaps even vanish, during the resuscitation attempt. We are left with a beating heart and moving lungs but little else. We must learn how to avoid this sad outcome. Rapid restoration of a beating heart remains the best way to restart a thinking brain. Yet many hospitals and communities have failed to develop strength in each link in the chain of survival. Every person who learns ACLS must ask whether his or her hospital and community has prepared itself to deal rapidly and effectively with sudden cardiac death.

Most of all, however, ACLS is about saving lives. ACLS is about "resuscitation." ACLS is about restoring life and turning back the catastrophe of sudden death or profound cardiac and respiratory compromise. ACLS is about people: with "foreign-body–obstructed trachea" comes a smiling child who insists on running with small toys in her mouth; with "lungs filled with pulmonary edema" comes a rheumatic young woman with three small children at home; with "coarse VF" comes a busy executive who forgot to hug his child that morning; with "profound vascular collapse" comes a grand matriarch whose anxious family is already filling the waiting room.

Finally, ACLS is about preparing yourself — preparing yourself to provide the best care possible for the most dramatic and emotional moment of a person's life. We think this book and the ACLS educational materials will prepare you for this moment, if you make the effort and devote the time. After all, the whole thing is about time — and about giving time back to your fellow man.

Richard O. Cummins, MD

Essentials of ACLS

Chapter 1

Introduction

People's hearts stop beating every day. For many people this cessation of pulse is premature—their hearts should be too good to die.[1] Resuscitative efforts can restore these hearts to spontaneous activity before the brain has been permanently injured. The core purpose of emergency cardiac care (ECC) is to provide effective care as soon as possible to these hearts that have stopped beating. Rapid restoration of a spontaneously beating heart produces the best chance of achieving the ultimate goal—a thinking, feeling, healthy human being.

This chapter presents "the essentials" of advanced cardiac life support (ACLS). Do not think the chapter provides everything a person must know about ACLS or even everything needed to successfully complete the skills stations and the written evaluation of the ACLS course. This textbook presents a way of thinking about people in cardiac arrest. This chapter will help participants in an ACLS course achieve a better understanding of a person in cardiac arrest and help them begin to learn the roles and interventions used by resuscitation teams.

Here are the core knowledge and skills needed for ACLS:

> For devices and procedures, participants must know
> - Indications (knowledge)
> - Precautions (knowledge)
> - Proper use (hands-on practice)
>
> For pharmacologic agents, participants must know
> - *Why* an agent is used (actions)
> - *When* to use an agent (indications)
> - *How* to use an agent (dosing)
> - *What to watch out for* (precautions)

Airway management and endotracheal intubation (core), including:

- Noninvasive airway techniques and devices (hands-on practice)
  — Rescue position
  — Nasal cannulae
  — Venturi masks
  — Oropharyngeal airways
  — Pocket face masks and barrier devices
  — Bag-valve mask
  — Tracheobronchial suctioning
  — Cricoid pressure

- Techniques to administer oxygen (hands-on practice)
  — Oxygen tanks
  — Cricothyrotomy (supplemental)
  — Transtracheal catheter ventilation (supplemental)
- Endotracheal intubation (hands-on practice)

Recognition and therapy of the major ACLS emergency conditions (core):

- Universal algorithm
- Ventricular fibrillation/pulseless ventricular tachycardia (VF/VT)
- Pulseless electrical activity (PEA)
- Asystole
- Bradycardia
- Tachycardias
- Acute myocardial infarction (MI)
- Hypotension/shock/acute pulmonary edema

Electrical therapy (core), including:

- Defibrillation with automated external defibrillators (AEDs) (hands-on practice)
- Defibrillation with conventional defibrillators (hands-on practice)
- Attachment of defibrillators (conventional and AED) as a cardiac monitor
- Electrical cardioversion with conventional defibrillators
- Transcutaneous pacemakers (hands-on practice)
  — Asynchronous pacing
  — Synchronous pacing

Intravenous (IV) and invasive therapeutic and monitoring techniques, including:

- Peripheral IV lines (core)
  — Hand, antecubital, saphenous, external jugular, femoral
- Central IV lines (supplemental)
  — Internal jugular (Seldinger technique and triple-lumen catheters)
  — Subclavian
- Pericardiocentesis (supplemental)
- Thoracentesis for tension pneumothorax (supplemental)

Recognition of the following rhythms (core):

- *Lethal rhythms*
  — VF
  — VT
  — Artifact from lead detachment, movement, electrical interference
  — Asystole
  — PEAs (narrow-complex and wide-complex)

- *Nonlethal arrhythmias*
  — Normal sinus rhythm
  — Bradycardias: sinus bradycardia, atrioventricular (AV) nodal blocks (first-, second-, third-degree)
  — Atrial tachycardia, atrial tachycardia with block, atrial flutter with various degrees of block, premature ventricular complexes (PVCs)
  — Tachycardias: sinus tachycardia, atrial fibrillation, atrial flutter, paroxysmal supraventricular tachycardia (PSVT), wide-complex tachycardias
  — Electrocardiographic (ECG) criteria for acute ischemia, acute injury, acute infarction (anterior, inferior)
  — Pacemaker spikes

ACLS cardiovascular pharmacology (core), including the *Why?* (actions), *When?* (indications), *How?* (dosing), and *Watch out for!* (precautions) of the following agents:

- Electricity
- Oxygen
- Epinephrine
- Lidocaine
- Bretylium
- Magnesium sulfate
- Procainamide
- Sodium bicarbonate
- Atropine
- Dopamine
- Isoproterenol
- Vagal maneuvers (used as a drug)
- Adenosine
- Verapamil
- Diltiazem
- A β blocker (atenolol, propranolol, or metoprolol)
- Nitroglycerin
- Nitroprusside
- Dobutamine
- Morphine sulfate
- Furosemide
- A thrombolytic agent (the one used in the provider's work setting)

Early management (first 30 minutes) of the following special resuscitation situations (supplemental):

- Stroke
- Hypothermia
- Drowning and near-drowning
- Cardiac arrest associated with trauma
- Electrocution and lightning strike
- Cardiac arrest of the pregnant patient
- Possible drug overdose

Megacode leadership (core) and full participation (core), including:

- Knowledge and skills to manage the core Megacode scenario: *the first 10 minutes of an adult VF cardiac arrest.*

- The core Megacode scenario covers the following areas:
  — Universal algorithm (for pulseless patient)
  — Basic adult CPR (primary ABCD survey)
  — VF/VT algorithm
  — Appropriate use of the secondary ABCD survey
  — Acceptable noninvasive airway management techniques
  — Endotracheal intubation (only if professional role requires)
  — IV techniques (peripheral line only)
  — Defibrillation with AEDs and conventional defibrillators
  — Use of pharmacologic agents: epinephrine, lidocaine, bretylium, procainamide, sodium bicarbonate, magnesium sulfate

Core ACLS Concepts

The Brain

- **Cerebral resuscitation is the most important goal.** ECC personnel must restart the heart as the first step toward that goal. Cerebral resuscitation—returning the patient to the prearrest level of neurological functioning—stands as the ultimate goal of ECC. Peter Safar has proposed the term *cardio-pulmonary-cerebral resuscitation* (CPCR) to replace the familiar CPR.[2] Many national and international experts support this proposal. Clinicians should always remember the term *cerebral*, for that word reminds us of our primary purpose: to return the patient to his or her best possible neurological outcome. Unless spontaneous ventilation and circulation are restored quickly, successful cerebral resuscitation cannot occur.[3]

The Patient

- **Never forget the patient.** Resuscitation challenges care providers to make decisions quickly, under pressure and in dramatic settings. Human nature can lead providers to focus on limited specific aspects of resuscitative attempts: getting the IV started, placing the tube, identifying the rhythm, remembering the "right" medication to use. Emergency care providers must constantly return to an overall view of each resuscitative attempt: is the airway adequate? are ventilations effective? what could have caused this arrest? what else could be wrong? what am I missing? The algorithms (flow diagrams) focus the provider on the most important aspects of a resuscitative effort: airway and ventilation, basic cardiopulmonary resuscitation (CPR), defibrillation of VF, and medications suitable for a particular patient and particular conditions.

Basic Life Support

• **The resuscitation continuum: Advanced cardiac life support (ACLS) is just the other end of basic life support (BLS).** BLS (ie, CPR) attempts to give a person in cardiopulmonary arrest an open airway, adequate ventilation, and (through chest compressions) mechanical circulation to the vital organs. ACLS attempts to restore spontaneous circulation. ACLS is interconnected with basic and intermediate life support. Traditionally we have considered ACLS interventions to be defibrillation, endotracheal intubation, and IV medications. These distinctions have been blurred, however, by automated defibrillation, invasive airway devices that do not extend into the trachea, and sublingual and endotracheal administration of medications. What is formally called *ACLS* should now be considered the latter end of a continuum that starts with recognition of a cardiopulmonary/cardiovascular emergency and moves through defibrillation, advanced airway management, and rhythm-appropriate IV medications.

Either in-hospital or prehospital emergency personnel cannot provide proper ACLS without constant and careful attention to the features of BLS and proper assessment of the patient. The interventions performed will vary according to the setting. Prehospital care systems have many combinations of personnel and skill levels.[4,5] Recognition of the importance of early defibrillation for witnessed adult cardiac arrest has led to use of defibrillation by traditional BLS providers. The curriculum recommended by the American Heart Association (AHA) for early defibrillation, for example, provides protocol recommendations for the simplest response level.[6-9] This would be two-rescuer response teams with two people trained to the BLS level plus defibrillation. Many systems prefer a three-person response team with all three responders trained to an advanced level.[10] In-hospital response teams display the same variety as prehospital teams.[11,12]

Time

• **Passage of time drives all aspects of ECC and determines patient outcomes.**[13-15] The probability of survival declines sharply with each passing minute of cardiopulmonary compromise. Some interventions, like basic CPR, slow the rate at which this decline in resuscitation probability occurs. Other interventions, such as opening an obstructed airway or defibrillating VF, can restore a beating heart. The longer it takes to perform these interventions, however, the lower the chances of benefit.

The Cause

• **Emergency personnel must identify medical conditions that lead to cardiac arrest as quickly as possible.** Once these conditions are identified, rescuers must start appropriate therapy rapidly. This textbook includes specific recommendations on the "prearrest" period, including conditions to look for and interventions to provide. AMI is the most dramatic example of a condition that may lead to a cardiac arrest but for which effective therapy now exists. Time is a critical factor, for the effectiveness of thrombolytic therapy dramatically declines the longer patients or medical personnel take to make the diagnosis and start therapy.

Postresuscitation Care

• **Emergency care providers must continue to provide appropriate evaluation and therapy in the period immediately after restoration of a spontaneous circulation.** The ACLS course concentrates on resuscitation during a cardiac arrest and on critical actions to take 30 minutes before and 30 minutes after a cardiac arrest. The ACLS recommendations during the postresuscitation period assume that invasive hemodynamic monitoring is *not* available. Emergency care providers are often on their own during this period while awaiting transport to an emergency department or to a critical care area of the hospital.

The Chain of Survival Applies in All Settings

• **Emergency care providers must never forget that the principles and recommendations for ECC apply to the prehospital cardiac arrest, the in-hospital cardiac arrest, and patients in emergency departments.** The sequence of BLS, intermediate life support, and advanced life support is a continuum that applies equally in the intensive care unit, the patient's home, and the local shopping mall. This fact supports inclusion of material on AEDs for all ACLS course participants and instruction in their use.

The Phased-Response Approach

• **Every resuscitative attempt possesses a structure, a time course, and a rich variety of intermediate stages.** These include anticipation by the rescuers, entry into the resuscitative efforts, the resuscitative effort itself, maintenance of the patient, family notification, transfer, and critique.[16,17] Every resuscitative attempt produces psychological effects on the rescuers.[18-20] This is true whether the cardiac arrest occurs in a rural community, an emergency department, a sophisticated urban emergency medical services (EMS) system, or the intensive care unit of a tertiary care medical center. Outcomes will be better if we recognize this architecture, plan for it, and follow the appropriate steps.

Expected Deaths and Futile Resuscitations

• **For many people the last beat of their heart should be the last beat of their heart.** They have simply reached the end of their life, and resuscitative efforts are inappropriate, futile, undignified, and demeaning to both the patient and the rescuers. Once started, resuscitative efforts can acquire this same mantle of futility and inappropriateness. Good ACLS requires careful thought about when to start and when to stop resuscitative efforts.

The Chain of Survival in Your Community

• **ACLS cannot exist in a vacuum.** We must examine closely the community in which cardiac arrests occur. We each may focus on an individual skill or role in resuscitative attempts—intubation, defibrillation, proper identification of rhythms, or sequencing of medications. Our success in these interventions, however, often depends on the performance of others. Successful outcomes depend on how well all these efforts are linked together in what has been termed the *chain of survival*.[14,15] The concept of a linked chain applies to cardiac arrests in-hospital as well as arrests in the prehospital arena. The chain of survival has four links:

- Early access—a cardiac emergency must be recognized and responded to
- Early CPR—some efforts at opening the airway, ventilation and blood circulation must occur as soon as possible
- Early defibrillation—identification and treatment of VF is the single most important intervention
- Early ACLS—advanced airway control and rhythm-appropriate IV medications must be administered rapidly

Failure to examine and strengthen all of these links condemns emergency personnel and the patient to inferior outcomes.

The Primary-Secondary Survey Approach to Emergency Cardiac Care

Taking an ACLS course for the first time makes some people anxious. They often focus on such psychomotor skills as intubation and starting central lines and worry about rhythm recognition and how to remember medications.

Emergency personnel need a systematic approach to resuscitation and cardiorespiratory emergencies. With an organized approach they will feel more comfortable about individual roles and about the tasks they face as a resuscitation team. Emergency medicine teaches a simple and familiar approach: **primary survey followed by the secondary survey.**[21] This approach provides a powerful conceptual tool for the ACLS provider to use when approaching cardiac care emergencies.

Key Points

In the primary survey, focus on basic CPR and defibrillation:

First "A-B-C-D"

- **A**irway: open the airway
- **B**reathing: provide positive-pressure ventilations
- **C**irculation: give chest compressions
- **D**efibrillation: shock VF/pulseless VT

In the secondary survey, focus on intubation, IV access, rhythms, and drugs and on why the cardiorespiratory arrest occurred:

Second "A-B-C-D"

- **A**irway: perform endotracheal intubation
- **B**reathing: assess bilateral chest rise and ventilation
- **C**irculation: gain IV access, determine rhythm, give appropriate agents
- **D**ifferential Diagnosis: search for, find, and treat reversible causes

---

The primary and secondary approach applies to more than just full cardiac arrests. Providers should learn to apply the primary ABCD survey and the secondary ABCD survey to all cardiac arrests, to all prearrest and postarrest patients, and during all major decision points in a difficult resuscitative effort.

The Primary Survey

In the primary survey, focus on basic CPR and defibrillation.

First "A-B-C-D"

Airway:
- Open the airway.

Breathing:
- Provide positive-pressure ventilation.

Circulation:
- Give chest compressions.

Defibrillation:
- Shock VF/pulseless VT.

In the primary ABCD survey personnel recognize that a person has experienced a cardiac arrest and start resuscitative efforts as follows: open the airway, initiate breathing, start chest compressions, and search for and shock VF if present (using either conventional or automated defibrillators).

All people involved in emergency care must master the primary survey. For example, the first person to discover a cardiac arrest in a general hospital floor would initiate the primary survey, in the course of which he or she would identify the cardiac arrest, call for help, and perform the basic ABCs of CPR. The first assistant to arrive would be asked to get the automated external defibrillator or the "crash cart." The first action to do when the cart arrives is complete the primary survey by looking for VF with the defibrillator. If VF or pulseless VT is present, shock it immediately with up to three shocks.

At this point, move to the secondary survey.

The Secondary Survey

The secondary survey repeats the same **A-B-C-D** mnemonic, but now each letter reminds the rescuer to perform more in-depth interventions and assessments.

Second "A-B-C-D"

Airway:

- Establish advanced airway control.
- Perform endotracheal intubation.

Breathing:

- Assess the adequacy of ventilation via endotracheal tube.
- Provide positive-pressure ventilations.

Circulation:

- Obtain IV access to administer fluids and medications.
- Continue CPR.
- Provide rhythm-appropriate cardiovascular pharmacology.

Differential Diagnosis:

- Identify the possible reasons for the arrest. Construct a differential diagnosis to identify reversible causes that have a specific therapy.

A. The Primary ABCD Survey

Preliminary First Actions

These are performed just before the "A" (Airway) of the primary ABCD survey.

- Assess responsiveness.
- "Call Fast."
- Appropriately position the victim.
- Appropriately position the rescuer.

Assess Responsiveness. "Man down—unconscious, unresponsive" is a familiar and riveting call in emergency care. Always assume that such people have cardiac arrest or respiratory arrest, or both, until proven otherwise. Establish unresponsiveness with the traditional "shake and shout": gently shake the person and shout, "Are you OK?" But for people with possible trauma the "shake" can aggravate traumatic injuries, and "touch and talk" is the better approach. These techniques distinguish the person who is asleep or who has a depressed sensorium from the person who is clinically comatose.

"Call Fast" for help. Once unresponsiveness is verified, the rescuer should immediately call for help. In the hospital or emergency department the rescuer should call out loudly for someone to help. Sometimes just step quickly to the doorway and shout, eg, "I need help at once in Room 3A!" The person who responds to this local call should be told to go activate the emergency response system. Inside a medical facility this call will go to the hospital paging operator or another designated operator. Outside the hospital the person who responds should be told to immediately call the local 911 system (activate EMS).

Personnel must always be filled with a great sense of urgency to get back to the patient to open the airway and verify that airway obstruction has not occurred. If and when someone arrives to help, send that person to activate the emergency response system, then return quickly to perform the A and B steps of CPR.

The AHA gives a high priority to a *call for help* once unresponsiveness is verified.[22] This approach underscores the principle that advanced care—in the form of electrical defibrillation, advanced airway management, and IV medications—must be brought to the patient as soon as possible. A rescuer should never forget that the prime chance for a successful resuscitation comes from decreasing the interval from the onset of the emergency to the restoration of an effective spontaneous circulation.

Special Case 1: the "Lone Rescuer"

What should the "lone rescuer" do when no one hears the local call for help? This question has stimulated much discussion in ECC. Do you begin full CPR with chest compressions, or do you leave the victim for the time it takes to activate emergency response personnel? A simple message—"Phone First"—has been adopted for the lone adult lay rescuer, but the professional trained rescuer can appreciate the subtleties involved and the need for judgment and individualized decision making. The AHA recommendations convey the need to provide a simple message to the lay rescuers.

The basic dilemma is whether the victim has experienced a respiratory arrest from an obstructed airway, a comatose state, a drug overdose, a postictal state, or any number of other causes of respiratory arrest. When rescuers suspect an obstructed airway, they should perform the AB sequence first. For example, the healthy adult who collapses in a restaurant while rushing to the bathroom should be evaluated first for an unobstructed airway.

Special Case 2: the "Lone Rescuer" With an Automated Defibrillator

An adult who is breathing normally may suddenly grasp his or her chest in severe pain and collapse in front of witnesses. Such a person is probably experiencing a lethal arrhythmia, such as VF. This person needs immediate defibrillation, and any delay in getting the defibrillator to this person will decrease the probability of successful return of spontaneous circulation. This includes, in particular, the delay involved in performing the traditional "1 minute of CPR" that has been recommended in the past for the "lone rescuer." For the lone rescuer with immediate access to a defibrillator, the recommended sequence is

- Assess responsiveness
- Call locally for help
- Open the airway **(A)**
- Confirm unobstructed airway with two breaths **(B)**
- Confirm pulselessness **(C)**
- Retrieve and operate the defibrillator **(D)**.

Note: This sequence omits the chest compressions.

Special Case 3: the "Lone Rescuer" With Remote Access to a Telephone

The other element for decision making is the time required to activate either the hospital's or the community's emergency response system. A delay of 1 to 2 minutes in CPR to activate the EMS system is acceptable for people with VF, assuming you return at once and begin the ABCs. If your jogging partner collapses on an isolated running trail, however, and there is a 15-minute run to the nearest telephone, you face some tough decisions. A 30-minute round trip on a deserted jogging trail to a telephone will leave the victim an intolerably long time without the benefits of CPR, yet CPR alone will be of little help if the adult, witnessed-collapse victim is in VF (80% to 90% probability in this scenario). Common sense would suggest that a trained health professional would ensure an open airway, provide several precordial thumps, and continue CPR for at least 10 to 15 minutes. The former recommendation to continue until the rescuer is exhausted is too severe since reasonably fit people can continue CPR well over 60 minutes before becoming exhausted.

Appropriately Position the Victim. If the cardiac arrest victim is not on a firm surface, roll the person over as one unit. If you suspect that trauma may have occurred in the collapse, maintain the head, neck, and trunk in a straight line to stabilize the cervical spine.

Do this by kneeling beside the person and placing one hand on the back of the head and neck. With the other hand roll the patient slowly toward you. Follow this method if there is any suspicion of cervical spine injury. Look for signs of bleeding around the head. Always think of associated trauma to the cervical spine when attempting CPR on people who fell from heights, who fell with great force when they collapsed, who had been diving head first, who were struck by lightning, or who were involved in a motor vehicle accident.

When two people are available to turn a prone victim over, the second person should be positioned at the head of the patient to maintain in-line head stabilization while the patient is turned. Do *not* apply firm traction on the head if you suspect a cervical spine injury. When the person is in bed, a firm support must be placed under the thoracic cage. Hospitals should maintain a plywood board for the purpose of CPR.

Appropriately Position the Rescuer. The most efficient position for a single rescuer is to kneel at the level of the victim's shoulders. In this position the single rescuer will not have to move his knees to move from the mouth to the chest of the victim.

THE PRIMARY ABCD SURVEY: Details of Performance

> **(A) Open the airway**
> **(B) Assess breathlessness**
> **(B) Ventilate the patient**
> **(C) Confirm pulselessness**
> **(C) Perform closed-chest compressions**
> **(D) Defibrillate VF/VT**

(A) Open the Airway. As a first step, the mouth should be opened and the upper airway inspected for foreign objects, vomitus, or blood. If present, these should be removed with the fingers covered with gauze or a piece of cloth or by turning the patient on the side, paying careful attention to the possibility of a cervical spine injury.

In addition to the head tilt–chin lift maneuver of basic CPR, all emergency personnel should learn the jaw-thrust technique of opening the airway. In the jaw thrust the rescuer stands or kneels at the head of the patient and grasps the mandible of the jaw with the fingertips while the hands are placed at the sides of the patient's face. The mandible is lifted forward. A position with the elbows on the stretcher or backboard is usually the most comfortable one for the rescuer. The jaw-thrust technique must be learned by all rescuers who may encounter patients with the combination of cervical spine injuries and respiratory compromise. It maintains a neutral position of the cervical spine while resuscitative attempts continue. This technique is used almost solely for trauma patients by out-of-hospital response teams.

(B) Assess Breathlessness. An assessment of the ability to move air is quickly made when the rescuer opens the airway with the head tilt–chin lift maneuver and then "looks, listens, and feels" for air movement. The look, listen, and feel technique is performed with the rescuer's head in a position with the ear placed almost touching the patient's mouth and the face turned toward the victim's chest. The rescuer "listens and feels" for breathing with his or her ear and simultaneously "looks" at the victim's chest for any respiratory movements. The rescuer may note that the victim has resumed breathing with the airway-opening maneuvers. Continued maintenance of an open airway may be the only rescue action required at this point.

When the rescuer confirms breathlessness by this basic CPR step, he or she enters the entire spectrum of airway management problems in cardiac arrest. The ACLS team leader will be responsible for all aspects of airway management throughout the resuscitative attempt. These topics are covered in more detail in chapter 2, "Adjuncts for Airway Control, Ventilation, and Oxygenation." Once breathlessness is confirmed, the rescuer must ask

- Is the absence of air movement due to an obstructed airway?
- What maneuver should I perform to check for an obstructed airway?
- If the airway is obstructed, what maneuver should I perform to clear it?
- If ventilations are needed, what ventilatory adjunct should I use?
- Are rate and volume of ventilations optimal?
- Are the ventilations effective?

(B) Ventilate the Patient. If immediately available, insert an oropharyngeal airway and begin ventilations with a pocket face mask. The professional emergency rescuer should always have some form of barrier ventilation device. Pocket face masks, preferably with a one-way valve, at a ratio of one mask per bed, should be ubiquitous in all patient care areas of a hospital. They can be placed in a wall-mounted holder at the head of the bed. They should be present on all code carts.

Provide two rescue ventilations over 2 to 4 seconds. Maintain proper head tilt to allow exhalation of the breath. Give adequate time (1 to 2 seconds per ventilation) to allow for exhalation. Ventilations with this slow inspiratory flow rate are recommended so that the esophageal opening pressure will not be exceeded and the chances of gastric distention, regurgitation, and aspiration are decreased.

At this point the rescuer must make several important observations. First, did the air of the first breath go in? Did the chest rise? Could the rescuer hear the sound of air escaping during passive exhalation? If air did not enter easily and the chest did not rise, then you must take steps to correct what may be an obstructed airway. In this situation the best first step is to repeat quickly the head tilt—chin lift maneuver and try again. If still unsuccessful, the person has, by definition, an obstructed airway, and you must then follow the protocols for the obstructed airway.

Remember that the next step, closed-chest compressions, will be completely ineffective if the patient cannot be successfully ventilated.

If experienced personnel are available, cricoid pressure should be applied continuously until definitive airway protection is achieved with endotracheal intubation. This effective but neglected technique uses the rigid cartilaginous tracheal rings to occlude the esophagus. When performed correctly it occludes the esophagus so that ventilations do not enter the stomach and produce gastric distention. It helps ensure that the ventilations enter the lungs. If gastric distention is avoided, the chances of regurgitation are decreased. If regurgitation does occur, cricoid pressure may prevent aspiration or airway obstruction. Airway management and ventilation techniques are discussed in detail in chapter 2.

(C) Confirm Pulselessness. Once breathlessness is established the rescuer should quickly check for a pulse at the carotid artery on the side closer to the rescuer. The pulse check should last for 5 to 10 seconds because the pulse may be present but difficult to detect if slow, irregular, weak, or rapid.

At this point the rescuer has confirmed a "full" cardiac arrest. Faced with a victim who is unconscious, unresponsive, breathless, and without a pulse, the rescuer must perform chest compressions and artificial ventilations at once. Activate the code team (if in a hospital) or the EMS system if outside the hospital. This may have occurred with the initial determination of unresponsiveness and local call for help.

(C) Perform Closed-Chest Compressions. The technique for chest compressions is discussed in the BLS texts. From the perspective of people learning ACLS, remember that it is your responsibility to check for the quality and effectiveness of chest compressions and ventilation throughout the resuscitative effort. ACLS personnel must be thoroughly familiar with basic CPR techniques, not only to supervise and monitor the performance of others but also to be ready for that inevitable day when the ACLS team leader arrives "first on the scene" of a cardiac arrest.

(D) Defibrillate VF and VT if Identified. The initial "call for help" or "phone fast" after assessing unresponsiveness should result in someone's arriving at the side of the cardiac arrest victim with a defibrillator. As soon as a defibrillator arrives, the rescuer should attach the device and "hunt for VF/VT."

Numerous clinical and epidemiological studies[5,23] have confirmed repeatedly two simple observations:

- Almost every adult (over 90% in most studies) who survives sudden nontraumatic cardiac arrest was resuscitated from VF.
- The success of defibrillation is remarkably time-dependent.

The probability of defibrillating someone back to a perfusing rhythm declines about 2% to 10% per minute, starting with an estimated probability of 70% to 80% survival at time zero. These depressing statistics mean that if you have not managed to shock a patient in VF within 10 minutes of the collapse, the probability of survival approaches zero.

Conceptually defibrillation no longer belongs solely to ACLS. The widespread availability of AEDs has rendered defibrillation an intermediate intervention between BLS and ACLS. Chapter 4 on defibrillation includes both conventional and automated external defibrillation and presents the rationale for early defibrillation.

Steps for Defibrillation Using Conventional (Manual) Defibrillators

1. Turn on defibrillator.
2. Select energy level at 200 J.
3. Set "lead select" switch on "Paddles" (or lead I, II, or III if monitor leads are used).
4. Position conductor pads on patient (or apply gel to paddles).
5. Position paddles on patient (sternum-apex).
6. Visually check the monitor display and assess the rhythm (subsequent steps assume VF/pulseless VT is present).
7. Announce to the team members, "Charging defibrillator—stand clear!"
8. Press "charge" button on apex paddle (right hand) on defibrillator controls.
9. When the defibrillator is fully charged, state firmly in a forceful voice the following chant (or some suitable equivalent) before each shock:
   - "I am going to shock on three. One, I'm clear." (Check and make sure you are clear of contact with the patient or the stretcher and equipment.)
   - "Two, you're clear." (Make a visual check to ensure that no one continues to touch the patient or stretcher. In particular, do not forget about the person doing ventilations. That person should not have hands on the ventilatory adjuncts, including the endotracheal tube!)
   - "Three, everybody's clear." (Check yourself one more time before pressing the shock buttons.)
10. Apply 25 lb pressure on both paddles.
11. Press the two "discharge" buttons simultaneously.
12. Check the monitor screen. If unquestionable VF/VT remains, recharge the defibrillator at once. Check a pulse if there is any question about the rhythm display (eg, a lead has been dislodged or the paddles are not displaying the correct signal).
13. Shock at 200 to 300 J, then at 360 J, repeating the same verbal statements noted above.

Steps for Defibrillation Using AEDs*

All AEDs operate using four basic steps:

1. *Power*: Turn power on.
2. *Attachment*: Attach to the patient.
3. *Analysis*: Place into "analyze" mode.
4. *Shock*: Press shock button.

1. *Power*: Turn power on.
2. *Attachment*:
   - Open adhesive defibrillator pads.
   - Attach defibrillator cables to the pads.
   - Expose adhesive surface.
   - Attach pads to the patient (upper right sternal border and cardiac apex).
3. *Analysis*:
   - Announce to the team members, "Analyzing rhythm—stand clear!" (Verify that there is no patient movement and that no one is in contact with the patient.)
   - Press the "analyze" control.
4. *Shock*: (If VF/VT is present, the device will charge to 200 to 360 J and signal that a shock is indicated.)
   - Announce, "Shock is indicated—stand clear!"
   - Verify that no one is touching the patient.
   - Press the "shock" button when signalled to do so.
5. Repeat these steps until VF/VT is no longer present. The device will signal "no shock indicated." In general, shock in sets of three without interposed CPR or pulse checks. After a set of three shocks, provide 1 minute of CPR and ventilations.

*Fully automated AEDs will require some variations in these steps.

B. The Secondary ABCD Survey

In the secondary ABCD survey the rescuers return to the ABCDs but at a more advanced level.

Airway
- Reassess the adequacy of the original airway-opening techniques.
- Direct personnel to secure the airway with further airway adjuncts, most definitively endotracheal intubation.

Breathing
- Assess status of ventilations after endotracheal intubation.
- Make necessary adjustments.
- Assess movement of the chest with ventilations.
- Examine for the presence of bilateral breath sounds.

Circulation
- Obtain IV access.
- Attach monitor leads.
- Identify rhythms and rates.
- Measure blood pressure (noninvasive blood pressure measurements).
- Provide rhythm-appropriate and vital-sign–appropriate medications.

  This rhythm-driven selection of medications has been the traditional emphasis in ACLS courses. Rescuers, however, must have a broader clinical perspective, and they can gain this perspective if they consider the full ABCD picture.

Differential Diagnosis

Consider the possible causes of the cardiac emergency and of the observed rhythms. This review provides help in refractory cardiac arrest or unstable postresuscitation conditions. This "D" of the secondary survey helps the team leaders refocus their thoughts and think in terms of "what caused or precipitated this arrest?" and "why have they not responded to our treatment?" Many patients will have responded to defibrillation. Patients in non–VF rhythms or those people who have not responded early present a more complicated challenge and require resuscitation teams to think of specific causes and possible corrective actions.

  The ABCD mnemonics for the secondary survey could have used "D" for drugs. As an aid to memory, however, we think cardiac medications (or "drugs") should be included under "C" for "circulation." "D" works better as a mental link to "differential diagnosis." Thinking about the "differential diagnosis" leads the resuscitation team to perform an important review of the causes of the original arrest and to review whether they should take other actions besides a narrow "rhythm-drug" response. The algorithms for asystole and PEA provide examples of the causes and cause-specific interventions that personnel must consider.

Additional Key Points to Remember About Defibrillation

1. As part of the primary survey and the ABCD approach you will deliver up to three "stacked" defibrillations (assuming persistent VF or VT). These three shocks are delivered consecutively, one after the other. You do not perform CPR between these shocks. You do not perform ventilations. You do not spend a long time feeling for a pulse after each shock. You do not take the paddles away from the chest if you are using defibrillators with conventional paddles.

2. You should recharge immediately after each shock. Push the charge control as soon as the first and second shock are delivered. Immediately look at the monitor screen (while recharging) to check for persistent VF.

3. If you see a non-VF rhythm, remove the paddles from the chest, disarm the defibrillator, and check for a pulse.

4. If you see persistent VF, keep the paddles on the chest and deliver the second (or third) shock.

5. Consider the "hunt for VF" one of your highest priorities during a resuscitative attempt. While the ABCs and CPR should not be neglected, there should always be a strong sense of urgency to attach the defibrillator and deliver the shock if the rhythm is VF.

6. A dead defibrillator means a dead patient. Learn about the proper care and maintenance of your defibrillators.

7. Never meet your defibrillator for the first time at a code! Learn about the location and controls of your defibrillator before you need to use it. Many code attempts go awry because personnel have not learned or do not remember the basic operational steps of a conventional defibrillator. Manufacturing standards have produced excellent devices with standardized controls and functions. Many locations, however, particularly code carts, have older devices that have been in place and seldom used for over 10 years! It is your obligation to learn to operate and maintain the defibrillators used in all locations where you have clinical responsibility.

8. Learn whether there are separate controls for the monitor and for the defibrillator. On most devices you can turn on the monitor independently of the defibrillator. If you then want to defibrillate the patient, you have to press separate "Power On" controls for the defibrillator portion. Most modern devices will automatically turn on the monitor screen if you press the defibrillator on first but not vice versa. Ask to see the defibrillator instruction manuals and the operator maintenance checksheets. Remember, this is *your* responsibility, not the responsibility of the engineering department or the manufacturer.

9. Learn how to attach the monitor cables correctly and without having to read the labels. Remember: "white goes to right, red goes to ribs, color left over goes to left shoulder."

10. Learn where the defibrillation gel or, even better, the adhesive defibrillation pads are kept.

11. Learn and always use the "clearing chant" to ensure safe defibrillation.

Note that remote defibrillation through adhesive patches and cable connections are available for many conventional defibrillators and all AEDs. Clinical experiences suggest that remote defibrillation is much safer for the operator, though you must still use the clearing chant.

Reasons for the Secondary Survey

At the simplistic level, the secondary ABCD survey translates into "tube 'em, start an IV, then try to remember which drug goes with which rhythm." Concentration on the ABCD paradigm, however, will help emergency personnel remember to always look at the whole patient and at what is going on with the entire resuscitative attempt.

Note that the assessments and actions of the secondary survey should be performed almost simultaneously. The roles of the team members should be defined *before* cardiac arrests occur. With proper planning the code leader should not even have to direct people to secure the airway with endotracheal intubation and to gain IV access through a large-gauge antecubital vein.

A problem may arise if personnel who can perform these advanced tasks are not available. In this case the team leader must step forward to perform the most essential next step. While airway and breathing always remain the highest priority, it may not be necessary to rush toward endotracheal intubation if the noninvasive ventilatory adjuncts (oropharyngeal airway, bag-valve mask, or the pocket face mask) appear to provide adequate oxygenation and ventilation or if regurgitation does not appear imminent (eg, absence of severe gastric distention). The AHA now recommends endotracheal intubation before gaining IV access. Stated unambiguously: *airway control and ventilation support is more important than medications.* Definitive scientific evidence to support the value of IV medications in full cardiac arrest is lacking. However, common sense should prevail: it is acceptable to gain IV access before endotracheal intubation *if* ventilation, oxygenation, and airway protection appear satisfactory.

THE SECONDARY ABCD SURVEY: *Details of Performance*

Airway

- Verify that someone is preparing to perform endotracheal intubation (getting out a tube of proper size, checking the laryngoscope, preparing a suction method). Endotracheal intubation provides definitive airway management—there is no equivalent substitute. Rescuers can delay endotracheal intubation for other interventions, however, if noninvasive ventilation techniques appear temporarily adequate.
- Insert a nasal trumpet or nasopharyngeal airway if not already done.
- Continuous cricoid pressure may be all that is needed to prevent regurgitation into the hypopharynx and aspiration of gastric contents.
- Check that a suction device (electrically powered, or hand or foot powered) is available, operating properly, and ready to be used.

Breathing

- Check that ventilations with the pocket face mask, the bag-valve mask, and through the endotracheal tube or other device are causing the chest to rise.

- Check that the patient has bilateral breath sounds by listening at the midaxillary line on each side.
- Auscultate over the epigastrium.
- Order a stat portable chest x-ray after the intubation. This will confirm tube placement (which you should have already confirmed clinically and by one other method) and provide information on pulmonary conditions.
- Confirm endotracheal tube placement by some means in addition to bilateral breath sounds. These techniques include end-tidal CO_2 indicators and measurements, endotracheal tube aspiration,[24] and chest radiograph.
- If there is any doubt about correct tube placement, use direct visualization with a laryngoscope. Consider removing the tube and starting over.

Circulation

- The antecubital vein should be the first target for IV access.
- Normal saline rather than D_5W is now recommended as the IV fluid vehicle. Normal saline expands the intravascular volume better than dextrose; the theoretic problem of pushing people into pulmonary edema has not turned out to be a frequent problem. Some studies have observed an association between high postresuscitation glucose level and poor neurological outcomes.[25,26] In addition, normal saline has longer shelf life and is less expensive. Control administered volume with smaller size bags and volumetric units.
- Remember that rescuers can administer the following medications down the endotracheal tube: A-L-E (atropine, lidocaine, epinephrine).
- The recommended technique for endotracheal drug administration is
  — Thread a long (35-cm) through-the-needle intracatheter rapidly down the inside of the endotracheal tube.
  — Stop CPR chest compressions.
  — Inject 2 to 2.5 times the normal dose of medication through the catheter.
  — Follow with 10 mL normal saline flush down the catheter.
  — Immediately attach the ventilation bag and forcefully ventilate 3 or 4 times. If an intracatheter is unavailable, it is possible to use a heparin lock with 20-gauge needle through the wall of the endotracheal tube to deliver and aerosolize medications during ventilations.[27]
- Be prepared to administer a 20- to 30-mL bolus of IV fluid and elevate the arm after each IV medication. This will enhance delivery of medications to the central circulation.

Differential Diagnosis

- The critical question that must be asked and answered is, what caused the arrest?
- The purpose of a differential diagnosis is to identify reversible causes—causes that have a specific therapy.
- Examine the rhythm. What is the rhythm? What could cause *this* rhythm? Each rhythm of arrest has many possible causes: VF/VT, asystole, PEA, severely symptomatic bradycardias, or tachycardias.
- The only possibility of successfully resuscitating a person may lie in searching for, finding, and treating reversible causes.
- Follow this same process for patients with *refractory cardiac arrests* that do not respond to the initial interventions. For example, transient postshock conversion rhythms in VF/VT may reveal an underlying bradycardia, in which case atropine can be added; or there may be a transient tachycardia, in which case a rapid-acting β blocker can be used.
- Follow this same process in the periarrest period for any severe cardiorespiratory emergency.

The Universal Algorithm for Adult ECC

The Algorithm Approach to Emergency Cardiac Care

For some years the AHA has used treatment algorithms as an educational tool. Table 1, "The Algorithm Approach to Emergency Cardiac Care," presents an overview of the algorithms and summarizes important points about their use.

Classification of Therapeutic Interventions in CPR and ECC

The 1992 National Conference on CPR and ECC used the following system of classifying interventions, based on the strength of the supporting scientific evidence.

Class I. — A therapeutic option that is usually indicated, always acceptable, and considered useful and effective.

Class II. — A therapeutic option that is acceptable, is of uncertain efficacy, may be controversial.

Class IIa. — A therapeutic option for which the weight of evidence is in favor of its usefulness and efficacy.

Class IIb. — A therapeutic option that is not well established by evidence but may be helpful and probably not harmful.

Class III. — A therapeutic option that is inappropriate, is without scientific supporting data, and may be harmful.

Table 1. The Algorithm Approach to Emergency Cardiac Care

The AHA guidelines for CPR and ECC use algorithms as an educational tool. They are an illustrative method to summarize information. Providers of emergency care should view algorithms as a summary and a memory aid. They provide a way to treat a broad range of patients. Algorithms by nature oversimplify. The effective teacher and care provider will use them wisely, not blindly. Some patients may require care not specified in the algorithms. When clinically appropriate, flexibility is accepted and encouraged. Many interventions and actions are listed as "considerations" to help providers think. These lists should not be considered endorsements or requirements or "standard of care" in a legal sense. Algorithms do not replace clinical understanding. Although the algorithms provide a good "cookbook," the patient always requires a "thinking cook."

The following clinical recommendations apply to all treatment algorithms:

- First, treat the patient, not the monitor.
- Algorithms for cardiac arrest presume that the condition under discussion continually persists, that the patient remains in cardiac arrest, and that CPR is always performed.
- Apply different interventions whenever appropriate indications exist.
- The flow diagrams present mostly Class I (acceptable, definitely effective) interventions. The footnotes present Class IIa (acceptable, probably effective), Class IIb (acceptable, possibly effective), and Class III (not indicated, may be harmful) interventions.
- Adequate airway, ventilation, oxygenation, chest compressions, and defibrillation are more important than administration of medications and take precedence over initiating an intravenous line or injecting pharmacologic agents.
- Several medications (epinephrine, lidocaine, and atropine) can be administered via the endotracheal tube, but the dosage should be 2 to 2.5 times the intravenous dose.
- With a few exceptions, intravenous medications should always be administered rapidly, by a bolus method.
- After each intravenous medication, give a 20 to 30 mL bolus of intravenous fluid and immediately elevate the extremity. This will enhance delivery of drugs to the central circulation, which may take 1 to 2 minutes.
- Last, treat the patient, not the monitor.

The Universal Algorithm for Adult Emergency Cardiac Care (Fig 1)

- **Assess responsiveness**
- **If not responsive, activate EMS system**
- **Call for defibrillator**
- **Assess breathing (open the airway, look, listen, and feel)**
- **If the patient is not breathing, give two slow breaths**
- **Assess the circulation**

Figure 1 presents the universal algorithm for adult emergency cardiac care (ECC). Rescuers should always start with this algorithm and concentrate on the major features illustrated.

The primary ABCD survey and the secondary ABCD survey described in the first part of this chapter incorporate all the steps and actions of the universal algorithm. Some people may find it easier to remember the steps of the universal algorithm; some may prefer the steps of the primary or secondary ABCD surveys. Whatever works best for each learner is acceptable.

The Primary ABCD Survey

The first steps in all emergency treatment are for the rescuer to quickly assess responsiveness, assess the ABCs, and if indicated start CPR (ABC of the primary survey). BLS training directs rescuers to immediately activate the EMS system when they determine that the patient is not responsive. They do this by placing a telephone call when outside the hospital or shouting to in-hospital colleagues "Bring the code cart!" or "Bring the defibrillator!"

The rescuer then assesses breathing by opening the airway and looking, listening, and feeling for respiration. If the patient is not breathing, the rescuer should give the victim two slow breaths.

- **Assess circulation: if no pulse, start CPR**

Some people in apparent cardiac arrest will respond to one or more of the initial actions of opening the airway and performing ventilations and chest compressions. These steps will also identify people with an obstructed airway. Rescuers should perform the appropriate actions for obstructed airways detailed in BLS.

The left branch of the first decision oval presents the sequence of actions to take for adults who are initially not in full cardiac arrest. They are not breathing, so they should receive full assessment and management of the airway and breathing with rescue breathing and endotracheal intubation. These patients are discussed later in this section and under the appropriate topics.

- **Ventricular fibrillation/tachycardia (VF/VT) present on the monitor/defibrillator?**

This step reflects the **"D"** part of the Primary ABCD Survey. The arrival of the defibrillator/monitor presents a major decision point in ECC. Instructors, students, and active care providers must recognize that defibrillation is the single most important intervention in adult ECC. Defibrillation, however, will work only with an adequate airway and effective ventilations. Rescuers must assess the ABCs repeatedly, perform CPR, and evaluate the effectiveness of those actions. The AED algorithm

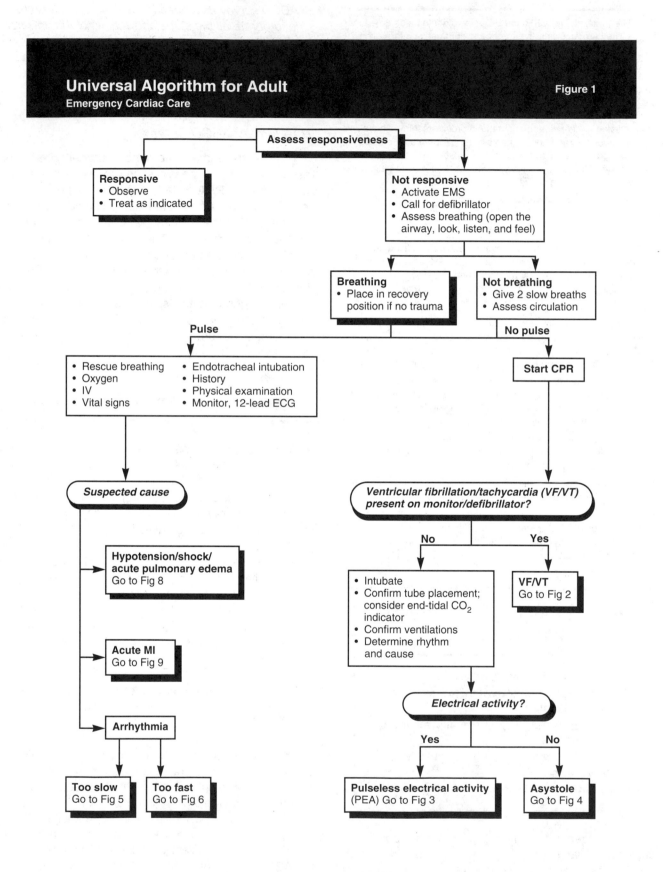

Universal Algorithm for Adult
Emergency Cardiac Care

Figure 1

Assess responsiveness

Responsive
• Observe
• Treat as indicated

Not responsive
• Activate EMS
• Call for defibrillator
• Assess breathing (open the airway, look, listen, and feel)

Breathing
• Place in recovery position if no trauma

Not breathing
• Give 2 slow breaths
• Assess circulation

Pulse

No pulse

• Rescue breathing
• Oxygen
• IV
• Vital signs
• Endotracheal intubation
• History
• Physical examination
• Monitor, 12-lead ECG

Start CPR

Suspected cause

Ventricular fibrillation/tachycardia (VF/VT) present on monitor/defibrillator?

No   Yes

Hypotension/shock/ acute pulmonary edema
Go to Fig 8

• Intubate
• Confirm tube placement; consider end-tidal CO_2 indicator
• Confirm ventilations
• Determine rhythm and cause

VF/VT
Go to Fig 2

Acute MI
Go to Fig 9

Electrical activity?

Yes   No

Arrhythmia

Too slow
Go to Fig 5

Too fast
Go to Fig 6

Pulseless electrical activity
(PEA) Go to Fig 3

Asystole
Go to Fig 4

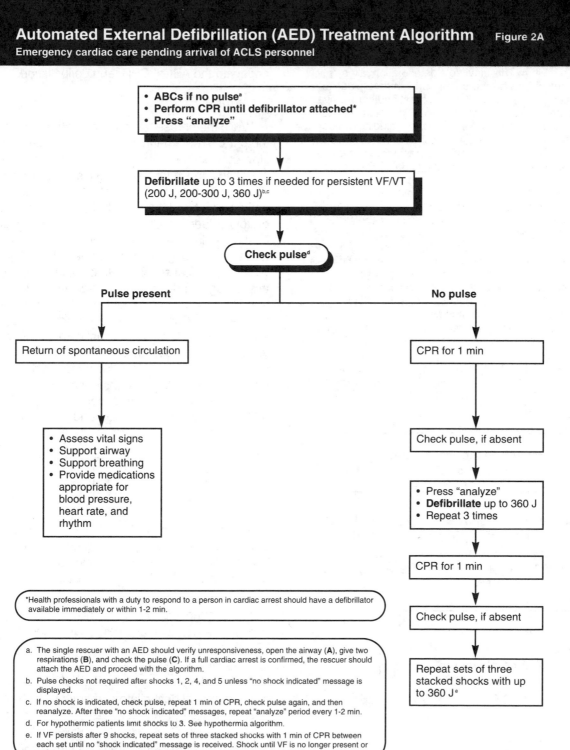

Automated External Defibrillation (AED) Treatment Algorithm   Figure 2A
Emergency cardiac care pending arrival of ACLS personnel

- **ABCs if no pulse**[a]
- **Perform CPR until defibrillator attached***
- **Press "analyze"**

↓

Defibrillate up to 3 times if needed for persistent VF/VT
(200 J, 200-300 J, 360 J)[b,c]

↓

Check pulse[d]

Pulse present / **No pulse**

Pulse present:

Return of spontaneous circulation

↓

- Assess vital signs
- Support airway
- Support breathing
- Provide medications appropriate for blood pressure, heart rate, and rhythm

No pulse:

CPR for 1 min

↓

Check pulse, if absent

↓

- Press "analyze"
- **Defibrillate** up to 360 J
- Repeat 3 times

↓

CPR for 1 min

↓

Check pulse, if absent

↓

Repeat sets of three stacked shocks with up to 360 J[e]

*Health professionals with a duty to respond to a person in cardiac arrest should have a defibrillator available immediately or within 1-2 min.

a. The single rescuer with an AED should verify unresponsiveness, open the airway (**A**), give two respirations (**B**), and check the pulse (**C**). If a full cardiac arrest is confirmed, the rescuer should attach the AED and proceed with the algorithm.

b. Pulse checks not required after shocks 1, 2, 4, and 5 unless "no shock indicated" message is displayed.

c. If no shock is indicated, check pulse, repeat 1 min of CPR, check pulse again, and then reanalyze. After three "no shock indicated" messages, repeat "analyze" period every 1-2 min.

d. For hypothermic patients limit shocks to 3. See hypothermia algorithm.

e. If VF persists after 9 shocks, repeat sets of three stacked shocks with 1 min of CPR between each set until no "shock indicated" message is received. Shock until VF is no longer present or the patient converts to a perfusing rhythm.

(Fig 2A) presents the recommendations for VF/VT pending arrival of ACLS personnel.

No matter what setting — home, community, or hospital — the majority of successful adult resuscitations depend on early defibrillation.[28] The focus on early defibrillation reflects the fact that an initial tachyarrhythmia causes 80% to 90% of nontraumatic cardiac arrests in adults.[29,30] The goal of early defibrillation is to get a defibrillator to these people before they deteriorate into a nonviable rhythm. This inevitable deterioration takes only a few minutes. This discouragingly brief interval leads to a constant emphasis on quick assessment and early arrival of personnel able to perform defibrillation. For in-hospital settings this means that nonphysicians, including all floor nurses, should be trained and equipped to perform defibrillation. Outside the hospital any emergency rescuers who are trained and expected to do CPR must be trained and allowed to perform defibrillation.

The Committee on Emergency Cardiac Care considers this principle of early defibrillation to be the standard of care in the community.[31] Every community should strive to reach this objective. The recommendation "a defibrillator on every ambulance" or "a defibrillator on every hospital floor" may not be possible to fulfill in all circumstances. However, failure of emergency personnel to maintain a functioning defibrillator and to provide someone who is trained to use it during a cardiac arrest is difficult to defend unless extenuating circumstances exist. This cannot be considered the responsibility of device manufacturing or service representatives. Consequently, the AHA has developed extensive educational material for training in the use of AEDs.[7-9] This technology makes possible widespread application of the principle of early defibrillation and should be known and understood by all ECC providers as core information.

VF/VT present on monitor/defibrillator?
• **VF/VT algorithm (Fig 2)**

If rescuers detect VF or pulseless VT, they should deliver up to three "stacked shocks" (200 J, 200 to 300 J, up to 360 J) for persistent or immediately recurrent VF/VT. The VF/VT algorithm (Fig 2) presents the full recommendations for VF/VT.

VF/VT absent
• **Intubate**
• **Confirm tube placement**
• **Confirm ventilations**
• **Determine rhythm and cause**

The Secondary ABCD Survey

The initial attachment of the defibrillator/monitor may reveal the absence of VF/VT. Rescuers should now turn to the ABCDs of the secondary ABCD survey:

- Intubate the patient (A)
- Confirm endotracheal tube placement (A)
- Confirm adequate chest rise and ventilations (B)
- Determine the rhythm (C)
- Consider the differential diagnosis and possible causes (D)

The universal algorithm makes no mention of IV access for patients without a pulse. This is intentional. Although medications play a major role in cardiac resuscitation, rescuers should consider medications secondary to the ABCs, CPR, and defibrillation.

Determine Rhythm and Cause

While the phrase "determine rhythm" appears obvious, the phrase "determine cause" may appear premature. How can rescuers determine the cause of the cardiac arrest so soon in the resuscitative attempt? The phrase, however, directs the rescuer to think at once about the entire patient and the overall clinical situation. Serum laboratory values may not return within the temporal window of success in a cardiac resuscitation. The astute clinician, however, can begin thinking immediately about the rich variety of clinical scenarios that could be taking place: Is this a drug overdose? What medications does the patient take? Is the patient in renal failure? Does the patient have a history that would suggest severe problems with acidosis or electrolyte abnormalities? What about hypovolemia? massive myocardial infarction (MI)? massive pulmonary embolism? cardiac tamponade? tension pneumothorax? dissecting aneurysm? Is the endotracheal tube still in the correct position? The wise rescuer will consider the entire patient and not just the cardiac monitor.

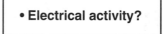

• **Electrical activity?**

The monitor display, however, does lead the rescue team to the next step in the algorithm. If the monitor reveals a flat line, the rescuer should remember that "flat line" has a differential diagnosis:

- Loose leads
- Not connected to the patient
- Not connected to the defibrillator/monitor
- No power
- Signal gain turned too low
- Isoelectric VF/VT or true asystole[32]

Older model defibrillators, many of which remain in use, display the rhythm and perform defibrillation in a variety of ways.[33] For example, power to the defibrillator and power to the monitor may require pressing two separate controls. Such defibrillators often lack the "quick look" feature of rhythm monitoring through the paddles/pads. VF/VT rarely may have a "vector of VF" that produces "false asystole" in one lead.[34,35] This rare phenomenon can be detected by checking two or more leads or by orienting the axis of the paddles 90°. Data have demonstrated, however, that operator mistakes in using the equipment are a more common cause of "false asystole" than an "isoelectric vector of VF."[32] Rescuers must know their defibrillator and must be ready to perform a quick troubleshooting checklist. In several studies errors in operator use, defibrillator care, and defibrillator maintenance have accounted for a high proportion of defibrillator failures.[33,36] Remember, if something appears wrong with your defibrillator, review its operation quickly. Operator error is the most common problem.

> • Go to PEA algorithm (Fig 3) if electrical activity is present
> • Go to asystole algorithm (Fig 4) if no electrical activity is present

If at this point in the resuscitative efforts the monitor displays true asystole, the rescuer proceeds to the asystole algorithm (see below and Fig 4). If, however, the monitor reveals some variety of organized electrical activity, the rescuer must check quickly for a pulse. If the pulse check indicates a pulseless state, the resuscitation team moves to the PEA algorithm (see below and Fig 3).

Ventricular Fibrillation/Pulseless Ventricular Tachycardia Algorithm (Fig 2)

> • Check ABCs
> • Perform CPR until defibrillator attached[a]
> • VF/VT present on defibrillator/monitor

[a]**Precordial Thump**. The precordial thump is a Class IIb action (acceptable, possibly helpful) in witnessed arrest, no pulse, and no defibrillator immediately available.[37] A forceful precordial thump can convert patients out of VF/VT and into a perfusing cardiac function. However, this thump can also convert patients from coordinated cardiac activity into VF/VT or asystole. The 1986 AHA guidelines recommended the precordial thump when a defibrillator/monitor was available to correct conversion into a worse rhythm. The 1992 guidelines recommend the precordial thump when a defibrillator/monitor is *not* available, following the rationale that the thump may help and there is no alternative method available to convert the arrhythmia. If a defibrillator is available, it makes sense to go directly to that therapy and not waste even a minimum of time with the precordial thump.

Figure 2 presents the algorithm for VF/VT. For adult resuscitation this is the most important sequence to know because the majority of people who collapse in cardiac arrest are in VF and the majority of survivors will regain their pulse during these interventions. Particularly in some prehospital settings, rescuers may seldom use the

VF/VT protocol because they seldom observe VF/VT. This does not mean infrequent VF/VT in those systems. They seldom observe VF/VT because they arrive late with the defibrillator. In addition, these patients may have received poor airway management and no basic CPR. The treatment of VF/VT cannot be presented in the AHA guidelines without discussing the contribution of the entire chain of survival.[14] Without a strong chain of survival, emergency personnel will see only asystole.[38] The section in chapter 16 on ensuring effectiveness of ECC in the community presents these important interrelationships in the chain of survival in more detail.

The treatment sequence for VF/VT is simple: defibrillate VF/VT, protect the airway, ventilate the patient. This sequence cannot be performed effectively if emergency personnel do not maintain their defibrillators in a state of constant readiness through the use of maintenance checklists.[36,39] The medications that clinicians administer are only adjuncts to defibrillation.

> • Defibrillate up to three times, if needed for persistent VF/VT (200 J, 200 to 300 J, 360 J)

The Purpose of Defibrillation

Defibrillation does not "jump start" the heart. The purpose of the shock is to produce temporary asystole. The shock attempts to completely depolarize the myocardium and provide an opportunity for the natural pacemaker centers of the heart to resume normal activity.[40-43] During asystole cardiac rhythmicity will resume if sufficient stores of high-energy phosphates remain in the myocardium.[44-46] The fibrillating myocardium consumes these stores at a greater rate than normal cardiac rhythms do.[45,47] Thus, early defibrillation — before fibrillation consumes all these energy stores — becomes critical.

Sequenced Shocks

These three shocks are delivered one after the other, in a "stacked shocks" sequence. Research has demonstrated that successive shocks are more important than adjunctive drug therapy and that delays between shocks to deliver medications are detrimental.[48-50] Clinicians should leave the paddles pressed to the chest or defibrillate "remotely" through adhesive defibrillation pads. Recharging the defibrillator and assessing the postshock rhythm should occur quickly.

Pulse Checks Between Shocks

Personnel should not resume CPR while they recharge the defibrillator and reassess the rhythm unless there is some unavoidable delay. At this point in the treatment sequence, do not pause for a pulse check if a properly connected monitor clearly displays persistent VF/VT. Push the charge control as soon as the first and second shocks are delivered. Look immediately at the monitor screen (while recharging) to check for persistent VF/VT. If a non–VF/VT rhythm appears on the monitor, remove the paddles from the chest (leave adhesive pads in place), disarm the charged defibrillator, and check for a pulse.

Nitroglycerin Patches

If the patient has placed a nitroglycerin patch on his or her chest, remove it or make sure the defibrillation electrode does not touch the patch. Despite concern about potential volatility, the nitroglycerin substrate will not burn or "explode."[51] However, the aluminized backing used on some old transdermal delivery systems can lead to electrical arcing during defibrillation, with explosive noises, smoke, visible arcing, and patient burns.[51-54] The patches may also impair the transmission of current.[51] Most aluminized backing systems have been discontinued.

Implanted Pacemakers/Cardioverters-Defibrillators

Rescuers should avoid placing defibrillator pads or paddles over the generator unit of an implanted pacemaker or automatic cardioverter-defibrillator. Defibrillation directly over an implanted pacemaker or automatic cardioverter-defibrillator may block a part of the defibrillation current and possibly misprogram, disable, or severely damage the implanted device. Discharges from automatic implanted defibrillators can be felt by rescuers if they touch the patient during the shock, though the chances of harm to the rescuer are extremely remote. Witnesses may report that the implanted defibrillator has discharged or is in the midst of a charge-discharge cycle.

Rescuers should monitor patients with implanted defibrillators and observe if the patient is in VF or refibrillates. Most implantable defibrillators will assess charge and shock within 20 to 30 seconds. If the patient appears in VF and the implanted defibrillator is not delivering a shock, proceed with defibrillation protocols.

Clearing Chant for Defibrillation

To ensure safe defibrillation, people who perform defibrillation must always announce when they are about to shock.[55] The person who controls the defibrillator should state, firmly and in a forceful voice, a "warning chant" before each shock, for example:

- *"I am going to shock on three. One, I am clear."* (The operator checks and makes sure he or she has no contact with the patient, the stretcher, or other equipment.)
- *"Two, you are clear."* (The operator checks the personnel doing ventilations and chest compressions, who should remove their hands from the ventilatory adjuncts, including the endotracheal tube and ventilation bags.)
- *"Three, everybody is clear."* (The operator makes a visual check to ensure that no one else has contact with the patient or stretcher.)

The person operating the defibrillator need not use these exact words but must warn others that he or she is about to defibrillate and that everyone needs to stand clear.

Rhythm after the first three shocks?[b]
Persistent or recurrent VF/VT

- **Continue CPR**
- **Intubate at once**
- **Obtain IV access**

---

[b]**Hypothermic cardiac arrest** is treated differently after this point. Do not continue to shock a person in hypothermic cardiac arrest if he or she remains in VF/VT after three defibrillations. This person needs rewarming according to the treatment guidelines in the section on hypothermia.

If VF/VT persists after three shocks, the treatment algorithm directs personnel to intubate the patient and obtain IV access. The effective team leader will have already assigned four tasks at the start of resuscitation:

- Airway and intubation
- Chest compressions
- Monitoring and defibrillation
- IV access

The flow diagram visually suggests that rescuers perform a linear sequence of events. Rescuers should realize, however, that a flow diagram conveys an order of priorities. The flow diagram assumes, for pedagogic reasons, that only one person performs the interventions. In well-organized resuscitative efforts, however, the other personnel (if available) prepare for and perform their assigned tasks in synchronization with the rhythm assessments and defibrillations.

- **Administer epinephrine 1 mg IV push[c,d]**
  (Repeat every 3 to 5 minutes)

---

[c]**The recommended dose of epinephrine** is 1 mg IV push every 3 to 5 minutes. If this approach fails, several Class IIb dosing regimens can be considered:

- Intermediate: epinephrine 2 to 5 mg IV push, every 3 to 5 minutes
- Escalating: epinephrine 1 mg-3 mg-5 mg IV push, 3 minutes apart
- High: epinephrine 0.1 mg/kg IV push, every 3 to 5 minutes

[d]**Sodium bicarbonate** 1 mEq/kg is Class I if patient has known preexisting hyperkalemia. (This is an excellent example of the "D" — for *differential diagnosis* — of the secondary ABCD survey. If the cardiac arrest is associated with hyperkalemia, the immediate use of sodium bicarbonate could be lifesaving.)

Ventricular Fibrillation/Pulseless Ventricular Tachycardia (VF/VT) Algorithm

Figure 2

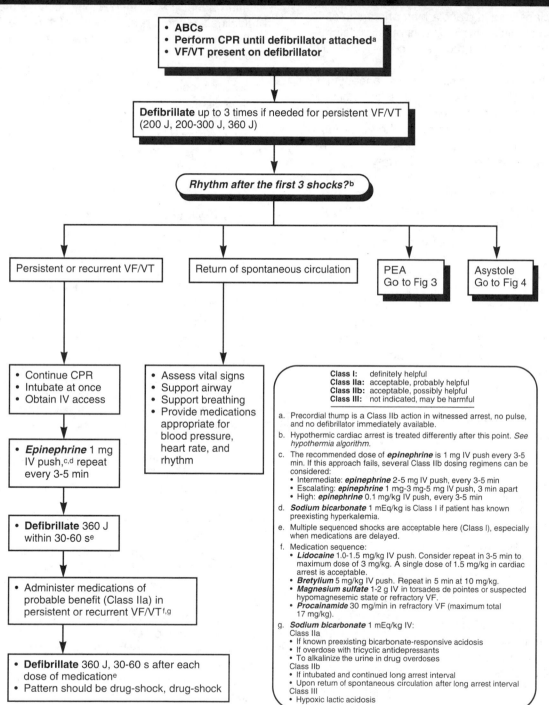

- **ABCs**
- **Perform CPR until defibrillator attached**[a]
- **VF/VT present on defibrillator**

Defibrillate up to 3 times if needed for persistent VF/VT (200 J, 200-300 J, 360 J)

Rhythm after the first 3 shocks?[b]

| Persistent or recurrent VF/VT | Return of spontaneous circulation | PEA Go to Fig 3 | Asystole Go to Fig 4 |

Persistent or recurrent VF/VT:
- Continue CPR
- Intubate at once
- Obtain IV access

- ***Epinephrine*** 1 mg IV push,[c,d] repeat every 3-5 min

- **Defibrillate** 360 J within 30-60 s[e]

- Administer medications of probable benefit (Class IIa) in persistent or recurrent VF/VT[f,g]

- **Defibrillate** 360 J, 30-60 s after each dose of medication[e]
- Pattern should be drug-shock, drug-shock

Return of spontaneous circulation:
- Assess vital signs
- Support airway
- Support breathing
- Provide medications appropriate for blood pressure, heart rate, and rhythm

Class I: definitely helpful
Class IIa: acceptable, probably helpful
Class IIb: acceptable, possibly helpful
Class III: not indicated, may be harmful

a. Precordial thump is a Class IIb action in witnessed arrest, no pulse, and no defibrillator immediately available.

b. Hypothermic cardiac arrest is treated differently after this point. *See hypothermia algorithm.*

c. The recommended dose of ***epinephrine*** is 1 mg IV push every 3-5 min. If this approach fails, several Class IIb dosing regimens can be considered:
   - Intermediate: ***epinephrine*** 2-5 mg IV push, every 3-5 min
   - Escalating: ***epinephrine*** 1 mg-3 mg-5 mg IV push, 3 min apart
   - High: ***epinephrine*** 0.1 mg/kg IV push, every 3-5 min

d. ***Sodium bicarbonate*** 1 mEq/kg is Class I if patient has known preexisting hyperkalemia.

e. Multiple sequenced shocks are acceptable here (Class I), especially when medications are delayed.

f. Medication sequence:
   - ***Lidocaine*** 1.0-1.5 mg/kg IV push. Consider repeat in 3-5 min to maximum dose of 3 mg/kg. A single dose of 1.5 mg/kg in cardiac arrest is acceptable.
   - ***Bretylium*** 5 mg/kg IV push. Repeat in 5 min at 10 mg/kg.
   - ***Magnesium sulfate*** 1-2 g IV in torsades de pointes or suspected hypomagnesemic state or refractory VF.
   - ***Procainamide*** 30 mg/min in refractory VF (maximum total 17 mg/kg).

g. ***Sodium bicarbonate*** 1 mEq/kg IV:
   Class IIa
   - If known preexisting bicarbonate-responsive acidosis
   - If overdose with tricyclic antidepressants
   - To alkalinize the urine in drug overdoses
   Class IIb
   - If intubated and continued long arrest interval
   - Upon return of spontaneous circulation after long arrest interval
   Class III
   - Hypoxic lactic acidosis

Epinephrine

Epinephrine, at the standard dose of 1 mg given IV every 3 to 5 minutes, remains the drug of choice for patients in cardiac arrest. Since the 1985 AHA national conference, clinicians and researchers have conducted extensive research on the use of adrenergic medications in cardiac arrest.[56-74] No agent has proven superior to epinephrine for increasing blood flow and improving outcomes. Clinicians should place a high priority on early administration of this agent. Epinephrine stimulates adrenergic receptors and produces increased blood flow to the brain and heart.

Pharmacologic principles support the concept that the dose of epinephrine, like most other agents, should be weight-adjusted. A wide variety of clinical situations, such as those discussed under bicarbonate therapy and PEA, demand variation in therapeutic actions. For example, patients with acidosis, fixed coronary artery lesions, and arrhythmogenic foci may respond adversely to higher and more frequent doses of epinephrine. Retrospective reviews, however, have observed no higher incidence of complications in survivors of higher dose epinephrine than survivors of standard doses of epinephrine.[63] "Rapid escalation" of epinephrine dose (1 mg-3 mg-5 mg given 3 to 5 minutes apart for those people who are "standard dose unresponsive") presents one example of this therapeutic variety. Intermediate doses (2 to 5 mg) combined with epinephrine infusions represents yet another approach, and clinicians have reported anecdotal successes.[56,57,66,70] See the discussion of high-dose epinephrine in chapter 7.

Defibrillate at 360 J, within 30 to 60 seconds[e]

---

[e]Multiple sequenced shocks (200 J, 200 to 300 J, 360 J) are acceptable here (Class I), especially when medications are delayed.

Rescuers should have delivered the first three defibrillation shocks quickly, one after another, in a "stacked" fashion, provided the monitor demonstrates persistent VF/VT. Next, rescuers should have intubated and hyperventilated the patient, started an IV, and given epinephrine 1 mg IV.

From 30 to 60 seconds after the first dose of epinephrine, the rescuers should reassess the rhythm and if VF/VT is present deliver additional shocks. These additional shocks that follow intubation and epinephrine may also be "stacked," one after another. The entire sequence may be

- Shock, shock, shock
- (Intubate, IV, epinephrine)
- Shock, shock, shock

Numerous reports confirm that the "sets of three" approach to defibrillation is effective and that successful defibrillations have occurred after six, nine, twelve, or more shocks, even in the absence of medications.[28,75-85] The 1992 national conference considers the use of stacked defibrillations to be a Class I recommendation (acceptable, definitely effective).

The resuscitation guidelines of the European Resuscitation Council, published within weeks of the AHA guidelines, recommend four sets of three defibrillations, with 1 mg of epinephrine after each set.[86] This approach results in 12 defibrillations and 3 mg of epinephrine before any other agent is added. The AHA guidelines, however, mostly because of established practice and clinical familiarity, continue to recommend a single shock at this point (after the first dose of epinephrine) if IV medications are immediately available. As noted above, persistent rapid shocks to persistent VF/VT are acceptable and definitely effective.

Administer medications of probable benefit in persistent or recurrent VF[f,g]

- **Defibrillate 360 J within 30 to 60 seconds after each dose of medication**
- **Pattern should be drug-shock, drug-shock**

---

[f]**Medications:**
- **Lidocaine** 1.0 to 1.5 mg/kg IV push. Consider repeat in 3 to 5 minutes to maximum dose of 3 mg/kg. A single dose of 1.5 mg/kg in cardiac arrest is acceptable; then use
- **Bretylium** 5 mg/kg IV push. Repeat in 5 minutes at 10 mg/kg
- **Magnesium sulfate** 1 to 2 g IV in torsades de pointes or suspected hypomagnesemic state or refractory VF
- **Procainamide** 30 mg/min in refractory VF (maximum total 17 mg/kg)

[g]**Sodium Bicarbonate** 1 mEq/kg IV: see comments below.

The guidelines of the European Resuscitation Council,[86] which recommend 12 defibrillations before adding any drug besides epinephrine, effectively underscore a critical point — other than epinephrine, no individual medication has clearly been demonstrated to make a difference in outcome for VF/VT arrest. The medications that clinicians can consider at this point in the VF/VT algorithm are the antiarrhythmic agents — lidocaine, bretylium, magnesium, procainamide — and the buffer agent sodium bicarbonate. It must be stated again, however, that we do not know the exact incremental value (over continued countershocks) of these agents in persistent VF/VT.[87]

Lidocaine

If VF/VT persists after basic CPR, intubation, ventilation, four defibrillations, and one or more doses of epinephrine, rescuers are dealing with refractory or persistent VF. In addition, minutes have passed during which the patient has likely received only modest blood flow (10% to 30% of normal) from conventional closed-chest CPR. The chances now of the patient's regaining spontaneous circulation and a successful neurological outcome are low. Typically at this point in the protocol, rescuers administer an antifibrillatory agent, such as lidocaine, bretylium, or procainamide. They should follow this within 30 to 60 seconds with a 360-J shock. Rescuers must understand that it is not the pharmacologic agent that defibrillates the heart but the direct current shock.

Which initial antifibrillatory agent should clinicians give? Recommendations from the last three national conferences vacillated between **lidocaine** and **bretylium,** based mainly on research in laboratory animals on fibrillation thresholds and changes in current levels needed for defibrillation.[88] Limited clinical trials in humans have not demonstrated a clear superiority of one agent over the other. One study from Seattle suggested that bretylium was slightly better,[89] and one study from Milwaukee suggested that lidocaine was slightly better.[90] Many emergency personnel favor **lidocaine** as the more familiar, presumably safer, and faster-acting agent. For these reasons the VF algorithm lists lidocaine first.

The Dosage of Lidocaine in Refractory VF/VT. The initial dosage of **lidocaine** recommended in the algorithm is 1.0 to 1.5 mg/kg IV push. There has been discussion about whether to give (and at what dose) a second dose of lidocaine.[87] It is acceptable, in treating the desperate problem of refractory VF, to give an additional bolus of 1.0 to 1.5 mg/kg in 3 to 5 minutes to a total of 3 mg/kg (an additional countershock should be administered between these doses). Some experts,[87] however, argue that a total of 3 mg/kg is excessive in the arrested patient with no spontaneous effective circulation because the lack of blood flow profoundly alters the pharmacokinetics and volume of distribution of lidocaine.[91,92] No human research data address this problem of the optimal dose of lidocaine late in the treatment of refractory VF/VT. Clinicians must be aware that the balance between optimal therapeutics and toxic overdose is narrow in cardiac arrest. Several clinical conditions, such as advanced age and compromised liver function, dictate lower loading doses of lidocaine. Such patients should receive a single loading dose of 1 mg/kg.

However, discussions of lidocaine toxicity are moot in patients who are dying because they cannot be converted from refractory VF/VT. Thus, for patients who remain in VF/VT despite multiple countershocks, epinephrine, and proper ventilations, the more aggressive dosing regimen remains rational and acceptable.

Clinicians must watch vigilantly for seizures, respiratory compromise, and other signs of lidocaine toxicity in those patients who do regain a spontaneous circulation after the use of higher doses of lidocaine.

Once a full loading dose of lidocaine has been administered, additional boluses of 0.5 mg/kg may be given but no more often than every 8 to 10 minutes. Only bolus therapy should be used in the setting of cardiac arrest. Upon return of spontaneous circulation, start a continuous infusion at 2 to 4 mg/min. When given in the nonarrest setting to conscious patients, lidocaine should be infused at no more than 1 to 4 mg/min.

Bretylium

Rescuers should use **bretylium** when **lidocaine** and defibrillation have failed to convert VF or when VF recurs despite lidocaine.[93] Administer 5 mg/kg of bretylium tosylate IV as a bolus (or a single 500-mg bolus), and then attempt defibrillation again. A second dose of 10 mg/kg can be given in 5 minutes (assuming persistent VF) with a maximum total dose of 30 mg/kg.

Rescuers should know the details of administration of the antifibrillatory agents and the cautions about altered pharmacokinetics in the arrested heart. The AHA Subcommittee on ACLS considers these agents to be Class IIa recommendations (acceptable, probably helpful). This reflects the clinical reality that in the latter stages of resuscitative attempts the effectiveness of pharmacologic agents, including adrenergic agents, remains unknown.[87]

Electricity vs Antiarrhythmics

The spread of early defibrillation programs represents a natural experiment about the relative effectiveness of early defibrillation alone versus defibrillation plus late medication. It is difficult in human clinical studies to confirm an independent positive benefit from IV medications.[48-50] Some research suggests that there may be special resuscitation situations where rescuers should administer medications, particularly adrenergic agents, before defibrillation.[71] There may be a point in the deterioration of VF to asystole where the shock has such a high probability of producing postshock asystole that medications should be administered first. In theory, giving medications first could decrease the chances of asystole as the postshock rhythm. New monitoring devices that can estimate the duration of VF through median frequency analysis may supply rescuers with information to help decide between medications and electric shock.[94-96] These promising data should not be misinterpreted. They do not resurrect the discredited concept of "sweetening up" or "coarsening" VF with medications.[48-50] Rescuers should continue to place their highest priority on airway, ventilation, and early defibrillation.

Refractory or Recurrent Ventricular Fibrillation

Procainamide and **magnesium sulfate** are two other medications to consider in VF/VT that persists after multiple shocks, epinephrine, lidocaine, and bretylium. Neither of these medications has been studied as extensively for cardiac arrest as lidocaine and bretylium. In refractory VF/VT, administer IV **procainamide** at a dose of 30 mg/min up to a total of 17 mg/kg. The poor likelihood of success at this low rate of infusion in the cardiac arrest patient (40 minutes for a 70-kg person to receive 17 mg/kg) leads many practitioners to administer procainamide at a faster rate, but there are no studies that address this specific question.

The success of **magnesium sulfate** in prevention of VF/VT in the setting of acute MI patients has generated great hope for magnesium sulfate as an antiarrhythmic to use in cardiac arrest due to refractory VF/VT.[97-99] In large doses, magnesium sulfate lowers the blood pressure,[100] but this may not necessarily compromise coronary perfusion pressure because it also dilates coronary arteries. The value of magnesium in human cardiac arrest has not been demonstrated in randomized controlled trials,[87] though encouraging anecdotal successes have been reported.[101-103] Therefore, the routine use of magnesium sulfate in VF/VT cardiac arrest is considered Class IIb (acceptable, possibly helpful). Magnesium sulfate, however, is a Class IIa agent (acceptable, probably helpful) in patients with low serum magnesium. Administer magnesium sulfate 1 to 2 g IV push in patients with known or suspected hypomagnesemia (eg, patients with alcoholism or other conditions associated with malnutrition). Use magnesium at the same dose or higher for patients with a torsades de pointes pattern of VF or VT.

The Value of Interposed Non–VF Rhythms During VF Treatment. Faced with persistent, refractory, or recurrent VF, astute clinicians will not continue with cycles of electric shocks and escalating drug doses. They should think in terms of the basics of resuscitation: adequate CPR, adequate airway and ventilation, and properly administered pharmacologic agents. The "D" of the Secondary ABCD Survey dictates consideration of the differential diagnosis of the cardiac arrest. Clinicians should consider coexisting electrolyte abnormalities and medication side effects. The non–VF cardiac rhythms that immediately follow shocks or that precede refibrillation may offer a clue to causes and interventions.

For example, epinephrine or excessive levels of endogenous catecholamines may be playing a role if a rapid tachycardia precedes the refibrillation. In these situations the team leader should consider withholding further doses of epinephrine, particularly if doses higher than 1 mg were used, and giving β **blockers**, such as **metoprolol** 5 mg IV.

If a sinus or AV bradycardia precedes the refibrillation, the clinician should consider the addition of **atropine** or the use of **transcutaneous pacing (TCP)**. Electrolyte abnormalities, particularly potassium and magnesium, may produce immediate postshock refibrillation or persistent VF.[101-103] Known or suspected hyperkalemia (serum potassium level higher than 6 mmol/L [6 mEq/L]) should be treated with calcium chloride 4 mg/kg acutely followed by insulin, glucose, and sodium bicarbonate. Hypokalemia is often associated with low magnesium (less than 0.7 mmol/L [1.4 mEq/L]) and should be treated with potassium chloride 10 mEq IV slowly over 10 to 15 minutes using a diluted solution.

gSodium Bicarbonate. Sodium bicarbonate has a variable status.[104] In specific situations sodium bicarbonate can be Class I (acceptable, definitely helpful), Class IIa (acceptable, probably effective), Class IIb (acceptable, possibly effective), or Class III (harmful).[105,106] Some researchers and clinicians have conducted the "bicarbonate debate" in absolute terms. Emergency personnel either give bicarbonate in cardiac arrest or completely avoid it. As with most areas in clinical medicine, however, bicarbonate therapy requires clinical judgment and modifications based on each clinical situation. In this regard there are clear indications for bicarbonate administration, and it should not be administered unless an appropriate indication exists.[104]

- Sodium bicarbonate (1 mEq/kg) is Class I (definitely helpful) if the patient is known to be hyperkalemic.
- Sodium bicarbonate therapy is Class IIa (acceptable and probably effective)
  — For patients with known or suspected preexisting bicarbonate-responsive acidosis and metabolic acidosis due to bicarbonate losses (gastrointestinal or renal)
  — To alkalinize the serum in severe tricyclic overdose
  — To alkalinize the urine in certain drug overdoses, such as phenobarbital or aspirin (this, of course, is an impractical therapeutic goal *during* cardiac arrest and applies in general to such overdoses)
- Sodium bicarbonate is Class IIb (acceptable and possibly effective)
  — For patients who are intubated and have been in protracted cardiac arrest
  — For patients with protracted cardiac arrest who experience return of spontaneous circulation
- Sodium bicarbonate is not indicated and is possibly harmful (Class III) in patients with hypoxic lactic acidosis, such as occurs in prolonged cardiopulmonary arrest. In such clinical situations the accumulation of metabolic byproducts, not bicarbonate deficits, has produced the acidosis. No evidence demonstrates that buffering the arterial pH with bicarbonate in such circumstances benefits the patient, and some evidence suggests it is harmful.[107]

Maintenance Antiarrhythmics After Return of Spontaneous Circulation

Once VF/VT has resolved after the sequence of treatment outlined above, clinicians should begin an IV infusion of the antiarrhythmic that appeared to aid in the restoration of a pulse. If defibrillation alone led to a restored circulation, the patient should be given a pharmacologic loading dose of **lidocaine** (not bretylium or procainamide) followed by a continuous infusion. These agents are administered as follows:

- **Lidocaine.** Loading dose of 0.5 to 1.5 mg/kg to a total of 2.0 mg/kg (if not already given lidocaine during the arrest); followed by a continuous infusion of 2 to 4 mg/min.
- **Bretylium.** Continuous infusion of 1 to 2 mg/min.
- **Procainamide.** Continuous infusion of 1 to 4 mg/min.

Pulseless Electrical Activity (PEA) Algorithm (Fig 3)

The PEA algorithm summarizes the treatment for a heterogeneous group of rhythms that includes electromechanical dissociation (EMD),[108-111] pseudo-EMD, idioventricular rhythms, ventricular escape rhythms, postdefibrillation idioventricular rhythms,[112] and bradyasystolic rhythms.[40,113-116] The major clinical point to remember about these arrhythmias is that they are often associated with specific clinical states that can be reversed when identified early and treated appropriately.

The absence of a detectable pulse and the presence of some type of electrical activity define this group of arrhythmias. When the electrical activity is narrow and no pulse is detectable, cardiologists traditionally have applied the term *electromechanical dissociation* or EMD.[116] This is a state in which organized electrical depolarization occurs throughout the myocardium but no synchronous shortening of the myocardial fiber occurs. Mechanical contractions are absent. Recent research with cardiac ultrasonography and indwelling pressure catheters, however, has led to a reconsideration of "electromechanical dissociation,"[117-119] and Paradis has proposed the term *pseudo-EMD*.[119] These data demonstrate that often the electrical activity is associated with mechanical contractions, only these contractions do not produce a blood pressure detectable by the usual methods of palpation or sphygmomanometer. This interesting group represents an intermediate state between bradycardia and cardiac arrest. If the electrical activity is rapid, the pulseless state may be a variation of tachycardia that is profoundly symptomatic. Countershock may be an appropriate intervention.

Hypovolemia is the most common cause of electrical activity without measurable blood pressure. Through prompt recognition and appropriate therapy clinicians can often correct the many causes of PEA and hypovolemia. These include hypovolemia from hemorrhage and other fluid losses, cardiac tamponade, tension pneumothorax, and massive pulmonary embolism. (See Fig 3 and Table 2.)

The other PEAs observed in cardiac arrest are arrhythmias that are broader than the narrow complexes of EMD. These rhythms are less likely to be associated with hypovolemia. Most clinical studies have observed poor survival rates from these rhythms, especially in the prehospital setting.[109,111,112,120-122] They often indicate malfunction of the myocardium or the cardiac conduction system, such as occurs with massive acute MI. These rhythms may represent the last electrical activity of a dying myocardium, or they may indicate specific critical rhythm disturbances. For example, severe hyperkalemia,

Table 2. Conditions That Cause Pulseless Electrical Activity

Condition	Clues	Management
Hypovolemia	History, flat neck veins	Volume infusion
Hypoxia	Cyanosis, blood gases, airway problems	Ventilations
Cardiac tamponade	History (trauma, renal failure, thoracic malignancy), no pulse with CPR, vein distention; impending tamponade-tachycardia, hypotension, low pulse pressure — changing to sudden bradycardia as terminal event	Pericardiocentesis
Tension pneumothorax	History (asthma, ventilator, chronic obstructive pulmonary disease, trauma) no pulse with CPR, neck vein distention, tracheal deviation	Needle decompression
Hypothermia	History of exposure to cold, central body temperature	See hypothermia algorithm (chapter 10, Fig 2)
Massive pulmonary embolism	History, no pulse felt with CPR, distended neck veins	Pulmonary arteriogram, surgical embolectomy, thrombolytics
Drug overdose (tricyclics, digoxin, β blockers, calcium channel blockers)	Bradycardia, history of ingestion, empty bottles at the scene, pupils, neurological exam	Drug screens, intubation, lavage, activated charcoal, lactulose per local protocols
Hyperkalemia	History of renal failure, diabetes, recent dialysis, dialysis fistulas, medications	Calcium chloride (immediate); then combination of insulin, glucose, sodium bicarbonate; then sodium polystyrene sulfonate/sorbitol; dialysis (long-term)
Preexisting acidosis	History of bicarbonate-responsive preexisting acidosis, renal failure	Sodium bicarbonate, hyperventilation
Acute, massive MI	History, ECG, enzymes	See algorithm on cardiogenic shock (Fig 8)

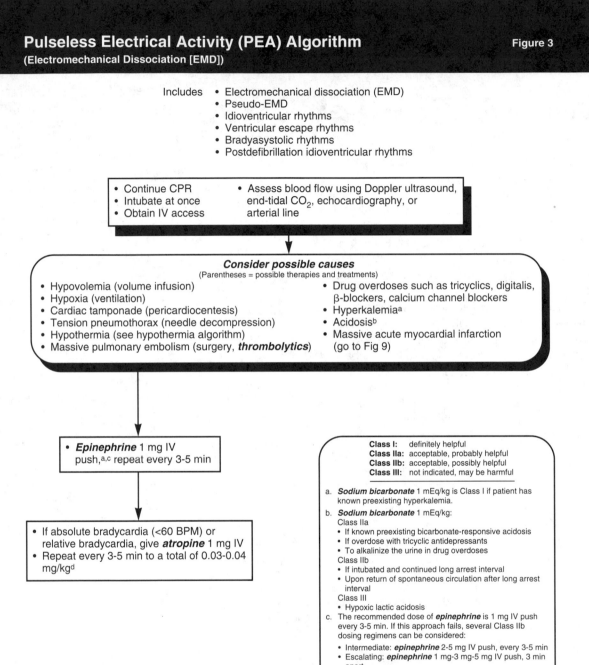

Pulseless Electrical Activity (PEA) Algorithm

Figure 3

(Electromechanical Dissociation [EMD])

Includes
- Electromechanical dissociation (EMD)
- Pseudo-EMD
- Idioventricular rhythms
- Ventricular escape rhythms
- Bradyasystolic rhythms
- Postdefibrillation idioventricular rhythms

- Continue CPR
- Intubate at once
- Obtain IV access

- Assess blood flow using Doppler ultrasound, end-tidal CO_2, echocardiography, or arterial line

Consider possible causes
(Parentheses = possible therapies and treatments)

- Hypovolemia (volume infusion)
- Hypoxia (ventilation)
- Cardiac tamponade (pericardiocentesis)
- Tension pneumothorax (needle decompression)
- Hypothermia (see hypothermia algorithm)
- Massive pulmonary embolism (surgery, **thrombolytics**)

- Drug overdoses such as tricyclics, digitalis, β-blockers, calcium channel blockers
- Hyperkalemia[a]
- Acidosis[b]
- Massive acute myocardial infarction (go to Fig 9)

- **Epinephrine** 1 mg IV push,[a,c] repeat every 3-5 min

- If absolute bradycardia (<60 BPM) or relative bradycardia, give **atropine** 1 mg IV
- Repeat every 3-5 min to a total of 0.03-0.04 mg/kg[d]

Class I: definitely helpful
Class IIa: acceptable, probably helpful
Class IIb: acceptable, possibly helpful
Class III: not indicated, may be harmful

a. **Sodium bicarbonate** 1 mEq/kg is Class I if patient has known preexisting hyperkalemia.
b. **Sodium bicarbonate** 1 mEq/kg:
   Class IIa
   - If known preexisting bicarbonate-responsive acidosis
   - If overdose with tricyclic antidepressants
   - To alkalinize the urine in drug overdoses
   Class IIb
   - If intubated and continued long arrest interval
   - Upon return of spontaneous circulation after long arrest interval
   Class III
   - Hypoxic lactic acidosis
c. The recommended dose of **epinephrine** is 1 mg IV push every 3-5 min. If this approach fails, several Class IIb dosing regimens can be considered:
   - Intermediate: **epinephrine** 2-5 mg IV push, every 3-5 min
   - Escalating: **epinephrine** 1 mg-3 mg-5 mg IV push, 3 min apart
   - High: **epinephrine** 0.1 mg/kg IV push, every 3-5 min
d. The shorter **atropine** dosing interval (3 min) is possibly helpful in cardiac arrest (Class IIb).

hypothermia, hypoxia, preexisting acidosis, and a large variety of drug overdoses can present as broad-complex PEA. Overdoses of tricyclic antidepressants, β blockers, calcium channel blockers, digitalis, and many other agents[123] can produce PEA. These overdoses have specific interventions.

Astute clinicians must take one major action when faced with any PEA: search for the possible causes. These rhythms, particularly when they are the presenting arrest rhythm, may be due to a number of problems. These must be learned and considered for every patient in PEA.

Nonspecific therapeutic interventions for PEA include epinephrine, and (if the rate is slow) atropine, administered as presented in Fig 3. In addition, personnel should provide proper airway management and aggressive hyperventilation since hypoventilation and hypoxemia are frequent causes of PEA. Clinicians also can give a fluid challenge since the PEA may be due to hypovolemia.

Clinicians should be aggressive when evaluating and treating patients with PEA. Bedside echocardiography, especially transesophageal, is invaluable in detecting good cardiac contractility.[124] Immediate use of Doppler ultrasound may reveal blood flow undetectable by simple arterial palpation. Such patients have a greater probability of survival since they are not truly in cardiac arrest.[119] Clinicians should aggressively treat patients who have detectable blood flow or good cardiac contractility, referring to the algorithm for severe hypotension (systolic blood pressure less than 70 mm Hg), Fig 8. These patients may need volume expansion, **norepinephrine, dopamine,** some combination of the three, or other interventions. Interventions may include β blockade, calcium channel blockade, or pacing, depending on unique clinical situations (eg, idiopathic hypertrophic subaortic stenosis). These patients may benefit from early TCP. Clinicians must identify possible reversible causes and institute cause-specific interventions.

Drug overdoses frequently produce PEA. In these situations a healthy myocardium exists, but a temporarily disturbed cardiac conduction system can cause death. Case reports confirm the success of specific interventions such as intra-aortic balloon pumping, cardiopulmonary bypass,[125] renal dialysis, and TCP[123,126-128] for patients with PEA. A rapid PEA may represent a variation of profoundly symptomatic tachycardia, and electrical countershock should be considered. While in general PEA has poor outcomes, clinicians should search for reversible causes.

Asystole Treatment Algorithm
(Fig 4)

A key point to remember about treatment of asystole is that the team leader must rapidly and aggressively consider the differential diagnosis.

Clinicians should treat asystole with

- Continued CPR
- Intubation
- Epinephrine
- Atropine

This treatment sequence is virtually identical to the treatment algorithm for PEA. Clinicians administer atropine routinely to all asystolic cardiac arrest patients, whereas they should administer atropine to PEA patients only when they have slow electrical activity. On rare occasions high levels of parasympathetic tone may lead to cessation of both ventricular and supraventricular pacemaker activity.[40,43] Electrical shocks also produce a "stunned heart" and profound parasympathetic discharge.[40,43] For this reason routine shocking of asystole because "it cannot make the rhythm any worse" should be strongly discouraged. Such shocks to asystole could eliminate any possibility for the return of spontaneous cardiac activity. EMS systems that instituted "shocks for asystole" detected no improvement in survival.[129-131] Rescuers should confirm asystole as the rhythm when faced with a "flat line" on the monitor. They can do this by changing to another lead on the lead-select switch or by changing placement of the defibrillation paddles by 90°. Operator errors that lead to "false asystole" are much more common than VF that masquerades as false asystole.[32]

The 1992 guidelines say "consider immediate transcutaneous pacing" with a number of caveats. Researchers have conducted many clinical trials of TCP since 1986.[42,126,127,132-147] This extensive clinical experience, numbering more than 1000 patients, has demonstrated that in the setting of prehospital cardiac arrest, the asystolic heart almost never responds to pacing. A recent controlled trial of early TCP by the first-responding personnel (emergency medical technicians) started pacing before intubation and IV medications. This study observed no benefit for early pacing either for patients initially found in asystole or for patients in postdefibrillation asystole.[139]

To have any chance of effectiveness, TCP must be performed early. Prehospital rescuers can rarely achieve this objective. The critical ingredient is the interval from the start of asystole to the start of pacing. Patients who have been in cardiac arrest for only a brief period may remain viable and capable of responding to pacing for a short while. This includes people who suddenly develop a bradyasystolic arrest, Stokes-Adams attacks, asystole due to vagal discharge, or myocardial "stunning" following prompt defibrillation.[138]

Therefore, the 1992 guidelines consider TCP a Class IIb intervention, with only rare, anecdotal success. There are no data to justify routine pacing in asystolic cardiac arrest or to justify placing free-standing transcutaneous pacemakers on all prehospital advanced life support vehicles.[139] Clinicians who decide to initiate pacing for asystole in particular clinical situations should do so early, simultaneously with CPR and administration of medications.

TCP, however, particularly when combined with defibrillator monitors, has emerged as a valuable intervention for non–cardiac arrest situations. The 1992 guidelines put forward stronger recommendations for pacing in bradycardic, nonarrest rhythms. In this text pacing interventions occupy an entire chapter.

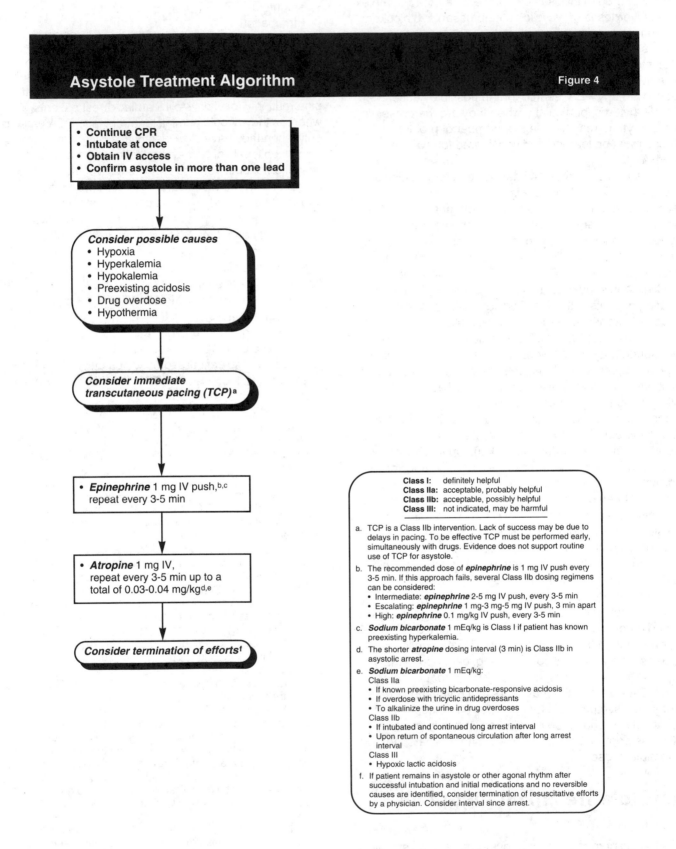

Asystole Treatment Algorithm

Figure 4

- **Continue CPR**
- **Intubate at once**
- **Obtain IV access**
- **Confirm asystole in more than one lead**

Consider possible causes
- Hypoxia
- Hyperkalemia
- Hypokalemia
- Preexisting acidosis
- Drug overdose
- Hypothermia

Consider immediate transcutaneous pacing (TCP)[a]

- ***Epinephrine*** 1 mg IV push,[b,c] repeat every 3-5 min

- ***Atropine*** 1 mg IV, repeat every 3-5 min up to a total of 0.03-0.04 mg/kg[d,e]

Consider termination of efforts[f]

Class I: definitely helpful
Class IIa: acceptable, probably helpful
Class IIb: acceptable, possibly helpful
Class III: not indicated, may be harmful

a. TCP is a Class IIb intervention. Lack of success may be due to delays in pacing. To be effective TCP must be performed early, simultaneously with drugs. Evidence does not support routine use of TCP for asystole.

b. The recommended dose of ***epinephrine*** is 1 mg IV push every 3-5 min. If this approach fails, several Class IIb dosing regimens can be considered:
   - Intermediate: ***epinephrine*** 2-5 mg IV push, every 3-5 min
   - Escalating: ***epinephrine*** 1 mg-3 mg-5 mg IV push, 3 min apart
   - High: ***epinephrine*** 0.1 mg/kg IV push, every 3-5 min

c. ***Sodium bicarbonate*** 1 mEq/kg is Class I if patient has known preexisting hyperkalemia.

d. The shorter ***atropine*** dosing interval (3 min) is Class IIb in asystolic arrest.

e. ***Sodium bicarbonate*** 1 mEq/kg:
   Class IIa
   - If known preexisting bicarbonate-responsive acidosis
   - If overdose with tricyclic antidepressants
   - To alkalinize the urine in drug overdoses
   Class IIb
   - If intubated and continued long arrest interval
   - Upon return of spontaneous circulation after long arrest interval
   Class III
   - Hypoxic lactic acidosis

f. If patient remains in asystole or other agonal rhythm after successful intubation and initial medications and no reversible causes are identified, consider termination of resuscitative efforts by a physician. Consider interval since arrest.

Termination of Efforts: Asystole as the Confirmation of Death

Usually asystole — the complete absence of electrical activity in the myocardium — represents extensive myocardial ischemia from prolonged periods of inadequate coronary perfusion. Such a status has a grim prognosis. Asystole most often represents a confirmation of death rather than a "rhythm" to be treated. Team leaders can cease efforts to resuscitate people from confirmed and persistent asystole when the patient has received successful endotracheal intubation, successful IV access, suitable basic CPR, and all rhythm-appropriate medications.

Once emergency personnel have performed these actions, how long should resuscitative efforts continue? The 1992 guidelines do not state a specific time limit beyond which rescuers can never have a successful resuscitation. Cardiac arrests in special situations such as hypothermia, electrocution, and drug overdoses present exceptions to any rules. Special situations call for common sense and clinical judgment. It is inappropriate, futile, and ethically unacceptable to routinely continue prehospital resuscitative efforts and require ambulance transport and ongoing CPR for all patients. Likewise, it is inappropriate for clinicians to routinely apply "stopping rules" without thinking about the particular clinical situation. Medical directors of prehospital care systems must develop criteria by which emergency personnel can, in coordination with medical control physicians, cease efforts to resuscitate asystole in the field. Chapter 15, "Ethical Aspects of CPR and ECC," provides a more detailed discussion of these issues. Cessation of efforts in the prehospital setting, following system-specific criteria and under direct medical control, should be standard practice in all EMS systems.

Postresuscitation Care of Patients Immediately After Cardiac Arrest

Key Points

1. Postresuscitation care refers to the period between restoration of a spontaneous circulation and transfer to the intensive care unit. In general, this period will be less than 30 minutes. Proper care in this period will make a critical difference in the eventual outcome, especially neurological function.

2. Patients may display a wide spectrum of responses to resuscitation, ranging from being awake and alert, with adequate spontaneous respirations and hemodynamic stability, to remaining comatose and apneic and having an unstable circulation.

3. In ACLS courses postresuscitation care does *not* cover invasive hemodynamic monitoring, as this topic more properly belongs in a discussion of critical care

medicine. Note, however, that most resuscitated patients will require invasive hemodynamic monitoring at some time for optimal management.

4. Personnel should continue to use the ABCDs of the primary and secondary surveys as a method to organize their evaluations and therapy. The immediate goal is to provide cardiorespiratory support to optimize tissue perfusion, especially to the brain. All patients require careful, repeated assessments to establish the status of their cardiovascular, respiratory, and neurological systems.

5. Do **not** apply the algorithms in reverse. That is, in the postresuscitation period do **not** use the tachycardia, bradycardia, and hypotension algorithms to treat postresuscitation tachycardia, bradycardia, and hypotension. As a general rule, most postresuscitation arrhythmias should be left untreated for the immediate postresuscitation period.

Critical Postresuscitation Actions to Take

1. Assess and treat following the **ABCD**s.

2. **Airway**
   - Secure the airway.
   - Verify endotracheal tube placement using physical examination (bilateral breath sounds and epigastric auscultation), end-tidal CO_2 indicators, endotracheal tube aspiration, and chest x-ray.

3. **Breathing**
   - Administer oxygen.
   - Supply positive-pressure ventilation through bag-valve mask or appropriate mechanical ventilation.
   - Verify bilateral chest movement.
   - Check pulse oximeter; order arterial blood gas analyses (unless the patient is a candidate for thrombolytic therapy).
   - Unless the patient resumes immediate spontaneous respirations, he or she will need to be mechanically ventilated. This will usually require paralysis and sedation. The level of mechanical ventilatory support is determined by the blood gas levels, respiratory rate, and perceived work of breathing. If high oxygen concentrations are needed, establish whether the cause is pulmonary or cardiac dysfunction.
   - Check for potential breathing complications from resuscitation, such as pneumothorax, rib fractures, sternal fractures, and improper endotracheal tube placement.

4. **Circulation**
   - Assess vital signs.
   - Start an IV line. Use normal saline. Glucose administration is reserved for patients with documented hypoglycemia.

- Apply an ECG monitor, pulse oximeter, and automatic sphygmomanometer.
- Monitor urine output.
- If the arrest rhythm was VF or VT and no antiarrhythmic treatment was given, lidocaine bolus followed by maintenance infusions should be initiated unless contraindicated, ie, in patients with ventricular escape rhythm.
- If an antiarrhythmic agent was used successfully during the code, a continuous infusion of that agent should be used.
- Consider thrombolytic therapy for patients with evidence of acute MI on their postresuscitation 12-lead ECG, provided that resuscitation duration was not prolonged and there was minimal trauma, no central line placement, and no other contraindications.

5. **Differential Diagnosis**

- Diagnose the precipitating causes of the arrest (MIs, primary arrhythmias, electrolyte disturbances).
- Diagnose complications (rib fracture, hemopneumothorax, pericardial tamponade, intra-abdominal trauma, misplaced endotracheal tube).
- Order a portable chest radiograph.
- Review the history, particularly the immediate pre-arrest period and current medications.
- Perform a physical examination.
- Order a 12-lead ECG.
- Order serum electrolytes, including magnesium and calcium, and cardiac enzymes.

Other Actions

- Change IV lines that were placed without proper sterile technique or those that cannot be maintained adequately.
- Insert a nasogastric tube.
- Insert a Foley catheter.
- Treat aggressively any electrolyte abnormalities identified, particularly potassium, sodium, calcium, or magnesium.
- Prepare the patient for transport to a special care unit with oxygen, ECG monitoring, and a full supply of resuscitation equipment and an adequate number of trained personnel. Maintain mechanical ventilation and oxygenation, along with ECG monitoring and blood pressure measurements.

Special Problems in the Immediate Postresuscitation Period

• **Central Nervous System.** A healthy brain is the primary goal of cardiopulmonary-cerebral resuscitation (CPCR). All efforts should be made to provide brain-oriented intensive care.[148] This topic is so critical that a separate chapter on cerebral resuscitation has been added to this edition of the ACLS textbook. The most important actions that ACLS providers can take in the immediate postresuscitation period to restore and protect cerebral function is to optimize the ABCs — oxygenation and perfusion. In particular this means providing adequately oxygenated arterial blood at a normal or slightly elevated mean arterial pressure. A growing body of evidence supports this concept of a "postresuscitation hypertensive bout."[148-150] Consider these specific actions in addition to maintaining oxygenation and blood pressure:

— Maintaining normothermia because hyperthermia increases the oxygen requirements of the brain[148]
— Controlling seizures because of similar increases in cerebral oxygen requirements (consider phenobarbital, phenytoin, or diazepam)
— Elevating the head to approximately 30° to increase cerebral venous drainage and decrease intracranial pressure

• **Hypotension.** Assess both circulating fluid volume and ventricular function. Even mild hypotension must be avoided because it can impair recovery of cerebral function. In the critically ill patient invasive hemodynamic monitoring will be necessary, including intra-arterial assessment of blood pressure and hydrostatic pressure measurements of the pulmonary circulation and cardiac output using a pulmonary artery flow-directed catheter. Invasive hemodynamic monitoring is beyond the scope of the ACLS Provider's Course.

Realistically ACLS providers will often have to deal with hemodynamic instability in the immediate postresuscitation period unassisted by invasive hemodynamic monitoring. Clinicians should consider whether the blood pressure instability arises from a problem with the cardiovascular triad — a volume, pump, or rate problem — as discussed in the section on problems of blood pressure, shock, and pulmonary congestion (Fig 8).

It is appropriate to administer a fluid bolus of 250 to 500 mL of normal saline unless known with certainty that the patient has volume overload. If hypotension with or without signs of shock persists after a fluid bolus, then inotropic (dobutamine) or vasopressor (dopamine, epinephrine, or norepinephrine) therapy may be indicated (Fig 8).

• **Recurrent VF/VT in the Postresuscitation Period.** Pulseless VF/VT may recur in the immediate postresuscitation period after return of spontaneous circulation. Lidocaine bolus (1 to 1.5 mg/kg) should routinely be administered after successful conversion from VF/VT even when lidocaine was not used during the cardiac arrest. Consider such recurrences as refractory VF/VT. Immediately review the therapy that successfully converted the original VF/VT. If lidocaine, procainamide, or bretylium was associated with the initial conversion to a spontaneous circulation, it can be repeated up to the maximum recommended dose. Consider magnesium sulfate 1 to 2 g IV. Follow the same drug-shock, drug-shock pattern used in the algorithm for VF/VT.

Quickly review the ABCDs: airway security, breathing and ventilation, circulation, and the differential diagnosis. Problems with poor ventilation, acid-base status, hypovolemia, and electrolyte abnormalities will often be the hidden culprits behind refractory or recurrent VF/VT. In this situation review of the ABCDs will produce better outcomes than more pharmacologic interventions.

• **Postresuscitation Tachycardias.** The rapid, supraventricular tachycardias rescuers may observe in the immediate postresuscitation period are best treated by leaving them alone. The high catecholamine state of cardiac arrest may be causing the tachycardia, particularly if high doses of epinephrine were administered. If the blood pressure drops or fails to increase reasonably soon after resuscitation, then the interventions listed in the tachycardia algorithm should be considered.

Again review the ABCDs. Thinking about the patient should take precedence over routine pharmacologic interventions. There is little experience with the use of adenosine in the treatment of postresuscitation tachycardias, so it should be considered a Class IIb recommendation. Lidocaine, bretylium, and procainamide should be considered Class IIa recommendations when administered for the appropriate arrhythmias.

• **Postresuscitation Bradycardias.** Poor ventilation and oxygenation play a major role in postresuscitation bradycardias. Clinicians should again attend to the ABCDs instead of asking immediately for atropine. If a profound bradycardia in the postresuscitation period is associated with hypotension and hypoperfusion, consider the use of pacing, atropine, and catecholamine infusions as directed in the bradycardia algorithm. TCP may be superior to atropine for postresuscitation bradycardias, although there is insufficient data to support pacing as the first intervention.

• **Postresuscitation Premature Ventricular Contractions.** Postresuscitation premature ventricular contractions may indicate problems with the secondary ABCDs. Clinicians should consider whether problems exist with the airway, breathing, or electrolytes. Watchful waiting is usually the most appropriate course of action, while improved oxygenation takes effect and the high levels of catecholamines and the acid-base status return to more normal levels. Lidocaine infusion is acceptable and probably helpful (Class IIa), especially if VF/VT originally precipitated the arrest.

Emergency Cardiac Care for Adults Not in Full Cardiac Arrest

The ECC provider should know how to manage cardiovascular and cardiopulmonary conditions in which the patient is not in full cardiac arrest. These are conditions which if not diagnosed and managed correctly could lead to a cardiac arrest in 30 to 60 minutes. The ECC provider must be able to care properly for patients *on their way* to a cardiac arrest. This section presents the initial approach to the major conditions that if identified and treated correctly may prevent deterioration to a cardiopulmonary arrest. These conditions are

- Serious, nonlethal arrhythmias ("too fast" or "too slow")
- Acute MI
- Hypotension/cardiogenic shock/acute pulmonary edema

The Universal Algorithm: Not in Full Cardiac Arrest

Figure 1, the universal algorithm for adult ECC, branches to the left when the provider determines that the patient is not in full cardiac arrest:

• **Rescue breathing**   • **Endotracheal** • **Oxygen**   **intubation** • **IV**   • **History** • **Vital signs**   • **Physical examination**   • **Monitor, 12-lead ECG**

• *Suspected Cause?*

As the algorithm is constructed, patients in this left branch have a pulse but are not breathing. For many of the conditions listed, however, the patients may have effective respirations. The **key point** is to repeatedly evaluate the adequacy of ventilations and breathing and to provide whatever support (rescue breathing, endotracheal intubation) is indicated.

Critical Actions to Take

- Learn *Oxygen-IV-monitor* as one word that should be memorized for easy recall and fast action in cardiac emergencies.[151]
  — *Oxygen*=provide supplemental oxygen to the patient.
  — *IV*=initiate an IV.
  — *Monitor*=attach the patient to a monitor.
- Continue to assess the status of the airways, the movement of air, and the status of ventilations.
- Provide rescue breathing and endotracheal intubation as indicated.
- Obtain the heart rate and blood pressure.
- Begin to take the history.
- Perform a primary and secondary physical examination survey.
- Obtain a 12-lead ECG within minutes, particularly if the patient complains of chest pain.

This initial evaluation, which concentrates on immediate patient assessment and collection of vital data, should lead the care providers to suspect one of several cardiovascular/pulmonary emergencies.[152] Figure 1 presents several conditions most likely to lead to a cardiac arrest if not rapidly diagnosed and treated correctly: a serious arrhythmia that is either too slow (Fig 5) or too fast (Fig 6); hypotension/shock/acute pulmonary edema (Fig 8); acute MI (Fig 9).

These conditions are complex. A full discussion exceeds the objectives of the AHA guidelines. The succinct recommendations presented in the treatment algorithms and discussed below provide a structure for thinking and a reminder of therapeutic possibilities. The algorithms are educational tools. They do not provide an in-depth review.

In addition, these conditions frequently overlap. For example, cardiogenic shock complicates 15% of acute MIs.[153] The following Venn diagram displays how multiple clinical conditions may occur simultaneously in ECC:

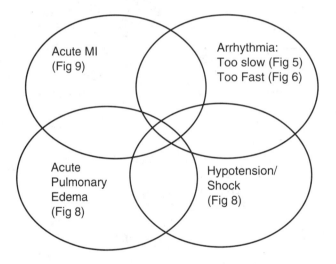

Acute MI (Fig 9)

Arrhythmia: Too slow (Fig 5) Too Fast (Fig 6)

Acute Pulmonary Edema (Fig 8)

Hypotension/ Shock (Fig 8)

The center of this Venn diagram reflects the critical state where acute MI leads simultaneously to cardiogenic shock (hypotension), acute pulmonary edema, and serious arrhythmias. This diagram also reminds care providers that they must always see the whole patient and not just the rhythm, the blood pressure, or the ECG. The ACLS algorithms present summaries of recommendations and cannot convey all clinical decision points.[152] Algorithms and guidelines are always a compromise between presenting complex clinical realities and useful clinical overviews.

- Arrhythmia
- Too slow: go to bradycardia algorithm
- Too fast: go to tachycardia algorithm

Overview of Rhythm Interpretation

Often emergency personnel can get lost in the complexities of rhythm identification, analysis, and the associated therapeutic interventions. All personnel should strive for an in-depth understanding of cardiac rhythms and the subtleties of treatment indications and contraindications. Complete mastery of rhythm analysis, however, could take an entire professional career. Even then there are cardiac conduction systems that can fool the most seasoned cardiologist.

In its simplest terms all rhythm diagnostics can be lumped into two classifications:

Simplified rhythm classification: cardiac arrest (lethal) rhythms and non–cardiac arrest (nonlethal) rhythms. This classification is easy to remember because there are, broadly speaking, only four cardiac arrest rhythms:

- VF
- VT
- Asystole
- Assorted PEAs (pulseless electrical activity, which includes EMD/bradyasystolic rhythms/pulseless idioventricular rhythms)

It could be argued that there is little need for ACLS providers to pay attention to the nonlethal, non–cardiac arrest rhythms, that all attention should be focused on the four lethal cardiac arrest rhythms. However, several of the non–cardiac arrest rhythms must be recognized because the rhythms may be pre-collapse or pre–cardiac arrest rhythms. These are easy to think about because, in the setting of ECC, there are only two non–cardiac arrest rhythms to consider:

- Too slow (less than 60 beats per minute)
- Too fast (more than 120 beats per minute)

The adjective *too* is used intentionally because it focuses attention on the next questions: How fast is "too fast"? And how slow is "too slow"? While it may seem overly simplistic to say "Is the rhythm too fast?" or "Is it too slow?" an emergency-care provider really does need to think at this level. To answer this question you must determine whether the rate problem is producing clinical symptoms.

Clinicians must consider whether the arrhythmia is causing the patient problems. Consider the rhythms dichotomously because there are simple "yes/no" (and perhaps "maybe") questions to ask: Is the rhythm causing the patient problems? Is the patient unstable? Is the rhythm causing signs and symptoms for the patient? The point is to not make decisions or take actions based only on the monitor display. Always concentrate on what is happening with the patient, using the ABCD surveys to review critical clinical parameters.

Bradycardia Treatment Algorithm

(Fig 5) (Patient is not in cardiac arrest)

Bradycardia, either absolute (<60 beats per minute) or relative

Serious signs or symptoms?[a,b]

Bradycardia Algorithm

(Patient is not in cardiac arrest)

Figure 5

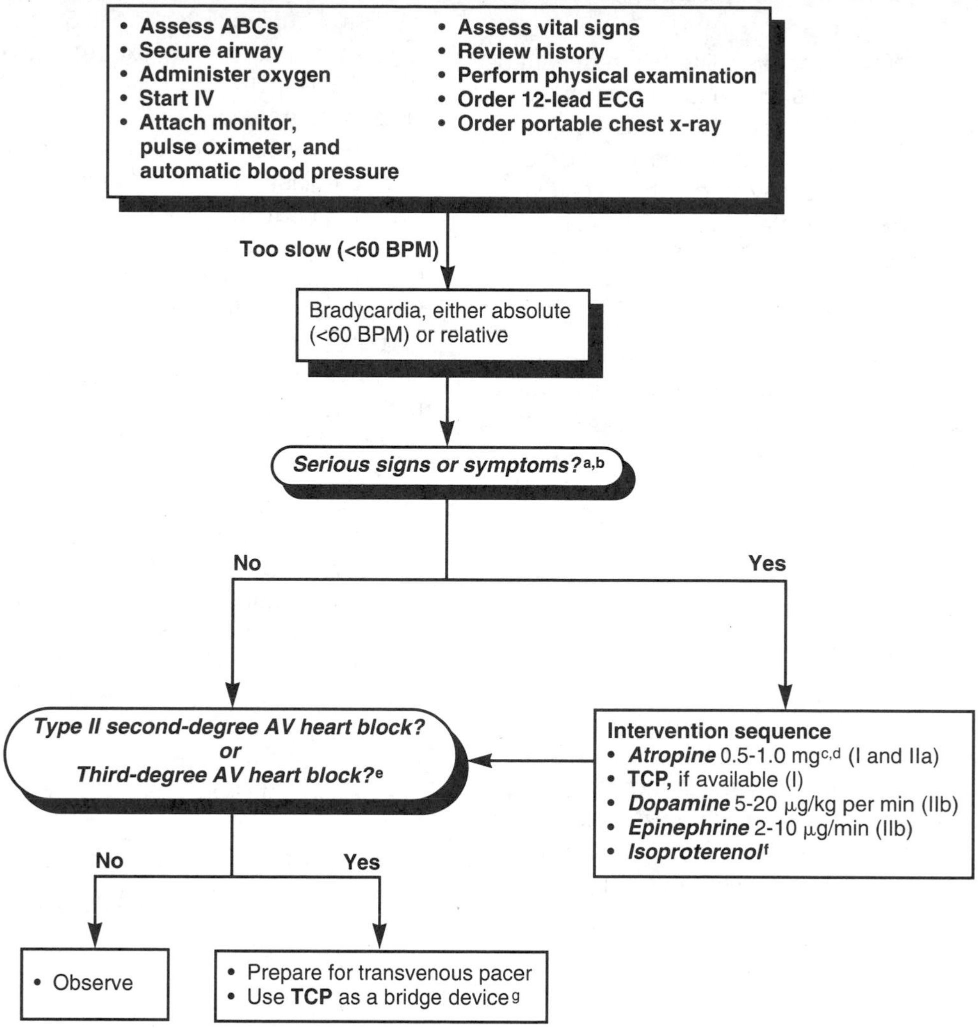

- **Assess ABCs**
- **Secure airway**
- **Administer oxygen**
- **Start IV**
- **Attach monitor, pulse oximeter, and automatic blood pressure**

- **Assess vital signs**
- **Review history**
- **Perform physical examination**
- **Order 12-lead ECG**
- **Order portable chest x-ray**

Too slow (<60 BPM)

Bradycardia, either absolute (<60 BPM) or relative

Serious signs or symptoms? [a,b]

No   **Yes**

Type II second-degree AV heart block?
or
Third-degree AV heart block? [e]

Intervention sequence
- ***Atropine*** 0.5-1.0 mg[c,d] (I and IIa)
- **TCP,** if available (I)
- ***Dopamine*** 5-20 μg/kg per min (IIb)
- ***Epinephrine*** 2-10 μg/min (IIb)
- ***Isoproterenol*** [f]

No   **Yes**

- Observe

- Prepare for transvenous pacer
- Use **TCP** as a bridge device [g]

---

a. Serious signs or symptoms must be related to the slow rate. Clinical manifestations include
   - Symptoms (chest pain, shortness of breath, decreased level of consciousness)
   - Signs (low BP, shock, pulmonary congestion, CHF, acute MI)
b. Do not delay TCP while awaiting IV access or for ***atropine*** to take effect if patient is symptomatic.
c. Denervated transplanted hearts will not respond to ***atropine.*** Go at once to pacing, ***catecholamine*** infusion, or both.
d. ***Atropine*** should be given in repeat doses every 3-5 min up to total of 0.03-0.04 mg/kg. Use the shorter dosing interval (3 min) in severe clinical conditions. It has been suggested that ***atropine*** should be used with caution in atrioventricular (AV) block at the His-Purkinje level (type II AV block and new third-degree block with wide QRS complexes) (Class IIb).
e. Never treat third-degree heart block plus ventricular escape beats with ***lidocaine.***
f. ***Isoproterenol*** should be used, if at all, with extreme caution. At low doses it is Class IIb (possibly helpful); at higher doses it is Class III (harmful).
g. Verify patient tolerance and mechanical capture. Use analgesia and sedation as needed.

[a]**Serious signs or symptoms** must be related to the slow rate. Clinical manifestations include

- Symptoms (chest pain, shortness of breath, decreased level of consciousness)
- Signs (low blood pressure, shock, pulmonary congestion, congestive heart failure, acute MI)

[b]Do not delay TCP while awaiting IV access or **atropine** to take effect if patient is symptomatic.

Key Points

1. The treatment of bradycardias, like the treatment of tachycardias, challenges the clinician to remember the admonition "treat the patient, not the monitor." Either autonomic influences or intrinsic cardiac conducting system disease may lead to bradycardia. In particular, acute MI can affect the cardiac conducting system and produce bradycardias ranging from sinus bradycardia to complete, third-degree heart blocks.

2. While cardiology usually defines bradycardia as a heart rate less than 60 beats per minute, the hearts of many people, particularly trained athletes, will beat at much slower rates. Clinicians must be aware of the concepts of absolute bradycardia (heart rate less than 60 beats per minute) and relative bradycardia. A person with a heart rate of 65 beats per minute and a blood pressure of 80 systolic may be experiencing a "relative" bradycardia: the pulse rate, relative to the blood pressure, is too low.

3. The key clinical questions to ask are, Does the slow rate make the patient ill? Are there "serious" signs or symptoms? Are the signs and symptoms related to the slow heart rate? Clinicians must look for several adverse clinical manifestations of the bradycardia: symptoms (chest pain, shortness of breath, decreased level of consciousness) and signs (hypotension, congestive heart failure, PVCs in the setting of acute MI).

Intervention Sequence

> - **Atropine** 0.5 to 1.0 mg[c,d] (Class I and IIa)
> - **Transcutaneous pacing** if available (Class I)
> - **Dopamine** 5 to 20 µg/kg per minute (Class IIb)
> - **Epinephrine** 2 to 10 µg per minute (Class IIb)
> - **Isoproterenol**[f]

[c]Denervated transplanted hearts will not respond to atropine. Go at once to pacing, **catecholamine** infusion, or both.

[d]**Atropine** should be given in repeat doses in 3 to 5 minutes up to a total of 0.03 to 0.04 mg/kg. Use the shorter dosing interval (3 minutes) in severe clinical conditions. It has been suggested that atropine should

be used with caution in AV block at the His-Purkinje level (type II AV block and new third-degree block with wide QRS complexes) (Class IIb).

[e]Never treat third-degree heart block plus ventricular escape beats with **lidocaine.**

[f]**Isoproterenol** should be used, if at all, with extreme caution. At low doses it is Class IIb (possibly helpful); at higher doses it is Class III (harmful).

Careful thought and clinical assessment should go into the decision to initiate treatment for symptomatic bradycardias. Atropine, listed in Fig 5 as the first pharmacologic agent to use, may exacerbate ischemia or induce VT or VF or both when used to treat bradycardia associated with an acute MI.[154-159]

To underscore the complexity of treating symptomatic bradycardias, clinicians should be aware of inconsistent recommendations on the use of atropine in bradycardia. A task force of the AHA and the American College of Cardiology on early management of patients with acute MI considered atropine to be Class III (possibly harmful) for patients with third-degree heart block and wide-complex ventricular escape beats and for patients with Mobitz type II second-degree heart block.[152] In type II second-degree heart block, atropine rarely may accelerate the atrial rate and produce increased AV nodal block. This increased block, in turn, may be accompanied by a paradoxical fall in the ventricular rate and blood pressure.[152]

The AHA Subcommittee on ACLS agrees with this recommendation for clinical caution and agrees that atropine is sometimes ineffective in higher level block or serious conduction system failure. The subcommittee does not agree, however, with the classification of atropine as a Class III (possibly harmful) agent. The subcommittee continues to recommend atropine as the initial pharmacologic intervention of choice for symptomatic bradycardia.[160]

Critical Points to Remember About the Treatment of Bradycardias

- Figure 5 suggests that a clinician might begin treatment with pharmacologic agents before determination of the specific type of bradycardia. In reality, diagnosis of the rhythm should proceed simultaneously with initiation of therapy. Figure 5 conveys the point that if the patient does have serious signs and symptoms from the bradycardia, the clinician must initiate treatment quickly.

- The specific treatment that clinicians initiate depends on the severity of the clinical situation. The sequence displayed in Fig 5 lists interventions in order of worsening clinical severity. In fact, 1-minute intervals can be used in severe conditions due to the bradycardia. Astute clinicians, however, know they cannot progress slowly, step-by-step through this intervention sequence when treating an unstable and severely bradycardic patient. Such a patient may be "pre–cardiac arrest" and merit multiple interventions, almost simultaneously. These may include preparation for pacing, IV atropine, and preparation of an epinephrine infusion. All algorithmic recommendations must be applied intelligently, by thinking clinicians, to individual patients.

- If the patient displays only mild problems due to the bradycardia, then **atropine** 0.5 to 1.0 mg IV can be given in a repeat dose every 3 to 5 minutes, up to a total of 0.03 mg/kg. This produces the familiar 2.0 mg total dose to a 70-kg person.[160] In the desperate condition of asystolic cardiac arrest, however, the maximum vagolytic dose, 0.04 mg/kg, is acceptable.[160] Choosing the interval of dosing (1 to 5 minutes) requires judgment about the severity of the patient's symptoms. The provider should repeat atropine at shorter intervals for more distressed patients. For example, clinicians should not wait 5 minutes between atropine doses for a severely hypotensive patient with a decreased sensorium. Similarly, an elderly, thin woman with a rate of 40 beats per minute and mild pulmonary congestion can be given an atropine trial at much longer dosing intervals.
- **Dopamine** (at rates of 5 μg/kg per minute) can be added and increased quickly if low blood pressure is associated with the bradycardia.
- If the patient displays severe clinical symptoms, clinicians can go directly to an **epinephrine** infusion instead of dopamine.
- **Lidocaine** can be **lethal** if the bradycardia is a ventricular escape rhythm and the unwary clinician thinks he or she is treating PVCs or slow VT.
- **Transcutaneous pacing (TCP)** can be extremely effective, but it is often painful and may fail to produce effective electrical capture or mechanical contractions.
- Sometimes the "symptom" the clinician treats when reacting to symptomatic bradycardia is not due to the bradycardia. For example, hypotension, associated with bradycardia, may be due to myocardial dysfunction or hypovolemia rather than to conducting system or autonomic problems.

Details on the Treatment of Symptomatic Bradycardias

Transcutaneous Pacing

TCP is a Class I intervention for all symptomatic bradycardias. If clinicians are concerned about the use of atropine in higher level blocks, they should remember that TCP is always appropriate, though not as readily available as atropine. In addition, if the bradycardia is severe and the clinical condition is unstable, clinicians should move immediately to perform TCP.

The clinician should prepare to administer TCP to patients who do not respond to atropine or who are severely symptomatic, especially when the block is at or below the His-Purkinje level. The technology for TCP is

an important therapeutic innovation that has matured over the past decade. Most recently manufactured defibrillator/monitors have the capability to perform TCP. This is an intervention, unlike insertion of transvenous pacemakers, that almost all ECC providers have available and can perform. Skill in operation of transcutaneous pacemakers is required for complete competency in ACLS. The AHA Subcommittee on ACLS, therefore, has added additional educational material on TCP to the ACLS textbook and the ACLS course.

TCP has several advantages over transvenous pacing. It can be started quickly and conveniently at the bedside and requires no special equipment such as fluoroscopy. There are common clinical impressions, however, that TCP fails more often to produce mechanical contractions than transvenous pacemakers. In addition, many patients may not tolerate the pacing stimulus to the skin that occurs with TCP. In these cases, IV analgesics or sedatives (short-acting benzodiazepines), or both, may afford relief and allow the patient to tolerate the stimuli.

Catecholamine Infusions (Epinephrine, Dopamine, and Isoproterenol)

Dopamine. Dopamine can also be used in severe, symptomatic bradycardia. Dopamine is a precursor of norepinephrine that stimulates dopaminergic, β-adrenergic and α-adrenergic receptors.

- *Low-dose dopamine:* 1 to 5 μg/kg per minute ("renal doses"). At low doses dopamine has a dopaminergic effect that causes renal, mesenteric, and cerebrovascular dilation. This tends to produce an increase in renal output.
- *Moderate-dose dopamine:* 5 to 10 μg/kg per minute ("cardiac doses"). At moderate doses dopamine has a β_1- and α-adrenergic effect, causing enhanced myocardial contractility, increased cardiac output, and a rise in blood pressure. Note that the bradycardia algorithm recommends starting at 5 μg/kg per minute for *symptomatic* bradycardias.
- *High-dose dopamine:* 10 to 20 μg/kg per minute ("vasopressor doses"). At high doses dopamine has an α-adrenergic effect, producing peripheral arterial and venous vasoconstriction. These doses are used to treat low blood pressures with signs and symptoms of shock.

Epinephrine. An epinephrine infusion can be started instead of dopamine for severe bradycardia with hypotension. These are generally patients close to the state of PEA or even asystole. For both of these groups of patients epinephrine is the agent of choice. Epinephrine infusions are easily prepared in the same manner as isoproterenol infusions: by mixing a 1-mg ampule in 500 mL D_5W to produce a concentration of 2 μg/mL. This can then be infused at 1 to 2 μg/min. Follow the recommendations for bradycardia, PEA, and asystole since epinephrine is the catecholamine common to the three algorithms.

Isoproterenol hydrochloride. Isoproterenol continues in disfavor for patients with severe symptomatic bradycardia. It was footnoted in the 1992 guidelines. The 1985 National Conference on CPR and ECC considered isoproterenol to be contraindicated in cardiac arrest patients. Isoproterenol produces negative effects of increased myocardial oxygen consumption and peripheral vasodilatation; its only positive effect is to provide chronotropic support. Isoproterenol would be relatively contraindicated if the patient were hypotensive, which is usually the case with severe symptomatic bradycardia. Thus, the only reason to use isoproterenol would be to speed up the rate of an asymptomatic patient, which is inappropriate. Isoproterenol requires a delicate risk-benefit balance: patients who are ill enough to need isoproterenol are probably too ill to tolerate it. Some experts, however, argue that at low doses that do not cause vasodilatation, isoproterenol can speed up the rate and thus elevate the blood pressure. Isoproterenol should be used, if at all, with extreme caution. At low doses it is a Class IIb (possibly helpful) intervention; at all other doses it is a Class III (harmful) intervention.

Right Ventricular Infarction

Although patients usually develop tachycardia in response to hypovolemia, excessive parasympathetic tone may be present in patients with inferior or right ventricular infarction. These patients may have bradycardia and hypotension, but the hypotension is due to hypovolemia rather than the bradycardia. A careful fluid challenge with normal saline may be lifesaving for these patients who possess what is in effect a relative bradycardia. An increase in right ventricular filling pressures will increase the strength of the right ventricular contractions based on the Starling mechanism. (See the discussion of right ventricular infarction in the section on acute MI.)

• **Type II second-degree AV block?** or • **Third-degree AV block?**[e]

---

[e]Never treat third-degree heart block plus ventricular escape beats with **lidocaine**.

Figure 5 singles out these two rhythms for particular attention even when the patient is asymptomatic. Type II second-degree AV block is a serious arrhythmia most often associated with anteroseptal MI. This infranodal block can rapidly convert to complete, third-degree AV block without warning.

- Prepare for transvenous pacer. Begin preparations for insertion of a transvenous pacemaker as soon as care providers identify this rhythm disturbance.
- Place the adhesive pads for the transcutaneous pacemaker while awaiting the transvenous pacemaker.
- Transcutaneous pacing can be used as a "bridge" intervention for third-degree AV heart block until the transvenous pacer becomes available.[g]

[g]Verify patient tolerance and mechanical capture. Use analgesia and sedation as needed.

When a patient develops third-degree AV block in association with anterior infarction, a transvenous pacemaker is indicated. An idioventricular escape pacemaker will produce wide QRS complexes. If the patient is symptomatic, clinicians should consider treatment with TCP, dopamine, and epinephrine, while awaiting insertion of the transvenous pacemaker. Atropine is relatively contraindicated[152] and should be used with care.

Importance of Infarct Location

Acute inferior MIs often produce second- or third-degree heart block with a narrow-complex junctional escape rhythm. If the patient remains hemodynamically stable, clinicians may not need to insert a transvenous pacemaker. Atropine can be used to increase the heart rate and blood pressure in these patients if they become symptomatic. Consider dopamine and epinephrine if there is no response to atropine. The conduction defect is often transient. A standby TCP should be placed on these patients (and tested) while awaiting transvenous insertion or resolution of the block.

Summary: Third-degree heart block with

Anterior acute MI

- Prepare to insert transvenous pacemaker.
- Be cautious with atropine.
- For severe symptoms use TCP (or catecholamines while preparing for pacing).

Inferior acute MI

- Apply standby TCP (verify patient tolerance and mechanical capture).
- Use atropine if symptoms necessitate.

Tachycardia Treatment Algorithms
(Figs 6 and 7)

At first glance the tachycardia algorithm (Fig 6) may appear intimidating and complicated. At second glance it is an overly simplistic algorithm that presumes to combine all tachycardia treatment guidelines on a single page. These rhythms are not usually grouped together. This educational grouping gives clinicians a broad overview of multiple related arrhythmias and their recommended treatments.

This algorithm also focuses the clinician on two important questions: Is the patient's tachycardia producing the serious signs or symptoms? Or are the signs and symptoms producing the tachycardia? For example, a patient with an acute MI may have a rapid heart rate in response to ischemic chest pain. Clinicians would err in this scenario if they cardioverted this patient thinking the tachycardia the source of the chest pain. Although the specific diagnosis is important, the critical therapeutic question is whether to perform cardioversion.

Tachycardia Algorithm

Figure 6

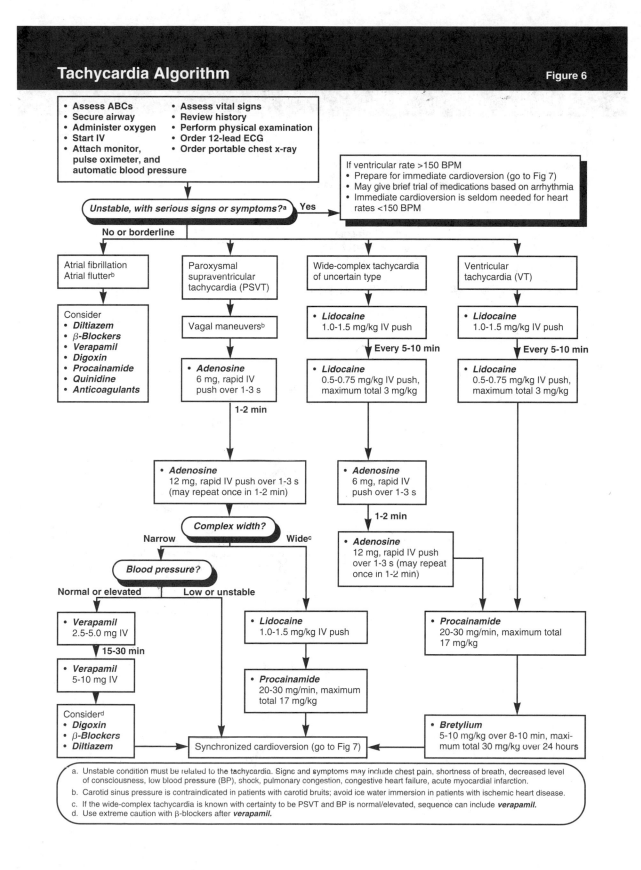

- Assess ABCs
- Secure airway
- Administer oxygen
- Start IV
- Attach monitor, pulse oximeter, and automatic blood pressure

- Assess vital signs
- Review history
- Perform physical examination
- Order 12-lead ECG
- Order portable chest x-ray

If ventricular rate >150 BPM
- Prepare for immediate cardioversion (go to Fig 7)
- May give brief trial of medications based on arrhythmia
- Immediate cardioversion is seldom needed for heart rates <150 BPM

Unstable, with serious signs or symptoms?[a] **Yes**

No or borderline

Atrial fibrillation Atrial flutter[b]

Consider
- *Diltiazem*
- *β-Blockers*
- *Verapamil*
- *Digoxin*
- *Procainamide*
- *Quinidine*
- *Anticoagulants*

Paroxysmal supraventricular tachycardia (PSVT)

Vagal maneuvers[b]

- *Adenosine* 6 mg, rapid IV push over 1-3 s

1-2 min

- *Adenosine* 12 mg, rapid IV push over 1-3 s (may repeat once in 1-2 min)

Complex width?

Narrow   **Wide**[c]

Blood pressure?

Normal or elevated   **Low or unstable**

- *Verapamil* 2.5-5.0 mg IV

15-30 min

- *Verapamil* 5-10 mg IV

Consider[d]
- *Digoxin*
- *β-Blockers*
- *Diltiazem*

Wide-complex tachycardia of uncertain type

- *Lidocaine* 1.0-1.5 mg/kg IV push

Every 5-10 min

- *Lidocaine* 0.5-0.75 mg/kg IV push, maximum total 3 mg/kg

- *Adenosine* 6 mg, rapid IV push over 1-3 s

1-2 min

- *Adenosine* 12 mg, rapid IV push over 1-3 s (may repeat once in 1-2 min)

- *Lidocaine* 1.0-1.5 mg/kg IV push

- *Procainamide* 20-30 mg/min, maximum total 17 mg/kg

Ventricular tachycardia (VT)

- *Lidocaine* 1.0-1.5 mg/kg IV push

Every 5-10 min

- *Lidocaine* 0.5-0.75 mg/kg IV push, maximum total 3 mg/kg

- *Procainamide* 20-30 mg/min, maximum total 17 mg/kg

- *Bretylium* 5-10 mg/kg over 8-10 min, maximum total 30 mg/kg over 24 hours

---

Synchronized cardioversion (go to Fig 7)

---

a. Unstable condition must be related to the tachycardia. Signs and symptoms may include chest pain, shortness of breath, decreased level of consciousness, low blood pressure (BP), shock, pulmonary congestion, congestive heart failure, acute myocardial infarction.
b. Carotid sinus pressure is contraindicated in patients with carotid bruits; avoid ice water immersion in patients with ischemic heart disease.
c. If the wide-complex tachycardia is known with certainty to be PSVT and BP is normal/elevated, sequence can include *verapamil*.
d. Use extreme caution with β-blockers after *verapamil*.

Electrical Cardioversion Algorithm

Figure 7

(Patient is not in cardiac arrest)

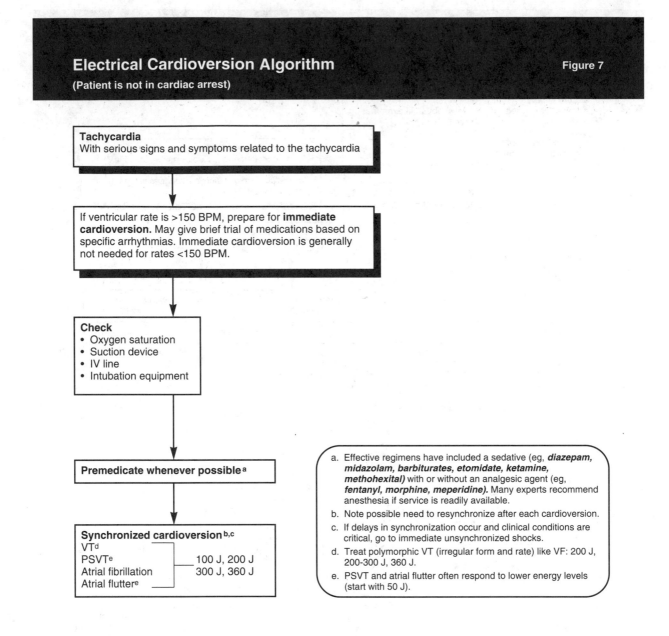

Tachycardia
With serious signs and symptoms related to the tachycardia

If ventricular rate is >150 BPM, prepare for **immediate cardioversion.** May give brief trial of medications based on specific arrhythmias. Immediate cardioversion is generally not needed for rates <150 BPM.

Check
• Oxygen saturation
• Suction device
• IV line
• Intubation equipment

Premedicate whenever possible[a]

Synchronized cardioversion[b,c]
VT[d]
PSVT[e]
Atrial fibrillation
Atrial flutter[e]

100 J, 200 J
300 J, 360 J

a. Effective regimens have included a sedative (eg, *diazepam, midazolam, barbiturates, etomidate, ketamine, methohexital)* with or without an analgesic agent (eg, *fentanyl, morphine, meperidine).* Many experts recommend anesthesia if service is readily available.

b. Note possible need to resynchronize after each cardioversion.

c. If delays in synchronization occur and clinical conditions are critical, go to immediate unsynchronized shocks.

d. Treat polymorphic VT (irregular form and rate) like VF: 200 J, 200-300 J, 360 J.

e. PSVT and atrial flutter often respond to lower energy levels (start with 50 J).

Tachycardias can produce the same adverse hemodynamic problems as bradycardias: hypotension, signs and symptoms of congestive heart failure, decreased level of consciousness, persistent chest pain, or continued PVCs in the setting of a possible acute MI.

• **Unstable, with serious signs or symptoms?**[a]

(Yes)

If the ventricular rate is more than 150 beats per minute:
• **Prepare for immediate cardioversion (go to Fig 7)**
• **May give brief trial of medications based on arrhythmia**
• **Immediate cardioversion is seldom needed for heart rate less than 150 beats per minute**

---

[a]Unstable condition must be related to the tachycardia. Signs and symptoms may include chest pain, shortness of breath, decreased level of consciousness, low blood pressure, shock, pulmonary congestion, congestive heart failure, acute MI.

For the hemodynamically unstable patient use cardioversion before antiarrhythmic therapy. Inexperienced ACLS providers sometimes misinterpret this approach and think that they should forego antiarrhythmics in unstable patients with a pulse. Delay is the issue. Clinicians should perform cardioversion first when it takes several minutes to locate, prepare, and administer medications. Once the clinician has made the decision to perform cardioversion, however, he or she may still administer medications if the medications are immediately available. One member of the resuscitation team can, for example, administer lidocaine (1 to 1.5 mg/kg IV push) while another member prepares the defibrillator.

When patients with symptomatic tachycardia are able to maintain a pulse and measurable blood pressure, the clinician can perform the cardioversion in a controlled manner.

• If the care providers have followed the universal algorithm (Fig 1), the patient will already be attached to a monitor and an oxygen source and have an IV line available or in progress.
• The team should take a few minutes to attach the patient to an oxygen saturation monitor and a non-invasive blood pressure device if available and should verify that they have access to an operational suction device.
• If the care providers are in a hospital setting, they should have qualified personnel assist with airway and anesthesia.
• If time and the clinical condition permit, give patients some combination of analgesia and sedation.

Clinicians can administer a variety of premedication regimens.[39] Some experts recommend near general anesthesia before cardioversion if readily available. Effective regimens have included sedatives with or without an analgesic agent. Clinicians should use such medications carefully, safely, and judiciously. The clinical goal is to alleviate the pain caused by the procedure without causing adverse effects.

• The sidebar "Steps for Synchronized Cardioversion" reviews the operation of a defibrillator/monitor in "sync" mode to perform cardioversion.[39]
• For ease of recall, the electrical cardioversion algorithm (Fig 7) recommends a standard sequence of energy levels for synchronized cardioversions: 100 J, 200 J, 300 J, 360 J.[11] The two exceptions to this are atrial flutter, which often responds to lower energy levels such as 50 J, and polymorphic VT (irregular morphology and rate), which often requires higher energy levels. The recommendation for polymorphic VT is to start with 200 J.

Steps for Synchronized Cardioversion

1. See electrical cardioversion algorithm (Fig 7) for sedation.
2. Turn on defibrillator.
3. Attach monitor leads to the patient ("white to right, red to ribs, what's left over to the left shoulder") and ensure proper display of the patient's rhythm.
4. Engage the synchronization mode by pressing the "sync" control button.
5. Look for markers on the R waves indicating sync mode.
6. If necessary adjust R wave gain until sync markers occur with each QRS complex.
7. Select appropriate energy level.
8. Position conductor pads on patient (or apply gel to paddles).
9. Position paddles on patient (sternum-apex).
10. Announce to the team members: "Charging defibrillator — stand clear!"
11. Press "charge" button on apex paddle (right hand).
12. When the defibrillator is charged, begin the final "clearing chant." State firmly in a forceful voice the following chant before each shock:

    • "I am going to shock on three. One, I'm clear." (Check to make sure you are clear of contact with the patient or the stretcher and equipment.)

    • "Two, you are clear." (Make a visual check to ensure that no one continues to touch the patient or stretcher. In particular, do not forget about the person providing ventilations. That person's hands should not be on the ventilatory adjuncts, including the endotracheal tube!)

    • "Three, everybody is clear." (Check yourself once more time before pressing the shock buttons.)

13. Apply 25 lb pressure on both paddles.
14. Press the "discharge" buttons simultaneously.
15. Check the monitor. If tachycardia persists, increase the joules according to the electrical cardioversion algorithm.

    • **Reset the sync mode after each synchronized cardioversion, because most defibrillators default back to unsynchronized mode.** This default to unsynchronized mode is to allow an immediate defibrillation if the cardioversion produces VF.

- **Atrial fibrillation**
- **Atrial flutter**[b]

Treatments to consider:

- Diltiazem
- β Blockers
- Verapamil
- Digoxin
- Procainamide
- Quinidine
- Anticoagulants

---

[b]Carotid sinus pressure is contraindicated in patients with carotid bruits; avoid ice water immersion in patients with ischemic heart disease.

Both of these rhythms can be stable and may not need treatment. If the patient experiences serious signs and symptoms, the clinician should prepare for immediate cardioversion as outlined in Fig 7. In the absence of serious signs and symptoms, observation may be the best immediate approach. Clinicians should consider acute conditions that might cause the atrial fibrillation/atrial flutter: acute MI, hypoxia, pulmonary embolism, electrolyte abnormalities, medication toxicity (particularly digoxin or quinidine) and thyrotoxicosis.[161] New onset atrial fibrillation can be due to acute myocardial infarction. In most cases other symptoms or signs (eg, ischemic ECG changes) are present. If there is a high index of suspicion for acute cardiac ischemia, the patient may require hospital admission.[162,163]

Clinicians should become more concerned, however, if the atrial fibrillation/atrial flutter produces a rapid ventricular response, even in the absence of hemodynamic instability. Atrial flutter is less stable than atrial fibrillation and demands more clinical attention, particularly when the ventricular response is rapid. Clinicians should heighten their sense of urgency if the tachycardia can lead to deleterious effects, such as precipitating angina in patients with ischemic heart disease. As their first priority clinicians should attempt to slow the ventricular response, not convert the patient to normal sinus rhythm. Spontaneous conversion to normal sinus rhythm often occurs once medications have achieved rate control. If not, then specific therapy can be given to produce pharmacologic conversion.

Clinicians should learn and become comfortable with a specific therapeutic sequence for atrial fibrillation/atrial flutter. For rate control, calcium channel blockers (such as diltiazem and verapamil), or β blockers (such as esmolol, metoprolol, atenolol, and propranolol) are recommended. Many experts now favor diltiazem as the agent of first choice.[164,165]

Experts have questioned the role of digoxin for urgent treatment of atrial fibrillation and flutter.[166,167] For chemical conversion, most experience has accumulated with IV or oral procainamide and oral quinidine. However, these agents can be proarrhythmic, and electricity is generally preferred. One caution to remember: IV propranolol should not be given soon after IV verapamil. Profound bradycardia and even asystole may occur when these two agents are given close together (less than 30 minutes apart).

While not an emergency decision, clinicians should remember that patients with atrial fibrillation of more than several days' duration may have developed intra-atrial emboli. Because of the risk of arterial embolization when converted, give these patients anticoagulant therapy for some time before attempting conversion. Atrial flutter need not be anticoagulated.

Vagal maneuvers may serve a diagnostic purpose in atrial flutter. Carotid sinus massage may render the flutter waves more apparent and thus confirm the diagnosis. The sections on VT and PSVT present several additional cautions and comments about carotid sinus massage, vagal maneuvers, and supraventricular versus ventricular tachycardia.

Key Points

- Atrial fibrillation may be a stable rhythm and not need treatment.
- Think of treatable conditions that might be causing the arrhythmia.
- Initial vagal maneuvers may serve both a diagnostic and therapeutic purpose.
- Use electrical cardioversion if the patient displays serious signs and symptoms.
- Consider admission for all patients with new onset atrial fibrillation or flutter. Most will need to be admitted.
- The first priority of treatment should be to slow the ventricular response with IV diltiazem, verapamil, or β blockers.
- After the immediate efforts to slow the ventricular response, use electrical cardioversion (preferred) or procainamide or quinidine to convert the patient to normal sinus rhythm. Consider the need for anticoagulation before cardioversion.

Paroxysmal supraventricular tachycardia (PSVT)

General treatment sequence:

- Vagal maneuvers[b]
- Adenosine 6 mg
- Adenosine 12 mg
- Adenosine 12 to 18 mg
- Verapamil 1.5 to 5 mg (if complex width is narrow and blood pressure is normal)
- Verapamil 5 to 10 mg

---

[b]Carotid sinus pressure is contraindicated in patients with carotid bruits or a history of vascular disease; avoid ice water immersion in patients with ischemic heart disease.

The distinctions between sinus tachycardia, VTs, non-paroxysmal supraventricular tachycardias, and PSVT are difficult yet important. People responsible for therapy must master these distinctions. Figure 6 may appear to oversimplify the complex challenge of supraventricular arrhythmias. This expanded tachycardia algorithm, however, conveys two critical points:

- If the patient displays serious signs and symptoms, prepare for immediate cardioversion.
- If the tachycardia complex appears wide, treat the rhythm like VT.

If remembered and acted upon, these two clinical rules should support clinicians in their management of the most difficult tachyarrhythmias.

Vagal Maneuvers

Therapy for PSVT aims to interrupt a cycle of impulses that goes supraventricular — to ventricles — back to the AV node. Vagal maneuvers increase parasympathetic tone and slow conduction through the AV node. Clinicians as well as patients have many vagal maneuvers in their armamentarium.[168,169] These range from the commonplace to the bizarre and include carotid sinus massage,[170] breath-holding, facial immersion in ice water, coughing,[171] nasogastric tube placement, gag reflex stimulation by tongue blades or fingers or oral ipecac, eyeball pressure, squatting, MAST garments,[172] Trendelenburg position,[173] and a circumferential digital sweep of the anus.[174] Many patients who experience recurrent episodes of PSVT learn to self-terminate their episodes. Eyeball massage should never be performed, encouraged, or taught. It may result in retinal detachment.

Clinicians should perform carotid sinus massage carefully, with ECG monitoring, avoiding its use in older patients. An IV line, atropine sulfate, and lidocaine should be available for immediate use. Case reports have identified numerous problems in association with carotid sinus massage, including cerebral emboli, stroke (embolic and occlusive), syncope, sinus arrest, asystole, increased degree of AV block, and paradoxical tachyarrhythmias in digoxin-toxic states.

Carotid sinus massage is a firm massage that lasts for no more than 5 to 10 seconds. Turn the patient's head to the left and massage the right carotid sinus. The massage can be repeated several times after brief pauses, and then the left carotid bifurcation near the angle of the jaw can be massaged. Never attempt simultaneous, bilateral massage.

Adenosine and Verapamil

These two agents are highly effective in converting PSVT to normal sinus rhythm. Clinical studies have confirmed that adenosine, which was not available in the United States until 1990, is as effective as verapamil in initial conversion of PSVT.[175-181] Because adenosine does not produce hypotension to the degree that verapamil does and because of its brief half-life, clinicians consider adenosine the safer agent.[176,179,181,182] Paramedics have administered adenosine successfully in the prehospital treatment of PSVT.[183] No clinical deteriorations have been reported even when paramedics gave adenosine to patients later identified as having VT,[183,184] and some VTs are adenosine-positive.

Adenosine

The AHA Subcommittee on ACLS recommends adenosine as the initial drug of choice for hemodynamically stable PSVT. Adenosine, however, does not replace verapamil in the PSVT armamentarium, for studies have observed a higher recurrence rate of PSVT after conversion by adenosine than after conversion by verapamil.[184-186] Thus, the clinician should think in terms of a sequence of agents for persistent PSVT: adenosine twice (or even three times), and then if the complex remains narrow and the blood pressure has not dropped, verapamil twice.

The success of adenosine depends on proper administration. Administer adenosine 6 mg by *rapid* IV push (3 to 5 seconds). Follow with a 20-mL fluid flush.[182] After 1 to 2 minutes a second dose of 12 mg should be administered rapidly. When given adenosine, patients frequently experience a few seconds of distressing chest pain similar to ischemic chest pain.[187,188] When conversion occurs the patient may display several seconds of asystole followed by resumption of normal sinus rhythm. The PSVT can recur up to 50% to 60% of the time,[184] and clinicians should be ready to move to verapamil if the complex remains narrow and the blood pressure remains acceptable.

Verapamil

Personnel should administer verapamil more slowly than adenosine. The recommended dose is 5 mg IV given over 2 minutes. Give smaller amounts (2 to 4 mg) over longer periods of time (3 to 4 minutes) when treating the elderly or when the blood pressure is within the lower range of normal. A second dose of 5 to 10 mg can be given in 15 to 30 minutes if the PSVT persists or recurs and if the blood pressure remains acceptable. Verapamil often produces a worrisome decrease in the blood pressure. This can be reversed with the Trendelenburg position, fluids, or calcium chloride, 0.5 to 1.0 g given slowly IV.[189] Many clinicians pretreat patients with an IV infusion of calcium chloride over 5 to 10 minutes before administration of verapamil. This approach may help patients with questionable hemodynamic suitability for verapamil. This cannot be made a routine recommendation because there are insufficient data to support such an action. If hemodynamic compromise develops and the PSVT continues, immediately cardiovert the patient. Use verapamil with caution in patients who receive chronic β-blocker therapy.

After Adenosine and Verapamil

Patients who fail to respond to adenosine and verapamil may be treated, according to the physician's judgment, with any of the following: digoxin, β blockade, sedation and rest, overdrive pacing, elective cardioversion, or a variety of other antiarrhythmic agents, including diltiazem (see Fig 6).

Wide-complex PSVT and wide-complex tachycardias of uncertain type

General treatment sequence:

- Lidocaine 1 to 1.5 mg/kg IV
- Lidocaine 0.5 to 0.75 mg/kg IV
- Adenosine 6 mg IV
- Adenosine 12 mg
- Procainamide 20 to 30 mg/min

Clinicians may be puzzled over whether a wide-complex tachyarrhythmia represents VT or wide-complex PSVT with aberrant conduction. Many textbooks and articles present lengthy, detailed guidelines to help distinguish between VT and PVCs from supraventricular tachycardias with aberrancy.[190-193] *The prudent clinician, faced with urgent care of an ill patient, should ignore these detailed criteria for ECG analysis and attend to the patient.*

Critical Points to Remember

1. Administration of verapamil to a patient with VT can be a **lethal error.** Verapamil can accelerate the heart rate and decrease the blood pressure, especially in patients with atrial fibrillation and Wolff-Parkinson-White syndrome.[194,195] Authors have reported numerous examples of adverse effects, including death.[193-196] Do not give verapamil to patients with a wide-complex tachycardia unless the tachycardia is known with certainty to be supraventricular in origin.

2. Clinicians should **not** use *clinical* criteria to distinguish between PSVT with aberrant conduction and VT.[193-197] Some clinicians have a misconception that the patient who is in VT will appear unstable and distressed and have a more rapid rate or a lower blood pressure. This misconception ignores the fact that many people in VT appear comfortable and stable.

3. Emergency clinicians should **not** use *ECG* criteria to distinguish between aberrant conduction and VT.[191,193] Unless they have extensive experience, these detailed distinctions are too esoteric and unreliable to be clinically useful in the immediate care setting, and the recommended therapy should not be changed.

Previous recommendations stated that whenever the clinician has doubts between stable supraventricular tachycardia and stable VT he or she should treat the patient as if the arrhythmia were VT. This recommendation is still valid, although it has confused many emergency care providers because of indecision over whether to use procainamide or lidocaine or any of a number of other suggested agents. The 1992 National Conference on CPR and ECC recommends the approach in Fig 6: **lidocaine** is the first agent to use for VT plus all wide-complex supraventricular arrhythmias not known with certainty to be supraventricular in origin. **Procainamide** is also acceptable, but it has a greater potential for lowering the blood pressure and takes longer to work.

Adenosine has demonstrated promise in this area because it produces little harm in patients with VT and converts many patients with wide–QRS-complex tachycardia.[177,178,182,198] Although Fig 6 recommends loading doses of lidocaine first, follow with **adenosine** in two rapid administrations if the tachycardia persists. Adenosine may successfully convert supraventricular tachycardias and will offer diagnostic help if the tachycardia persists. In this setting lidocaine and procainamide are Class I agents (acceptable and definitely effective), adenosine is a Class IIa agent (acceptable and probably effective), and verapamil is a Class III agent (possibly or probably harmful).

The tachycardia algorithm was carefully constructed to restrict the use of verapamil to only patients with narrow-complex PSVT with normal or elevated blood pressures. Verapamil can, however, successfully convert wide-complex tachycardias known to be supraventricular in origin. Consequently, the use of verapamil is acceptable if the blood pressure is normal or elevated and the wide-complex tachycardia is known with certainty to be PSVT. Some experts, however, argue that electrophysiological stimulation testing is necessary to confirm this diagnosis, and thus they always withhold verapamil from patients with wide-complex tachycardias.

- **Ventricular tachycardia (stable)**

General treatment sequence:

- **Lidocaine** 1 to 1.5 mg/kg IV
- **Lidocaine** 0.5 to 0.75 mg/kg IV
- **Procainamide** 20 to 30 mg/min
- **Bretylium** 5 to 10 mg/kg

Full Cardiac Arrest

Clinicians must never forget that persistent VT without a pulse, with signs of a full cardiac arrest, must be treated like VF. The treatment is

- Three unsynchronized stacked **shocks** (200 J, 300 J, 360 J)
- Intubate and start an IV
- Epinephrine-**shock**

- Lidocaine-**shock**
- Lidocaine-**shock**
- Bretylium-**shock**
- Bretylium-**shock**
- Procainamide-**shock**

See Fig 1, the universal algorithm, and Fig 2, the VF/VT algorithm, for full cardiac arrest.

VT: Hemodynamically Unstable (Not Full Cardiac Arrest)

When the patient with VT has low blood pressure, shortness of breath, chest pain, altered consciousness, or pulmonary edema, the clinician should prepare for **immediate cardioversion** as presented in Fig 7 and discussed earlier in this section.

VT: Patient Is Clinically Stable

Clinicians should use lidocaine as the drug of choice in this clinical situation. As noted above, it is also the first drug to use for wide-complex tachycardias of uncertain type. Lidocaine requires an initial loading dose of 1 to 1.5 mg/kg. If needed, a second dose of 0.75 to 1.5 mg/kg can be administered 5 to 10 minutes later. The total loading dose is 3 mg/kg. If lidocaine appears to convert the arrhythmia, then continue a lidocaine drip of 2 to 4 mg/min. There are many other clinical "recipes" for lidocaine administration, most of which are acceptable and effective (Class IIa). Clinicians must be aware, however, of the necessary careful balance between ineffective levels of medication and toxicity.

Procainamide

Clinicians should use procainamide as the second-line agent for stable VT. Procainamide is not given as a bolus but as a steady IV infusion. Figure 6 recommends an infusion rate of procainamide at 20 to 30 mg/min. Pharmacologic studies have established 17 mg/kg as the proper loading dose. While difficult to remember and calculate, this will result in more accurate doses than the former recommendation of "a total loading dose of 1000 mg" given without reference to the patient's size. The end points of procainamide therapy are hypotension, more than 50% widening of the QRS complex, a maximum of 17 mg/kg, or termination of the arrhythmia. If procainamide terminates the VT, start a continuous infusion at 1 to 4 mg/min to maintain the suppression.

Bretylium

Clinicians should administer bretylium as the third agent for the treatment of sustained VT. Bretylium displays more effectiveness as an antifibrillatory agent than as an antiarrhythmic agent for tachycardias. Administer bretylium 5 mg/kg, not as a bolus as with VF but in a continuous infusion over 8 to 10 minutes. If bretylium appears to convert the arrhythmia, complete the loading dose (5 mg/kg) and begin a continuous infusion at a rate of 1 to 2 mg/min.

> ### Synchronized Cardioversion

Synchronized vs Unsynchronized Shocks

With unsynchronized shocks the capacitors discharge whenever the operator presses the shock controls. The shocks have no relation to the cardiac cycle. A properly connected defibrillator/monitor placed in synchronization ("sync" mode) searches for the peak of the QRS complex (or R-wave deflection) and delivers the shock a few milliseconds after the highest part of the R wave. This programmed approach thus avoids delivery of the shock during the "vulnerable period" of cardiac repolarization (the T wave). Such shocks are more likely to induce VF.

A problem occurs, however, during some rapid tachycardias when the defibrillator program may be unable to discriminate between the peak of the QRS complex and the peak of a T wave. This can produce delays and failure of shock delivery when using synchronization mode, especially when the arrhythmia presents as a polymorphic VT. Clinicians should therefore attempt synchronized cardioversion when the patient is relatively stable. They should perform unsynchronized cardioversion whenever the patient has a rapid tachycardia combined with clinical instability or whenever there are delays with synchronization.

Torsades de Pointes

This special form of VT displays a gradual alteration in the amplitude and direction of the electrical activity.[199,200] The true frequency of torsades is unknown because many clinicians do not look for or recognize this arrhythmia. However, clinicians who may not immediately recognize torsades should consider it when patients not in cardiac arrest display VT refractory to the recommended agents lidocaine, procainamide, and bretylium.

Torsades requires different treatment than the other VTs. Clinicians have employed a wide variety of agents and reported anecdotal success. Electrical pacing has been the treatment of choice,[199,200] though variable capture rates has led many clinicians to prefer magnesium sulfate. Transcutaneous pacemakers can easily supply immediate pacing (up to rates of 180 beats per minute) while preparations are made for a transvenous pacemaker. In addition, isoproterenol (2 to 8 μm/min) can overdrive the ventricular rate and break the triggered arrhythmic mechanism. Recent reports have demonstrated that magnesium sulfate can effectively abolish runs of torsades de pointes.[201,202] Magnesium sulfate can be given 1 to 2 g IV over 1 to 2 minutes, followed by the same amount infused over 1 hour. Up to 4 to 6 g may be required to suppress torsades. Quinidine and other drugs that prolong repolarization (procainamide, phenothiazines, tricyclic antidepressants, disopyramide) are contraindicated because they can exacerbate torsades.[203] Direct defibrillator shocks should be used if pharmacologic interventions are unsuccessful.

Clinicians must understand that torsades is often due to various offending circumstances, such as hypokalemia, tricyclic agents, and drug overdoses. Although torsades can be suppressed by magnesium and transvenous pacing, it will often recur unless the precipitating mechanisms are removed.

Hypotension/Shock/Acute Pulmonary Edema

> • **Acute Pulmonary Edema/Hypotension/Shock Go to Fig 8**

ECC providers often care for patients with low blood pressures. Clinicians must consider whether the reduced blood pressure produces clinical signs of tissue hypoperfusion. *Shock* indicates a syndrome of diverse causes and variable presentations. The common denominator for all shock states is inadequate cellular perfusion and inadequate oxygen delivery for existing metabolic demands.[204-206] Clinical manifestations differ according to the underlying cause and the compensatory mechanisms that have occurred. For example, cool, mottled skin and oliguria may indicate the compensatory mechanism of increased vascular resistance. Tachycardia may indicate an effort to increase cardiac output. Adrenergic mediators may produce diaphoresis, anxiousness, nausea, vomiting, and diarrhea. Altered mentation and myocardial ischemia may occur when compensatory mechanisms become inadequate and hypotension ensues.

Approaches to hypotension and shock have been developed from different perspectives.[204-206] One common approach is to categorize shock based on the cause:

- Cardiogenic shock: myocardial, valvular, and dysrhythmic diseases
- Hypovolemic shock: hemorrhagic and other volume losses
- Distributive shock: septic and neurogenic
- Flow obstruction shock: embolism, tamponade, valvular stenoses, atrial myxomata
- Anaphylactic shock

The clinician must always attempt to determine and correct underlying causes. A variety of historical, clinical, hemodynamic, and laboratory features can be combined to identify the cause of shock, but advanced diagnosis and treatment requires a critical care unit and invasive hemodynamic monitoring.

This causal approach, however, is helpful mostly in retrospect. The initial ECC provider needs a conceptual tool to help understand and treat hypotension and shock during the first 30 to 60 minutes of clinical contact before invasive monitoring is usually available. The *cardiovascular triad* (consisting of the electrical system, the myocardium, and the vascular system) can provide such a tool.[151,204-207] From this perspective all forms of hypotension result from one of the following mechanisms or some combination of these mechanisms: a rate problem, a pump problem, or a volume problem (Table 3).

A fourth element to consider is *vascular resistance*. Decreased vascular resistance leads to volume problems through vasodilation and to pump problems through vasoconstriction. For simplicity it is often useful to think in terms of just the three problems of pump, rate, or volume. For many patients, however, vascular resistance should be considered a separate sign to evaluate.

Understanding these mechanisms can be a powerful aid to patient assessment, clinical problem solving, and medical decision making. In addition, this approach can help clinicians integrate difficult clinical problems, eg, the patient with arrhythmias that lead to hypotension by being too fast (Fig 6) or too slow (Fig 5) or the patient with acute pulmonary edema (Fig 8) and hypotension.[151,204-207]

To use these concepts properly, practitioners should follow a two-step process:

- First, consider each individual component *separately,* as a *distinct functional entity.*
- Second, consider the overall clinical picture and integrate the information by putting it all together.

Table 3. The Cardiovascular Triad

Rate Problems	Pump Problems	Volume (Includes Vascular Resistance) Problems
Too slow (Fig 5)	*Primary*	*Volume loss*
• Sinus bradycardia	• Myocardial infarction	• Hemorrhage
• Type I and II second-degree heart block	• Cardiomyopathies	• Gastrointestinal loss
	• Myocarditis	• Renal losses
• Third-degree heart block	• Ruptured chordae	• Insensible losses
	• Acute papillary muscle dysfunction	• Adrenal insufficiency (aldosterone)
• Pacemaker failures	• Acute aortic insufficiency	
	• Prosthetic valve dysfunction	
	• Ruptured intraventricular septum	
Too fast (Fig 6)	*Secondary*	*Vascular resistance*
• Sinus tachycardia	• Drugs that alter function	(Vasodilatation or redistribution):
• Atrial flutter		• Central nervous system injury
• Atrial fibrillation	• Cardiac tamponade	• Spinal injury
• PSVT	• Pulmonary embolus	• Third space loss
• Ventricular tachycardia	• Atrial myxomata	• Adrenal insufficiency (cortisol)
	• Superior vena cava syndrome	• Sepsis
		• Drugs that alter tone

Acute Pulmonary Edema/Hypotension/Shock Algorithm   Figure 8

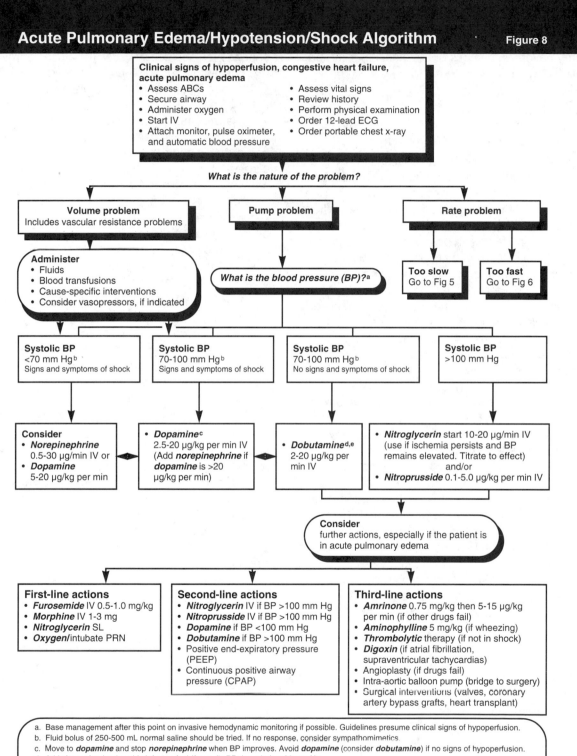

Clinical signs of hypoperfusion, congestive heart failure, acute pulmonary edema
- Assess ABCs
- Secure airway
- Administer oxygen
- Start IV
- Attach monitor, pulse oximeter, and automatic blood pressure
- Assess vital signs
- Review history
- Perform physical examination
- Order 12-lead ECG
- Order portable chest x-ray

What is the nature of the problem?

Volume problem
Includes vascular resistance problems

Pump problem

Rate problem

Administer
- Fluids
- Blood transfusions
- Cause-specific interventions
- Consider vasopressors, if indicated

What is the blood pressure (BP)?[a]

Too slow
Go to Fig 5

Too fast
Go to Fig 6

Systolic BP
<70 mm Hg[b]
Signs and symptoms of shock

Systolic BP
70-100 mm Hg[b]
Signs and symptoms of shock

Systolic BP
70-100 mm Hg[b]
No signs and symptoms of shock

Systolic BP
>100 mm Hg

Consider
- *Norepinephrine* 0.5-30 µg/min IV or
- *Dopamine* 5-20 µg/kg per min

- *Dopamine*[c] 2.5-20 µg/kg per min IV (Add *norepinephrine* if *dopamine* is >20 µg/kg per min)

- *Dobutamine*[d,e] 2-20 µg/kg per min IV

- *Nitroglycerin* start 10-20 µg/min IV (use if ischemia persists and BP remains elevated. Titrate to effect) and/or
- *Nitroprusside* 0.1-5.0 µg/kg per min IV

Consider
further actions, especially if the patient is in acute pulmonary edema

First-line actions
- *Furosemide* IV 0.5-1.0 mg/kg
- *Morphine* IV 1-3 mg
- *Nitroglycerin* SL
- *Oxygen*/intubate PRN

Second-line actions
- *Nitroglycerin* IV if BP >100 mm Hg
- *Nitroprusside* IV if BP >100 mm Hg
- *Dopamine* if BP <100 mm Hg
- *Dobutamine* if BP >100 mm Hg
- Positive end-expiratory pressure (PEEP)
- Continuous positive airway pressure (CPAP)

Third-line actions
- *Amrinone* 0.75 mg/kg then 5-15 µg/kg per min (if other drugs fail)
- *Aminophylline* 5 mg/kg (if wheezing)
- *Thrombolytic* therapy (if not in shock)
- *Digoxin* (if atrial fibrillation, supraventricular tachycardias)
- Angioplasty (if drugs fail)
- Intra-aortic balloon pump (bridge to surgery)
- Surgical interventions (valves, coronary artery bypass grafts, heart transplant)

a. Base management after this point on invasive hemodynamic monitoring if possible. Guidelines presume clinical signs of hypoperfusion.
b. Fluid bolus of 250-500 mL normal saline should be tried. If no response, consider sympathomimetics.
c. Move to *dopamine* and stop *norepinephrine* when BP improves. Avoid *dopamine* (consider *dobutamine*) if no signs of hypoperfusion.
d. Add *dopamine* (and avoid *dobutamine*) if systolic BP drops below 90 mm Hg.
e. Start with *nitroglycerin* if initial blood pressures are in this range.

This *systematic approach* will often clarify the mechanisms of shock, identify the factors that may be producing hypotension, provide a problem list, suggest appropriate therapy, and help prevent errors. For example, an unsophisticated clinician might treat a hypotensive rate problem with fluid or a hypotensive volume problem with pressors. These are common, serious errors.

For every patient with shock or hypotension, clinicians should ask four questions:

- Is there a rate problem?
- Is there a pump problem?
- Is there a volume problem?
- Is there a vascular resistance problem?

It is acceptable to answer these questions in terms of probabilities (ie, a patient might be judged to have a probable pump problem or a probable volume problem). Heart rate can easily be determined by taking the pulse or from a cardiac monitor. Pump, volume, and vascular resistance problems, however, can be more difficult to assess unless the patient is being monitored with a Swan-Ganz catheter. Nevertheless, experienced clinicians can make a reasonable assessment of the probability of a pump, volume, or vascular resistance problem based on history, physical examination, and other available information.

It is also important to ask *why* each component may be failing and whether there may be an underlying problem that can be corrected, such as hypoventilation, hypoxia, or a fluid deficit. In the absence of obvious fluid loss, a clinician might assume that a hypotensive patient with an acute MI does not have a volume problem. A more sophisticated clinician would realize that many patients with acute MI, particularly patients with inferior wall or right ventricular infarcts, do in fact have a concurrent volume problem leading to suboptimal ventricular filling pressures. Such patients may improve dramatically following an IV fluid challenge. These kinds of diagnosis and selection of treatment require invasive monitoring techniques and a clinician familiar with the management of severely ill patients. When such patients are being treated in the emergency setting, the directing physician must make appropriate arrangements to ensure that necessary equipment and clinical expertise are made available.

Volume problem
Administer:

- Fluids
- Blood transfusions
- Cause-specific interventions
- Consider vasopressors, if indicated

Volume problems can be of two types: *absolute* (due to an actual fluid deficit) or *relative* (the circulatory blood volume is inadequate relative to the vascular tone). Absolute volume problems include bleeding, vomiting, diarrhea, polyuria, insensible losses, and dehydration. Relative volume problems occur when the systemic vascular resistance is too low, causing vasodilation, or when there is redistribution of fluid to third spaces. Anaphylactic shock provides an example of a relative volume problem caused by a decrease in systemic vascular resistance (vasodilation) and redistribution of fluid.

In most patients, volume problems are treated with either fluid (to "fill the tank") or vasopressors (to increase vascular resistance and thus decrease the volume of the tank). Volume replacement is the treatment of choice for hemorrhagic and hypovolemic shock.[204-207] For many etiologies the clinician should accomplish volume replacement with blood, blood products, or balanced crystalloid solutions. Precise treatment of these conditions often requires invasive hemodynamic monitoring, which is beyond the scope of this text.

ECC providers also should consider unique volume or vascular resistance problems that require, in addition to volume replacement, specific vasoactive agents[204-207]:

- Septic shock: dopamine, norepinephrine, phenylephrine, dobutamine
- Spinal shock: dopamine, phenylephrine
- Anaphylactic shock: epinephrine, dopamine, norepinephrine, phenylephrine
- β-Blocker overdose: epinephrine, atropine, glucagon, dopamine, isoproterenol
- α-Blocker overdose: epinephrine, norepinephrine

Volume problems may be subtle, and the clinician should consider both primary and secondary causes of hypovolemia. Most patients in shock will, in time, develop a secondary volume problem due to vasodilation and the eventual collapse of vasomotor tone. *This may occur even if the primary cause of the shock is a rate or a pump problem.* When one system fails, others may follow. Clinicians should be alert for occult volume or vascular resistance problems and should provide a fluid challenge when their suspicions are high. In general:

- *The first priority is to provide adequate volume (fluid) replacement*
- *Vasopressors play a secondary (though often important) role in hypovolemic states* (Fig 8).

Do not treat hypovolemia with vasopressors unless combined with adequate volume replacement. Vasopressors alone may cause cardiac decompensation and hemodynamic deterioration, particularly in patients with ischemic heart disease. Vasopressors should be used to increase the systemic vascular resistance only when the circulating blood volume is thought to be adequate or simultaneously with fluids.

Rate problem?
Too slow?
• Go to Fig 5
Too fast?
• Go to Fig 6

If a significant rate problem exists, and it is not clear that a significant pump, volume, or resistance problem coexists, then the heart rate should be treated first (Fig 8).[151] For example, a patient with a low blood pressure and bradycardia should have the heart rate corrected before receiving an inotrope, a vasopressor, or a fluid challenge. If pump or volume problems *are* thought to coexist, they should be treated concurrently. Rate problems that produce hypotension are discussed in the sections on bradycardias (Fig 5) and tachycardias (Fig 6).

Pump problem?
What is the blood pressure?[a]

---

[a]Base management after this point on invasive hemodynamic monitoring if possible. Guidelines presume clinical signs of hypoperfusion.

A pump problem can produce either "backwards" signs (pulmonary congestion — acute pulmonary edema) or "forward" signs (increased peripheral vascular resistance with clinical signs of hypoperfusion).

The concepts of intravascular volume and systemic vascular resistance are often referred to as cardiac *preload* and *afterload*. Think of *preload* as how far the myocardium is stretched ("loaded") by the cardiac volume just before it begins a contraction. Once a contraction begins, the heart encounters resistance ("load") to the contraction. This is called *afterload*.

Pump problems can produce clinical signs of low cardiac output (hypotension, weak pulses, fatigue, weakness, dermatologic signs of hypoperfusion) or pulmonary congestion (tachypnea, labored respirations, rales, jugular venous distention, frothy sputum, cyanosis, dyspnea).

Many conditions can produce cardiac pump failure. Clinicians must try to determine the specific cause of pump failure because appropriate therapy can be lifesaving. For example, emergency surgery can reverse acute rupture of the chordae tendineae, rupture of the intraventricular septum, or acute valvular dysfunction, but only if identified early. Clinicians can also reverse certain drug toxicities such as β-blocker or calcium channel blocker overdoses.

Pump problems can also be primary or secondary. Table 3 lists a number of primary and secondary causes. Primary pump problems, such as those caused by MI, drug overdose, or poisoning, tend to be readily diagnosed if an adequate history is available. Secondary pump problems, however, can easily be overlooked. In addition to evaluating each component, practitioners must consider the clinical setting and the complete clinical picture. Remember that virtually all patients in shock will develop a secondary pump problem as the heart is depleted of essential substrates such as oxygen, glucose, and adenosine triphosphate (ATP).

Patients in pump failure may require (1) treatment of any coexisting rate or volume problem; (2) correction of any other underlying problem, such as hypoxia, hypoglycemia, drug overdose, or poisoning; and (3) support for the failing pump. Pump support may require one or more agents to improve contractility, such as dopamine, dobutamine, or other inotropes; vasodilator therapy to reduce abnormally high systemic vascular resistance (afterload); vasodilator, diuretic, or other therapy to reduce preload; mechanical assistance in the form of an intra-aortic balloon; or even surgery.

Figure 8 presents clinical guidelines that focus on two severe conditions: cardiogenic shock and acute pulmonary edema. Detailed appropriate treatment depends upon invasive hemodynamic monitoring that measures ventricular filling pressures and cardiac output. For the ECC provider, however, Fig 8 provides a therapeutic overview to use while awaiting placement of devices for invasive hemodynamic measurements. These guidelines are based on recommendations from the American College of Cardiology and the American Heart Association for the early management of patients with acute MI[152] and others.[151,152,207]

Clinicians must first be certain that the filling pressure of the ventricles is adequate. If the left ventricular filling pressure is less than 15 mm Hg, hypotension is more likely due to volume problems than pump failure. An intravascular volume challenge sufficient to raise the filling pressure of the left ventricle to more than 18 mm Hg is appropriate.[152] In acute emergencies, however, hemodynamic monitoring takes time to establish, and measurements of left ventricular filling pressure are often not available. In the absence of acute pulmonary edema, a fluid bolus of 250 to 500 mL of normal saline, infused over a short period, can be tried. If there is little or no response then clinicians can begin pressor agents. Repeat volume challenges should be considered for patients who show some improvement after an initial fluid bolus. Conceptually, clinicians divide the treatment of cardiogenic shock or heart failure into hemodynamic subsets.[152,207] Patients may change clinically and move from one subset to another as they respond to therapy. Clinicians must constantly consider and change the therapeutic regimen.[208]

Remember, 250 mL is only one cup of fluid. It may be necessary to use several times this volume.

**Systolic blood pressure
<70 mm Hg[b]**
Signs and symptoms of shock

> **Consider:**
> • *Norepinephrine* 0.5 to 30 µg/min
>   or
> • *Dopamine* 5 to 20 µg/kg per minute

[b]Fluid bolus of 150 to 500 mL normal saline should be tried. If no response, consider sympathomimetics.

Patients in this subset are severely ill and have a high mortality rate. Often both pump (cardiogenic) and volume problems cause this level of profound hypotension. Because it has both inotropic and vasoconstrictive properties, **norepinephrine** 0.5 to 30 µg/min IV may be used until systolic arterial pressure rises to the range of 70 to 100 mm Hg.[152,208] **Dopamine** at 2.5 to 20 µg/kg per minute should be started at that level of blood pressure.

Clinicians should consider angioplasty and intra-aortic balloon counterpulsation in patients with acute MI and cardiogenic shock since these offer the best chances of survival.[209] This group of patients has a high mortality rate. If these patients are seen in the first 12 to 24 hours, consider transferring them to a facility capable of catheterization, angioplasty, and cardiovascular surgery.[152]

> **Systolic blood pressure**
> **70 to 100 mm Hg**[b]
> Signs and symptoms of shock

> **Consider:**
> • *Dopamine*[c]
>   2.5 to 20 µg/kg per minute IV
>   (Add *norepinephrine* if *dopamine* is
>   >20 µg/kg per minute)

[b]Fluid bolus of 150 to 500 mL normal saline should be tried. If no response, consider sympathomimetics.
[c]Move to *dopamine* and stop *norepinephrine* when blood pressure improves. Avoid *dopamine* (consider *dobutamine*) if no signs of hypoperfusion.

These patients have signs and symptoms of shock. The detailed management of these patients with severe hypotension and shock is beyond the scope of the basic ACLS provider. Some helpful guidelines are listed below, but effective management requires individualized therapy and expert consultation.

- Attempt to switch to dopamine and stop norepinephrine as soon as blood pressure responds to initial treatment and rises above 70 mm Hg.
- In the range of 70 to 100 mm Hg, **dopamine** is usually the agent of choice if the patient has signs and symptoms of shock. Dopamine should be started at 2.5 µg/kg per minute and titrated as needed to 20 µg/kg per minute.

- Dobutamine and dopamine can be given together, but dobutamine should not be used alone in the seriously ill patient with systolic blood pressure less than about 90 mm Hg.
- If more than 20 µg/kg per minute of dopamine is required to maintain arterial pressure, the clinician should consider switching to norepinephrine, which has fewer chronotropic effects (though it may be less effective as an inotrope).
- Clinicians should be alert to patients with acute right ventricular infarction. These patients are sensitive to volume depletion and often respond to volume infusion, which rapidly increases right ventricular filling pressure. Dobutamine is preferred over dopamine as a pressor agent in right ventricular infarction. Avoid nitroglycerin and other venodilators, as well as diuretics such as furosemide. Patients with right ventricular infarction respond to angioplasty and intra-aortic balloon counterpulsation and can have excellent outcomes.[209]

> **70 to 100 mm Hg**[b]
> No signs and symptoms of shock

[b]Fluid bolus of 150 to 500 mL normal saline should be tried. If no response, consider sympathomimetics.

> **Consider:**
> • **Dobutamine**[d,e] 2 to 20 µg/kg per minute IV

[d]Add *dopamine* (and avoid *dobutamine*) if systolic blood pressure drops below 90 mm Hg.
[e]Start with *nitroglycerin* if initial blood pressures are in this range.

The key point in these patients is their combination of low blood pressure but no signs or symptoms of shock. In this range of blood pressures, **dobutamine** provides good inotropic and vasoactive effect. If systolic blood pressures are dropping and fall below 90 mm Hg, dopamine can be added, especially if signs and symptoms of shock develop. The initial dobutamine dose is 2 µg/kg per minute titrated upward to a maximum of 20 µg/kg per minute.

Footnote **e** refers specifically to patients in acute pulmonary edema who have blood pressures in the 70 to 100 mm Hg range with no signs and symptoms of shock. This represents one of those complicated clinical "overlap" situations where the pulmonary congestion requires the "unloading" effects of nitroglycerin but the patient may not tolerate the blood pressure–lowering effects of nitroglycerin. These patients require invasive hemodynamic monitoring and expert consultation for proper clinical management.

> **Systolic blood pressure
> >100 mm Hg[b]**

[b]Fluid bolus of 150 to 500 mL normal saline should be tried. If no response, consider sympathomimetics.

> **Consider:**
> - *Nitroglycerin* start 10 to 20 μg/min IV
>   (Use if ischemia persists and
>   blood pressure remains elevated.
>   Titrate to effect)
>   and/or
> - *Nitroprusside* 0.1 to 5.0 μg/kg per minute IV

Some patients may have pump failure manifested by elevated ventricular filling pressures with associated pulmonary congestion and edema. The clinical setting is most often that of acute MI. Clinicians should consider **nitroprusside** and **nitroglycerin** in this clinical situation.

In the early minutes of acute infarction, when ischemia produces the pump failure, nitroglycerin can be administered (10 to 20 μg/min). Most emergency departments have become familiar with IV nitroglycerin for the acute treatment of MI. With acute pulmonary edema and hypertensive emergencies, most emergency physicians prefer IV nitroglycerin, reserving nitroprusside for the intensive care unit. Nitroprusside produces more active afterload reduction. Nitroprusside (0.5 to 5 μg/kg per minute) is the agent of choice when ischemia is not prominent. Nitroprusside requires more complex hemodynamic monitoring than nitroglycerin.

> **Consider:**
> Further actions, especially if the patient is in acute pulmonary edema

Figure 8 directs the clinician who manages pump problems to *categorize* patients by their blood pressure level. The *diagnosis* of a "pump" problem should occur first, and then the blood pressure is reviewed. Pump problems are not defined by the blood pressure only. The pump problem that produces the acute pulmonary edema may be associated with either hypotension and shock or with a marked elevation of the blood pressure. In the presence of a severe pump problem like acute pulmonary edema, the blood pressure becomes a critical initial decision point. *In acute pulmonary edema the blood pressure must be raised if it is too low and lowered if it is too high.* If the patient has normal or elevated blood pressures, the clinician has more room in which to work because these patients can tolerate the drop in blood pressure that several agents produce.

First-line Actions

Emergency personnel should place the patient in the sitting position, with the legs dependent. This increases lung volume and vital capacity, diminishes the work of respiration, and decreases the venous return to the heart. Personnel should immediately institute oxygen therapy, IV access, and cardiac monitoring. Pulse oximetry provides a display of clinical changes over time and helps evaluate the response to therapy. Oxygen saturation measurements may be inaccurate because of decreased peripheral perfusion. Only arterial blood gases provide information on ventilation and acidosis.

> **First-line actions**
> - *Furosemide* IV 0.5 to 1.0 mg/kg
> - *Morphine* IV 1 to 3 mg
> - *Nitroglycerin* SL
> - *Oxygen*/ intubate PRN

An oxygen mask should be placed (if not already accomplished) and high-flow oxygen started at a rate of 5 to 6 L/min. Nonrebreather masks with reservoir bags can yield a concentration of 90% to 100% oxygen. Positive end-expiratory pressure (PEEP) can be used to prevent alveolar collapse and improve gas exchange. The bag-valve mask can replace the simple face mask if hypoventilation is suspected clinically. Continuous positive airway pressure (CPAP) can be applied during spontaneous respirations with a tight-fitting mask or endotracheal tube. A person capable of intubation should be available if intubation appears imminent: if Pao_2 cannot be maintained above 60 mm Hg despite 100% oxygen delivery, if the patient displays signs of cerebral hypoxia (advancing lethargy and obtundation), if the patient displays progressive increase in Pco_2 or increasing acidosis.

If patients in acute pulmonary edema have signs and symptoms of shock and an initial systolic blood pressure less than 70 to 100 mm Hg, order **dopamine** infusion at 2.5 to 20 μg/kg per minute. If more than 20 to 30 μg/kg per minute of dopamine needed, add **norepinephrine** and decrease the dose of dopamine to 10 μg/kg per minute. If acute pulmonary edema patients with initial systolic blood pressure from 70 to 100 mm Hg do not have signs and symptoms of shock, start **dobutamine** infusion at 2.0 to 20 μg/kg per minute.

Once systolic blood pressure exceeds 100 mm Hg, **nitroglycerin** can be started. Most clinicians now consider nitroglycerin to be the most effective agent for acute pulmonary edema. Nitroglycerin inhibits venous return to the heart by its effect on the venous capacitance vessels (reduces preload). At the same time nitroglycerin decreases systemic vascular resistance and facilitates cardiac emptying (reduces afterload). Sublingual **nitroglycerin** tablets, nitroglycerin oral spray, or **isosorbide** oral spray permits the initiation of nitrate therapy before personnel can start an IV line. Two of the standard 0.4 mg tablets can be given every 5 to 10 minutes as long as the systolic blood pressure is greater than 90 to 100 mm Hg. Sublingual nitroglycerin is preferred over nitro paste or oral isosorbide dinitrate because patients with peripheral vasoconstriction will have inconsistent skin absorption.

Intravenous **furosemide** has long been a mainstay of treatment of acute pulmonary edema. Furosemide has a biphasic action. First, it causes an immediate decrease in venous tone and thus an increase in venous capacitance. This leads to a fall in left ventricular filling pressure and improves the clinical symptoms.[210] This effect occurs within 5 minutes. Second, furosemide produces the familiar diuresis several minutes later, which reaches a peak in 30 to 60 minutes. This diuresis need not be massive to be effective. If the patient is already taking oral furosemide, then the clinical rule of thumb is to administer an initial dose that is twice the daily oral dose. If no effect occurs within 20 minutes, clinicians should double the initial dose and use higher doses if the patient has massive fluid retention or renal insufficiency or both.

Morphine sulfate (2 to 8 mg IV if blood pressure is greater than 100 mm Hg) also remains part of the therapeutic armamentarium for acute pulmonary edema, though recent research questions its effectiveness, especially in the prehospital setting.[211] Morphine dilates the capacitance vessels of the peripheral venous bed. This reduces venous return to the central circulation and diminishes the preload of the heart.

Morphine decreases the afterload of the heart by mild arterial vasodilatation and conveys a sedative effect, thus decreasing musculoskeletal and respiratory activity. Now, however, there are superior vasodilators and clearly more effective inotropes. Morphine administration in acute pulmonary edema will probably fade from use as clinicians become more familiar with these newer agents. Some observers have questioned the value of giving a potent sedative to people who are clinically drowning and acutely struggling for breath.[212] Clinical evaluations have demonstrated that the outdated approach of rotating tourniquets provides no positive benefit.[213]

Second-line actions

- *Nitroglycerin* IV if blood pressure
  >100 mm Hg
- *Nitroprusside* IV if blood pressure
  >100 mm Hg
- *Dopamine* if blood pressure <100 mm Hg
- *Dobutamine* if blood pressure >100 mm Hg
- Positive end-expiratory pressure (**PEEP**)
- Continuous positive airway pressure (**CPAP**)

Second-line Actions

Patients may respond to the first-line actions and may not require additional measures. Clinicians can institute the second-line actions with a bit less urgency than the first-line actions, especially in normotensive patients. Intravenous **nitroglycerin** is listed as a second-line action only because it takes time to start an IV line. The sublingual form is more convenient and more readily available. As a potent vasodilator nitroglycerin is the mainstay of treatment. Clinicians can accurately titrate the amount of IV nitroglycerin while monitoring the hemodynamic effects. The other second-line vasoactive agents are administered to patients according to the hemodynamic subsets noted above: nitroprusside (pressure too high), dopamine (pressure too low), and dobutamine (normotensive pump failure).

Third-line actions

- *Amrinone* 0.75 mg/kg then
  5 to 15 µg/kg per minute IV (if other drugs fail)
  if blood pressure >100 mm Hg
- *Aminophylline* 5 mg/kg (if wheezing)
- *Thrombolytic* therapy (if not in shock)
- *Digoxin* (if atrial fibrillation, supraventricular tachycardias)
- Angioplasty (if drugs fail)
- Intra-aortic balloon pump (bridge to surgery)
- Surgical interventions (valves, coronary artery bypass grafts, heart transplant)

Third-line Actions

The third-line actions are reserved for those patients with pump failure and acute pulmonary edema who are resistant to the first- and second-line actions or who experience specific complications. Most of the third-line actions require invasive hemodynamic monitoring in intensive care units or specialized tertiary care facilities. They are only briefly mentioned in these guidelines.

Amrinone (loading dose of 0.75 mg/kg over 2 to 3 minutes, followed by 2 to 20 µg/kg per minute) has inotropic and vasodilatory effects similar to dobutamine.[214] **Aminophylline** (loading dose of 5 mg/kg given over 10 to 20 minutes, followed by 0.5 to 0.7 mg/kg per hour) has been effective in patients with acute bronchospasm ("cardiac asthma"), though it should be reserved for severe bronchospasm and should be avoided in patients with supraventricular arrhythmias, especially when they have ischemic heart disease. **Thrombolytics** have a limited role in patients with acute MI and pump failure. Such patients are usually better candidates for angioplasty and **intra-aortic balloon pumping**.[152]

Angioplasty has been performed in many patients in cardiogenic shock. If it is used within the first 18 hours of symptom onset, researchers have reported survival rates of 50%,[215] which is much higher than reports using thrombolytic therapy or counterpulsation or both. Selected patients will be candidates for acute surgical procedures, such as coronary artery bypass grafts,[216] repair of mitral insufficiency,[217] or cardiac transplantation.[218] Intra-aortic balloon counterpulsation[219] and even total artificial hearts[220,221] can successfully "bridge" these patients over until their operation or a nonsurgical recovery.[152]

Acute Myocardial Infarction (Fig 9)

Chapter 9 discusses acute MI in detail. This section presents key points and the major critical actions to take in treating patients with acute MI.

Key Points

1. The algorithm for acute MI (Fig 9) summarizes the recommendations for early treatment of patients with chest pain and possible acute MI. Four components must coordinate well to produce the best clinical outcomes: the community, the EMS system, the emergency department, and the coronary care unit.

2. All citizens in a community must place a strong emphasis on "call first/call fast/call 911" at the first signs of chest pains and possible acute MI. The National Heart Attack Alert Program is developing a number of professional and community education programs that will help increase the percentage of people with an acute MI who call 911 and seek help soon. Patients and health providers must work together to help decrease the "patient–decision-making interval" between the onset of symptoms and the decision to seek help. The current average time of 3 to 4 hours between the onset of symptoms and seeking help must be reduced.

   The National Heart, Lung, and Blood Institute publication *Emergency Department: Rapid Identification and Treatment of Patients With Acute Myocardial Infarction* (NIH publication 93-3278; September 1993) provides an excellent series of protocols and recommendations consistent with the AHA guidelines and should be reviewed by all providers who treat patients with chest pain.

3. Managers, medical program directors, and emergency personnel in every EMS system must consider a system approach to people with acute MI. Although the AHA does not recommend specific actions that EMS systems must take in regard to the patient who is "myocardially infarcting," the AHA does recommend that each EMS system develop specific policies regarding the following aspects of care:

   • Standing orders for oxygen–IV–cardiac monitor–vital signs
   • Nitroglycerin and narcotics for pain relief
   • Notification of the emergency department

• Rapid transport to the emergency department
• Prehospital identification of patients who may need thrombolytic therapy (review of inclusion and exclusion criteria)
• Prehospital use of 12-lead ECGs, computerized ECG interpretation with transmission of the ECG to the base emergency department
• Initiation of thrombolytic therapy

4. Every emergency department must establish a defined protocol approach for patients who present with chest pain and suspected acute MI. Clinicians have referred to the interval from the patient's arrival in the emergency department to the start of thrombolytic agents as the "door-to-drug" interval. Emergency departments should take no more than 30 to 60 minutes to assess and begin thrombolytic treatment for patients with evidence of coronary thrombosis and no reasons for exclusion.

Critical Actions to Take

1. Immediate assessment should include the following:

   • Vital signs — automated blood pressure measurements are helpful
   • Measurement of oxygen saturation level
   • 12-lead ECG review, with review by physician within 3 to 5 minutes
   • Brief, targeted history and physical
   • Early decision on eligibility for thrombolytic therapy
   • Chest x-ray
   • Blood studies (electrolytes, enzymes, coagulation studies)
   • Request for cardiology consultation for complicated situations

2. Remember to use the four triads as a memory aid for this early assessment:

   • Airway–Breathing–Circulation
   • Oxygen–IV–monitor
   • Pulse–respirations–blood pressure
   • Volume problem–pump problem–rate problem

3. Consider the following treatments if there is evidence of coronary thrombosis plus no reasons for exclusion (some but not all may be appropriate):

   • **Oxygen** at 4 L/min. Use mask or nasal cannula.

   • **Nitroglycerin** sublingual, paste, or spray (if the systolic blood pressure is greater than 90 mm Hg). Followed by:
   Nitroglycerin IV. Limit the systolic blood pressure drop to 10% if normotensive and 30% if hypertensive; never drop the blood pressure below 90 mm Hg systolic. Do *not* delay thrombolytic therapy, when indicated, for a full therapeutic dose of nitroglycerin. Consider giving nitroglycerin and thrombolytics simultaneously.

   • **Morphine** IV. Use small (1- to 3-mg) IV doses of morphine sulfate, repeated at 5-minute intervals

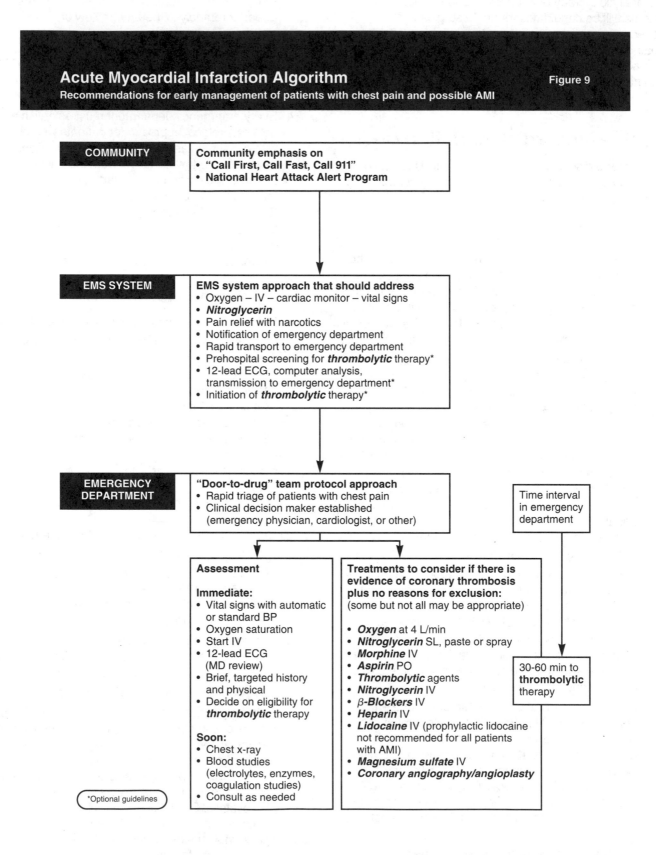

Acute Myocardial Infarction Algorithm

Recommendations for early management of patients with chest pain and possible AMI

Figure 9

COMMUNITY

Community emphasis on
- "Call First, Call Fast, Call 911"
- National Heart Attack Alert Program

EMS SYSTEM

EMS system approach that should address
- Oxygen – IV – cardiac monitor – vital signs
- *Nitroglycerin*
- Pain relief with narcotics
- Notification of emergency department
- Rapid transport to emergency department
- Prehospital screening for *thrombolytic* therapy*
- 12-lead ECG, computer analysis, transmission to emergency department*
- Initiation of *thrombolytic* therapy*

EMERGENCY DEPARTMENT

"Door-to-drug" team protocol approach
- Rapid triage of patients with chest pain
- Clinical decision maker established (emergency physician, cardiologist, or other)

Time interval in emergency department

Assessment

Immediate:
- Vital signs with automatic or standard BP
- Oxygen saturation
- Start IV
- 12-lead ECG (MD review)
- Brief, targeted history and physical
- Decide on eligibility for *thrombolytic* therapy

Soon:
- Chest x-ray
- Blood studies (electrolytes, enzymes, coagulation studies)
- Consult as needed

Treatments to consider if there is evidence of coronary thrombosis plus no reasons for exclusion:
(some but not all may be appropriate)

- *Oxygen* at 4 L/min
- *Nitroglycerin* SL, paste or spray
- *Morphine* IV
- *Aspirin* PO
- *Thrombolytic* agents
- *Nitroglycerin* IV
- *β-Blockers* IV
- *Heparin* IV
- *Lidocaine* IV (prophylactic lidocaine not recommended for all patients with AMI)
- *Magnesium sulfate* IV
- *Coronary angiography/angioplasty*

30-60 min to **thrombolytic** therapy

*Optional guidelines

as needed. Pain relief is a high priority. Morphine should be used in conjunction with increasing doses of nitroglycerin and a β-blocking agent and should not be relied on as the sole agent to treat pain, which is an indication of ongoing ischemia.

- **Aspirin** by mouth. The routine use of aspirin (150 to 325 mg) is strongly recommended for all acute MI patients (Class I), including those who receive thrombolytic therapy. Patients should chew one chewable aspirin and then take one by mouth.

- **Thrombolytic agents.** These agents are Class I for patients with acute transmural MI, those treated within 6 hours of symptoms, and those with new left bundle branch block. Thrombolytics are Class IIa for patients seen more than 6 hours after onset of symptoms and should be considered for all patients with symptoms and ECG findings of acute MI (excluding non–Q wave infarctions).

- **Heparin** IV. This may prevent recurrence of thrombosis after thrombolysis has occurred. Use a bolus of 5000 U followed with 1000 U/h for 24 to 48 hours. Adjust dose to maintain activated partial thromboplastin time (aPTT) 1.5 to 2.0 times the control values.

- **β Blockers**. Intravenous followed by oral β blockers (metoprolol, propranolol, esmolol) given within the first 4 to 6 hours of a patient's presentation with acute MI and continued for 1 to 2 years after acute MI reduces mortality by about 33%. β Blockers are contraindicated by hypotension, bradycardia, heart failure, or asthmatic condition.

- **Magnesium sulfate** infusion (prophylactic). Give when hypomagnesemia is detected (serum magnesium level of less than 0.7 mmol/L [1.4 mEq/L]) or suspected on the basis of the patient's history (malnutrition, etc). There is contradictory evidence about the benefit of routine magnesium in normomagnesemic patients.[222]

- **Percutaneous transluminal coronary angioplasty (PTCA)**. The need for emergent coronary catheterization with possible angioplasty must be considered early in the following situations:

  — Patients with signs and symptoms of a large acute MI for less than 6 hours who should get thrombolytic therapy but for whom for some reason the thrombolytic therapy is contraindicated (eg, recent surgery, tumors, history of gastrointestinal bleeding) (Class I)

  — Patients with possible "stuttering" infarction, with ECG changes, but without clear indication for thrombolytic therapy (Class IIa)

  — Patients with acute MI who develop cardiogenic shock or pump failure within 18 hours (Class IIa)

  — Patients with a history of previous coronary artery bypass graft surgery in whom a recent occlusion of a vein graft may have occurred (Class IIa)

  — Availability of institutions that can offer 24-hour availability of PTCA

- Routine prophylactic **lidocaine** administration is not recommended for patients with acute MI. Clinicians should withhold lidocaine until the acute MI patient displays a specific indication, such as symptomatic PVCs or VT. The algorithms for tachycardias and VF/VT should be followed.

Treatments to Consider in Acute MI: Details

The Subcommittee on ACLS recommends using the following format when thinking about medications and treatments in ECC:

- **Why?** (actions)
- **When?** (indications)
- **How?** (dosing regimens)
- **Watch out!** (precautions)

The treatments to consider in acute MI are presented in this format.

Oxygen

Why?

The therapeutic goal is to increase the supply of oxygen to ischemic tissues. Oxygen should be thought of as a drug, just like the other oral and IV agents. The only difference is it is administered in a different manner. Oxygen is the most important and effective agent in ECC.

When?

- Always use oxygen when acute MI is suspected. Some experts say the quality of emergency care can be judged by how fast personnel administer supplemental oxygen.
- Remember *oxygen-IV-monitor* as one word.

How?

- Start with a nasal cannula at 4 L/min. Use an oxygen saturation monitor to check that the oxygen saturation exceeds 97% to 98%.
- If you are unable to maintain this level, increase the delivery of oxygen to 6 to 8 L/min.
- Switch to a Venturi mask if oxygen saturation remains low.

Watch out!

Very rarely you may encounter patients with chronic obstructive pulmonary disease (COPD) who are dependent on a hypoxic ventilatory drive. Do not deprive any patient of oxygen just because of a suspicion that oxygen will induce severe hypoventilation. The frequency of this problem is grossly overestimated. Remember that most patients with severe chronic obstructive pulmonary disease are already on supplemental home oxygen. Start with low-flow oxygen (1 to 2 L/min) and observe whether significant hypoventilation ensues. Adjust oxygen delivery accordingly.

Nitroglycerin

Why?

- Nitroglycerin is an important drug to use early for suspected acute MI patients. Multiple clinical trials have observed that the effect of nitroglycerin on infarct size and mortality from acute MI is as powerful as that of thrombolytics.[223-228]
- Nitroglycerin is well known to decrease the pain of ischemia. It is important to realize that nitroglycerin also produces positive altered hemodynamics and through this mechanism limits the size of the infarct and subsequent mortality.
- Nitroglycerin produces the following actions:
  — Decreases the pain of ischemia
  — Increases venous dilation
  — Decreases venous blood return to the heart
  — Decreases preload and oxygen consumption
  — Dilates coronary arteries
  — Increases cardiac collateral flow

When?

- In 1990 the AHA/ACC task force on the early management of patients with acute MI stated, "There are inadequate data at present to recommend infusion of intravenous nitroglycerin in all patients with uncomplicated acute myocardial infarction."[152] However, informal surveys of cardiology practice at the time of this writing (1993) suggest that most cardiologists do administer routine nitroglycerin infusions in people with high suspicion of acute MI.
- The indications for nitroglycerin are
  — Suspected ischemic chest pain
  — Unstable angina (change in angina pattern)
  — Acute pulmonary edema (if blood pressure is greater than 100 systolic)
  — Routine use in acute MI (not just for continuing pain)
  — Elevated blood pressure in the setting of acute MI (especially with signs of left ventricular failure)

How?

- The clinical goal in nitroglycerin administration (particularly IV infusion) is not just to relieve pain but to produce improved hemodynamics.[223,227] Changes in blood pressure are desired and indicate that these altered hemodynamics are taking place.

- Several dosing approaches are acceptable:
  — Sublingual: 0.3 to 0.4 mg. Repeat every 5 minutes.
  — Spray inhaler: repeat every 5 minutes.
  — Paste: apply 1 to 2 inches with backing pad.
  — IV infusion: 10 to 20 µg/min; increase by 5 to 10 µg/min every 5 to 10 minutes.
  — Goal: pain relief *plus* lowered blood pressures.

Watch out!

In patients with evidence of acute MI:

- Use with extreme caution if systolic blood pressure is less than 90 mm.
- Limit mean blood pressure drop to 10% if the patient is normotensive.
- Limit mean blood pressure drop to 30% if the patient is hypertensive.
- Watch for headache, drop in blood pressure, syncope, tachycardia.
- Do not delay thrombolytics while waiting to eradicate pain with nitroglycerin.
- Instruct the patient to sit or lie down.
- Be especially cautious in patients who may have a right ventricular infarction (up to one in five inferior myocardial infarctions!).

Morphine Sulfate

Why?

- Pain in patients who are myocardially infarcting can be so severe that the patients produce high levels of catecholamines. These catecholamines increase blood pressure, heart rate, and oxygen demands on the heart. It is important to control these demands on the infarcting heart, and morphine is a key agent for this purpose.
- The major actions of morphine are
  — Reduces pain of ischemia
  — Reduces anxiety
  — Increases venous capacitance
  — Decreases systemic vascular resistance.
- These actions lead to reduced oxygen demands on the heart, which leads to less ischemia and infarct extension.
- Both morphine and nitroglycerin have a purpose beyond pain relief. Both alter hemodynamics in a positive manner and are indicated even if the ischemic pain is minimal or has disappeared.

When?

- The indications for morphine are
  — Continuing pain
  — Evidence of vascular congestion (acute pulmonary edema)
  — Blood pressure greater than 90 systolic
  — No hypovolemia

- Morphine is losing favor as a major agent to be used in acute pulmonary edema (Class IIb). This topic is discussed further in the section on hypotension/shock/acute pulmonary edema.

How?

- Morphine dosing is 1 to 3 mg IV at frequent intervals (as often as every 5 minutes).
- Most EMS systems, emergency departments, and critical care units use a "titrated to pain" approach. This allows the paramedic or nurse to identify when the pain is relieved and when the next dose should be administered.
- While complete pain relief is the clinical goal, the amount of morphine is constrained by the blood pressure and by respiratory depression.

Watch out!

- Observe the following precautions with morphine:
  - Drop in blood pressure, especially with
    Volume-depleted patients
    Patients with increased systemic resistance
    Patients receiving β blockers
  - Depression of ventilation
  - Nausea and vomiting (common)
  - Bradycardia
  - Itching and bronchospasm (uncommon)
- Use the Trendelenburg position as the first response to moderate-to-severe drops in blood pressure.
- Use naloxone 0.4 to 0.8 mg IV to reverse respiratory depression.

Aspirin

Why?

- The ISIS-2 study surprised the cardiology community by observing that aspirin alone, started within 24 hours of the onset of acute MI, reduced overall mortality to almost the same degree as thrombolytic agents.[229]
- For acute MI and unstable angina, aspirin is the most cost-effective agent available.[152]
- Mechanism of action of aspirin:
  - Among other actions, aspirin blocks formation of thromboxane A_2. Thromboxane A_2 causes platelets to aggregate and arteries to constrict.
  - This action will
    Reduce overall mortality from acute MI
    Reduce nonfatal reinfarction
    Reduce nonfatal stroke

When?

- As soon as possible!
- Standard therapy for all patients with new pain suggestive of acute MI
- Give within minutes of arrival

The AHA/ACC task force on early management of acute MI makes this recommendation.[152] However, it has not been fully implemented.[224,225]

How?

- 160 mg to 325 mg tablet taken as soon as possible
- Most emergency departments keep a supply of aspirin in the examination and treatment rooms to allow immediate administration of aspirin to patients suspected of having an acute MI.
- Some EMS systems have paramedics administer aspirin in the prehospital setting.

Watch out!

- Some precautions with aspirin:
  - It is relatively contraindicated in patients with active ulcer disease or asthma.
  - It is contraindicated in patients with known hypersensitivity to aspirin.
  - Higher doses can interfere with prostacyclin production and interfere with positive benefits.

Thrombolytic Therapy[152,230]

Why?

- Thrombolytic therapy has revolutionized the treatment of patients with acute MI. Research has established that the majority of acute MIs occur in people with coronary arteries narrowed by the slow buildup of atheromatous plaques.
  - The acute event is caused by the sudden rupture of an arterial plaque.
  - The raw surfaces of the ruptured plaque stimulate the formation of a blood clot or thrombus at the site of the rupture.
  - This thrombus leads to further narrowing of the artery and often to complete blockage.
  - This narrowing and blockage slows or even stops the flow of blood to the myocardium.
  - The area of the heart supplied by the blocked artery in Q-wave infarction rapidly develops first ischemia (tall or inverted T waves), then injury (ST segment elevation), and soon actual infarction (Q waves).
  - The emphasis in thrombolytic therapy is to use thrombolytic agents to dissolve the clot as quickly as possible to reopen the blocked artery and prevent this progression of ischemia to injury and infarction.
  - The goal of thrombolytic therapy is to "salvage" as much as possible of the injured myocardium and prevent its deterioration to actual infarction and death ("myocardial salvage" concept).
  - Thrombolytic therapy must be used as quickly as possible ("time-is-muscle" concept, and the concept of a short "door-to-drug" interval).

- Thrombolytic therapy has the remarkable ability to actually reopen coronary arteries that have been blocked by a blood clot.
- The term to keep in mind is that these patients are *myocardially infarcting*. An analogous clinical situation would be patients who are experiencing status epilepticus. The same sense of urgency should prevail.
- One of the critical teaching points in ACLS is the need to identify patients who should receive thrombolytic therapy.

When?

- One small point of semantics must be understood. Thrombolytics are used for people who are presumed to be myocardially infarcting. This is a presumption, not an actual diagnosis. Definitive diagnosis of an acute MI depends on characteristic serum enzyme changes and the development of Q waves on the ECG. The evolution of Q waves takes hours, even days. However, the clinician cannot wait for enzyme results to return or for Q waves to evolve. A person qualifies for thrombolytic therapy if he or she has a characteristic history plus ECG changes of *injury* (elevated ST segments), not necessarily of *infarction* (Q waves).
- Qualifications for thrombolytic therapy:
  — History (nature, location of pain) consistent with acute MI
  — ECG consistent with acute MI (acute injury)
  — No absolute contraindication
  — Few or no relative contraindications
- ECG criteria for acute MI:
  — More than 1 to 2 mm ST elevation in two contiguous V (precordial) leads
  — More than 1 to 2 mm ST elevation in two contiguous limb (frontal) leads
  Note: Measure the ST deviation 0.04 second after the J point using the PQR segment as the isoelectric line.
- ECG criteria for location of infarction:
  1. Anterior infarction (injury)
     — ST elevation in leads V_1 through V_4
     — Indicates occlusion of the left anterior descending branch of the left coronary artery
  2. Inferior infarction (injury)
     — ST elevation in leads II, III, AVF
     — Indicates occlusion of the right coronary artery
  3. Right ventricular infarction (injury)
     — ST elevation in leads II, III, AVF *plus*
     — ST elevation in right precordial leads (V_{4R})

     Note: Recent studies have indicated a growing awareness of the frequency of right ventricular infarction and the high rate of associated complications.[231] If an inferior infarction is identified (ST elevation in II, III, AVF), obtain a second ECG with the six precordial leads arrayed to the right rather

than the left.[232] Look for ST segment elevation in V_{4R}.
  4. Lateral infarction (injury)
     — ST elevation in leads I, AVL, V_5, V_6
     — Indicates occlusion of a left circumflex artery
     — May be part of multiple-site infarction (eg, anterolateral infarction)
  5. Posterior infarction (injury)
     — ST depression in V_1 and V_2 with tall R wave (represents reciprocal changes)
     — Indicates occlusion of right coronary artery or left circumflex artery or both
     — May be part of multiple-site infarction, including inferior MI

- Absolute contraindications for thrombolytic therapy:
  — Active internal bleeding
  — Suspected aortic dissection
  — Known traumatic CPR (rib fractures, pneumothorax, traumatic endotracheal intubation, etc)[233]
  — Severe persistent hypertension despite pain relief and initial drugs (greater than 180 systolic or 110 diastolic)
  — Recent head trauma or known intracranial neoplasm
  — History of cerebrovascular accident in the past 6 months
  — Pregnancy

- Relative contraindications:
  — Recent trauma or major surgery in the past 2 months
  — Initial blood pressure greater than 180 systolic or 110 diastolic that is controlled by medical treatment
  — Active peptic ulcer or guaiac-positive stools
  — History of cerebrovascular accident, tumor, injury, or brain surgery
  — Known bleeding disorder or current use of warfarin
  — Significant liver dysfunction or renal failure
  — Exposure to streptokinase or anistreplase during the preceding 12 months (these agents only)
  — Known cancer or illness with possible thoracic, abdominal, or intracranial abnormalities
  — Prolonged CPR[233]

Note: Defibrillation is never a contraindication to lytic therapy.

How?

Currently approved agents are

- *Anisoylated plasminogen streptokinase activator complex*
  (APSAC) Anistreplase: 30 U IV over 2 to 5 minutes
- *Tissue Plasminogen Activator* (TPA)
  Alteplase: 100 mg IV, given 60 mg in first hour (6 to 10 mg IV push initially) then 20 mg/h for 2 additional

hours. An "accelerated" regimen (not yet FDA-approved) is used by many clinicians as follows:
— Give 15-mg bolus IV
— Then 0.75 mg/kg over next 30 min (not to exceed 50 mg)
— Then 0.50 mg/kg over next 60 min (not to exceed 35 mg)
— Total dose ≤100 mg
- *Streptokinase*: 1.5 million U in a 1-hour infusion
- *Urokinase*
  Abbokinase: 1.5 million U IV over 2 minutes, then 1.5 million U IV over 90 minutes (FDA approval pending)

Heparin

Why?

- Heparin has received increasing attention as part of the "thrombolytic package" administered to patients with acute MI (along with aspirin and thrombolytic agents). Much of the scientific debate about the many thrombolytic therapy trials centers on whether, when, and how heparin is used with thrombolytic agents.
- Independent of the question of giving heparin with thrombolytic agents has been the increasing practice of giving heparin to all patients with large anterior acute MIs.[224,225] This is because these patients are at increased risk from mural ventricular thrombi and cerebral emboli. The ACC/AHA guidelines on the early management of AMIs grade this use of heparin a Class IIa recommendation (acceptable, probably helpful).[152]
- The reasons for using heparin in acute MI:
  — Acute coronary thrombosis comes from thrombus formation over ruptured plaque.
  — Even after thrombolysis the following remain: residual thrombus, vascular injury, active (thrombogenic) surfaces.
  — These active surfaces stimulate more thrombus formation.
  — Heparin prevents recurrence of thrombosis after thrombolysis has occurred.
  — Maintains patency of infarct-related artery.
  — Heparin prevents mural thrombus formation in patients with a large anterior acute MI.
- IV heparin is mandatory with alteplase (TPA).
- Subcutaneous heparin is probably the optimal route with streptokinase.
- Heparin is unnecessary with anistreplase (APSAC).

When?

- Responsible staff in every hospital and emergency department should establish specific directions for when to use heparin.
- Use of heparin to prevent mural thrombi is often based on echocardiography that shows a large hypokinetic area of the ventricles (thus setting up the site for thrombus formation).

- The options for *when* to give heparin:
  — Option 1: at the same time as the thrombolytic agent.
  — Option 2: on completion of thrombolytic infusion.
  — Option 3: empirically in patients with large anterior acute MIs without thrombolytics.

How?

Obtain a blood sample for control of partial thromboplastin time (PTT), then administer heparin:
- Bolus IV: 5000 U (other regimens, such as 100 to 150 U/kg are also acceptable)
- Continue: 1000 U/h for 24 to 48 hours
- Then adjust to maintain activated PTT time: 1.5 to 2.0 times the control values

Watch out!

The same contraindications to using thrombolytics apply to the use of heparin:
- Active bleeding
- Recent intracranial, intraspinal, or eye surgery
- Severe hypertension
- Bleeding tendencies

β Blockers

Why?

- Many studies support the use of β blockers for patients with acute MI.[224,225] Through multiple mechanisms β blockers help reduce the amount of MI. The concepts to understand are "myocardial salvage" in the anatomic area of the "infarct-related artery" and the "penumbra" of ischemic tissue that surrounds an area of infarcted tissue. Despite thrombolytic therapy certain ischemic areas may deteriorate into dead, infarcted areas. One goal of β blocker therapy is to prevent as much of this deterioration as possible by reducing the oxygen consumption and the demands on the ischemic areas so that they are "salvaged."
- The therapeutic actions of β blockers in acute MI:
  — Decrease arrhythmias by decreasing catecholamine levels
  — Reduce sinus node discharge
  — Lower blood pressure
  — Reduce myocardial contractility
  — Block catecholamine stimulation
  — Reduce myocardial oxygen consumption
  Net effect: Reduce size of infarction

When?

- Administration of IV β blockers to patients with acute MI can have significant side effects. Initiate IV β blockers with caution and usually in consultation with cardiologists who have or will assume care of patients in critical care units.

- The major indications:
  — Acute MI (anterior) with excess sympathetic activity (elevated heart rate and blood pressure)
  — Large MIs treated early (less than 6 hours of pain)
  — Refractory chest pain or tachycardias due to excessive sympathetic tone

How?

The following regimens have been adopted by many institutions and clinicians. Other approaches are possible and acceptable.

- Metoprolol: 5 mg IV infusion (slow), every 5 minutes to a total of 15 mg

or

- Atenolol: 5 mg IV infusion (over 5 minutes); wait 10 minutes then give a second dose of 5 mg IV (over 5 minutes)

or

- Propranolol: 1 mg IV (slow) every 5 minutes to a total of 5 mg

Watch Out!

- β Blockers can cause marked myocardial depression and therefore must always be used with care and close observation.
- Contraindications are:
  — Congestive heart failure/pulmonary edema
  — Bronchospasm or history of asthma
  — Bradycardia (less than 50 to 60 beats per minute)
  — Hypotension (blood pressure less than 100 systolic)

Lidocaine

Why?

- The major reasons to use lidocaine in patients with acute MI are to
  — Suppress ventricular irritability
  — Decrease excitability in ischemic tissue
  — Elevate the VF threshold
  — Prevent the patient from going into VF/VT
- By reducing tissue excitability and elevating the VF threshold, lidocaine reduces PVCs. These PVCs have the potential to set off "reentry" VT which in turn could degenerate into fatal VF.
- There now exists, however, a great deal of discussion surrounding the routine use of lidocaine to prevent PVCs in the setting of acute MI.[87,224,225,234] Lidocaine can cause seizures, neurological problems, hypotension, and even fatal asystole.[235] Lidocaine indications are confusing, particularly regarding prophylactic versus therapeutic use (are you preventing VT or treating PVCs?).[87] Some authors recommend lidocaine only for symptomatic VT, implying that there is a form of asymptomatic VT

that should not be treated with lidocaine.[87,234] Lidocaine pharmacokinetics are complex and change in the cardiac arrest patient.[91,92]

When?

- Routine *prophylactic* lidocaine to prevent VF/VT is **not** recommended for acute MI patients.[236] This recommendation represents a change from the previous AHA recommendations. This question has now been extensively studied, and the weight of the evidence is that the number of deaths prevented by lidocaine is matched by the deaths caused by lidocaine.[224,234,237-239]
- Routine *prophylactic* lidocaine before thrombolytic therapy is **not** recommended.[87]
- Treatment of lone PVCs (especially asymptomatic) in acute MI is **not** recommended.
- The proper treatment of PVCs in acute MI is proper treatment of the acute MI:
  — Oxygen
  — Nitroglycerin
  — Morphine
  — β Blockers
  — Thrombolytic agents
- We now have more effective direct treatments for acute MIs than in the past. PVCs serve as a warning that these other treatments are needed or may not have been used effectively.
- Patients with new onset, symptomatic ventricular ectopy (runs, couplets, salvos) who are myocardially infarcting may benefit from treatment (not prophylaxis) with lidocaine. Post-thrombolysis arrhythmias are usually self-limited and do not often require treatment.

How?

- There are four features to remember about administration of lidocaine: bolus, repeat bolus, total dose, and continuous infusion.
  — Bolus: 1 to 1.5 mg/kg IV
  — Repeat in 2 to 10 minutes at 0.5 to 0.75 mg/kg
  — Total: 3 mg/kg
  — Continue: 2 to 4 mg/min
- Use the lower doses and longer intervals for
  — Patients aged more than 70 years
  — Liver failure
  — Heart failure
  — Smaller body size
  — Bradycardias
  — Conduction disturbances (particularly blocks)

Watch out!

- The clinical indications of lidocaine toxicity are usually related to the central nervous system. The following signs and symptoms are listed in order of increasing severity, reflecting increasing blood levels:
  — Paresthesias
  — Dizziness

— Slurred speech
— Drowsiness
— Altered consciousness
— Decreased hearing
— Muscle twitching
— Seizures
— Respiratory arrest

Magnesium Sulfate

Why?

- By 1993 there was increased interest and research in the benefits of magnesium in acute MI.[224,225] Several large scale randomized, controlled trials suggested a significant overall reduction in mortality from acute MI.[98,99,224,240,241] A recent major study was the 1992 LIMIT-2 trial that included over 2000 patients and showed a mortality decrease of 24% when magnesium was administered.[98] The ISIS-4 study did not confirm this benefit.[222]
- The known effects of magnesium are
  — Antiarrhythmic
  — Vasodilatory
  — Spasmolytic
  — Affects electrical stability in myocardium
  — Magnesium deficiency is associated with arrhythmias and sudden death
  — Possesses "cardioprotective" effect due to unknown mechanism
- The exact mechanism of benefit of magnesium is unknown. In the randomized clinical trials people who did not receive magnesium died from cardiogenic shock and PEA. These observations suggest that the benefit arises from a "cardioprotective effect" rather than a specific antiarrhythmic effect.

When?

- The current recommendations for the use of magnesium are
  — To suppress torsades de pointes (Class I) until the offending circumstances are removed
  — Cardiac arrest with known or suspected magnesium deficiency (Class I)
  — Acute MI with known or *suspected magnesium deficiency* (Class I)
  — Routine prophylactic administration in acute MI is considered Class IIb (acceptable, possibly helpful). Data presented in late 1993 from the ISIS-4 Collaborative Group suggest no benefit from routine use of magnesium in acute MI.[222]
- The key term here is *suspected magnesium deficiency*, which should be suspected in patients who use diuretics and in patients with poor nutrition (such as alcoholics), chronic diseases, poor dietary intake, and poor dietary habits. When treating such people do not hesitate to use magnesium. (Absent deep tendon reflexes may indicate people who do *not* need magnesium.)

How?

Administer magnesium in the following regimens:
- Cardiac arrest: 1 to 2 g (2 to 4 mL of 50% $MgSO_4$) IV push
- Torsades: 1 to 2 g (2 to 4 mL of 50% $MgSO_4$) over 1 to 2 minutes
- Acute MI prophylaxis: 1 to 2 g (2 to 4 mL of 50% $MgSO_4$) diluted in 100 mL of normal saline; over 5 to 60 minutes. Follow with 0.5 to 1.0 g/h up to 24 hours.

Watch out!

- In general, magnesium is a safe drug that can be given quickly in large quantities. Obstetricians have administered large doses of magnesium to pre-eclamptic women for years without serious side effects. Side effects include
  — Hypotension
  — Hyporeflexia
  — Diaphoresis and drowsiness
- Magnesium is excreted by the kidney, so caution is warranted in renal failure patients. However, even renal failure patients can tolerate a reduced (<16 g) first bolus and will experience clinical difficulties only with more prolonged infusions.
- Calcium chloride can be used to counteract the deleterious effects of magnesium. Follow deep tendon reflexes in nonarrest patients for early clues to possible toxic levels.

Percutaneous Transluminal Coronary Angioplasty (PTCA)

Why?

- PTCA is an important intervention to consider early in the course of evaluating patients with known or suspected acute MI.[152] There are specific indications for PTCA, and emergency personnel must know and look for these indications early.[242]
- ACLS providers should know whether PTCA can be performed at the health centers where they work. Recent publications have observed superior outcomes in patients who receive early PTCA compared with patients who receive early thrombolytic therapy.[243-245] These PTCA patients had better restoration of arterial patency and less reocclusion of the infarct-related artery. These results are highly dependent, however, on sophisticated centers with well-equipped laboratories and staff experienced in invasive cardiovascular procedures.[246] ACLS participants also should know how to refer patients to centers with PTCA capability if their professional setting lacks that capability.[246]

- The rationale for early PTCA:
  — It provides a method for mechanical reperfusion of the infarct-related artery.
  — It addresses the true problem (chronically narrowed artery) more directly than thrombolytics (acute clot in the narrowed artery).
  — Some patients with acute MI have contraindications to thrombolytic therapy.
  — It provides the best outcome for acute MI patients with cardiogenic shock or pump failure.
  — It provides the best outcome for patients with occluded vein grafts from coronary artery bypass.

When?

- The major indications for consideration of PTCA are[152]
  — Patients with signs and symptoms of a large acute MI for less than 6 hours for whom thrombolytic therapy is contraindicated (Class I)
  — Patients with "stuttering" infarction and ECG changes but no clear indication for thrombolytic therapy (Class IIa)
  — Patients with acute MI who develop cardiogenic shock or pump failure within 18 hours (Class IIa)
  — Patients with a history of previous coronary artery bypass graft (CABG) plus possible recent occlusion of a vein graft (Class IIa)
  — Patients with in-hospital acute MIs (Class IIb)
- The three most common indications will be
  — Patients with acute MI and contraindications to thrombolytic agents
  — Patients with cardiogenic shock[215]
  — Patients with a history of previous CABG and suspected new occlusion of vein graft

How?

PTCA should be performed only in centers with[152]
- Rapid access to a catheterization laboratory
- Personnel experienced in expeditious angioplasty (completion within 1 hour)

Watch out!

The following uses of PTCA are considered Class III (possibly harmful)[152]:
- Severe left main coronary artery disease plus instrumentation of a more distal occluded artery
- Involvement of only a small area of myocardium
- Dilation of vessels other than the infarct-related artery during the early hours of acute MI

Evaluation and Treatment of Arrhythmias Associated With Acute MI

1. A critical point to remember about arrhythmias associated with acute MI is that they often do not require antiarrhythmic agents. The principle "treat the patient, not the monitor" dictates that the prudent clinician think of possible treatable causes of the arrhythmia. For example, bradycardias due to inadequate ventilation or tachycardias due to pain and anxiety do not require antiarrhythmic agents.

2. One helpful approach to arrhythmias in acute MI is to ask, as suggested earlier, a series of questions about the rhythm:
   - Lethal or nonlethal?
   - VF or not VF?
   - Shock indicated or no shock indicated?
   - Too fast or too slow?

3. The *too* of *too fast* or *too slow* can be determined only by looking at the patient, not the monitor. The critical question about all arrhythmias is simple: is the patient stable or unstable? The answer can be determined only by close clinical attention. With these questions in mind, here are the major arrhythmias to look for in acute MI:
   - Lethal:
     — VF/pulseless VT
     — PEA (same as profound cardiogenic shock)
   - Too slow:
     — First-degree heart block
     — Second-degree heart block (types I and II)
     — Third-degree (complete) heart block
   - Too fast:
     — VT with a pulse
     — PVCs in salvos and runs
     — Sinus tachycardia (rarely gets "too" fast)
     — Atrial flutter/atrial fibrillation
     — PSVT
     — Wide-complex tachycardias of undetermined origin

Each of these arrhythmias is discussed in other sections of this chapter and in other sections of this book. The following section provides some comments on these arrhythmias in the context of acute MI.

"Too Slow": Bradycardias

1. Bradycardias are common during the first hour of symptoms and may include sinus bradycardia, junctional escape rhythms, and AV block at the level of the AV node.

2. Treat these bradycardias if the ventricular rate is slow (eg, below 60 beats per minute) *and* the patient appears to be experiencing symptoms from the slow rate. These symptoms may include chest pain, shortness of breath, hypotension, or PVCs. In the absence of symptoms, bradycardias do not need antiarrhythmic treatment. Pharmacologic interventions, such as atropine or catecholamine infusions, may make the patient worse by exacerbating ischemia or inducing VT or VF.

3. It is critical to understand two potentially conflicting concepts about bradycardias:

- *Slow rates* may lead to diminished coronary flow on the basis of the rate alone. This will increase ischemia and injury and lead to increased development of ventricular escape arrhythmias (eg, PVCs and VT).
- *Slow rates* may protect against rate-related ischemia and injury that occur when faster rates put more demands on the injured myocardium. The myocardium responds to tachycardia with increased ischemia and increased arrhythmias (eg, PVCs and VT).

4. Therefore, leaving symptomatic (eg, with pain) acute MI bradycardia patients in a slow rate can be *bad*. However, speeding up the heart rate of patients with acute MI can be *very bad*. Faster rates may induce cardiac strain, which produces more ischemia, more injury, more cardiac damage, more irritability, and more lethal arrhythmias.

5. Remember, do not treat bradycardias in acute MI unless forced to do so by the severity of symptoms. Even then remember that you are treading a narrow path between helping and hurting.

6. **Second-degree Heart Block Type I**

   This block usually indicates dysfunction high in the AV node. The vagal discharge associated with acute MI, rather than conduction system injury, may be the culprit. This arrhythmia is usually transient and resolves as the vagal effects dissipate. No treatment is indicated unless the patient is significantly symptomatic. Again there is a dilemma that must be considered with symptomatic bradycardia: leave the rate slow, the ischemia gets worse; speed the rate up, the ischemia gets worse. In general, watchful waiting is the best course.

7. **Second-degree Heart Block Type II**

   This block usually indicates injury below the AV node, either at the bundle of His (uncommon) or the bundle branch level (more common). This is a serious arrhythmia, for it indicates significant ischemic pathology of the conduction system. There is a high risk of progression to complete heart block, which has a high risk of mortality.

   The major point is that these patients are displaying signs of severe injury to the conduction system at the infranodal region. Emergency personnel must prepare for pacing with both transvenous and transcutaneous pacing. This preparation means
   - Call a cardiologist or other person who will be responsible for insertion of a transvenous pacer
   - Attach a transcutaneous pacer prophylactically
   - Always give a brief trial of TCP to make sure that it will capture (cause mechanical beats of the heart) and that the patient can tolerate the pacing stimulus
   - If pacing pain appears to pose a major problem, be prepared to give IV analgesics and muscle relaxants/anxiolytics

8. **Third-degree AV Blocks at the Level of the AV Node (Normal QRS)**
   - In patients with a normal-looking QRS and a rate usually between 40 to 60 beats per minute, a stable junctional escape pacemaker has probably taken over.
   - These are often transient blocks and have a good prognosis.
   - These patients still need close observation and consultation with a cardiologist. Consider prophylactic placement of a transvenous pacemaker.

9. **Third-degree AV Blocks at the Level of the Bundle Branches (Wide QRS)**
   - The major clue in these patients is the wide QRS complex and the slow rate — less than 40 beats per minute. This represents an infranodal block with the only escape mechanism coming from the ventricles below the block.
   - This indicates extensive damage from the acute MI. The escape pacemaker is not stable.
   - These patients should have a temporary transvenous pacemaker inserted as soon as possible. The same preparations for pacing noted above should be made.
   - In the setting of an acute MI these patients may suddenly develop catastrophic asystole, so that transcutaneous pacing pads should be placed and tested to determine if the pacing stimulus produces a mechanical contraction.

"Too Fast": Tachycardias

1. **Supraventricular tachycardias associated with acute MI**. Rapid supraventricular tachycardias (such as sinus tachycardia, atrial flutter and fibrillation, and atrial tachycardia) may occur with acute MI. The major clinical concern is that they may increase the area of infarction or exacerbate the ischemia.
   - Clinicians should first ensure that oxygenation and pain control are adequate and that all other appropriate interventions noted in the algorithm for acute MI are being initiated.
   - Sinus tachycardia in acute MI patients is a sign that something else is going on with the patient. The clinical challenge is to identify and treat that "something else."
     — Pain: use appropriate analgesia
     — Anxiety: use sedation and anxiolytics
     — Hyperdynamic state secondary to high catecholamines: use β-blockers
     — Extensive myocardial damage: use thrombolytics, nitroglycerin, oxygen, analgesics, β-blockade
   - Clinicians should have a low threshold to perform immediate synchronized cardioversion for unstable conditions clearly related to the tachycardia (increased chest pain, shortness of breath, decreased level of consciousness, low blood pressure, shock,

pulmonary congestion, congestive heart failure). However, this is an area of decision making that demands sharp clinical judgment. Are the acute MI and ischemic chest pain causing the tachycardia? Or is the tachycardia producing excessive demands on the damaged myocardium and thus increasing pain and myocardial damage? Therapy will differ based on this clinical decision.

- The tachycardia algorithm and the earlier discussion in this chapter present the major assessment and treatment points to consider when treating symptomatic tachycardias in patients.
- The electrical cardioversion algorithm (Fig 7) presents the critical points for performing this intervention.

2. **Electrolyte abnormalities**

- Electrolyte abnormalities may contribute to several arrhythmias observed in acute MI patients, in particular PVCs. These should be identified as quickly as possible and treated appropriately.
- *Hypokalemia* (<3.5 mmol/L [3.5 mEq/L]). Administer 10 mEq of potassium chloride diluted in 50 to 100 mL of D_5W, over 30 minutes. This dosage can be repeated as necessary, rechecking serum potassium every hour until it measures 4.0 to 4.5 mmol/L (4.0 to 4.5 mEq/L). Correct lesser degrees of hypokalemia with oral replacement therapy.
- *Hypomagnesemia* (less than 0.7 mmol/L [1.4 mEq/L]). Administer 1 to 2 g (8 to 16 mEq) of magnesium sulfate diluted in 50 to 100 mL of D_5W over 5 to 60 minutes. An infusion of 0.5 to 1.0 g (4 to 8 mEq) per hour should follow for up to 24 hours. The rate and duration of the infusion should be determined by the clinical situation or the level of hypomagnesemia. Magnesium supplementation is safe and reduces the incidence of ventricular arrhythmias.
- *Hypocalcemia*. Administer 10 to 20 mL of 10% calcium gluconate (96 mg elemental calcium per 10-mL ampule) or 10% calcium chloride (273 mg elemental calcium per 10-mL ampule) at an IV infusion rate of 1 to 2 mL/min. If hypocalcemia is severe give constant IV infusion of 15 to 20 mg of elemental calcium per kilogram of body weight every 4 to 8 hours, at a rate of 15 to 20 mg/min or less.

3. **PVCs**. In the setting of acute MI consider whether the PVCs are due to an associated problem with oxygenation, hypotension, electrolyte or acid-base abnormalities, other medications, or increased catecholamine state from unrelieved ischemic pain or anxiety. The best approach to PVCs in acute MI is to provide excellent treatment of the acute MI with oxygen, pain relief, and alteration of hemodynamics with nitroglycerin and β blockers. As noted above, routine prophylactic lidocaine administration is not recommended for patients with acute MI.

4. **Acute myocardial infarction associated with hypotension**

- Hypotension associated with acute MI may represent the ominous problem of cardiogenic shock.[209] The management of acute MI with hypotension is presented in the section on hypotension, cardiogenic shock, and acute pulmonary edema and in algorithm Fig 8. This algorithm presents the "cardiovascular triad," which can be used to treat patients with acute MI associated with hypotension.
- The major interventions to use will be volume replacement (normal saline, lactated Ringer's solution), especially for right ventricular infarction; **pressor** agents (dopamine, norepinephrine, and epinephrine); **inotropic** agents (dobutamine, amrinone); and **angioplasty** (PTCA).

5. **Acute myocardial infarction associated with hypertension**

- Clinicians should consider taking specific actions if patients with a possible acute MI display systolic blood pressure higher than 140 mm Hg or diastolic blood pressure higher than 90 mm Hg. These pressure levels may begin to increase myocardial oxygen demand and exacerbate ischemia or infarction.
- Therapy should include administration of oxygen and relief of pain and anxiety with morphine or sublingual nitroglycerin. Intravenous furosemide should be administered if the patient shows signs of fluid overload or pulmonary congestion.
- Figure 8 provides recommendations for patients with elevated diastolic blood pressures. For patients whose elevated blood pressures fail to respond to morphine and sublingual nitroglycerin, start **nitroglycerin** 10 to 20 µg/min IV and titrate to effect. **Nitroprusside**, 0.1 to 5.0 µg/kg per minute IV can be added as a second-line agent if needed.

Special Resuscitation Situations

Several special situations associated with cardiopulmonary arrest require rescuers to change their approach to resuscitation. Such situations include cardiorespiratory emergencies and cardiac arrest associated with

- Stroke
- Hypothermia
- Near-drowning
- Trauma
- Electric shock and lightning strike
- Toxicology (drug overdoses)
- Pregnancy

Chapter 10, "Special Resuscitation Situations," reviews each of these situations in detail. This section summarizes the key points and critical actions for each of these situations. Emergency personnel should carefully note the differences in triage, emphasis, and technique.

Stroke: Key Points

- The major emphasis with stroke simply is to think of the possibility that a neurological catastrophe has occurred. Sudden alterations in consciousness, breathing, and cardiac function can indicate a central nervous system event, in particular a central nervous system hemorrhage.
- Intracranial hemorrhage may be amenable to neurosurgical intervention but only if initiated in a timely fashion. The concept "time is muscle" applied to MI and thrombolytic therapy[247] is also being applied to the central nervous system with the phrase "time is brain."[248] ACLS providers must not forget either of these admonitions.
- Emergency personnel should consider early consultation with neurosurgical specialists and neurologists and the early use of diagnostic evaluations such as CT scans or arteriograms. Although such consultation and evaluations are not indicated in every cardiopulmonary emergency, ACLS providers should recognize the possibility of potentially reversible neurological events if rapid action is taken in appropriate cases.

Drowning: Key Points[249]

- Prevention
- Rescuer safety
- Possibility of associated trauma (particularly cervical)
- Possibility of associated hypothermia
- Knowledge of techniques for rewarming the victim
- Primary role of rapid advanced airway control and management (rather than early defibrillation)

Hypothermia: Key Points

(See the hypothermia algorithm, chapter 10, Fig 2.)
- Prevention
- Rescuer safety
- Techniques and actions to stop further heat loss
- Knowledge of techniques for rewarming the victim
- Withholding additional defibrillation attempts for persistent VF if initial shocks are unsuccessful in restoring circulation (until further central rewarming has occurred)
- Withholding aggressive drug therapy if initial efforts are unsuccessful (until further central rewarming has occurred)
- Proper equipment for assessing the core temperature
- Recognition of the need for rapid transport of victims to facilities that can perform rapid, advanced core rewarming (eg, extracorporeal bypass, mediastinal lavage)
- Proper setting-specific equipment for rewarming the victim (prehospital vs emergency department vs operating room vs intensive care facility)

- Recognition of the need to distinguish between normothermic cardiac arrest in a cold environment versus cardiac arrest caused by progressive cooling of the heart (eg, the person who suffers "warm" VF while shoveling snow versus the improperly protected person in a cold environment)

Trauma: Key Points

- Prevention
- Rescuer safety
- Rapid advanced airway control and management
- Aggressive fluid resuscitation
- Diminished emphasis on defibrillation and medications
- Recognition of the need to distinguish between cardiac arrest caused by trauma and trauma that occurs after a cardiac arrest (eg, the person who suffers VF while driving then suffers trauma when the car runs off the highway)
- Need for rapid alerting of, and transport to, advanced trauma centers for definitive intraoperative treatment. Cardiac arrest associated with trauma has a dismal outcome without early intraoperative intervention.

Electrocution and Lightning Strike: Key Points

- Prevention
- Rescuer safety
- Possibility of associated trauma, particularly cervical spine trauma, entrance and exit point burns, and deep thermal burns
- Knowledge of techniques for removing victim from source of electricity
- Knowledge of principles of "reverse triage" (treat the most severely injured victims first)
- Asystole has a better prognosis in electrocution victims than in other conditions.
- Because reversible respiratory arrest may persist after restoration of spontaneous circulation, victims' respirations must be aggressively supported for longer periods to allow recovery.

Toxicology (Drug Overdoses): Key Points

- The primary approach to cardiac arrest associated with drug overdoses is the same as that for metabolic and electrolyte abnormalities:
  — Proper maintenance of the airway and ventilations
  — Defibrillation when indicated
  — Pharmacologic interventions (pressors, inotropes, rate control)
- The emphases in toxicology:
  — Early diagnosis
  — Specific antidotes for specific overdoses

— Adjustment of ACLS medications when indicated for certain overdoses
— Early use of interventions such as TCP, dialysis, and extracorporeal bypass
— Need to persist for longer periods of CPR and ACLS while awaiting metabolism or dissipation of the offending agent (eg, some people have survived overdoses by being sustained for hours with basic CPR chest compressions)

Cardiac Arrest in the Pregnant Woman: Key Points

• The pregnant woman in cardiac arrest poses unique problems, the most obvious being that there are two victims, the mother and the fetus. This means that emergency personnel must consider questions of fetal viability and emergency cesarean section.
• The different emphases in cardiac arrest in the pregnant woman:
— Perform CPR in a different manner. Use either a human or mechanical wedge that partially rolls the mother to her left side. This relieves vena caval compression from the gravid uterus, thus permitting more blood return to the heart.[250]
— Medications (type and doses) and defibrillation are performed exactly as in the recommended ACLS guidelines. This is a change from previous guidelines, which recommended reduced doses and longer dosing intervals.
— Personnel should think early about performing an emergency cesarean section. "Emptying the uterus" for persistent cardiac arrest in the mother offers the best hope for a positive outcome for both the mother and the fetus.
— Emergency cesarean section is indicated when
  1. Personnel with the appropriate skill and equipment to perform the procedure are involved
  2. The mother fails to develop return of spontaneous circulation in 5 minutes and there is a potential for fetal viability
  3. Appropriate facilities and personnel are available to care for the mother and baby after the procedure

Pediatric Advanced Life Support

This section compares the emergency care of critically ill or injured children with the care required by adults and provides an introduction to the care of children. Children constitute a small but significant portion of the victims who require BLS and advanced life support (ALS). They account for 5% to 10% of all ambulance runs and approximately 25% to 30% of all emergency department visits.[251] The principles, equipment, and drugs used for pediatric BLS and ALS are similar to those used for adult BLS and ACLS. The care of seriously ill or injured children, however, requires specific knowledge of pediatric anatomy and physiology plus practical pediatric expertise.

The AHA strongly recommends that all ECC providers gain this knowledge and expertise by taking a course in pediatric ALS. Comprehensive instruction in pediatric ALS is beyond the scope of adult ACLS courses, and the material does not substitute for a pediatric ALS provider course. It is included here for providers who may experience some delay in attending a pediatric ALS course.

Epidemiology of Pediatric Cardiopulmonary Arrest

The epidemiology of cardiopulmonary arrest in children differs dramatically from cardiopulmonary arrest in adults. Adults suffer primarily *cardiac* emergencies; children suffer primarily *respiratory* emergencies. Primary cardiac problems, mainly sudden cardiac arrest, are the most common indications for ALS in the adult. Hence the term "Advanced *Cardiac* Life Support." For infants and children, however, *sudden* cardiopulmonary arrest is uncommon. Instead they experience respiratory distress or failure that leads to a progressive deterioration in respiratory or circulatory function. Cardiopulmonary failure and cardiopulmonary arrest are final rather than initiating events in children.

In children respiratory arrest is far more common than cardiac arrest[252] and is associated with a much higher survival rate than cardiac arrest. If respiratory arrest is detected and treated while a child still has a perfusing cardiac rhythm (central pulses), survival is 60% to 70% or higher,[252-255] and most survivors are neurologically intact.

In adults, cardiopulmonary arrest typically develops with the sudden onset of VT or VF.[256] Prompt provision of bystander CPR and prompt defibrillation will maximize the victim's chance of survival.[256,257] In contrast, pediatric cardiac arrest typically occurs as a *secondary* event, following the development of progressive shock or respiratory failure, with associated hypoxemia and acidosis. In one study 40 children of 93 requiring CPR upon initial presentation demonstrated respiratory arrest that progressed to cardiac arrest when ventilation could not be adequately supported.[252]

The *terminal* rhythm of children who develop pulseless prehospital cardiac arrest is most often bradycardia that deteriorates to asystole. Ventricular fibrillation has been documented in fewer than 15% of pediatric cardiac arrest victims less than 10 years of age,[258-260] even in the first minutes of resuscitation.[261] In children mortality following prehospital cardiac arrest averages 90%, and most survivors are neurologically devastated.[251,252,259,262,263] Higher survival rates have been reported in pulseless pediatric submersion victims if prompt BLS[264] and ALS with intubation are provided.[252,265]

These differences between adult and pediatric cardiopulmonary arrest lead to two important conclusions:

- The major intervention for pediatric resuscitation is *prevention*. Once cardiac arrest occurs the outcome is dismal.
- The key to *prevention* of cardiac arrest in children is support of oxygenation and ventilation.

These conclusions account for important differences between adult and pediatric ALS. The major focus of adult ALS is to respond to a cardiopulmonary arrest that has already occurred. The major focus in pediatric ALS is to detect the early signs of cardiopulmonary compromise and to prevent cardiopulmonary arrest through the support of oxygenation, ventilation, and perfusion.

Anatomic and Physiological Differences Between Children and Adults

Respiratory Differences

The causes of respiratory failure are the same in children and adults. However, several factors make the compromised infant and child more likely to develop respiratory failure.

Oxygen Consumption. The high metabolic rate in the child creates a high oxygen demand per kilogram of body weight, particularly during the first months of life. Oxygen consumption in infants is approximately 6 to 8 mL/kg per minute, compared with 3 to 4 mL/kg per minute in adults.[266] Therefore, with the onset of apnea or inadequate alveolar ventilation, hypoxemia develops more rapidly in the child.

Airways. Pediatric airways are much smaller and different in orientation and function than adult airways.[267]

- The upper and lower airways of the infant or child are much smaller in caliber than those of the adult.
- The tongue in the infant is relatively large compared with the oropharynx.
- The larynx in infants and toddlers is more cephalad in position.
- The epiglottis in infants and toddlers is short, narrow, and angled away from the axis of the trachea.
- The vocal cords have a lower anterior attachment.
- In infants and children less than 10 years of age, the narrowest portion of the airway is below the vocal cords at the level of the nondistensible cricoid carti-

lage. This creates a funnel-shaped larynx during childhood (Fig 10). In adolescents and adults, the larynx is cylinder-shaped with the narrowest portion at the vocal cords.

- The trachea is much shorter in children.

These pediatric anatomic differences have important clinical consequences:

- Small amounts of edema or obstruction can reduce airway radius and increase resistance to airflow and the work of breathing.
- Posterior displacement of the tongue readily causes complete airway obstruction. Control of the tongue's position with the laryngoscope blade may be difficult during intubation.
- The high position of the larynx makes the angle for laryngoscopy (and intubation) more acute. As a result, straight laryngoscope blades are more useful than curved blades in creating a visual plane from the mouth to the glottis in infants and toddlers.
- Control of the epiglottis with a laryngoscope blade may be more difficult.
- A blindly placed endotracheal tube may become caught at the anterior commissure.
- The selection of endotracheal tube size must be determined by the size of the cricoid ring rather than the glottic opening. Evaluate the tube size following intubation. If the endotracheal tube is sized correctly, an air leak will be observed when a positive inspiratory pressure of 20 to 30 cm H_2O is provided. If no air leak is detected at these inspiratory pressures, the tube is probably too large and may produce post-extubation complications, such as subglottic stenosis or edema.
- In the intubated infant, even minor displacement of an endotracheal tube can result in extubation or main bronchus intubation. Orotracheal tubes can displace

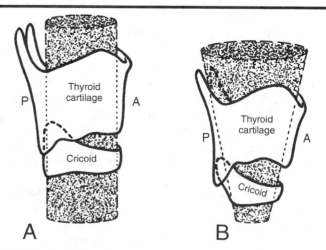

Fig 10. Configuration of the adult (A) and the infant larynx (B). Note cylinder shape of adult larynx: infant larynx is funnel-shaped because of narrow, undeveloped cricoid cartilage. A, anterior; B, posterior. From Coté and Todres.[268]

simply from head movement.[269] Neck flexion can displace an orotracheal tube further into the trachea, and extension or rotation of the neck can move the orotracheal tube out of the trachea.

The lower airways of infants and children also differ from the lower airways of adults. In infants and young children, these airways are smaller and more compliant and their supporting cartilage is less developed. The airways can therefore easily become obstructed by mucus, blood, pus, edema, active constriction, or external compression (eg, by a vascular ring or tumor). When upper or lower airway obstruction is present, intrathoracic pressure changes produced during spontaneous respiratory effort contribute to dynamic airway collapse.

Even a minor reduction in diameter of the small pediatric airway can increase resistance to airflow and the work of breathing. The infant or child with airway obstruction should be kept as calm and quiet as possible to prevent turbulent airflow and further increases in airway resistance.

The high compliance of pediatric airways makes them very susceptible to collapse. Upper airway obstruction (eg, epiglottitis, croup, or extrathoracic foreign body) may cause tracheal collapse with inspiration. An intrathoracic foreign body or a disease such as bronchiolitis or asthma often causes lower airway obstruction during exhalation.

Chest Wall. In older children and adults, the ribs and sternum support the lungs and help them remain expanded. In infants and toddlers, the ribs and intercostal cartilages are highly compliant and fail to adequately support the lungs. As a result, functional residual capacity is reduced when respiratory effort is diminished or absent. If airway obstruction is present, active inspiration often results in paradoxical chest movement (sternal and intercostal retractions) rather than chest and lung expansion. In addition, the lack of lung support makes the tidal volume of infants and toddlers almost totally dependent on diaphragm movement.

The high compliance of the child's chest means that the chest should readily expand when positive-pressure ventilation (via bag and mask or mechanical ventilation) is provided. *If the chest wall does not rise visibly during positive-pressure ventilation, ventilatory support is inadequate.*[270] Because the chest wall is compliant, it will readily expand, and excessive positive pressure can produce a pneumothorax. Thus, positive-pressure ventilatory support should produce visible chest expansion without hyperexpansion.

Breath sounds are easily transmitted through the thin chest wall of the infant or young child. As a result, breath sounds may sound normal even over areas of lung pathology such as pneumothorax, hemothorax, or chylothorax. Often such pathology produces a change in *pitch* rather than a change in intensity of breath sounds. Auscultation of both lungs must be performed carefully, particularly under the axillae. Breath sounds of one lung should be compared with those of the other so that differences can be detected.

Respiratory Muscles. The intercostal muscles are incapable of lifting the chest wall of the infant or young child. As a result, when movement of the diaphragm is impeded by high intrathoracic pressure (eg, pulmonary hyperinflation such as occurs in asthma) or gastric or abdominal distention, respiration and tidal volume are compromised. Children with respiratory distress often swallow air during breathing. This swallowed air may contribute to gastric distention, limitation of diaphragm movement, and further respiratory deterioration.

Lung Tissue. Lung compliance is very low in the neonate but increases during childhood. The combination of low lung compliance and high chest wall compliance makes ventilation inefficient during periods of respiratory distress or failure.

The closing lung volume (the minimum lung volume required to maintain peripheral airway patency) constitutes a higher percentage of total lung volume in the child than in the adult.[270] Some of the infant's airways may remain closed during normal breathing.[271,272] As a result infants are more susceptible to the development of atelectasis.

Control of Ventilation. Depression of central control of ventilation may compromise ventilation. Some causes of central nervous system depression are hypoxemia, hypothermia, street drugs or drug intoxication, medications, metabolic derangements (eg, hypoglycemia), or central nervous system injury or dysfunction. Apnea is common in ill infants and in children with drug intoxication or head injury. Respiratory rate and effort must be carefully monitored in these patients.

When spinal injury is associated with head injury, the spine injury is typically high in the cervical spine (C_4 or above) and may cause apnea by disrupting the innervation of the diaphragm.

Respiratory Rate. The respiratory rate of the infant and child is normally more rapid than that of the adult. Always evaluate the child's respiratory rate in terms of age and clinical condition. Children in cardiorespiratory distress or pain or those with fever should be tachypneic. A "normal" respiratory rate in such patients often indicates deterioration. Slowing of respirations is an ominous sign that may indicate that respiratory arrest is imminent.

Cardiovascular Function

Children have a higher cardiac output per kilogram of body weight than adults. However, since the child's oxygen demand is high, oxygen reserve is limited. Thus, anything that compromises oxygen delivery or increases oxygen demand in the child can result in cardiopulmonary compromise and deterioration.

Heart Rate and Rhythm. The heart of the infant and child beats faster than the heart of the adult, and stroke volume is smaller. Neonates, infants, and children increase their cardiac output principally by increasing heart rate rather than stroke volume. *This makes the infant and child extremely dependent on an adequate heart rate to maintain effective cardiac output.* Heart rate should always be evaluated in light of the child's age and clinical condition. The younger and more distressed the child, the higher should be the heart rate.

Sinus tachycardia is the normal response to many types of stress, including anxiety, fever, pain, trauma, hypoxemia, hypercapnia, hypovolemia, and cardiac dysfunction. When tachycardia fails to maintain adequate tissue oxygenation, tissue hypoxia and hypercapnia produce acidosis, and bradycardia develops.

Tachyarrhythmias. Occasionally infants and young children develop tachyarrhythmia that compromise cardiac output. Supraventricular tachycardia (SVT) is the most common tachyarrhythmia. It typically occurs during infancy or in children with congenital heart disease. SVT resulting in ventricular rates exceeding 180 to 220 per minute can produce signs of shock. If signs of shock are observed, synchronized cardioversion or treatment with adenosine (if vascular access is already established) should be performed emergently.

Bradycardia. Bradycardia is the most common arrhythmia in seriously ill infants or children. It is usually associated with a fall in cardiac output.[273] Bradycardia in a seriously ill or injured child should be presumed to be caused by hypoxia or acidosis unless these conditions have been ruled out or effectively treated. Thus, initial therapy for the *symptomatic* child with bradycardia is administration of oxygen and support of airway and ventilation. Next, epinephrine may be administered if the child fails to respond. Note another difference here between adult and pediatric ALS: atropine is the first drug used in symptomatic adult bradycardia, whereas oxygen administration, ventilatory support, and epinephrine administration are the treatments for pediatric patients. *The development of bradycardia in an infant or child with cardiorespiratory distress is an ominous sign, usually indicating that cardiac arrest is imminent.*

Pulseless rhythms (including pulseless VT and VF and PEA) are treated much the same as these pulseless rhythms are treated in adults. In the child as in the adult, reversible causes of PEA, including hypoxia, hypovolemia, and tension pneumothorax, must be detected and treated. If pulseless VT or VF is present, countershock immediately.

Epinephrine is the drug of choice for the resuscitation of pulseless patients of any age. If the pulseless child fails to respond to an initial standard IV dose of epinephrine (0.01 mg/kg, administered as 0.1 mL/kg of 1:10 000 dilution), use a higher dose and concentration of epinephrine for all subsequent doses (0.1 mg/kg administered as 0.1 mL/kg of 1:1000 dilution). Whenever epinephrine is administered by the endotracheal route for children, the higher dose and concentration are used.

Blood Pressure. Children in shock initially maintain their cardiac output and blood pressure through compensatory mechanisms such as vasoconstriction, tachycardia, and increased myocardial contractility. In fact, children with trauma will not demonstrate hypotension until acute blood loss totals approximately 25% of the child's circulating blood volume. Thus, *the presence of a normal blood pressure does not rule out the presence of shock.* The development of hypotension is an ominous finding, indicating that cardiovascular decompensation has developed and cardiorespiratory arrest is imminent.

Blood Volume. The circulating blood volume in the child is 75 to 80 mL/kg. All blood lost or drawn for laboratory analysis should be considered as a percentage of this circulating blood volume. Since the blood volume of the child is much smaller than that of the adult, small volumes of blood loss may be significant.

Response to Catecholamines. There are several reasons why children may respond in unique ways to the administration of exogenous catecholamines.[274] Children often develop tachycardia during catecholamine administration, which may limit the dose of catecholamine. These drugs are often provided to redistribute blood flow (eg, improve renal blood flow) or increase heart rate. Whether caring for an adult or a pediatric patient, the healthcare provider should always titrate drug therapy based on the individual patient's clinical response.

Neurological Function

All major structures of the brain and all cranial nerves are present and developed at birth, although dendritic arborization is incomplete until childhood. The infant's neurological system functions largely at a subcortical level. Brainstem functions and spinal cord reflexes are present, but cortical functions, such as memory and fine motor coordination, are incompletely developed and are impossible to assess. Cortical damage sustained during early infancy may not be clinically detectable until the infant is 6 months of age or older. The infant will function largely at a reflexive level until that time.

The skull offers inadequate protection for the brain of the infant or young child, and head trauma may produce severe brain injury during the first year of life. The head of the infant and young child is large in relation to the rest of the body. As a result, if the infant falls some distance or is thrown out of an automobile after impact or is struck by an automobile, it is likely that the infant will fly head-first and sustain a severe head injury. Although spinal cord injuries are less common in children than in adults, such injuries should still be suspected in children with head injuries and multisystem trauma. Children often sustain *S*pinal *C*ord *I*njury *W*ith*O*ut *R*adiographic *A*bnormality (SCIWORA). When spinal cord injury does occur in infants, the ligamentous laxity and the shape of the vertebrae contribute to injuries high in the cervical spine. Injuries at the C_1-C_2 level may be observed in infants, while the lower cervical spine is more likely to be injured in older children.

The brain of the infant and young child has higher water content and is incompletely myelinated during early childhood. Since the myelin helps provide structure to the brain, the lack of myelin makes the brain much more homogeneous and much more susceptible to diffuse injury and gliding contusions with blunt head trauma. Signs of diffuse head injury and diffuse brain swelling in children may include initial loss of consciousness and fixed and dilated pupils. Although these signs are usually associated with severe brainstem injury and poor prognosis (or extremely high blood alcohol levels) in adults, they may be associated with mild, moderate, or severe head injury and complete recovery in children. For this reason, children with Glasgow Coma Scores of 5 through 8 have lower mortality (≤35%) and a lower morbidity than do adults with the same Glasgow Coma Score. The reason for this lower mortality remains controversial. It may be related to the fact that the dendritic arborization continues throughout early childhood and may enable compensation for injured areas of the brain. Alternatively, the child with a low Glasgow Coma Score may have a relatively less severe injury than an adult with the same Glasgow Coma Score.[275-279] In any event, the lower mortality associated with a low Glasgow Coma Scale in children explains the aggressive resuscitation undertaken for many children with head injury.

Fluid and Electrolyte Requirements

The child has smaller fluid requirements than the adult, and excessive fluid administration can rapidly produce fluid overload in the small child. For this reason, fluid administered to infants and children should always be measured and totaled. If at all possible, fluids should be administered using a syringe or a volume-controlled infusion pump.

Fluid Boluses. Rapid expansion of circulating blood volume may be necessary if the child demonstrates inadequate intravascular volume related to acute blood loss, severe dehydration, or extravascular fluid shifts. Under these conditions, boluses of isotonic crystalloid totaling 20 mL/kg should be administered over 20 minutes or less. It may be necessary to repeat these boluses several times. If blood administration is needed, boluses of 10 mL/kg of packed red blood cells or 20 mL/kg of whole blood or 5% albumin are administered.

Intravascular Access. With the seriously ill infant or child, support of airway, oxygenation, and ventilation must take first priority. However, vascular access should also be accomplished, particularly during resuscitation. Vascular access should be attempted in the largest vein with the largest catheter that can be inserted; however, any vascular access is better than none during resuscitation. Rescuers should use the catheter size and site with which they are most comfortable.

Intraosseous Access. If reliable intravascular access cannot be achieved within minutes during the resuscitation of children (particularly those under the age of 6 years), use the intraosseous route to administer crystalloid, colloid, or drugs such as epinephrine. This method of vascular access can be achieved within seconds and may be lifesaving. Many emergency departments use the rule "no IV in three tries, then go to intraosseous."

Endotracheal Access. Lipid-soluble drugs, including epinephrine, atropine, and lidocaine (A-L-E), may be administered by endotracheal route in children or adults, although the precise doses and absorption of resuscitation drugs by this route are not yet determined. In general, IV doses of resuscitation medications are increased by a factor of 2 to 3 times and diluted to 3 to 5 mL before instillation via the endotracheal tube. All doses of epinephrine administered by endotracheal route are "high dose," and the higher concentration is used (0.1 mg/kg, which results in a volume of 0.1 mL/kg of 1:1000 concentration).

Glucose. Neonates and young infants have high glucose needs and low glycogen stores. During periods of stress such as hypoxia or cardiac arrest, these very young children may develop hypoglycemia rather than hyperglycemia. If at all possible, rapid methods of evaluating blood glucose through heel-stick sample and reagent strips should be used to monitor blood glucose levels during resuscitation and postresuscitation stabilization. Because *hyperglycemia* has been linked with poor outcome following trauma and resuscitation in patients of all ages, glucose administration should be reserved for infants and children with documented hypoglycemia. For this reason dextrose solutions should not be routinely used during resuscitation of children. Hypoglycemic children should receive 2 mL/kg of $D_{25}W$.

Temperature Control

Infants and children have larger ratios of surface area to volume than adults have. As a result, the small child will lose heat rapidly to the environment. Young infants cannot shiver to generate heat but must break down brown fat, which requires energy. Cold stress can complicate cardiorespiratory distress or deterioration and subsequent resuscitation, because it increases oxygen demand, produces peripheral vasoconstriction, and makes assessment of systemic perfusion difficult. The young infant and child must be kept warm, using heat lamps and blankets.

Assessment of the Seriously Ill or Injured Infant or Child

General Assessment

The child's color, perfusion of extremities, activity, and responsiveness should be evaluated continuously. Early signs of cardiorespiratory failure can be more subtle in children than in adults, so the healthcare provider should be alert for the development of small changes. Evaluation of trends over time will enable detection of either deterioration or improvement in response to therapy.

Color. With cardiorespiratory distress, the child's color and perfusion deteriorate. The child may become pale, mottled, or grey in the presence of shock or respiratory distress. Central cyanosis is often an inconsistent or late sign of hypoxemia.

Perfusion of Extremities. When ambient temperature is warm the child's extremities should be warm, with rapid (less than 2 seconds) capillary refill. Shock, respiratory failure, or a cold environmental temperature may result in cooling of extremities and prolonged capillary refill.[280] When systemic oxygenation or perfusion is compromised, the extremities often become mottled, grey, or pale.

Peripheral Pulses. Peripheral pulses should be easily palpable when the child is well perfused. When cardiorespiratory distress is present, however, peripheral vasoconstriction decreases the intensity of these pulses. It may become impossible to feel pulses in the hands and feet. As in the adult, if central pulses (brachial, carotid, femoral) are not palpable, start CPR.

Activity and Responsiveness. The hypoxemic or hypercarbic child or the child with inadequate systemic perfusion at first is extremely irritable. As cerebral oxygenation and perfusion deteriorate, the child becomes lethargic. This lethargy is an ominous finding and may indicate that cardiorespiratory arrest is imminent. *In any child, a decreased response to painful stimulus is abnormal and usually indicates severe cardiorespiratory or neurological compromise.*[270]

The child's activity and responsiveness should always be evaluated in light of normal cognitive and psychosocial development. An infant should visually track brightly colored objects and should maintain eye contact and demonstrate a social smile beyond 4 weeks of age. The infant older than 5 to 6 months of age and the toddler should not separate willingly from parents and should protest vigorously if separation is attempted. Preschool children should be frightened of strangers but should be able to respond to simple questions regarding pain and sensation and should be able to follow simple commands. School-age children and adolescents should be oriented to time and place and should be able to identify painful body parts and respond to simple questions and commands.

Vital Signs. Monitor vital signs, including blood pressure, closely in the critically ill or injured infant or child (see Tables 4 through 6). *Heart rate and respiratory rate in particular should be appropriate for age and clinical condition.* The presence of a normal or slowed heart rate and respiratory rate in the child with cardiorespiratory distress is an ominous clinical finding and usually indicates that cardiorespiratory arrest is imminent.

Table 4. Normal Heart Rates in Children*

Age	Awake Heart Rate (per min)	Sleeping Heart Rate (per min)
Neonate	100-180	80-160
Infant (6 months)	100-160	75-160
Toddler	80-110	60-90
Preschooler	70-110	60-90
School-age child	65-110	60-90
Adolescent	60-90	50-90

*Always consider patient's normal range and clinical condition. Heart rate will normally increase with fever or stress. Adapted from Gillette PC, et al. Dysrhythmias. In: Adams FH, Emmanouilides GC, eds. *Moss' Heart Disease in Infants, Children, and Adolescents.* 4th ed. Baltimore, Md: Williams & Wilkins; 1989. Reproduced with permission from Hazinski.[270]

Table 5. Normal Respiratory Rates in Children*

Age	Rate (breaths per min)
Infant	30-60
Toddler	24-40
Preschooler	22-34
School-age child	18-30
Adolescent	12-16

*Always consider patient's normal range. The child's respiratory rate is expected to increase in the presence of fever or stress. From Hazinski.[270]

Table 6. Normal Blood Pressures in Children*

Age	Systolic Pressure (mm Hg)	Diastolic Pressure (mm Hg)
Birth (12 h, <1000 g)	39-59	16-36
Birth (12 h, 3 kg weight)	50-70	25-45
Neonate (96 h)	60-90	20-60
Infant (6 mo)	87-105	53-66
Toddler (2 y)	95-105	53-66
School age (7 y)	97-112	57-71
Adolescent (15 y)	112-128	66-80

*Blood pressure ranges for neonates are from Versmold H, et al. Aortic blood pressure during the first 12 hours of life in infants with birth weight 610-4220 gms. *Pediatrics.* 1981;67:107. 10th through 90th percentile ranges used. Blood pressure ranges for others are from Horan MJ, chairman. Task Force on Blood Pressure Control in Children. Report of the Second Task Force on Blood Pressure in Children. *Pediatrics.* 1987;79:1. 50th through 90th percentile ranges indicated. From Hazinski.[270]

Measure the blood pressure with a cuff of appropriate size. The cuff width should equal approximately two thirds the length of the child's upper arm, and the bladder should not wrap more than once around the child's arm. *Shock may be present despite a normal blood pressure in the child, and hypotension typically develops only in children with decompensated shock.* For this reason, normotension may not be reassuring, and hypotension is cause for alarm.

Airway and Breathing

Evaluate the child's respiratory rate, air entry, mechanics, and color continuously. If there is any sign of deterioration, consider ventilatory support.

Respiratory Rate. The child's respiratory rate should be rapid when cardiorespiratory distress is observed. Slowing of the respiratory rate or apnea indicates the need for ventilatory assistance.

Air Entry. Although the child normally breathes more rapidly than the adult, the breathing should be quiet and unlabored. Stridor or wheezing indicates airway obstruction in the adult or child, which increases the work of breathing.

The child's chest should expand during ventilation, and breath sounds should be heard easily over all lung fields. Signs of respiratory distress include chest retractions and a decrease in intensity or change in pitch of breath sounds.

Mechanics. Normal breathing is quiet breathing. The chest expands during inspiration, and the child appears calm. The child's cry is loud and strong. In contrast, when respiratory distress is present the child may have chest wall or intercostal muscle retractions, head bobbing, and nasal flaring. As the work of breathing increases, the child may grimace and appear frightened. Grunting and a weak cry are signs of *severe* distress and the need for ventilatory support. Gasping respirations indicate the need for immediate intervention.

Color. The child's color should be consistent, and the mucous membranes should be pink. Circumoral cyanosis may be normal in the neonate or very young infant, particularly if exposed to a cold environment. The child in cardiorespiratory distress often demonstrates pallor or a mottled color over the extremities or trunk. Central cyanosis is a late and serious sign of hypoxemia, particularly in children who have experienced blood loss.

Pulse oximetry is an important noninvasive tool to detect hypoxemia and to monitor the child's response to therapy. It may provide an early indication of respiratory deterioration and should be used during stabilization and transport. The accuracy of pulse oximeters during resuscitation is unacceptable because these devices require pulsatile blood flow to determine hemoglobin saturation.

Circulation

Evaluate the circulation during the general assessment. The child's heart rate, perfusion of extremities, quality of peripheral pulses, and activity and general responsiveness all reflect the effectiveness of the child's cardiac output and oxygen delivery.

Heart Rate. The child's heart rate should be rapid, particularly if the child is anxious, in pain, or in cardiorespiratory distress. A "normal" heart rate or bradycardia are ominous findings under these conditions.

Perfusion and Pulses. The child's skin should be warm with consistent color and temperature over trunk and extremities. In the presence of cardiorespiratory distress, cooling of the skin in a peripheral to proximal fashion may be noted, and capillary refill time may become prolonged. Capillary refill must always be evaluated in light of ambient temperature. A cold ambient temperature may result in prolonged capillary refill even in normal children.[280] Peripheral vasoconstriction may make peripheral pulses difficult to detect.

Oliguria may be an early sign of compromise in systemic perfusion. However, evaluation of urine output requires observation over time, so it may not be helpful on the initial encounter with the child.

Color. Shock generally produces mottling of skin tones or pallor. The skin may also appear grey.

Activity and General Responsiveness. The child in shock is often irritable and then becomes lethargic as cerebral perfusion is compromised. This change in level of consciousness will be appreciated if the child is closely monitored. The child's responsiveness should be classified via the AVPU scale as one of the following (listed as indicating decreasing responsiveness):

1. Awake (provides good eye contact, response to questions and therapy)
2. Responsive to Voice
3. Responsive to Pain
4. Unresponsive

Blood Pressure. Hypotension in the child is a late sign of cardiovascular deterioration. A useful reference systolic blood pressure is the fifth percentile systolic blood pressure for the child beyond 1 year of age, which is estimated using the following formula:

$$\leq 70 \text{ mm Hg} + [2 \times age (y)]$$

The systolic blood pressure derived from this equation is normal in only approximately 5% of children that age. It will constitute hypotension for 95% of children of that age. For example, the fifth percentile systolic blood pressure for a 5-year-old child is 70 mm Hg + (2 x 5), or 80 mm Hg. Only 5% of normal 5-year-olds will have a systolic blood pressure less than 80 mm Hg. Thus, a systolic blood pressure of 80 mm Hg or less is worrisome in a 5-year-old.

Assessment of Neurological Function

Normal infants will make good eye contact with adults and will respond to voice and painful stimuli. Beyond 2 to 3 years of age, the child should be able to follow commands such as "Hold up two fingers," "Wiggle your toes," or "Stick out your tongue." The normal child is reluctant to be separated from parents, is frightened of painful stimuli, and will react to venipunctures or other painful procedures.

Signs of neurological deterioration in infants may be subtle. Spontaneous bicycling movements of the legs or random eye opening may be incorrectly interpreted to be purposeful movements. In infants eye deviation to the side or bicycling movements are often signs of seizure activity.

Children who are seriously ill or injured generally act it. As neurological function deteriorates, the child becomes irritable, then lethargic. The child will stop following commands, and progressive deterioration will render the child unresponsive to all but painful stimuli. If the previously normal child fails to respond to even painful stimuli, severe compromise in cardiorespiratory or neurological function is present, and the child requires urgent intervention.

Although the Glasgow Coma Scale has not been prospectively validated in children, it may still be a useful tool to quantify the child's responsiveness and to identify trends over time. Modified Glasgow Coma Scales have been developed for use in infants and preverbal children.

Signs of increased intracranial pressure in children include decreased responsiveness, decreased spontaneous movement, decreased response to painful stimuli, and pupil dilation with decreased constrictive response to light. Any or all of the findings of Cushing's triad — hypertension (often only systolic), bradycardia, and apnea — are indications of elevated intracranial pressure and may signal impending cerebral herniation. Unfortunately these findings may appear quite late in a child's course.

Initial Stabilization

Airway and Breathing

Effective support of oxygenation and ventilation is the single most important aspect of pediatric emergency care. The goals of emergency management of airway and ventilation include *anticipation* and *recognition* of respiratory problems and support or replacement of those functions when compromised or lost. In an emergency it may be impossible and unnecessary to determine the cause of respiratory dysfunction. Initial steps of emergency airway management and support of ventilation must still be completed.

Administer oxygen, in the highest concentration possible, to all seriously ill or injured patients with respiratory insufficiency, shock, or trauma, even if measured arterial oxygen tension is high. In these patients, oxygen delivery to tissues may be limited either by inadequate pulmonary gas exchange or by inadequate circulatory volume, cardiovascular function, or blood volume distribution. Add humidification to inspired oxygen as soon as practical to prevent obstruction of the small airways by dried secretions. Heated humidification systems are preferable to cool mist systems since the latter can produce hypothermia in young infants.

Allow alert children in respiratory difficulty to remain in a position of comfort since they usually assume a position that promotes optimal airway patency and minimizes respiratory effort. Anxiety increases oxygen consumption and possibly respiratory distress. Allow *alert* children in

respiratory distress to remain with their parents, and introduce airway equipment, including oxygen, in a nonthreatening manner. If the *alert* child is upset by one method of oxygen support (such as a mask), attempt alternative methods of oxygen administration (such as a "blow-by" stream of humidified oxygen held by a parent toward the child's mouth and nose or a face tent).

If the child is somnolent or unconscious, the airway may be obstructed by a combination of neck flexion, relaxation of the jaw, posterior displacement of the tongue against the roof of the mouth, and collapse of the hypopharynx. Use noninvasive methods of opening the airway before using adjuncts. If necessary clear the airway by removal of secretions, mucus, or blood from the oropharynx and nasopharynx with suction.

Provide assisted ventilation if ventilation is inadequate (as judged by evaluation of respiratory rate, chest movement, and breath sounds) despite a patent airway. In the vast majority of respiratory emergencies, infants and children can be successfully ventilated with a bag-valve–mask device, even in the presence of airway obstruction.[281] Use positive-pressure breaths administered with a bag-valve–mask device to augment the child's spontaneous inspiratory efforts. Time these breaths with the child's breathing. If the breaths are not coordinated with the child's spontaneous efforts, ventilation may be ineffective and may result in coughing, vomiting, and gastric distention.

If bag-mask ventilation does not provide effective ventilation or if transport or diagnostic tests necessitate control of the airway, intubation should be performed by providers skilled in pediatric intubation. Monitor the child's heart rate and color (and, if possible, pulse oximetry readings) continuously during intubation. Interrupt intubation attempts to provide oxygenation and bag-mask ventilation if a fall in heart rate or deterioration in color or hemoglobin saturation develops.

Circulation

Provide fluid resuscitation *if shock is present*. Boluses of isotonic crystalloid at volumes of 20 mL/kg should be administered in less than 20 minutes if evidence of hypovolemia is observed. The trauma patient with hemorrhagic shock will require crystalloids plus blood (bolus of 10 to 20 mL/kg). Administration of large volumes of fluid is unnecessary if systemic perfusion is adequate, and repeated bolus fluid therapy for trauma victims who have no evidence of shock may, in fact, be harmful.

Epinephrine is the drug of choice for the child with refractory shock, particularly if hypotension or bradycardia is present (1 mg in 500 mL D_5W titrated to effect). Dopamine or dobutamine may also be useful, depending on the etiology of the shock. Whenever any catecholamine is administered, ensure that the drug is delivered to the patient (rather than "lost" in the IV tubing), and titrate the drug dose to patient response (heart rate, blood pressure, or perfusion).

Warming

The infant or child should be kept warm during resuscitation and transport. Use of warming overbed lights or heated blankets may be helpful. If large quantities of IV fluids or blood products are administered, first warm these fluids using a blood warmer.

Equipment

Equipment used to stabilize the infant or child is provided in Table 7. The sizing of equipment can be based on the child's body length using a resuscitation tape.

Table 7. Pediatric Emergency Department Supplies*

Color on Broselow Pediatric Resuscitation Tape	Infant (3-7 kg) RED	Small Child (8-11 kg) PURPLE	Child (12-14 kg) YELLOW	Child (14-17 kg) WHITE	Child (18-22 kg) BLUE	Small Adult (24-30 kg) ORANGE	Adult (32-34 kg +) GREEN
Bag-valve device	Infant	Child	Child	Child	Child	Child/adult	Adult
O$_2$ mask	Newborn	Pediatric	Pediatric	Pediatric	Pediatric	Adult	Adult
Oral airway	Infant/small child	Small child	Child	Child	Child/small adult	Child/small adult	Medium adult
Laryngoscope blade	0-1 straight	1 straight	2 straight or curved	2 straight or curved	2 straight or curved	2-3 straight or curved	3 straight or curved
ET tubes (mm)	Premature infant 2.5 Term 3.0 Infant 3.5 uncuffed	4.0 uncuffed	4.5 uncuffed	5.0 uncuffed	5.5 uncuffed	6.0 cuffed	6.5 cuffed
ET tube length (cm at lip)	10-10.5	11-12	12.5-13.5	14-15	15.5-16.5	17-18	18.5-19.5
Stylet (F)	6	6	6	6	14	14	14
Suction (F)	8	8	8-10	10	10	10	12
BP cuff	Newborn-infant	Infant-child	Child	Child	Child	Child-adult	Adult
IV: Catheter (G)	22-24	20-24	18-22	18-22	18-20	18-20	16-20
Butterfly (G)	23-25	23-25	21-23	21-23	21-23	21-22	18-21
NG tube (F)	5-8	8-10	10	10-12	12-14	14-18	18
Urinary catheter (F)	5-8	8-10	10	10-12	10-12	12	12
Chest tube (F)	10-12	16-20	20-24	20-24	24-32	28-32	32-40

*Adapted from the Broselow Pediatric Resuscitation Tape, with permission from Broselow Medical Technologies, Hickory, NC. From Hazinski.[270]

ACLS Code Organization

People perform best in a resuscitative attempt with planning and organization. Traditionally ACLS provider courses have focused on the "team leader." This is the person who is supposed to "know it all," "take charge," and direct all aspects of the resuscitation. While ACLS providers are still encouraged to know and experience the role of team leader, the ACLS courses now emphasize more of the team aspects of ECC.

Therefore, ACLS providers should know the principles of management for the ACLS team, Megacode organization, and the chain of survival. The chain-of-survival concept links all members of the team. Consider the team in a broad context that includes the family members who recognize the collapse and call 911, the citizen who starts CPR, the ambulance technician who performs defibrillation, the paramedic who intubates and transports, the emergency department personnel who stabilize the patient, and the intensive care unit personnel who assume responsibility for prolonged life support.

The course of resuscitative attempts may be complex and unpredictable. It is not easy to maintain organization, leadership, and a cool head. Authors have likened a good resuscitation team to a fine symphony orchestra.[16,17] The maestro (team leader) is recognized for broad skills of organization and performance; the individual artists (team members) are recognized for specific performance skills. All are playing the same orchestrated piece, polished by practice and experience, with attention to both detail and outcome. There are no excuses for a disorganized and frenetic Megacode scene. Both the team leader and team members must remain calm and collected.

The Phased-Response Format

The phased-response format should be applied to any resuscitation.[16,17] No matter where it occurs (field, emergency department, critical care unit) and no matter how many personnel are involved, the principles of phased-response resuscitation remain the same:

- **Phase I: Anticipation.** This phase occurs as rescuers either move to the scene of a possible cardiac arrest or await the arrival of a possible cardiac arrest from outside the hospital. The steps to perform are
  — Analyze initial data
  — Gather the team
  — State leadership
  — Delineate duties
  — Prepare and check equipment
  — Position oneself

- **Phase II: Entry.** At this phase the team leader quickly introduces himself or herself to the prehospital or floor resuscitation team. The steps to perform are
  — Obtain entry vital signs
  — Perform orderly transfer
  — Consider baseline arterial blood gas (ABG) levels and other laboratory values if necessary
  — Gather a concise history
  — Repeat vital signs

- **Phase III: Resuscitation.** The team leader should be decisive, professional, and unflappable. The team should keep to the ABCs and keep the resuscitation room quiet so that personnel can hear the leader's voice. The team members should
  — State the vital signs every 5 minutes or with any change in the monitored parameters
  — State when procedures and medications are completed
  — Request clarification of any orders
  — Provide primary and secondary assessment information

The team leader should communicate her or his observations and should always be open to and actively seek suggestions from team members.

Whenever the vital signs are unstable and when treatment appears to be failing, a focus on "Airway-Breathing-Circulation" should guide the efforts before any procedures are initiated. The Airway-Breathing-Circulation sequence also should organize routine and periodic updates during the resuscitation.

- **Phase IV: Maintenance.** In this phase vital signs that were once unstable have settled down. The team should stabilize and secure the patient and stay ahead. The team must realize that the anticipatory rush will subside and that this is a vulnerable period. Maintain attention by repeatedly returning to the ABCs.

- **Phase V: Family Notification.** "Telling the living" — either good news or bad news — must be done with honesty, sensitivity, and promptness. The section "Psychological Aspects of Resuscitation" at the end of this chapter discusses this topic.

- **Phase VI: Transfer.** The resuscitation team must transfer the patient to a team of equal or greater expertise. They should transfer the patient and information in a manner that is complete, concise, and well organized.

- **Phase VII: Critique Process.** Every team should perform a code critique, no matter how brief. This activity provides feedback to prehospital and in-hospital personnel, an avenue to express grieving, and an opportunity for education. The section "Psychological Aspects of Resuscitation" provides information on the techniques of critical incident stress debriefing.

CPR: The Human Dimension. The Psychological Aspects of CPR and Resuscitation

We now recognize the importance of the psychological effects resuscitative efforts may have on emergency personnel. The AHA encourages all resuscitation teams to use the model presented in this chapter, which was developed by experts in critical incident debriefing.

Since 1973 over 50 million people have learned CPR. Although CPR is considered by some to be the most successful public health initiative in recent times, the survival rate to hospital discharge may range from 3% to 20%. This means that even in the best system or hospital more than four out of five times rescuers who were taught to save lives are unsuccessful and fail in their attempts.

Serious, long-lasting physical and emotional symptoms may occur in rescuers who attempt CPR unsuccessfully. Rescuers may undergo grief reactions. Performance of CPR is also stressful, often leaving the rescuer feeling fatigued and uncertain, which may result in chronic anxiety, depression, and burnout.

To allow rescuers to work through their feelings and their grief, a critical incident debriefing is recommended. Debriefings should be held after any unsuccessful CPR attempt. In these sessions rescuers discuss their thoughts, feelings, and performance. Ideally all members of the resuscitation team should be present at the debriefing. A detailed analysis of what was done and why should occur, with a discussion of things that went right and things that went wrong. The critical incident debriefing is also a time for learning things that may be useful next time. The "human dimension" of CPR is often not discussed. Because of its importance it should be incorporated into CPR training and practice.

The Impact of Providing Help: Emergency Workers and CPR Attempts

An unsuccessful CPR attempt may lead to persistent psychological dysfunction in volunteer emergency personnel. Personnel may experience vivid, involuntary, and uncontrollable thoughts, feelings, or mental images concerning the CPR attempt. Some rescues are particularly stressful for emergency personnel, and these tend to cause distress (including nightmares, involuntary daytime recollections, anxiety, and ruminations) for years afterward. Deaths of young people and accidents involving major trauma are most difficult.

A major coping strategy for emergency personnel is to focus on the technical details of a rescue and the clinical details of the patient, not on bystanders, friends, and relatives. Ongoing research suggests that emergency personnel find "routine CPR" relatively unstressful.[19]

Death, Grieving, and Families

Physicians and other healthcare workers may not receive proper training on how to convey the death of a patient to the family. The initial contact with the family will have a significant impact on the grief response. Bad news conveyed in an inappropriate, incomplete, or uncaring manner may have long-lasting psychological effects on the family.[20] It may be difficult for the healthcare professional to switch from medical trauma to family trauma, from the highly technical aspects of directing a resuscitation — a "no time for feelings" situation — to the post-resuscitation situation where feelings, thoughts, and empathetic communication are essential for the beginning of a healthy grief reaction.[18] Feelings of failure and inadequacy may also make it difficult for the healthcare professional to initially support and counsel the patient's family.[18] The physician may feel isolated and may second-guess actions and decisions. Some suggestions for conveying news of a sudden death to family members is found in Table 8. Similar recommendations can be followed in the event of a critical illness or injury.

Table 8. Conveying News of a Sudden Death to Family Members

- Remember: the moment you stop resuscitative efforts on a person you acquire a new set of patients — the family and loved ones.
- Call the family if they have not been notified. Explain that their loved one has been admitted to the emergency department and that the situation is serious. In general, survivors should be told of a death face-to-face, not over the telephone.
- Obtain as much information as possible about the patient and the circumstances surrounding the death. Carefully go over the events as they happened in the emergency department.
- Ask someone to take family members to a private area. Walk in, introduce yourself, and sit down. Address the closest relative.
- Briefly describe the circumstances leading to the death. Go over the sequence of events in the emergency department. Avoid euphemisms such as "he's passed on," "she is no longer with us," or "he's left us." Instead use the words "death," "dying," or "dead."
- Allow time for the shock to be absorbed. Make eye contact. Consider touching the family member and sharing your feelings. Convey your feelings with a phrase such as "You have my (our) sincere sympathy" rather than "I am (we are) sorry."
- Allow as much time as necessary for questions and discussion. Go over the events several times to make sure everything is understood and to facilitate further questions.
- Allow the family the opportunity to see their relative. If equipment is still connected, let the family know in advance.
- Know in advance what happens next and who will sign the death certificate. Physicians may impose burdens on staff and family if they fail to understand policies about death certification and disposition of the body. Know the answers to these questions before meeting the family. One of the survivors will surely ask, "What do we do next?" Be prepared with a proper answer.
- Enlist the aid of a social worker or the clergy if not already present.
- Offer to contact the patient's attending or family physician and be available if there are further questions. Arrange for follow-up and continued support during the grieving period.

Helping the Helpers: Methods and Insights

Some authorities regard emergency medicine as a high-stress occupation.[282] The stress of emergencies and their sequelae frequently leaves emergency workers in a state of chronic psychological dysfunction. This may manifest itself as chronic anxiety, reactive depression, and burnout. Burnout is a phenomenon resulting from the cumulative effects of stress in a work-related environment. It leads to job dissatisfaction, decreased job performance, and a loss of enjoyment of life in general.[282] Burnout can affect anyone, but those in the helping professions are particularly vulnerable. The condition must be distinguished from major depression and post-traumatic stress disorder.

Therapeutic interventions after stressful emergency events, like unsuccessful resuscitations, may significantly decrease the probability of burnout. The most important intervention is a critique or debriefing of the critical incident.[17] Suggested guidelines for a critical incident debriefing are shown in Table 9. Debriefings should occur after any event in which emergency workers are exposed to significant stress. During debriefings the workers involved discuss their thoughts, feelings, and performance. With the support of their coworkers, they work through and express their anxiety, guilt, anger, and other emotions. In this manner their "grief work" is facilitated and resolution accomplished. In addition, debriefing allows a review of critical responsibility and provides continuing education or "practice reflection."

Psychological issues in CPR, which have not been satisfactorily addressed, are important to both emergency medical workers and their families in times of death and critical illness. With proper knowledge of issues and interventions, both professionals and their families will be able to work through the grieving process that is part of death and critical illness.

Table 9. Recommendations for a Modified Critical Incident Debriefing

---

- The debriefing should occur as soon as possible after the event, with all team members present.
- Call the group together, preferably in the resuscitation room. State that you want to have a "code debriefing."
- Review the events and conduct of the code. Include the contributory pathophysiology leading to the code, the decision tree followed, and any variations.
- Analyze the things that were done wrong and especially the things that were done right. Allow free discussion.
- Ask for recommendations/suggestions for future resuscitative attempts. All team members should share their feelings, anxieties, anger, and possible guilt.
- Team members unable to attend the debriefing should be informed of the process followed, the discussion generated, and the recommendations made.
- The team leader should encourage team members to contact him or her if questions arise later.

Ethical Aspects of Emergency Cardiac Care

Several recent Supreme Court decisions and the Self-determination Act of 1991 have ushered in a new period in resuscitation where much more emphasis is placed on the ethics of resuscitation and less on the medicolegal aspects. We are at the point where ECC acknowledges explicitly that resuscitative efforts should not be started for some patients and if started should not be continued.

For many people the last beat of the heart should be the last beat of the heart. ECC attempts to restore those "hearts too good to die."[1] It should not attempt to restore "hearts too sick to live."[148] CPR and ECC are meant to reverse premature death. They should restore the process of living, not prolong the process of dying. When people reach the end of life, continued resuscitative efforts are inappropriate, futile, undignified, and demeaning to both the patient and the rescuers. Once started, resuscitative efforts can quickly become futile and inappropriate.

Chapter 15, "Ethical Aspects of CPR and Emergency Cardiac Care," provides an ethical framework with which to consider the key questions of starting and stopping resuscitative efforts and presents specific recommendations for prehospital and in-hospital care providers. All personnel whose work involves resuscitation should read this chapter, for it is truly part of the "essentials of ACLS."

Summary: Ten Commandments for ACLS

1. **Do good CPR.** Make sure personnel do CPR when indicated, and make sure they do CPR well.
2. **Place the highest priority on the primary ABCD survey:** Airway, Breathing, Circulation, and Defibrillation. The "hunt for VF" is one of your major tasks.
3. **Place the next highest priority on the secondary ABCD survey:** intubation, effective ventilations, IV access and drugs, and differential diagnoses.
4. **Know your defibrillator!** Never meet your defibrillator for the first time at a patient's cardiac arrest. Know how to perform the daily maintenance check. A working defibrillator is *your* responsibility: a "dead" defibrillator can mean a dead patient.
5. **Search for reversible and treatable causes.** Always ask yourself: "Why did this arrest occur?" "What is going on?" "What cause or complication am I missing?" If you do not try to learn what caused the arrest, you will seldom save the patient.
6. **Know the "Why?", "When?", "How?", and "Watch Out!" for all ECC medications.** Use your medications accurately and effectively.

7. **Be a good team captain.** Be a master conductor. Be a good team member.

8. **Know and practice the phased response format for resuscitations:** anticipation, entry, resuscitation, maintenance, family notification, transfer, critique.

9. **Determine "code status" and "DNAR status" in advance, when your patients are medically stable.** Many resuscitation attempts are futile, not wanted, and unnecessary. Do not neglect to discuss this topic with your patients and family members. They want this topic discussed and will appreciate your care.

10. **Learn and practice the most difficult resuscitation skills:** when not to start CPR, when to stop CPR, how to tell the living, the need to talk with your colleagues. These skills are more important, and more challenging, than any others in ACLS.

References

1. Beck C, Leighninger D. Reversal of death in good hearts. *J Cardiovasc Surg.* 1962;3:357-375.

2. Safar P, Bircher N. *Cardiopulmonary Cerebral Resuscitation: World Federation of Societies of Anaesthesiologists International CPCR Guidelines.* 3rd ed. Philadelphia, Pa: WB Saunders Co; 1988.

3. Abramson NS, Safar P, Detre K. Brain Resuscitation Clinical Trial II Study Group. Factors influencing neurologic recovery after cardiac arrest. *Ann Emerg Med.* 1989;18:477-478. Abstract.

4. Braun O, McCallion R, Fazacherley J. Characteristics of midsized urban EMS systems. *Ann Emerg Med.* 1990;19:536-546.

5. Eisenberg MS, Horwood BT, Cummins RO, Reynolds-Haertle R, Hearne TR. Cardiac arrest and resuscitation: a tale of 29 cities. *Ann Emerg Med.* 1990;19:179-186.

6. Cummins RO. EMT-defibrillation: national guidelines for implementation. *Am J Emerg Med.* 1987;5:254-257.

7. Cummins RO, Thies WH. Encouraging early defibrillation: the American Heart Association and automated external defibrillators. *Ann Emerg Med.* 1990;19:1245-1248.

8. Cummins RO, Thies WH. Automated external defibrillators and the advanced cardiac life support program: a new initiative from the American Heart Association. *Am J Emerg Med.* 1991;9:91-93.

9. Automated external defibrillation. In: Jaffe AS, ed. *Textbook of Advanced Cardiac Life Support.* 2nd ed. Dallas, Tex: American Heart Association; 1991:287-299.

10. Abarbanell NR. Problems with prehospital cardiac resuscitation: the two-rescuer response. *Am J Emerg Med.* 1992;10:166-167. Letter.

11. Lowenstein SR, Sabyan EM, Lassen CF, Kern DC. Benefits of training physicians in advanced cardiac life support. *Chest.* 1986;89:512-516.

12. Skinner DV, Camm AJ, Miles S. Cardiopulmonary resuscitation skills of preregistration house officers. *Br Med J.* 1985;290: 1549-1550.

13. Cummins RO, Chamberlain DA, Abramson NS, Allen M, Baskett P, Becker L, Bossaert L, Delooz H, Dick W, Eisenberg M, et al. Recommended guidelines for uniform reporting of data from out-of-hospital cardiac arrest: the Utstein Style. Task Force of the American Heart Association, the European Resuscitation Council, the Heart and Stroke Foundation of Canada, and the Australian Resuscitation Council. *Ann Emerg Med.* 1991;20:861-874.

14. Cummins RO, Ornato JP, Thies WH, Pepe PE. Improving survival from sudden cardiac arrest: the 'chain of survival' concept. *Circulation.* 1991;83:1833-1847.

15. Cummins RO. The 'chain of survival' concept: how it can save lives. *Heart Dis Stroke.* 1992;1:43-45.

16. Burkle FJ. Code organization. In: Eisenberg MS, Cummins RO, Ho MT, eds. *Code Blue: Cardiac Arrest and Resuscitation.* Philadelphia, Pa: WB Saunders Co;1987:26-31.

17. Burkle M Jr, Rice MM. Code organization. *Am J Emerg Med.* 1987;5:235-239.

18. Robinson MA. Informing the family of sudden death. *Am Fam Phys.* 1981;23:115-118.

19. Genest M, Levine J, Ramsden V, Swanson R. The impact of providing help: emergency workers and cardiopulmonary resuscitation attempts. *J Trauma Stress.* 1988;1:353-372.

20. Dubin W, Sarnoff JR. Sudden unexpected death: intervention with the survivors. *Ann Emerg Med.* 1986;15:54-57.

21. Ramenofsky M, Aprahamian C, Brown R, et al. *Advanced Trauma Life Support Student Manual.* Chicago, Ill: American College of Surgeons; 1989:1-298.

22. Emergency Cardiac Care Committee and Subcommittees, American Heart Association. Guidelines for cardiopulmonary resuscitation and emergency cardiac care, Part II: Adult basic life support. *JAMA.* 1992;268:2184-2198.

23. Eisenberg MS, Cummins RO, Damon S, Larsen MP, Hearne TR. Survival rates from out-of-hospital cardiac arrest: recommendations for uniform definitions and data to report. *Ann Emerg Med.* 1990;19:1249-1259.

24. O'Leary JJ, Pollard BJ, Ryan MJ. A method of detecting oesophageal intubation or confirming tracheal intubation. *Anaesth Intensive Care.* 1988;16:299-301.

25. Longstreth WT Jr, Invi TS. High blood glucose level on hospital admission and poor neurological recovery after cardiac arrest. *Ann Neurol.* 1984;15:59-63.

26. Longstreth WT Jr, Diehr P, Cobb LA, Hanson RW, Blair AD. Neurologic outcome and blood glucose levels during out-of-hospital cardiopulmonary resuscitation. *Neurology.* 1986;36:1186-1191.

27. Dick T, Todd C. Injection port for an endotracheal tube. *J Emerg Med Serv.* 1988;13:34.

28. Hargarten KM, Stueven HA, Waite EM, et al. Prehospital experience with defibrillation of coarse ventricular fibrillation: a ten-year review. *Ann Emerg Med.* 1990;19:157-162.

29. Greene HL. Sudden arrhythmic cardiac death: mechanisms, resuscitation and classification. *Am J Cardiol.* 1990;65:4B-12B.

30. De Luna AB, Coumel P, Leclercq JF. Ambulatory sudden cardiac death: mechanism of production of fatal arrhythmia on the basis of data from 157 cases. *Am Heart J.* 1989;117:151-159.

31. Kerber RE. Statement on early defibrillation from the Emergency Cardiac Care Committee, American Heart Association. *Circulation.* 1991;83:2233.

32. Cummins RO, Austin D Jr. The frequency of 'occult' ventricular fibrillation masquerading as a flat line in prehospital cardiac arrest. *Ann Emerg Med.* 1988;17:813-817.

33. Cummins RO, Chesemore K, White RD. Defibrillator Working Group. Defibrillator failures: causes of problems and recommendations for improvement. *JAMA.* 1990;264:1019-1025.

34. Ewy GA, Dahl CF, Zimmerman, M, Otto C. Ventricular fibrillation masquerading as ventricular standstill. *Crit Care Med.* 1981;9: 841-844.

35. McDonald JL. Coarse ventricular fibrillation presenting as asystole or very low amplitude ventricular fibrillation. *Crit Care Med.* 1982; 10:790-791.

36. White RD. FDA recommendations for maintaining defibrillator readiness: defibrillator daily checklists. *J Emerg Med Serv.* 1992;4:70-82.

37. Kerber RE. Electrical treatment of cardiac arrhythmias: defibrillation and cardioversion. *Ann Emerg Med.* 1993;22:296-301.

38. Becker LB, Pepe PE. Ensuring the effectiveness of community-wide emergency cardiac care. *Ann Emerg Med.* 1993;22:354-365.

39. White RD. Maintenance of defibrillators in a state of readiness. *Ann Emerg Med.* 1993;22:302-306.

40. Brown DC, Lewis AJ, Criley JM. Asystole and its treatment: the possible role of the parasympathetic nervous system in cardiac arrest. *J Am Coll Emerg Phys.* 1979;8:448-452.

41. Eysmann SB, Marchlinski FE, Buxton A, Josephson ME. Electrocardiographic changes after cardioversion of ventricular arrhythmias. *Circulation.* 1986;73:73-81.

42. Niemann JT, Haynes KS, Garner D, Rennie CJ III, Jagels G, Storm O. Postcountershock pulseless rhythms: response to CPR, artificial cardiac pacing, and adrenergic agonists. *Ann Emerg Med.* 1986;15:112-120.

43. Vassalle M. On the mechanisms underlying cardiac standstill: factors determining success or failure of escape pacemakers in the heart. *J Am Coll Cardiol.* 1985;5:35B-42B.

44. Klein GJ, Ideker RE, Smith WM, Harrison LA, Kasell J, Wallace AG, Gallagher JJ. Epicardial mapping of the onset of ventricular tachycardia initiated by programmed stimulation in the canine heart with chronic infarction. *Circulation*. 1979;60:1375-1384.

45. Neumar RW, Brown CG, Robitaille PM, Altschuld RA. Myocardial high energy phosphate metabolism during ventricular fibrillation with total circulatory arrest. *Resuscitation*. 1990;19:199-226.

46. Neumar RW, Brown CG, Van Ligten P, Hoekstra J, Altschuld RA, Baker P. Estimation of myocardial ischemic injury during ventricular fibrillation with total circulatory arrest using high-energy phosphates and lactate as metabolic markers. *Ann Emerg Med*. 1991;20: 222-229.

47. Kern KB, Garewal HS, Sanders AB, et al. Depletion of myocardial adenosine triphosphate during prolonged untreated ventricular fibrillation: effect on defibrillation success. *Resuscitation*. 1990;20:221-229.

48. Weaver WD, Fahrenbruch CE, Johnson DD, Hallstrom AP, Cobb LA, Copass MK. Effect of epinephrine and lidocaine therapy on outcome after cardiac arrest due to ventricular fibrillation. *Circulation*. 1990;82:2027-2034.

49. Martin TG, Hawkins NS, Weigel JA, Rider DE, Buckingham BD. Initial treatment of ventricular fibrillation: defibrillation or drug therapy. *Am J Emerg Med*. 1988;6:113-119.

50. Cummins RO, Graves JR, Horan S, Larsen MP, Crump K. The relative contributions of early defibrillation and ACLS interventions to resuscitation and survival from prehospital cardiac arrest. *Ann Emerg Med*. 1989;18:468-469. Abstract.

51. Panacek E, Munger M, Rutherford W, Gardner S. Report of nitropatch explosions complicating defibrillation. *Am J Emerg Med*. 1992;10:128-129.

52. Parke JD, Higgins SE. Hazards associated with chest application of nitroglycerin ointments. *JAMA*. 1982;248:427. Letter.

53. Pride H, McKinley D. Third degree burns from the use of an external cardiac pacing device. *Crit Care Med*. 1990;18:572-573.

54. Babka JC. Does nitroglycerin explode? *N Engl J Med*. 1983;309:379. Letter.

55. Gibbs W, Eisenberg M, Damon SK. Dangers of defibrillation: injuries to emergency personnel during patient resuscitation. *Am J Emerg Med*. 1990;8:101-104.

56. Barton C, Callaham M. High-dose epinephrine improves the return of spontaneous circulation rates in human victims of cardiac arrest. *Ann Emerg Med*. 1991;20:722-725.

57. Beless D, Otsuki A, Davis W. Neurologically intact survivor of prolonged ventricular fibrillation: a case for intermediate dose epinephrine and postresuscitation infusion. *Am J Emerg Med*. 1992;10: 133-135.

58. Brown CG, Werman HA, Davis EA, Hamlin R, Hobson J, Ashton JA. Comparative effect of graded doses of epinephrine on regional brain blood flow during CPR in a swine model. *Ann Emerg Med*. 1986;15:1138-1144.

59. Brown CG, Werman HA, Davis EA, Hobson J, Hamlin RL. The effects of graded doses of epinephrine on regional myocardial blood flow during cardiopulmonary resuscitation in swine. *Circulation*. 1987;75:491-497.

60. Brown CG, Tayor RB, Werman HA, Luu T, Spittler G, Hamlin RL. Effect of standard doses of epinephrine on myocardial oxygen delivery and utilization during cardiopulmonary resuscitation. *Crit Care Med*. 1988;16:536-539.

61. Brown CG, Martin DR, Pepe PE, Stueven H, Cummins RO, Gonzalez E, Jastremski M. A comparison of standard-dose and high-dose epinephrine in cardiac arrest outside the hospital: The Multicenter High-Dose Epinephrine Study Group. *N Engl J Med*. 1992;327:1051-1055.

62. Callaham M. Epinephrine doses in cardiac arrest: is it time to outgrow the orthodoxy of ACLS? *Ann Emerg Med*. 1989;18: 1011-1012.

63. Callaham M, Barton CW, Kayser S. Potential complications of high-dose epinephrine therapy in patients resuscitated from cardiac arrest. *JAMA*. 1991;265:1117-1122.

64. Callaham M, Madsen CD, Barton CW, Saunders CE, Daley M, Pointer J. A randomized clinical trial of high-dose epinephrine and norepinephrine versus standard-dose epinephrine in prehospital cardiac arrest. *Ann Emerg Med*. 1992;21:606-607. Abstract.

65. Ditchey RV, Lindenfeld J. Failure of epinephrine to improve the balance between myocardial oxygen supply and demand during closed-chest resuscitation in dogs. *Circulation*. 1988;78:382-389.

66. Koscove EM, Paradis NA. Successful resuscitation from cardiac arrest using high-dose epinephrine therapy: report of two cases. *JAMA*. 1988;259:3031-3034.

67. Kosnik JW, Jackson RE, Keats S, Tworek RM, Freeman SB. Dose-related response of centrally administered epinephrine on the change in aortic diastolic pressure during closed-chest massage in dogs. *Ann Emerg Med*. 1985;14:204-208.

68. Lindner KH, Ahnefeld FW, Bowdler IM. Comparison of different doses of epinephrine on myocardial perfusion and resuscitation success during cardiopulmonary resuscitation in a pig model. *Am J Emerg Med*. 1991;9: 27-31.

69. Lindner KH, Ahnefeld FW, Grünert A. Epinephrine versus norepinephrine in prehospital ventricular fibrillation. *Am J Cardiol*. 1991;67:427-428.

70. Martin D, Werman HA, Brown CG. Four case studies: high-dose epinephrine in cardiac arrest. *Ann Emerg Med*. 1990;19:322-326.

71. Niemann JT, Cairns CB, Sharma J, Lewis RJ. Treatment of prolonged ventricular fibrillation: immediate countershock versus high-dose epinephrine and CPR preceding countershock. *Circulation*. 1992;85:281-287.

72. Otto C, Yakaitis R. The role of epinephrine in CPR: a reappraisal. *Ann Emerg Med*. 1987;16:743-748.

73. Paradis NA, Koscove EM. Epinephrine in cardiac arrest: a critical review. *Ann Emerg Med*. 1990;19:1288-1301.

74. Stiell IG, Hebert PC, Weitzman BN, Wells GA, Raman S, Stark RM, Higginson LA, Ahuja J, Dickinson GE. High-dose epinephrine in adult cardiac arrest. *N Engl J Med*. 1992;327:1045-1050.

75. Eisenberg MS, Copass MK, Hallstrom AP, et al. Treatment of out-of-hospital cardiac arrest with rapid defibrillation by emergency medical technicians. *N Engl J Med*. 1980;302:1379-1383.

76. Weaver WD, Hill D, Fahrenbruch CE, et al. Use of the automatic external defibrillator in the management of out-of-hospital cardiac arrest. *N Engl J Med*. 1988;319:661-666.

77. Bocka JJ. Automatic external defibrillators. *Ann Emerg Med*. 1989;18:1264-1268.

78. Cummins RO, Eisenberg MS, Litwin PE, Graves JR, Hearne TR, Hallstrom AP. Automatic external defibrillators used by emergency medical technicians: a controlled clinical trial. *JAMA*. 1987;257:1605-1610.

79. Cummins RO. From concept to standard-of-care? review of the clinical experience with automated external defibrillators. *Ann Emerg Med*. 1989;18:1269-1275.

80. Haynes BE, Mendoza A, McNeil M, Schroeder J, Smiley D. A statewide early defibrillation initiative including laypersons and outcome reporting. *JAMA*. 1991;266:545-547.

81. Jaggarao NS, Heber M, Grainger R, Vincent R, Chamberlain DA. Use of an automated external defibrillator-pacemaker by ambulance staff. *Lancet*. 1982;2:73-75.

82. Cobe SM, Redmond MJ, Watson JM, Hollingworth J, Carrington DJ. 'Heartstart Scotland' — initial experience of a national scheme for out of hospital defibrillation. *Br Med J*. 1991;302:1517-1520.

83. Olsen DW, LaRochelle J, Fark D, Aprahamian C, Aufderheide TP, Mateer JR, Hargarten KM, Stueven HA. EMT-defibrillation: the Wisconsin experience. *Ann Emerg Med*. 1989;18:806-811.

84. Stults KR, Brown DD, Kerber RE. Efficacy of an automated external defibrillator in the management of out-of-hospital cardiac arrest: validation of the diagnostic algorithm and initial clinical experience in a rural environment. *Circulation*. 1986;73:701-709.

85. Walters G, D'Auria D, Glucksman EE. Controlled trial of automated external defibrillators in the London ambulance service. *J R Soc Med*. 1990;83:563-565.

86. Guidelines for advanced life support: a statement by the Advanced Life Support Working Party of the European Resuscitation Council, 1992. *Resuscitation*. 1992;24:111-121.

87. Jaffe AS. The use of antiarrhythmics in advanced cardiac life support. *Ann Emerg Med*. 1993;22:307-316.

88. Anderson JL, Rodier HE, Green LS. Comparative effects of beta-adrenergic blocking drugs on experimental ventricular fibrillation threshold. *Am J Cardiol*. 1983;51:1196-1202.

89. Haynes RE, Chinn TL, Copass MK, Cobb LA. Comparison of bretylium tosylate and lidocaine in management of out of hospital ventricular fibrillation: a randomized clinical trial. *Am J Cardiol*. 1981;48:353-356.

90. Olson DW, Thompson BM, Darin JC, Milbrath MH. A randomized comparison study of bretylium tosylate and lidocaine in resuscitation of patients from out-of-hospital ventricular fibrillation in a paramedic system. *Ann Emerg Med*. 1984;13:807-810.

91. Chow MS, Ronfeld RA, Ruffet D, Fieldman A. Lidocaine pharmacokinetics during cardiac arrest and external cardiopulmonary resuscitation. *Am Heart J.* 1981;102:799-801.

92. Chow MS, Ronfeld RA, Hamilton RA, Helmink R, Fieldman A. Effect of external cardiopulmonary resuscitation on lidocaine pharmacokinetics in dogs. *J Pharmacol Exp Ther.* 1983;224:531-537.

93. Hanyok JJ, Chow MS, Kluger J, Fieldman A. Antifibrillatory effects of high dose bretylium and a lidocaine-bretylium combination during cardiopulmonary resuscitation. *Crit Care Med.* 1988;16:691-694.

94. Martin DR, Brown CG, Dzwonczyk R. Frequency analysis of the human and swine electrocardiogram during ventricular fibrillation. *Resuscitation.* 1991;22:85-91.

95. Brown CG, Griffith RF, Van Ligten P, et al. Median frequency: a new parameter for predicting defibrillation success rate. *Ann Emerg Med.* 1991;20:787-789.

96. Brown CG, Dzwonczyk R, Werman HA, Hamlin RL. Estimating the duration of ventricular fibrillation. *Ann Emerg Med.* 1989;18:1181-1185.

97. Ceremuzynski L, Jurgiel R, Kulakowski P, Gîbalska J. Threatening arrhythmias in acute myocardial infarction are prevented by intravenous magnesium sulfate. *Am Heart J.* 1989;118:1333-1334.

98. Woods KL, Fletcher S, Roffe C, Haider Y. Intravenous magnesium sulphate in suspected acute myocardial infarction: results of the second Leicester Intravenous Magnesium Intervention Trial (LIMIT-2). *Lancet.* 1992;339:1553-1558.

99. Shechter M, Hod H, Marks N, Behar S, Kaplinsky E, Rabinowitz B. Beneficial effect of magnesium sulfate in acute myocardial infarction. *Am J Cardiol.* 1990;66:271-274.

100. Brown C, Griffith R. The effect of magnesium administration on aortic pressures during CPR in swine. *Resuscitation.* 1992;24:173. Abstract.

101. Cannon LA, Heiselman DE, Dougherty JM, Jones J. Magnesium levels in cardiac arrest victims: relationship between magnesium levels and successful resuscitation. *Ann Emerg Med.* 1987;16:1195-1199.

102. Craddock L, Miller B, Clifton G, Krumbach B, Pluss W. Resuscitation from prolonged cardiac arrest with high-dose intravenous magnesium sulfate. *J Emerg Med.* 1991;9:469-476.

103. Tobey RC, Birnbaum GA, Allegra JR, Horowitz MS, Plosay JJ III. Successful resuscitation and neurologic recovery from refractory ventricular fibrillation after magnesium sulfate administration. *Ann Emerg Med.* 1992;21:92-96.

104. von Planta M, Bar-Joseph G, Wiklund L, Bircher NG, Falk JL, Abramson NS. Pathophysiologic and therapeutic implications of acid-base changes during CPR. *Ann Emerg Med.* 1993;22:404-410.

105. Federiuk CS, Sanders AB, Kern KB, Nelson J, Ewy GA. The effect of bicarbonate on resuscitation from cardiac arrest. *Ann Emerg Med.* 1991;20:1173-1177.

106. Aufderheide TP, Martin DR, Olson DW, et al. Prehospital bicarbonate use in cardiac arrest: a 3-year experience. *Am J Emerg Med.* 1992;10:4-7.

107. Kette F, Weil M, Gazmuri R, et al. Buffer solutions may compromise cardiac resuscitation by reducing coronary perfusion pressure. *JAMA.* 1991;266:2121-2126.

108. Stueven HA, Aufderheide T, Thakur RK, Hargarten K, Vanags B. Defining electromechanical dissociation: morphologic presentation. *Resuscitation.* 1989;17:195-203.

109. Stueven HA, Aufderheide T, Waite EM, Mateer JR. Electromechanical dissociation: six years prehospital experience. *Resuscitation.* 1989;17:173-182.

110. Aufderheide TP, Thakur RK, Stueven HA. Electrocardiographic characteristics in EMD. *Resuscitation.* 1989;17:183-193.

111. Charlap S, Kahlan S, Lichstein E, Frishman W. Electromechanical dissociation: diagnosis, pathophysiology, and management. *Am Heart J.* 1989;118:355-360.

112. Hoffman JR, Stevenson LW. Postdefibrillation idioventricular rhythm: a salvageable condition. *West J Med.* 1987;146:188-191.

113. Harrison EE, Amey BD. Use of calcium in electromechanical dissociation. *Ann Emerg Med.* 1984;13:844-845.

114. Thijs LG, Vincent JL, Weil MH, Michaels WS, Carlson R. A closed-chest model for the study of electromechanical dissociation of the heart in dogs. *Resuscitation.* 1982;10:25-32.

115. Vincent JL, Thijs LG, Weil MH, Michaels S, Silverberg RA. Clinical and experimental studies on electromechanical dissociation. *Circulation.* 1981;64:18-27.

116. Ewy GA. Defining electromechanical dissociation. *Ann Emerg Med.* 1984;13:830-832.

117. Berryman CR. Electromechanical dissociation with a directly measurable arterial blood pressure. *Ann Emerg Med.* 1986;15:625-626.

118. Bocka JJ, Overton DT, Hauser A. Electromechanical dissociation in human beings: an echocardiographic evaluation. *Ann Emerg Med.* 1988;17:450-452.

119. Paradis NA, Martin GB, Goetting MG, Rivers EP, Feingold M, Nowak RM. Aortic pressure during human cardiac arrest: identification of pseudo-electromechanical dissociation. *Chest.* 1992;101:123-128.

120. Lindner KH, Ahnefeld FW, Prengel AW. Comparison of standard and high-dose adrenaline in the resuscitation of asystole and electromechanical dissociation. *Acta Anaesthesiol Scand.* 1991;35:253-256.

121. Stueven H, Troian P, Thompson B, et al. Bystander/first responder CPR: ten years experience in a paramedic system. *Ann Emerg Med.* 1986;15:707-710.

122. Vanags B, Thakur RK, Stueven HA, Aufderheide T, Tresch DD. Interventions in the therapy of electromechanical dissociation. *Resuscitation.* 1989;17:163-171.

123. Cummins RO, Haulman J, Quan L, Graves JR, Peterson D, Horan S. Near-fatal yew berry intoxication treated with external cardiac pacing and digoxin-specific FAB antibody fragments. *Ann Emerg Med.* 1990;19:38-43.

124. Hwang JJ, Shyu KG, Chen JJ, Tseng YZ, Kuan P, Lien WP. Usefulness of transesophageal echocardiography in the treatment of critically ill patients. *Chest.* 1993;104:861-866.

125. Reichman RT, Joyo CI, Dembitsky WP, Griffith LD, Adamson RM, Daily PO, Overlie PA, Smith SC Jr, Jaski BE. Improved patient survival after cardiac arrest using a cardiopulmonary support system. *Ann Thorac Surg.* 1990;49:101-104.

126. Kenyon CJ, Aldinger GE, Joshipura P, Zaid GJ. Successful resuscitation using external cardiac pacing in beta adrenergic antagonist-induced bradyasystolic arrest. *Ann Emerg Med.* 1988;17:711-713.

127. Paris PM, Stewart RD, Kaplan RM, Whipkey R. Transcutaneous pacing for bradyasystolic cardiac arrests in prehospital care. *Ann Emerg Med.* 1985;14:320-323.

128. Tachakra SS, Jepson E, Beckett MW, Barrie R. Successful transcutaneous external pacing for asystole following cardiac arrest. *Arch Emerg Med.* 1988;5:184-185.

129. Thompson BM, Brooks RC, Pionkowski RS, Aprahamian C, Mateer JR. Immediate countershock treatment of asystole. *Ann Emerg Med.* 1984;13:827-829.

130. Stults K, Brown D, Kerber R. Should ventricular asystole be cardioverted? *Circulation.* 1987;76(suppl IV):IV-12. Abstract.

131. Stults K, Brown D. Converting asystole. *J Emerg Med Serv.* 1984;9:38-39.

132. Olson CM, Jastremski MS, Smith RW, Tyndall GJ, Montgomery GF, Daye MC. External cardiac pacing for out-of-hospital bradyasystolic arrest. *Am J Emerg Med.* 1985;3:129-131.

133. O'Toole KS, Paris PM, Heller MB, Stewart RD. Emergency transcutaneous pacing in the management of patients with bradyasystolic rhythms. *J Emerg Med.* 1987;5:267-273.

134. Syverud SA, Dalsey WC, Hedges JR. Transcutaneous and transvenous cardiac pacing for early bradyasystolic cardiac arrest. *Ann Emerg Med.* 1986;15:121-124.

135. Syverud S. Cardiac pacing. *Emerg Med Clin North Am.* 1988;6:197-215.

136. Vukov LF, Johnson DQ. External transcutaneous pacemakers in interhospital transport of cardiac patients. *Ann Emerg Med.* 1989;18:738-740.

137. Zoll PM, Zoll RH, Falk RH, Clinton JE, Eitel DR, Antman EM. External noninvasive temporary cardiac pacing: clinical trials. *Circulation.* 1985;71:937-944.

138. Bocka JJ. External transcutaneous pacemakers. *Ann Emerg Med.* 1989;18:1280-1286.

139. Cummins RO, Graves JR, Larsen MP, Hallstrom AP, Hearne TR, Ciliberti J, Nicola RM, Horan S. Out-of-hospital transcutaneous pacing by emergency medical technicians in patients with asystolic cardiac arrest. *N Engl J Med.* 1993;328:1377-1382.

140. Berliner D, Okun M, Peters RW, Carliner NH, Plotnick GD, Fisher ML. Transcutaneous temporary pacing in the operating room. *JAMA.* 1985;254:84-86.

141. Eital DR, Guzzardi LJ, Stein SE, Drawbaugh RE, Hess DR, Walton SL. Noninvasive transcutaneous cardiac pacing in prehospital cardiac arrest. *Ann Emerg Med.* 1987;16:531-534.

142. Hedges JR. Prehospital external pacing for treating cardiac arrest. *Arrhythmias and Conduction Disturbances.* 1988;5:39-46.

143. Hedges JR, Syverud SA, Dalsey WC, Feero S, Easter R, Schultz B. Prehospital trial of emergency transcutaneous cardiac pacing. *Circulation.* 1987;76:1337-1343.

144. Hedges JR, Syverud SA, Dalsey WC. Developments in transcutaneous and transthoracic pacing during bradyasystolic arrest. *Ann Emerg Med.* 1984;13:822-827.

145. Kelly JS, Royster RL, Angert KC, Case LD. Efficacy of noninvasive transcutaneous cardiac pacing patients undergoing cardiac surgery. *Anesthesiology.* 1989;70:747-751.

146. Madsen JK, Meibom J, Videbak R, Pedersen F, Grande P. Transcutaneous pacing: experience with the Zoll noninvasive temporary pacemaker. *Am Heart J.* 1988;116:7-10.

147. McNeil EL. Successful resuscitation using external cardiac pacing. *Ann Emerg Med.* 1985;14:1230-1232.

148. Safar P. Cerebral resuscitation after cardiac arrest: research initiatives and future directions. *Ann Emerg Med.* 1993;22:324-349.

149. Spivey WH, Abramson NS, Safar P, Tyrell KS, Schoffstaff JM. Correlation of blood pressure with mortality and neurologic recovery in comatose postresuscitation patients. *Ann Emerg Med.* 1991;20:453. Abstract.

150. Sterz F, Leonov Y, Safar P, Radovsky A, Tisherman SA, Oku K. Hypertension with or without hemodilution after cardiac arrest in dogs. *Stroke.* 1990;21:1178-1184.

151. Miller S. The cardiovascular triad: a conceptual tool. In: Miller S, ed. *Basic Principles of Resuscitation.* Boston, Mass: Boston Medical Education Group Inc; 1991.

152. Gunnar RM, Bourdillon PO, Dixon DW, et al. ACC/AHA guidelines for the early management of patients with acute myocardial infarction. *Circulation.* 1990;82:664-707.

153. Genton R, Jaffe AS. Management of congestive heart failure in patients with acute myocardial infarction. *JAMA.* 1986;256: 2556-2560.

154. Chadda KD, Lichstein E, Gupta PK, Kourtesis P. Effects of atropine in patients with bradyarrhythmias complicating myocardial infarction: usefulness of an optimal dose for overdrive. *Am J Med.* 1975;63:503-510.

155. Scheinman MM, Thorburn D, Abbott JA. Use of atropine in patients with acute myocardial infarction and sinus bradycardia. *Circulation.* 1975;52:627-633.

156. Massumi RA, Mason DT, Amsterdam EA, et al. Ventricular fibrillation and tachycardia after intravenous atropine for treatment of bradycardias. *N Engl J Med.* 1972;287:336-338.

157. Lunde P. Ventricular fibrillation after intravenous atropine for treatment for sinus bradycardia. *Acta Med Scand.* 1976;199:369-371.

158. Knoebel SB, McHenry PS, Phillips JF, Widlansky S. Atropine-induced cardioacceleration and myocardial blood flow in subjects with and without coronary artery disease. *Am J Cardiol.* 1974;33: 327-332.

159. Cooper MJ, Abinader EG. Atropine-induced ventricular fibrillation: case report and review of the literature. *Am Heart J.* 1979;97: 225-228.

160. Gonzalez ER. Pharmacologic controversies in CPR. *Ann Emerg Med.* 1993;22:317-323.

161. Pritchett EL. Management of atrial fibrillation. *N Engl J Med.* 1992;326:1264-1271.

162. Friedman HZ, Goldberg SF, Bonema JD, Cragg DR, Hauser AM. Acute complications associated with new-onset atrial fibrillation. *Am J Cardiol.* 1991;67:437-439.

163. Sugiura T, Iwasaka T, Ogawa A, Shiroyama Y, Tsuji H, Onoyam H, Inada M. Atrial fibrillation in acute myocardial infarction. *Am J Cardiol.* 1985;56:27-29.

164. Ellenbogen KA, Dias VC, Plumb VJ, Heywood JR, Mirvis DM. A placebo-controlled trial of continuous intravenous diltiazem infusion for 24-hour heart rate control during atrial fibrillation and atrial flutter: a multicenter study. *J Am Coll Cardiol.* 1991;18:891-897.

165. Salerno DM, Dias VC, Kleiger RE, et al. Efficacy and safety of intravenous diltiazem for treatment of atrial fibrillation and atrial flutter. *Am J Cardiol.* 1989;63:1046-1051.

166. Ewy GA. Urgent parenteral digoxin therapy: a requiem. *J Am Coll Cardiol.* 1990;15:1248-1249.

167. Falk RH, Leavitt JI. Digoxin for atrial fibrillation: a drug whose time has gone? *Ann Intern Med.* 1991;114:573-575.

168. Mehta D, Wafa S, Ward DE, Camm AJ. Relative efficacy of various physical manoeuvers in the termination of junctional tachycardia. *Lancet.* 1988;1:1181-1185.

169. Waxman MB, Wald RW, Sharma AD, Huerta F, Cameron DA. Vagal techniques for termination of paroxysmal supraventricular tachycardia. *Am J Cardiol.* 1980;46:655-664.

170. Hess DS, Hanlon T, Scheinman M, Budge R, Desai J. Termination of ventricular tachycardia by carotid sinus message. *Circulation.* 1982;65:627-630.

171. Wei JY, Greene HL, Weisfeldt ML. Cough-facilitated conversion of ventricular tachycardia. *Am J Cardiol.* 1980;45:174-176.

172. Walker LA III, MacMath TL, Chipman H, Bayne E. MAST application in the treatment of paroxysmal supraventricular tachycardia in a child. *Ann Emerg Med.* 1988;17:529-531.

173. Hauswald M, Tandberg D. The effect of patient position and MAST inflation on carotid sinus diameter. *Ann Emerg Med.* 1985;14:1065-1068.

174. Roberge R, Anderson E, MacMath T, Rudolf J, Luten R. Termination of paroxysmal supraventricular tachycardia by digital rectal massage. *Ann Emerg Med.* 1987;16:1291-1293.

175. Rankin AC, McGovern BA. Adenosine or verapamil for the acute treatment of supraventricular tachycardia? *Ann Intern Med.* 1991;114:513-515.

176. Viskin S, Belhassen B. Acute management of paroxysmal atrioventricular junctional reentrant supraventricular tachycardia: pharmacologic strategies. *Am Heart J.* 1990;120:180-188.

177. Rankin AC, Oldroyd KG, Chong E, Rae AP, Cobbe SM. Value and limitations of adenosine in the diagnosis and treatment of narrow and broad complex tachycardias. *Br Heart J.* 1989;62:195-203.

178. Griffith MJ, Linker NJ, Ward DE, Camm AJ. Adenosine in the diagnosis of broad complex tachycardia. *Lancet.* 1988;1:672-675.

179. DiMarco JP, Miles W, Akhtar M, et al. Adenosine for paroxysmal supraventricular tachycardia: dose ranging and comparison with verapamil: assessment in placebo-controlled, multicenter trials: the Adenosine for PVST Study Group. *Ann Intern Med.* 1990;113: 104-110.

180. DiMarco JP, Sellers TD, Lerman BB, Greenberg ML, Berne RM, Belardinelli L. Diagnostic and therapeutic use of adenosine in patients with supraventricular tachyarrhythmias. *J Am Coll Cardiol.* 1985;6:417-425.

181. Garratt C, Linker N, Griffith M, Ward D, Camm AJ. Comparison of adenosine and verapamil for termination of paroxysmal junctional tachycardia. *Am J Cardiol.* 1989;64:1310-1316.

182. Camm AJ, Garratt CJ. Adenosine and supraventricular tachycardia. *N Engl J Med.* 1991;325:1621-1629.

183. McCabe J, Adhar GC, Menegazzi JJ, Paris PM. Intravenous adenosine in the prehospital treatment of paroxysmal supraventricular tachycardia. *Ann Emerg Med.* 1992;21:358-361.

184. Cairns CB, Niemann JT. Intravenous adenosine in the emergency department management of paroxysmal supraventricular tachycardia. *Ann Emerg Med.* 1991;20:717-721.

185. Caruso A. Supraventricular tachycardia: changes in management. *Postgrad Med.* 1991;90:73-76,79-82.

186. Ros SP, Fisher EA, Bell TJ. Adenosine in the emergency management of supraventricular tachycardia. *Pediatr Emerg Care.* 1991; 7:222-223.

187. Sylvën C, Beerman NB, Jonzon B, Brandt R. Angina pectoris-like pain provoked by intravenous adenosine in healthy volunteers. *Br Med J.* 1986;293:227-230.

188. Crea F, Pupita G, Galassi AR, el-Tamimi H, Kaski JC, Davies G, Masseri A. Role of adenosine in pathogenesis of anginal pain. *Circulation.* 1990;81:164-172.

189. Weiss AT, Lewis BS, Halon DA, Hasin Y, Gotsman MS. The use of calcium with verapamil in the management of supraventricular tachyarrhythmias. *Int J Cardiol.* 1983;4:275-284.

190. Grauer KN, Cavallaro DL. Differentiation of PVCs from aberrancy. In: *ACLS: A Comprehensive Review.* 3rd ed. St Louis, Mo: Mosby Lifeline; 1993:489-546.

191. Brugada P, Brugada J, Mont L, Smeets J, Andries EW. A new approach to the differential diagnosis of a regular tachycardia with a wide QRS complex. *Circulation.* 1991;83:1649-1659.

192. Wellens HJ, Bär FW, Lie KI. The value of the electrocardiogram in the differential diagnosis of a tachycardia with a widened QRS complex. *Am J Med.* 1978;64:27-33.

193. Stewart RB, Bardy GH, Greene HL. Wide complex tachycardia: misdiagnosis and outcome after emergent therapy. *Ann Intern Med.* 1986;104:766-771.

194. McGovern B, Garan H, Ruskin JN. Precipitation of cardiac arrest by verapamil in patients with Wolff-Parkinson-White syndrome. *Ann Intern Med.* 1986;104:791-794.

195. Jacob AS, Nielsen DH, Gianelly RE. Fatal ventricular fibrillation following verapamil in Wolff-Parkinson-White syndrome with atrial fibrillation. *Ann Emerg Med.* 1985;14:159-160.

196. Dancy M, Camm AJ, Ward D. Misdiagnosis of chronic recurrent ventricular tachycardia. *Lancet.* 1985;2:320-323.

197. Rankin AC, Rae AP, Cobbe SM. Misuse of intravenous verapamil in patients with ventricular tachycardia. *Lancet.* 1987;2:472-474.

198. Sharma AD, Klein GJ, Yee R. Intravenous adenosine triphosphate during wide QRS complex tachycardia: safety, therapeutic efficacy, and diagnostic utility. *Am J Med.* 1990;88:337-343.

199. Vukmir RB. Torsades de pointes: a review. *Am J Emerg Med.* 1991;9:250-255.

200. Kossman CE. Torsades de pointes: an addition to the nosography of ventricular tachycardia. *Am J Cardiol.* 1978;42:1054-1056.

201. Tzivoni D, Banai S, Schuger C, et al. Treatment of torsades de pointes with magnesium sulfate. *Circulation.* 1988;77:392-397.

202. Perticone F, Adinolfi L, Bonaduce D. Efficacy of magnesium sulfate in treatment of torsades de pointes. *Am Heart J.* 1986;112:847-849.

203. Khan MM, Logan KR, McComb JM, Adgey AAJ. Management of recurrent ventricular tachyarrhythmias associated with Q-T prolongation. *Am J Cardiol.* 1981;47:1301-1308.

204. Dronen S, Birrer P. Shock. In: Tintinalli J, Krome RL, Ruiz E, eds. *Emergency Medicine: A Comprehensive Study Guide.* 3rd ed. New York, NY: McGraw-Hill Book Co; 1992:132-140.

205. Saunders C. Vasoactive agents. In: Barsan WG, Jastremski MS, Syverud SA, eds. *Emergency Drug Therapy.* Philadelphia, Pa: WB Saunders Co; 1991:224-261.

206. Sypniewski EJ, Ornato J. Circulatory shock. In: Ornato JP, Gonzalez ER, eds. *Drug Therapy in Emergency Medicine.* New York, NY: Churchill Livingstone Inc; 1990:49-62.

207. Forrester JS, Diamond G, Chatterjee K, Swan HJC. Medical therapy of acute myocardial infarction by application of hemodynamic subsets: parts 1 and 2. *N Engl J Med.* 1976;295:1356-1362, 1404-1413.

208. Gunnar RM, Lambrew CT, Abrams W, et al. Task Force IV: pharmacologic interventions: emergency cardiac care. *Am J Cardiol.* 1982;50:393-408.

209. Johnson SA, Scanlon PJ, Loeb HS, Moran JM, Pifarre R, Gunnar RM. Treatment of cardiogenic shock in myocardial infarction by intraaortic balloon counterpulsation and surgery. *Am J Med.* 1977;62:687-692.

210. Kraus PA, Lipman J, Becker PJ. Acute preload effects of furosemide. *Chest.* 1990;98:124-128.

211. Hoffman JR, Reynolds S. Comparison of nitroglycerin, morphine and furosemide in treatment of presumed prehospital pulmonary edema. *Chest.* 1987;92:586-593.

212. Bukata R. Cardiogenic acute pulmonary edema. *Emerg Med Acute Care Essays.* 1990;14:1-5.

213. Roth A, Hochenberg M, Keren G, Terdiman R, Laniado S. Are rotating tourniquets useful for left ventricular preload reduction in patients with acute myocardial infarction and heart failure? *Ann Emerg Med.* 1987;16:764-767.

214. Mancini D, LeJemtel T, Sonneblick E. Intravenous use of amrinone for the treatment of the failing heart. *Am J Cardiol.* 1985;56:8B-15B.

215. Lee L, Bates ER, Pitt B, Walton JA, Laufer N, O'Neill WW. Percutaneous transluminal coronary angioplasty improves survival in acute myocardial infarction complicated by cardiogenic shock. *Circulation.* 1988;78:1345-1351.

216. Kahn JK, Rutherford BD, McConahay DR, et al. Outcome following emergency coronary artery bypass grafting for failed electric balloon coronary angioplasty in patients with prior coronary bypass. *Am J Cardiol.* 1990;66:285-288.

217. Tepe NA, Edmunds LH Jr. Operation for acute postinfarction mitral insufficiency and cardiogenic shock. *J Thorac Cardiovasc Surg.* 1985;89:525-530.

218. Bolman RN III, Cance C, Spray T, et al. The changing face of cardiac transplantation: the Washington University program, 1985-1987. *Ann Thorac Surg.* 1988;45:192-197.

219. DeWood MA, Notske RN, Hensley GR, et al. Intraaortic balloon counterpulsation with and without reperfusion for myocardial infarction shock. *Circulation.* 1980;61:1105-1112.

220. Emery RW, Joyce LD, Prieto M, Johnson K, Goldenberg IF, Pritzker MR. Experience with the symbion total artificial heart as a bridge to transplantation. *Ann Thorac Surg.* 1992;53:282-288.

221. Griffith B. Interim use of the Jarvik-7 artificial heart: lessons learned at Presbyterian-University Hospital of Pittsburgh. *Ann Thorac Surg.* 1989;47:158-166.

222. ISIS Collaborative Group. ISIS-4: randomised study of intravenous magnesium in over 50,000 patients with suspected acute myocardial infarction. *Circulation.* 1993;88(suppl):I-292. Abstract.

223. Jugdutt BI. Intravenous nitroglycerin unloading in acute myocardial infarction. *Am J Cardiol.* 1991;68:52D-63D.

224. Antman EM, Lau J, Kupelnick B, Mosteller F, Chalmers TC. A comparison of results of meta analyses of randomized control trials and recommendations of clinical experts: treatments for myocardial infarction. *JAMA.* 1992;268:240-248.

225. Lau J, Antman EM, Jimenez-Silva J, Kupelnick B, Mosteller F, Chalmers TC. Cumulative meta-analysis of therapeutic trials for myocardial infarction. *N Engl J Med.* 1992;327:248-254.

226. Yusuf S, Collins R, MacMahon S, Peto R. Effect of intravenous nitrates on mortality in acute myocardial infarction: an overview of the randomized trials. *Lancet.* 1988;1:1088-1092.

227. Jugdutt BI, Warnica JW. Intravenous nitroglycerin therapy to limit myocardial infarct size, expansion, and complications: effect of timing, dosage, and infarct location. *Circulation.* 1988;78:906-919.

228. Yusuf S. Interventions that potentially limit myocardial infarct size: overview of clinical trials. *Am J Cardiol.* 1987;60:11A-17A.

229. ISIS (Second International Study of Infarct Survival) Collaborative Group. Randomized trial of intravenous streptokinase, oral aspirin, both, or neither among 17 187 cases of suspected acute myocardial infarction: ISIS-2. *Lancet.* 1988;2:349-360.

230. Eisenberg MS, Aghababian RV, Bossaert L, Jaffe AS, Ornato JP, Weaver WD. Thrombolytic therapy. *Ann Emerg Med.* 1993;22:417-427.

231. Zehender M, Kasper W, Kauder E, Schionthaler M, Geibel A, Olesehewski M, Just H. Right ventricular infarction as an independent predictor of prognosis after acute inferior myocardial infarction. *N Engl J Med.* 1993;328:981-988.

232. Wellens HJ. Right ventricular infarction. *N Engl J Med.* 1993;328:1036-1038.

233. Merriman CS, Kalbfleisch ND. Thrombolysis in acute myocardial infarction following prolonged cardiopulmonary resuscitation. *Acad Emerg Med.* 1994;1:61-66.

234. Jaffe AS. Prophylactic lidocaine for suspected acute myocardial infarction? *Heart Dis Stroke.* 1992;1:179-183.

235. Applebaum D, Halperin E. Asystole following a conventional therapeutic dose of lidocaine. *Am J Emerg Med.* 1986;4:143-145.

236. Hargarten K, Chapman PD, Stueven HA, Waite EM, Mateer JR, Haecker P, Aufderheide TP, Olson DW. Prehospital prophylactic lidocaine does not favorably affect outcome in patients with chest pain. *Ann Emerg Med.* 1990;19:1274-1279.

237. MacMahon S, Collins R, Peto R, Koster RW, Yusuf S. Effects of prophylactic lidocaine in suspected acute myocardial infarction: an overview of results from randomized controlled trials. *JAMA.* 1988;260:1910-1916.

238. Berntsen RF, Rasmussen K. Lidocaine to prevent ventricular fibrillation in the prehospital phase of suspected acute myocardial infarction: the North-Norwegian Lidocaine Intervention Trial. *Am Heart J.* 1992;124:1478-1483.

239. Wyse DG, Kellen J, Rademaker AW. Prophylactic versus selective lidocaine for early ventricular arrhythmias of myocardial infarction. *J Am Coll Cardiol.* 1988;12:507-513.

240. Teo KK, Yusuf S, Collins R, Held PH, Peto R. Effects of intravenous magnesium in suspected acute myocardial infarction: overview of randomized trials. *BMJ.* 1991;303:1499-1503.

241. Rasmussen HS, McNair P, Norregard P, Backer V, Lindeneg O, Balslev S. Intravenous magnesium in acute myocardial infarction. *Lancet.* 1986;1:234-236.

242. Ryan T, Faxon D, Gunnar R, et al. Guidelines for percutaneous transluminal coronary angioplasty: a report of the American College of Cardiology/American Heart Association Task Force on assessment of Diagnostic and Therapeutic Cardiovascular Procedures. *J Am Coll Cardiol.* 1988;12:529-545.

243. Gibbons RJ, Holmes DR, Reeder GS, Bailey KR, Hopfenspirger MR, Gersh BJ. Immediate angioplasty compared with the administration of a thrombolytic agent followed by conservative treatment for myocardial infarction. *N Engl J Med.* 1993;328:685-691.

244. Grines CL, Browne KF, Marco J, et al. A comparison of immediate angioplasty with thrombolytic therapy for acute myocardial infarction. *N Engl J Med.* 1993;328:673-679.

245. Zijlstra F, de Boer MJ, Hoorntje JC, Reiffers S, Reiber JH, Suryapranata H. A comparison of immediate coronary angioplasty with intravenous streptokinase in acute myocardial infarction. *N Engl J Med.* 1993;328:680-684.

246. Lange RA, Hillis LD. Immediate angioplasty for acute myocardial infarction. *N Engl J Med.* 1993;328:726-728.

247. Eisenberg MS, Smith M. The farmer and the cowman should be friends: emergency physicians and cardiologists must work together to ensure rapid initiation of thrombolytic therapy. *Ann Emerg Med.* 1988;17:653-654. Editorial.

248. Gomez C. Time is brain! *J Stroke Cerebrovasc Dis.* 1993;3:1-20.

249. Modell JH. Drowning. *N Engl J Med.* 1993;328:253-256.

250. Goodwin AP, Pearce AJ. The human wedge: a manoevre to relieve aortocaval compression during resuscitation in late pregnancy. *Anaesthesia.* 1992;47:433-434.

251. Tsai A, Kallsen G. Epidemiology of pediatric prehospital care. *Ann Emerg Care.* 1987;16:284.

252. Zaritsky A, Nadkarni V, Getson P, Kuehl K. CPR in children. *Ann Emerg Med.* 1987;16:1107-1111.

253. Lewis JK, Minter MG, Eshelman SK, et al. Outcome of pediatric resuscitation. *Ann Emerg Med.* 1983;12:297-299.

254. Torphy DE, Minter MG, Thompson BM, et al. Cardiopulmonary arrest and resuscitation of children. *Am J Dis Child.* 1984;138:1099-1102.

255. Ludwig S, Kettrick RC, Parker M. Pediatric cardiopulmonary resuscitation. *Clin Pediatr.* 1984;23:71-75.

256. Bayes de Luna A, Coumel P, Leclercq JF. Ambulatory sudden cardiac death: mechanisms of production of fatal arrhythmia on the basis of data from 157 cases. *Am Heart J.* 1989:117:151-159.

257. Weaver WD, Hill D, Fahrenbruch CE, et al. Use of automatic external defibrillator in the management of out-of-hospital cardiac arrest. *N Engl J Med.* 1988;319:661-666.

258. Walsh CK, Krongrad E. Terminal cardiac electrical activity in pediatric patients. *Am J Cardiol.* 1983;51:557-561.

259. Eisenberg M, Bergner L, Hallstrom A. Epidemiology of cardiac arrest and resuscitation in children. *Ann Emerg Med.* 1983;12:672-674.

260. Chandra NC, Krischer JP. The demographics of cardiac arrest support "phone fast" for children. *Circulation.* 1993;88(suppl):I-193. Abstract.

261. Coffing CR, Quan L, Graves JR, Cummins RO, et al. Etiologies and outcomes of the pulseless, nonbreathing pediatric patient presenting with ventricular fibrillation. *Ann Emerg Med.* 1992;21:1046. Abstract.

262. O'Rourke PP. Outcome of children who are apneic and pulseless in the emergency room. *Crit Care Med.* 1986;14:466-468.

263. Applebaum D. Advanced prehospital care for pediatric emergencies. *Ann Emerg Med.* 1985;14:7.

264. Kyriacou DN, Kraus JF, Arcinire E. Effect of immediate resuscitation on childhood outcomes after aquatic submersion injury. *Ann Emerg Med.* 1992;21:1046. Abstract.

265. Quan L, Wentz KR, Gore EJ, Copass MK. Outcome and predictors of outcome in pediatric submersion victims receiving prehospital care in King County, Washington. *Pediatrics.* 1990;86:586-593.

266. Lister G. Oxygen delivery in lambs: cardiovascular and hematologic development. *Am J Physiol.* 1979;237:H668-H681.

267. Eckenhoff JE. Some anatomic considerations of the infant larynx influencing endotracheal anesthesia. *Anesthesiology.* 1951;12:401-413.

268. Coté CJ, Todres ID. The pediatric airway. In: Coté CJ, Todres ID, Goudsouzian NG, eds. *A Practice in Pediatric Anesthesia.* Philadelphia, Pa: WB Saunders Co; 1993.

269. Donn SM, Kuhns LR. Mechanisms of endotracheal tube movement with change of head position in the neonate. *Pediatric Radiol.* 1980;9:39-43.

270. Hazinski MF. Children are different. In: Hazinski MF, ed. *Nursing Care of the Critically Ill Child.* 2nd ed. St Louis, Mo: Mosby Year Book; 1992.

271. Chernick V, Avery ME. The functional basis of respiratory pathology. In: Kendig EL, ed. *Disorders of the Respiratory Tract in Children.* Philadelphia, Pa: WB Saunders Co; 1977.

272. Davis GM, Cureau MA. Pulmonary mechanics in newborn respiratory control. *Clin Perinatol.* 1987;14:551-558.

273. Rudolph AM, Heymann MA. Cardiac output in the fetal lamb: the effects of spontaneous and induced changes of heart rate on right and left ventricular output. *Am J Obstet Gynecol.* 1976;124:183-189.

274. Zaritsky A. Pharmacokinetics of catecholamines in critically ill children: 'You pays your money and you takes your choice.' *Crit Care Med.* 1993;21:645-647. Editorial.

275. Bruce DA. Head injuries in the pediatric population. *Curr Probl Pediat.* 1990;20:61-107.

276. Hennes H, Lee M, Smith D, Sty JR, Losek J. Clinical predictors of severe head trauma in children. *Am J Dis Child.* 1988;142:1045-1047.

277. Kraus JF, Fife D, Conroy C. Pediatric brain injuries: the nature, clinical course, and early outcomes in a defined United States' population. *Pediatrics.* 1987;79:501-507.

278. Luerssen TG, Klauber MR, Marshall LF. Outcome from head injury related to patient's age: a longitudinal prospective study of adult and pediatric head injury. *J Neurosurg.* 1988;68:409-416.

279. Tepas JJ III, DiScala C, Ramenofsky ML, Barlow B. Mortality and head injury: the pediatric perspective. *J Pediatr Surg.* 1990;25:92-96.

280. Gorelick MH, Shaw KN, Baker MD. Effect of ambient temperature on capillary refill in healthy children. *Pediatrics.* 1993;92:699-702.

281. Davis HW, Gartner JC, Galvis AG, Michaels RH, Mestad PH. Acute upper airway obstruction: croup and epiglottitis. *Pediatr Clin North Am.* 1981;28:859-880.

282. Graham N. Done in, fed up, burned out: too much attrition in EMS. *J Emerg Med Serv.* 1981;6:24-31.

Adjuncts for Airway Control, Ventilation, and Oxygenation

Chapter 2

The objectives of respiratory support are to ensure a patent airway, provide supplemental oxygen, and institute positive-pressure ventilation when spontaneous breathing is inadequate or absent. Special devices can help control the airway, ventilate the patient, and provide oxygenation. This chapter describes these devices and the techniques for their use.

Overview

In the patient who is breathing spontaneously, supplemental oxygen may prevent cardiac or respiratory arrest. Anyone in respiratory distress or cardiovascular crisis with the potential for decreased blood oxygen content or compromised oxygen transport should receive supplemental oxygen.

A patient can make spontaneous respiratory efforts but still have inadequate alveolar ventilation because of respiratory depression or fatigue. Inadequate ventilation may also result because of upper airway obstruction from foreign material such as food, vomit, or blood clots or from a posterior displacement of the tongue or epiglottis, occluding the pharynx or larynx. In the person who is not breathing, airway obstruction may be more difficult to recognize. In the breathing patient, significant partial upper airway obstruction is recognized when the patient has noisy airflow during inspiration (stridor or "crowing") and becomes cyanotic (late sign). Also, in the breathing patient, the contractions of the accessory muscles of respiration cause retractions of the suprasternal, supraclavicular, and intracostal spaces. This condition should be treated as if the airway were completely obstructed. The management of foreign-body airway obstruction includes basic techniques, such as subdiaphragmatic abdominal thrusts (the Heimlich maneuver), and advanced techniques, such as direct laryngostomy or removal of the foreign body with forceps or suction. However, for airway obstruction produced by the tongue and epiglottis, head tilt with anterior displacement of the mandible (chin lift or jaw thrust) may be all that is needed to relieve the obstruction. If this is insufficient, an oropharyngeal or nasopharyngeal airway should be inserted.

If spontaneous ventilation is present after clearing the airway, the patient should receive supplemental oxygen. If spontaneous breathing is inadequate or absent, positive-pressure ventilation must be provided. The preferred technique depends on the circumstances, but a technique that also provides the best oxygenation should be used. Ventilation techniques include mouth-to-mouth (with barrier protection) and mouth-to-mask rescue breathing and the use of a bag-valve device, an oxygen-powered, manually triggered device, or an automatic transport ventilator.

Tracheal intubation is the preferred method for advanced airway control. Once the airway is protected by an endotracheal tube, ventilations need not be synchronized with chest compressions.[1] The recommended rate for ventilation during CPR in the adult is 12 to 15 per minute, using a tidal volume of 10 to 15 mL/kg. Alternative, but markedly less preferable, methods of airway control include the esophageal obturator airway, the esophageal gastric tube airway, the pharyngotracheal lumen airway, and the esophageal-tracheal Combitube (recommended only when endotracheal intubation is unavailable). Rarely, transtracheal catheter ventilation or cricothyrotomy is indicated. After intubation, positive-pressure ventilation should be continued.

Airway Control: Head and Jaw Position[2-6]

During acute airway obstruction of any cause, attempts to open the airway have the highest priority. Upper airway obstruction in the unconscious person most commonly is the result of the loss of tonicity of the submandibular muscles, which provide direct support to the tongue and indirect support to the epiglottis. Posterior displacement of the tongue occludes the airway at the level of the pharynx, and the epiglottis may occlude the airway at the level of the larynx. The basic technique for opening the airway is head tilt with anterior displacement of the mandible (chin lift and, if necessary, jaw thrust). In the trauma victim with suspected neck injury, the initial step for opening the airway is the chin lift or jaw thrust without head tilt. If the airway remains obstructed, then head tilt is added slowly and gently until the airway is open (Fig 1).

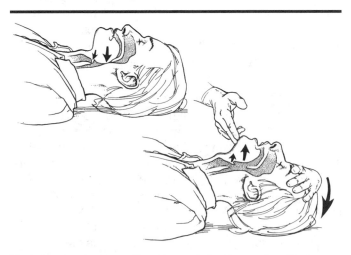

Fig 1. Opening the airway. Top, Airway obstruction produced by tongue and epiglottis. Bottom, Relief by head tilt–chin lift.

These maneuvers should be attempted before any airway adjunct is used, and if the patient is capable of spontaneous respiration, proper airway positioning may be all that is required. In some instances, an oropharyngeal or nasopharyngeal airway may be needed to maintain airway patency.

Airway Adjuncts

Oropharyngeal Airways

The oropharyngeal airway is a semicircular device to hold the tongue away from the posterior wall of the pharynx. Oropharyngeal airways facilitate suctioning of the pharynx and prevent the patient from biting and occluding an endotracheal tube. The most frequently used airways are plastic and disposable. The two common types are the Guedel and Berman. The Guedel is tubular, and the Berman has channels along its sides.[7]

Sizes for Adults

The size reflects the distance, in millimeters, from the flange to the distal tip. The following sizes are recommended:

Large adult: 100 mm (Guedel size 5)
Medium adult: 90 mm (Guedel size 4)
Small adult: 80 mm (Guedel size 3)

Techniques of Insertion

The mouth and pharynx should be cleared of secretions, blood, or vomit, using a rigid pharyngeal suction-tip (Yankauer) catheter. An easy way to place the airway is to turn it so that it is inserted backward as it enters the mouth. As the airway transverses the oral cavity and approaches the posterior wall of the pharynx, the operator rotates the airway into proper position. Another method is to move the tongue out of the way with a tongue blade depressor before the airway is inserted. The airway is in the proper position and of proper size when there are clear breath sounds on auscultation of the lungs during ventilation. Even with the use of this airway, proper head position must be maintained (Fig 2).

Complications

If the airway is too long, it may press the epiglottis against the entrance of the larynx, producing complete airway obstruction.[8] If the airway is not inserted properly, it may push the tongue posteriorly, aggravating upper airway obstruction. To prevent trauma, the operator should make sure that the lips and the tongue are not between the teeth and the airway. The airway should be used only in the unconscious patient because it may stimulate vomiting and laryngospasm in the conscious or semiconscious patient.

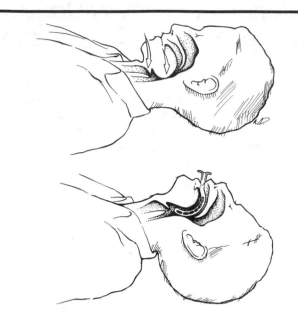

Fig 2. Placement of correctly inserted oropharyngeal airway. Top, Before insertion, incorrect head position. Bottom, After insertion, showing head tilted and oropharyngeal airway in place.

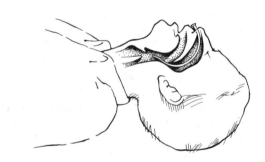

Fig 3. Nasopharyngeal airway in place. Note head tilted back for proper insertion.

Nasopharyngeal Airways

Nasopharyngeal airways are uncuffed tubes made of soft rubber or plastic. Their use is indicated when the insertion of an oropharyngeal airway is technically difficult or impossible (because of trismus, massive trauma around the mouth, mandibulo-maxillary wiring, etc) (Fig 3). They are also of value in the breathing semiconscious patient who does not tolerate an oropharyngeal airway.

Sizes for Adults

Size for this type of airway indicates the internal diameter (i.d.) in millimeters. The larger the internal diameter, the longer the tube. The following sizes are recommended:

Large adult: 8.0 to 9.0 i.d.
Medium adult: 7.0 to 8.0 i.d.
Small adult: 6.0 to 7.0 i.d.

Technique of Insertion

The proper-sized airway is lubricated with a water-soluble lubricant or anesthetic jelly and gently inserted close to the midline along the floor of the nostril into the posterior pharynx behind the tongue. If resistance is encountered, slight rotation of the tube may facilitate insertion at the angle of the nasal passage and the nasopharynx.

Complications

If the tube is too long, it may enter the esophagus, causing gastric distention and hypoventilation during artificial ventilation. This type of airway is better tolerated by the semiconscious patient. However, its use may also precipitate laryngospasm and vomiting in these patients. The insertion of the airway may injure the nasal mucosa with bleeding and possible aspiration of clots into the trachea. Suction may be needed to remove secretions or blood. It is still important to maintain head tilt with anterior displacement of the mandible by chin lift and, if necessary, jaw thrust when using this airway.

Immediately after insertion of the pharyngeal airway (oral or nasal), check for respirations. If respirations are absent or inadequate, artificial positive-pressure ventilation should be initiated with an appropriate device. If adjuncts are not available, mouth-to-mouth ventilation should be used.

Endotracheal Intubation

As a matter of necessity, oxygenation and ventilation of the lungs by exhaled-air methods or by the use of simple airway adjuncts usually precede attempts at endotracheal intubation. In the absence of a protected airway, however, attempts to provide adequate lung inflations may result in the generation of pharyngeal pressure high enough to cause gastric distention. In turn, gastric insufflation promotes regurgitation with the potential for aspiration of gastric contents into the lungs and may on occasion elevate the diaphragm enough to interfere with lung inflation. Therefore, as soon as possible during the resuscitative effort, the trachea should be intubated by properly trained personnel. This procedure isolates the airway, keeps it patent, reduces the risk of aspiration, permits suctioning of the trachea, ensures delivery of a high concentration of oxygen, provides a route for administration of certain drugs, and most important, ensures delivery of a selected tidal volume (10 to 15 mL/kg) to maintain adequate lung inflation.[9]

Because of the advanced skill required to place an endotracheal tube and the possibility of complications, its use should be restricted to medical and other healthcare personnel who are well trained and who either intubate frequently or are retrained frequently.[9] During endotracheal intubation, the maximum interruption of ventilation should be 30 seconds. Adequate ventilation and oxygenation must be provided between attempts.

Whenever possible, cricoid pressure should be applied by a second rescuer during endotracheal intubation *in adults* to protect against regurgitation of gastric contents and to ensure placement in the tracheal orifice. Pressure should be applied to the anterolateral aspects of the cricoid cartilage just lateral to the midline with the thumb and index finger.[10,11] Overzealous pressure should be avoided. Cricoid pressure should be maintained until the cuff of the endotracheal tube is inflated and proper tube position verified.

Indications for endotracheal intubation include

- Cardiac arrest with ongoing chest compressions
- Inability of a conscious patient to ventilate adequately
- Inability of the patient to protect the airway (coma, areflexia, or cardiac arrest)
- Inability of the rescuer to ventilate the unconscious patient with conventional methods

Once an endotracheal tube is in place, ventilation need not be synchronized with chest compressions. Rather, it should be performed asynchronously at 12 to 15 ventilations per minute while providing a tidal volume of 10 to 15 mL/kg.[1] Using a tidal volume of 15 mL/kg, a rate of 12 ventilations per minute is usually sufficient to provide mild to moderate hyperventilation. Also, using 100% inspired oxygen ($FIO_2 = 1.0$) and a tidal volume of 10 to 15 mL/kg, desaturation of hemoglobin should be avoided in most cases, no matter how severe the lung impairment.

Equipment

All equipment should be checked before attempting to intubate. Equipment checks should be done at least daily.

Laryngoscope (Fig 4). This device is used to expose the glottis. It has two parts: the handle, which holds the batteries for the light source, and the blade, with a bulb in the distal third. The connection point between the blade and the handle is called the fitting. This is where electrical contact is made. To check for adequate light,

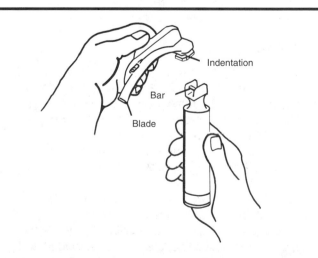

Fig 4. Attaching the laryngoscope blade to the handle. The blade locks into place when it is properly engaged.

the indentation of the blade is attached to the bar of the handle. When the blade is elevated to the point of making a right angle to the blade, the light should go on. If it does not, the bulb or the batteries may have malfunctioned. There are two common types of blades: a curved blade (MacIntosh design) and a straight blade (Miller, Wisconsin, Flagg, et al). Choice of blade is a matter of personal preference. However, different designs usually alter the technique used by the operator.

Endotracheal Tube. The tube is open at both ends. The proximal end has a standard 15-mm connector that will fit the devices for positive-pressure ventilation. The distal end has a cuff attached by the inflating tube to a one-way inflating valve designed to accept a syringe for inflation. A pilot balloon between the one-way valve and the inflating tube helps indicate that the cuff is inflated. The cuff must always be tested for integrity before insertion.

Tubes come in several sizes. Size markings indicate the internal diameter of the tube in millimeters (eg, 3.5 mm). The marking *IT* or *Z79* indicates that the tube has met certain tests or standards. The length of the tube, measuring from the distal end, is indicated at several intervals in centimeters. When the tube is properly placed, the depth marking in adults will usually lie between the 20- and 22-cm mark at the front teeth.

Stylet. A malleable stylet, preferably plastic coated, may be inserted through the tube. This device will help conform the endotracheal tube to any desired configuration, facilitating insertion of the tube into the larynx and trachea. The end of the stylet must always be recessed at least ½ inch from the distal end of the tube. It is often preferable to lubricate the stylet with a water-soluble lubricant before insertion into the endotracheal tube.

Additional Equipment:
- 10-mL syringe for cuff inflation
- Magill forceps, for removing foreign material or directing the tip of the tube into the larynx
- Water-soluble lubricant
- Suction unit with one pharyngeal rigid suction-tip (Yankauer) and one tracheal suction catheter

Technique

After checking all equipment, select the appropriate size tube. The proper endotracheal tube sizes for women usually are 7.0 to 8.0 mm i.d., and for men, 8.0 to 8.5 mm i.d. However, in an emergency a good standard-size tube for both women and men is 7.5 mm i.d.

Before insertion, the tube should be lubricated with a water-soluble lubricant. However, if this procedure delays intubation, it may be waived.

Next, obtain the proper head position (Fig 5). Three axes, those of the mouth, the pharynx, and the trachea, must be aligned to achieve direct visualization of the larynx. To accomplish this, the head is extended and the neck flexed (ie, the "sniffing position"). The head must not be allowed to hang over the end of a bed or table

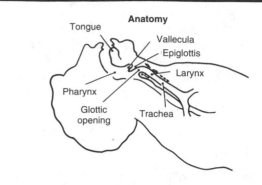

Fig 5. Essential anatomical landmarks in direct laryngoscopy.

because in that position intubation is virtually impossible. In many cases it is helpful to place several layers of toweling under the patient's occiput to elevate it a few inches above the level of the bed for proper flexion of the neck. Extension of the head is effected by the person performing the intubation.

It may be necessary to suction the mouth and pharynx before attempting intubation, but if proper procedure is used, this is often unnecessary.

The mouth is opened with the fingers of the right hand. The laryngoscope is held in the left hand and the blade inserted in the right side of the mouth, displacing the tongue to the left. Then the blade is moved toward the midline and advanced to the base of the tongue. Simultaneously the lower lip is moved away from the blade, using the right index finger. Gentleness and the avoidance of pressure on the lips and teeth are essential. When the curved blade is used (Fig 6), the tip of the blade is advanced into the vallecula (ie, the space between the base of the tongue and the pharyngeal surface of the epiglottis). When a straight blade is used, the tip of the blade (Fig 7) is inserted under the epiglottis. The glottic opening (Fig 8) is exposed by exerting upward traction on the handle. The handle must not be used with a prying motion, and the upper teeth must not be used as

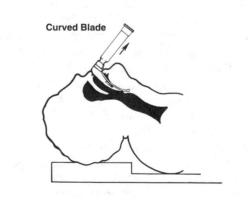

Fig 6. When a curved blade is used, the epiglottis is displaced anteriorly by upward traction, with the tip of the blade in the vallecula.

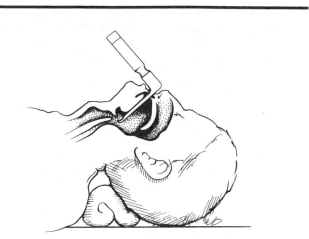

Fig 7. Laryngoscopic technique with a straight blade; the epiglottis is elevated anteriorly to expose the glottic opening.

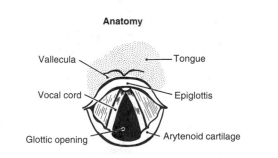

Anatomy

Vallecula — Tongue
Vocal cord — Epiglottis
Glottic opening — Arytenoid cartilage

Fig 8. Anatomical structures seen during direct laryngoscopy.

a fulcrum. It is best to point and firmly direct the end of the handle at a 30° to 45° angle toward and above the patient's feet. This will create a "sniffing position" and best facilitate visualization of the vocal cords.

An assistant, if available, may retract the right corner of the mouth. The tube is advanced through the right corner of the mouth and, under direct vision, through the vocal cords. If a stylet has been used, it should be removed from the tube at this time. The person performing the intubation should view the proximal end of the cuff at the level of the vocal cords and advance the tube about ½ to 1 inch (1 to 2.5 cm) farther into the trachea. This will place the tip of the tube about halfway between the vocal cords and the carina. In the average adult, this position usually results in the depth marking on the side of the tube lying between the 19- and 23-cm mark at the front teeth. The tube is then inflated with enough air to occlude the airway (usually 10 to 20 mL). This position will allow for some displacement of the tip of the tube during flexion or extension of the neck without extubation or movement of the tip into a main bronchus. Attempts at endotracheal intubation should take no longer than 30 seconds and preferably less than 15 seconds.

Tube placement must be confirmed simultaneously with delivery of the first manual breath by auscultating the epigastrium while observing the chest wall for evidence of thoracic inflation. If stomach gurgling occurs and chest wall expansion is not evident, inadvertent esophageal intubation should be assumed and no further breaths delivered. Proper placement should be reattempted after the victim has been well oxygenated (15 to 30 seconds of basic ventilatory techniques using $FIO_2 = 1.0$). If the chest wall rises appropriately and stomach insufflation is not suspected, auscultation of the left and right lung fields, at both the apices and anterior bases, should be performed and the status of breath sounds documented. When in doubt, ventilation through the tube should be suspended. If the location of the tube is difficult to confirm, direct visualization of the tube passing through the vocal cords should be performed to reconfirm its proper placement. After reconfirming the position of the marker at the front teeth, as originally noted during placement of the tube just past the cords, the tube should be secured. Once the tube is secured, an oropharyngeal airway should be placed. In the meantime, the patient should be ventilated with a tidal volume of 10 to 15 mL/kg. Slightly more volume can be provided for very obese patients and slightly less for patients with fragile intrathoracic airways or diminished lung volumes. Using 15 mL/kg, the respiratory rate during cardiac or respiratory arrest should be 10 to 12 breaths per minute (one breath every 5 to 6 seconds). During the initial phases after resuscitation from cardiac arrest, when spontaneous circulation has been restored, 12 to 15 breaths per minute (one every 4 to 5 seconds) should be provided. Each breath should be delivered into the lungs over a 2-second period using 100% oxygen during the early resuscitative phases.

Whenever feasible, a chest x-ray should be obtained to confirm proper placement. In patients suspected of having hypovolemia, severe obstructive lung disease, or asthma with increased resistance to exhalation, care should be taken to not induce air-trapping, which may result in a positive end-expiratory pressure (PEEP) effect.[12] In cases of hypovolemia, intravascular volume should be restored. With obstructive lung disease, lower respiratory rates should be used, allowing more complete exhalation of intrathoracic gas while bronchospasm is treated.

Devices that measure the concentration of exhaled carbon dioxide (end-tidal carbon dioxide detectors) should be used to assess proper endotracheal tube placement. A lack of carbon dioxide on the detector generally means that the tube is in the esophagus, particularly in patients with spontaneous circulation. Occasionally carbon dioxide may not be detected in cardiac arrest patients with extremely low blood flow to the lungs or in those with a large amount of dead space (eg, significant pulmonary embolus).[13-15]

A variety of electronic as well as simple, inexpensive, carbon dioxide detectors are available for both in-hospital and prehospital use.[16] The use of such devices as an adjunct to assessment of endotracheal tube position is strongly encouraged. However, no device or adjunct is a substitute for proper visualization of the endotracheal tube passing through the vocal cords. Proper training, supervision, and frequency of performance are the keys to guaranteeing successful intubation.[9]

Complications[17-19]

Without careful technique, trauma can easily occur during intubation. Lips or tongue can be compressed and lacerated between the blade of the laryngoscope and the teeth. The teeth themselves may be chipped. The tip of the tube or stylet may lacerate the pharyngeal or tracheal mucosa, resulting in bleeding, hematoma, or abscess formation. Rupture of the trachea has been reported.[20] Avulsion of an arytenoid cartilage and injury to the vocal cords is also possible. Other complications include pharyngeal-esophageal perforation[21] and intubation of the pyriform sinus.[22] In the semiconscious patient, vomiting and aspiration of gastric contents into the lower airway may occur. In the patient who is not in circulatory arrest, the stimulation of endotracheal intubation produces a significant release of epinephrine and norepinephrine, which may be manifested by hypertension, tachycardia, or arrhythmias.[23]

Insertion of the endotracheal tube into a main bronchus is perhaps the most frequent complication. The chest should be auscultated to check for bilateral breath sounds and examined for equal expansion of both sides during ventilation. Intubation of a bronchus can result in hypoxemia due to underinflation of the other lung. Accidental insertion of the endotracheal tube into the esophagus will result in no ventilation or oxygenation (unless the patient is still breathing spontaneously).[24]

To minimize complications, these recommendations should be followed:

- Tracheal intubation should be performed only by properly trained personnel.
- Endotracheal tubes and laryngoscopes should be immediately available to rescuers, and patients in cardiac arrest should be immediately intubated to diminish the risk of gastric insufflation.
- If a laryngoscope and tube are not readily available or if the attempt to place the tube is not successful within 20 to 30 seconds, rescuers should provide other basic ventilatory techniques with 100% oxygen until the next attempt is made, 20 to 30 seconds later. Cricoid pressure may decrease the incidence of gastric distention and pulmonary aspiration during positive-pressure ventilation before placement of the tube.[10,25,26] It should be applied if an assistant is available and familiar with the technique. To find the cricoid cartilage, the depression below the thyroid cartilage (Adam's apple) is palpated (Fig 9). This corresponds to the cricothyroid membrane. The prominence inferior to that is the cricoid cartilage. Firm backward pressure is applied with the thumb

and index finger to the anterolateral aspects of the cricoid. The pressure is released when the endotracheal tube cuff has been inflated and proper tube position verified.
- Because of the possible need for prolonged intubation after resuscitation, a tube with a high-volume, low-pressure cuff is recommended for use during CPR. The intracuff pressure is measured and adjusted to 25 to 35 cm H_2O. The minimum intracuff pressure to prevent aspiration appears to be 25 cm H_2O,[27] and the pressure that produces a decrease in capillary mucosal blood flow (ischemia) is higher than 40 cm H_2O.[28]

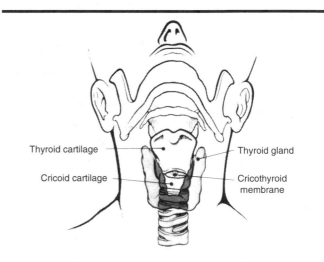

Thyroid cartilage

Cricoid cartilage

Thyroid gland

Cricothyroid membrane

Fig 9. Landmarks for locating the cricothyroid membrane.

Patients With Severe Trauma

The trauma victim poses special problems in airway control. If there is a known or suspected cervical spine injury, excessive movement of the spine, which may produce or exacerbate spinal cord injury, must be avoided. All patients with multiple trauma, head injury, or facial trauma should be presumed to have a cervical spine injury until proper evaluation can be made to rule it out. In other instances, a high index of suspicion for spinal injury may be triggered by the type of accident (eg, motor vehicle accident, fall from a height), and precautions should be taken.

The first step in airway control in the victim with a suspected neck injury is chin lift or jaw thrust, without head tilt. If the airway remains obstructed, head tilt is added slowly and carefully until the airway is open. A trained rescuer should stabilize the head in a neutral position during airway manipulation to prevent excessive flexion, extension, or lateral movement of the head during airway control. To avoid having to manipulate the head and neck during intubation, "blind" nasal intubation may be used in breathing patients, but this technique should be performed only by an experienced person and spinal immobilization still maintained manually because the stimulus may result in spontaneous neck movement. Nasal intubation is relatively contraindicated in a patient with facial fractures and fractures at the base of the skull. In this instance, direct orotracheal intubation should be attempted while a second person provides spinal immobilization. Suctioning of the upper airway should be provided if necessary. If endotracheal intubation cannot be performed, cricothyrotomy or tracheotomy may be necessary. The use of paralytic drugs is recommended in those with trismus and clenched jaws. Again, these techniques should be used only by persons experienced in these procedures.

Administering Supplemental Oxygen

Most acute cardiac patients without respiratory distress should receive 2 liters of oxygen per minute by a nasal cannula to provide comfort. In those with mild respiratory distress, 5 to 6 L/min should be administered. Because oxygen content and oxygen delivery are compromised during severe respiratory distress, acute congestive heart failure, or cardiac arrest, a system that provides a high inspired oxygen concentration (preferably 100%) should be used during artificial ventilation. Once it is feasible, oxygen should be titrated according to the PaO_2, or oxygen saturation value, considering the patient's potential for respiratory deterioration (eg, suspected aspiration of vomitus or congestive heart failure). Early on, however, endotracheal intubation and 100% oxygen are advised in the most serious cases.

The person caring for a patient needing supplemental oxygen should understand the oxygen delivery system, which consists of

- Oxygen supply (cylinder or piped wall oxygen)
- Valve handles to open the cylinder, pressure gauge, and flowmeter
- Tubing connecting the oxygen supply to the patient's oxygen administration device
- Humidifier

Four devices are commonly used to administer supplemental oxygen.[29]

Nasal Cannula

A nasal cannula is a low-flow system that does not provide sufficient gas to supply an entire inspired tidal volume. Thus, a large part of the tidal volume will be mixed with ambient gas (room air). The inspired oxygen concentration depends on the flow of oxygen in the unit and the tidal volume of the patient. For every liter per minute of flow increase, the inspired oxygen concentration will be increased by approximately 4%. In turn, the oxygen concentration supplied by the nasal cannula with a flow of 1 to 6 L/min to a patient with a normal tidal volume

is 24% to 44%. This system is acceptable for patients with minimal or no respiratory distress or oxygenation problem, particularly when they find a face mask bothersome.

Face Mask

The face mask is usually well tolerated by the adult patient. However, to avoid accumulation in the mask reservoir of exhaled air that might be rebreathed, the oxygen flow should be higher than 5 L/min. The recommended flow is 8 to 10 L/min. As with the nasal cannula, inspired oxygen is diluted by room air. This system can provide oxygen concentrations as high as 40% to 60%. It should be provided to those who may require higher concentrations of inspired oxygen.

Face Mask With Oxygen Reservoir

This system, in which there is a constant flow of oxygen into an attached reservoir, will provide oxygen concentrations higher than 60%. A flow of 6 L/min will provide approximately 60% oxygen concentration, and each liter per minute increase in flow will increase the inspired oxygen concentration by 10%. When used properly, at 10 L/min the oxygen concentration is almost 100%. This system is most appropriate for spontaneously breathing patients who require the highest possible oxygen concentrations, at least initially, but who cannot be tracheally intubated immediately because of an intact gag reflex or clenched teeth (eg, in head injury, carbon monoxide poisoning, or near-drowning). Such patients may have diminished levels of consciousness and a risk for nausea and vomiting. A tight-fitting mask always requires close monitoring. Suctioning devices should be immediately available.

Venturi Mask

The Venturi mask provides a high gas flow but with a more fixed oxygen concentration. Oxygen under pressure is passed through a narrow orifice and, after leaving the orifice, provides a subatmospheric pressure that entrains room air into the system. The oxygen concentration is adjusted by changing the size of the orifice and oxygen flow. This type of oxygen delivery, which offers more control over inspired oxygen fractions, is used frequently in patients with chronic hypercarbia (COPD) and moderate to severe hypoxemia because the administration of high oxygen concentrations in this type of patient may produce respiratory depression. In these cases, a sudden increase in PaO_2 blocks the stimulant effect of hypoxemia on the respiratory centers. However, *never* withhold oxygen from patients who have respiratory distress simply because you suspect hypoxic ventilatory drive. With the Venturi mask, oxygen concentrations can be adjusted to 24%, 28%, 35%, and 40%. The mask with 24% oxygen concentration is used initially. The patient is observed for respiratory depression, and PaO_2 is evaluated. The oxygen concentration is then titrated to the preferred level of PaO_2. Pulse oximeters can be useful to quickly titrate the oxygen concentration before arterial blood gas analysis.

Techniques for Oxygenation and Ventilation

Mouth-to-Mouth[30] and Mouth-to-Nose[31]

The basic technique of expired air ventilation can provide adequate volumes of air to the victim. The only limitation is the vital capacity of the rescuer and the oxygen concentration because the concentration of oxygen in exhaled air is approximately 17%. However, the average person's vital capacity is several liters larger than the 10 to 15 L/min tidal volume needed to provide adequate lung inflation. Also, if a simple oxygen source is available (eg, nasal cannula or simple face mask delivery system), the rescuer can breathe the oxygen source and deliver a breath that is only 5% less than what the rescuer inspires. Remember, professional rescuers should always have a barrier device available to perform mouth-to-mouth breathing.

Mouth-to-Mask[32-34]

A well-fitting mask can be an effective, simple adjunct for use in artificial ventilation by appropriately trained rescuers.

Masks should be made of transparent material to allow detection of regurgitation; capable of a tight fit on the face, with an oxygen inlet; and available in one average size for adults and additional sizes for infants and children.

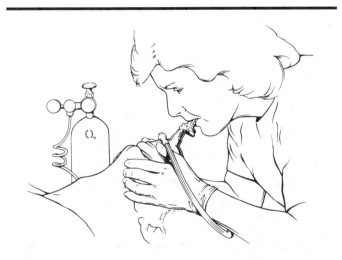

Fig 10. Mouth-to-mask ventilation with a one-way valve.

The mouth-to-mask technique (Fig 10) has many advantages:

- It eliminates direct contact with the victim's mouth and nose.
- It makes possible administration of supplemental oxygen.
- It eliminates exposure to exhaled gas if the unit has a one-way valve.
- It is easy to teach and easy to learn.
- It can provide effective ventilation and oxygenation.
- It has been shown to be superior to bag-valve–mask technique in delivering adequate tidal volume (on manikins).

With mouth-to-mask ventilation an oxygen flow rate of 10 L/min will provide an inspired oxygen concentration of about 50%. A mask can also be used to enrich the oxygen mixture delivered to a spontaneously breathing patient. An oxygen flow rate of 15 L/min will provide an inspired oxygen concentration of approximately 80%.

A one-way valve should be connected to the mask and oxygen tubing connected to the inlet with an oxygen flow rate of 10 L/min. An oropharyngeal airway can be inserted if needed. Head tilt should be applied, and the mask is placed on the victim's face. With the thumb side (thenar) of the palm of both hands, pressure should be applied to the sides of the mask. Upward pressure can then be applied to the mandible, just in front of the ear lobes, using the index, middle, and ring fingers of both hands while maintaining head tilt. If no oropharyngeal airway is in place, the rescuer should keep the mouth open. The operator should then blow in through the opening of the mask, observing the rise and fall of the chest.

If a trained assistant is available, cricoid pressure should be applied. This will prevent gastric inflation during positive-pressure ventilation and reduce the possibility of regurgitation and aspiration. Delivery of the breath should be slow and steady (minimum inspiratory time of 2 seconds).

Bag-Valve Devices[35-37]

Bag-valve devices, which consist of a self-inflating bag and a nonrebreathing valve, may be used with a mask, an endotracheal tube, or other invasive airway devices.

Most commercially available adult bag-valve–mask units have a volume of approximately 1600 mL, which is usually adequate for proper lung inflation with endotracheal intubation. However, in several studies many rescuers were unable to deliver adequate tidal volumes (10 to 15 mL/kg) to unintubated manikins.[38-42] In adults bag-valve units may provide less ventilatory volume than mouth-to-mouth or mouth-to-mask ventilation. Also, a single rescuer may have difficulty providing a leakproof seal to the face while squeezing the bag adequately and maintaining an open airway. For this reason, manually operated, self-inflating bag-valve–mask units are used most effectively by at least two well-trained and experienced rescuers working together.

An adequate bag-valve unit should have these features:

- A self-refilling bag that is easily cleaned and sterilized
- A nonjam valve system allowing for a minimum oxygen inlet flow of 15 L/min
- A no–pop-off valve
- Standard 15-mm/22-mm fittings
- A system for delivering high concentrations of oxygen through an ancillary oxygen inlet at the back of the bag or by an oxygen reservoir[36]
- A true nonrebreathing valve
- Ability to perform satisfactorily under all common environmental conditions and extremes of temperature
- Availability in both adult and pediatric sizes

As with mouth-to-mask systems, oral airways, head position, rate of delivery of the breath, and the option of cricoid pressure are important considerations.

Technique

The rescuer is positioned at the top of the victim's head. If there is no concern about neck injury, the victim's head is tilted back if possible and raised on a towel or pillow to better achieve a sniffing position. If the victim is unconscious, an oropharyngeal airway is inserted. The victim's mouth should remain open under the mask.

While maintaining the head in extension, the selected tidal volume (preferably 10 to 15 mL/kg) should be delivered over 2 seconds. Effective ventilation is more likely when two rescuers use these devices, one to hold the mask and one to squeeze the bag. A third person may provide cricoid pressure. This can be attempted with two rescuers, but it is often awkward.

If only one rescuer is available for respiratory support, the mask is applied to the face with the rescuer's left hand. The last two or three fingers are placed on the mandible while the remaining fingers are placed on the mask. The rescuer must maintain head tilt, keeping the anterior displacement of the mandible (jaw lift), while finding the optimum mask fit.

The bag is then compressed with the right hand and the chest observed to make certain that the lungs are being ventilated. The rescuer may want to use his or her body to compress the bag to achieve a larger tidal volume.

Complications

The most frequent problem with this type of device is the inability to provide adequate ventilatory volumes to a patient who is not intubated. Proper use of a bag-valve device with certain invasive airways (EOA or EGTA) also depends on a proper mask fit and requires training, practice, and demonstrated proficiency.

Esophageal Obturator Airway

The esophageal obturator airway (EOA)[43-47] is a Class IIb intervention (acceptable, possibly helpful) compared with the endotracheal tube, which is Class I (definitely helpful). The EOA is a large-bore tube, 37 cm in length, with a high-volume cuff close to the distal end. When inflated in the lower part of the adult esophagus, the cuff helps prevent regurgitation and gastric insufflation during positive-pressure ventilation. The tube is mounted through a clear face mask. It has multiple openings at the level of the pharynx through which air or oxygen is delivered by artificial ventilation into the lungs via the larynx and trachea. When properly applied to the victim's face, the mask helps prevent leaks around and through the nose. The single-length tube is designed for adults only.

The EOA is a proposed alternative to tracheal intubation. It has been suggested for use in situations where the rescuer cannot (or is not permitted to) intubate the trachea, when equipment for endotracheal intubation is not available or is not working properly, and in patients for whom tracheal intubation is technically unfeasible.[44,45] Visualization is not required for insertion, nor is there any need for hyperextension of the head and flexion of the neck. However, it is often difficult to maintain an adequate seal between the mask and the face, so ventilatory volumes can be inadequate. Also, inadvertent tracheal intubation as well as other serious complications can occur.[48-50] Thus, esophageal airways must be used only by persons properly trained and proficient in their use.[51] Practice and retraining are mandatory to maintain proficiency.

Technique of Insertion (Fig 11)

Before insertion, the tube should be attached to the mask and the cuff tested for leaks. The cuff is then deflated before insertion and the tube lubricated.

With the head in midposition or slight flexion, the rescuer elevates the tongue and jaw with one hand and with the other inserts the tube through the mouth and into the esophagus. The tube is advanced until the mask is seated on the face. When this is accomplished, the cuff should lie below the level of the carina (Fig 12). If the cuff is above the carina, when inflated it may compress the posterior membranous portion of the trachea and cause tracheal obstruction. If it is difficult to advance the tube during insertion, withdraw the tube slightly, improve the tongue-jaw lift, and readvance the tube.

Because the tube may enter the trachea, the rescuer should first deliver one or two positive-pressure ventilations before inflating the cuff while auscultating the epigastrium. If the chest rises, indicating that the obturator is not in the trachea, the cuff is inflated with 35 mL of air. After inflation of the cuff, the epigastrium is again auscultated, and if the tube is improperly placed in the trachea, gurgling sounds will be heard. In such cases the tube should be carefully removed and the patient given

Insertion of Esophageal Airway

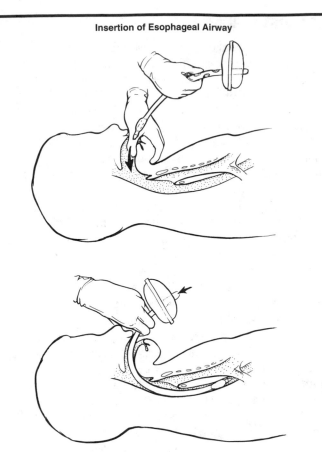

Fig 11. An obturator is introduced into the esophagus by elevating the tongue and jaw from the corner of the mouth with one hand, with head and neck flexed forward.

Final Position of Esophageal Airway and Mask

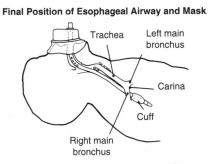

Trachea

Left main bronchus

Carina

Cuff

Right main bronchus

Fig 12. Properly positioned obturator airway. The rim of the face mask must be sealed tightly against the face to effect an airtight seal.

positive-pressure (oxygenated) breaths by other means until a second attempt at placement. If the chest wall still rises and no epigastric sounds are heard, breath sounds are auscultated bilaterally in the midaxillary line.

Final Position of Esophageal Airway and Mask

The trachea should be intubated with a cuffed endotracheal tube before the EOA is removed because regurgitation frequently follows removal. If the patient is conscious and no longer requires intubation, he or she should be turned onto the side and suction provided. The EOA should be removed within 2 hours after its insertion. This will reduce the incidence of necrosis of the esopha-

geal mucosa secondary to ischemia in the area of the cuff.

Complications [48-51]

A number of studies have demonstrated that ventilation and oxygenation with the EOA may be inferior to that achieved with tracheal intubation and that there may be an increased risk of complications. Esophageal injuries, including rupture, have been reported. In the semiconscious victim, the insertion of the EOA could produce laryngospasm, vomiting, and aspiration. The EOA does not protect the patient against aspiration of foreign material in the mouth and pharynx into the trachea and bronchi.

To minimize complications, these recommendations should be followed:

- The EOA should be used only by properly trained and supervised personnel.[51]
- It should not be used in persons younger than 16 years, conscious persons, those who are breathing spontaneously, those who have esophageal disease, or those who have swallowed caustic material.
- It should not be left in place for longer than 2 hours.
- Force should not be used during insertion.
- Suction should be immediately available during insertion and removal.
- Before removal of the EOA, the patient should be fully conscious or tracheal intubation should be performed.

Esophageal Gastric Tube Airway[52]

The esophageal gastric tube airway (EGTA) is a modified EOA (Fig 13). The EGTA is open throughout its length, allowing passage of a gastric tube for decompression of the stomach. Because of this added advantage, it may be preferred to the EOA. Ventilation is carried out by way of an additional port in the mask. The technique of insertion and complications are the same as those for the EOA.

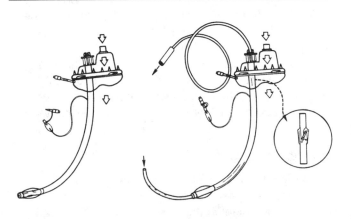

Fig 13. Esophageal gastric tube airway (EGTA). The gastric tube can be passed through the lumen of the airway. Ventilation is carried out by standard mask technique, with the mask held securely against the face.

Several other devices similar to the EOA have been developed and marketed:

- Esophageal pharyngeal airway (EPA)[51]
- Pharyngotracheal lumen airway (PTL)[53]
- Laryngeal mask airway (LMA)[54]
- Tracheal-esophageal airway (TEA)[55]
- Berman intubating-pharyngeal airway (BIPA)[56]
- Esophageal-tracheal Combitube (ETC)[57]

These devices are *not* equivalent to endotracheal intubation for airway control and ventilation. In some instances, however, they are acceptable and helpful.

Laryngeal Mask Airway

This device is widely used in Europe for airway control during elective anesthesia. It consists of a tube similar to an endotracheal tube, with a small mask with an inflatable circumferential cuff intended for placement in the posterior pharynx, sealing the region of the base of the tongue and laryngeal opening.

Although this device is effective under controlled operating room conditions, its use requires considerable training and skill. No studies have evaluated its effectiveness for emergency situations. A recent study performed in the operative setting showed it could be placed safely and successfully by paramedics.[58]

Pharyngotracheal Lumen Airway

The PTL is a double-lumen tube (shorter than the EOA or EGTA) that is inserted blindly into the oropharynx.[53] As a result, either an esophageal or a tracheal placement is possible. Assessment of the placement is made, and the patient is then ventilated through the port (lumen) that provides lung inflation. An airway seal is obtained with a large proximal balloon that fills the oropharynx. A smaller distal balloon is then inflated and the device secured to the patient with a strap fastened around the neck. In the trachea, the distal balloon provides a tracheal seal similar to that provided by the cuff of an endotracheal tube. In the esophagus, the cuff acts like an obturator.

The PTL was designed specifically to address two major concerns reported with the use of the EOA — inadvertent tracheal intubation and improper face-to-mask seal. With the PTL, the problem of inadvertent tracheal intubation is not considered a complication because it is expected in many cases. Also, the pharyngeal balloon theoretically helps to avoid the problems of proper face-to-mask seal observed with EOA and EGTA devices. Some authors, however, still describe an inadequate seal with the pharyngeal balloon.[59] Also, replacement of the PTL with a tracheal tube can pose problems. To date, however, these complications have not been frequent. Most available studies indicate that the PTL device can provide adequate oxygenation and ventilation.[60] However, further study is necessary before its widespread use can be endorsed. Although the PTL may be better than properly performed basic airway techniques

(eg, mouth-to-mask), this comparison has not been evaluated directly.

Combination Esophageal-Tracheal Tube

The esophageal-tracheal double-lumen airway is an invasive device structurally and functionally similar to the PTL.[51,57,61-63] The twin-lumen tube is inserted without visualization of the vocal cords. Its location is then assessed, and the patient is ventilated through the opening that provides inflation of the lungs. Technically the ETC is similar to the PTL except for a modified pharyngeal balloon and a simpler basic structure.

The reported advantages of the ETC include those proposed for the PTL, but because of a difference in design (no stylet in the distal lumen), it provides for immediate suctioning of gastric contents. Also, in an undiagnosed tracheal placement, the spontaneously breathing patient may breathe through multiple small ports in the unused lumen. Unlike the PTL, the ETC has a self-adjusting, self-positioning posterior pharyngeal balloon.[57]

To date, the overall complication rate reported with ETC use is low. However, experience with this device has been limited primarily to the hospital setting. More experience is necessary before this device can be recommended for widespread use. Available data show that ventilation and oxygenation with the ETC compare favorably with that achieved with the endotracheal tube. At times oxygenation has been greater with the ETC, which is thought to be due to a PEEP effect induced by the higher resistance of the ETC compared with the endotracheal tube. However, this same elevated resistance to airflow or air-trapping may also account for the higher $PaCO_2$ seen with ETC use.[61]

Considerable training is required for safe and appropriate use of any of the alternative invasive airway devices described above. Despite such training, serious complications with such devices occur.[46,48,64-66] The endotracheal tube remains the optimal adjunct to achieve adequate airway protection and ventilation during CPR.[9,51]

Transtracheal Catheter Ventilation[67-71]

Transtracheal catheter ventilation is a temporary emergency procedure to provide oxygenation when airway obstruction cannot be relieved by other methods. The technique consists of insertion of an over-the-needle catheter through the cricothyroid membrane and intermittent jet ventilation. It is only used as a temporizing emergency technique when airway obstruction cannot be immediately relieved.

Equipment (Fig 14)

- Over-the-needle catheter with a 5- or 10-mL syringe
- Pressure-regulating valve and a pressure gauge attached to a high-pressure (30 to 60 psi) oxygen supply

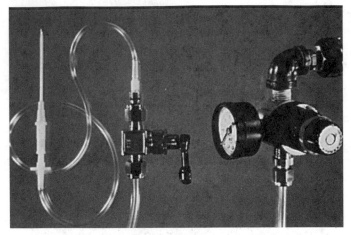

Fig 14. Equipment used in transtracheal catheter ventilation.

- High-pressure tubing connecting the pressure-regulating valve to a hand-operated release valve
- Relief valve connected by tubing to the catheter

Technique

The small depression below the thyroid cartilage (Adam's apple) corresponds to the cricothyroid membrane (Fig 9). The catheter-needle combination attached to the syringe is directed in the midline downward and caudally at an angle of 45°. Negative pressure is applied to the syringe during insertion. Entrance of air into the syringe indicates that the needle is in the trachea (Fig 15).

The catheter is advanced over the needle, the needle and syringe are withdrawn, and the distal end of the tubing is attached to the catheter (Fig 16). An assistant holds the hub of the catheter to prevent accidental removal during tracheostomy or endotracheal intubation. The release valve is opened, and oxygen under pressure is introduced into the trachea. The pressure is adjusted to levels that allow adequate lung expansion. The chest must be observed carefully and the release valve turned off as soon as the chest rises. Exhalation then occurs passively.

The chest is observed during exhalation for deflation. If the chest remains inflated, a complete proximal airway obstruction may be present. In this case a second large-bore catheter is inserted next to the first catheter. If the chest continues to remain distended, cricothyrotomy should be performed.

Complications [72]

The high pressure used during ventilation and the possibility of air entrapment may produce a pneumothorax. Hemorrhage may occur at the site of the needle insertion, especially if the thyroid is perforated. If the needle is advanced too far, the esophagus may be perforated. This technique does not allow direct suctioning of secretions — some secretions are expelled by the retrograde flow during jet ventilation into the pharynx. Subcutaneous or mediastinal emphysema may occur. A disadvantage of the technique is that while it can provide oxygenation, it

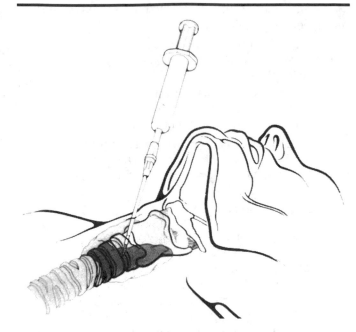

Fig 15. Insertion of a catheter with an attached syringe into the trachea across the cricothyroid membrane.

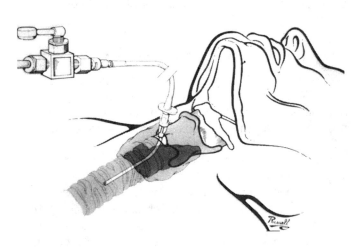

Fig 16. Attachment of a transtracheal ventilation system to an intratracheal catheter.

usually does not allow enough ventilation to adequately eliminate carbon dioxide.

Cricothyrotomy[73-78]

The cricothyrotomy technique allows rapid entrance to the airway for temporary ventilation and oxygenation in patients in whom airway control is not possible by other methods. In surgical cricothyrotomy the cricothyroid membrane is opened with a scalpel (Fig 17) and a tube is inserted as described below.[74] Percutaneous dilational cricothyrotomy is performed by making a small vertical incision and advancing a cricothyrotomy tube over a guidewire and dilator.[78]

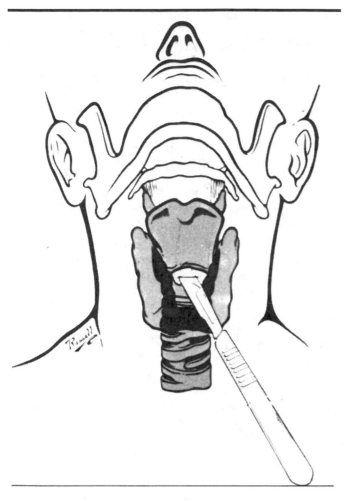

Fig 17. Cricothyrotomy performed with a scalpel.

Surgical Technique

- If possible, the area is cleaned with alcohol or another antiseptic solution.
- A horizontal incision is made with a knife at the level of the cricothyroid membrane.
- The handle is inserted through the incision and rotated 90°.
- A pediatric tube, the largest possible, is inserted through this opening.
- Ventilation is done with a bag-valve unit, and the highest available oxygen concentration is provided.

Complications

Hemorrhage, false passage, perforation of the esophagus, and subcutaneous or mediastinal emphysema are possible complications.

Tracheostomy

Surgical opening of the trachea and insertion of the tracheostomy tube should ideally be performed under controlled conditions in the operating room by a skilled person after the airway has first been secured by an endotracheal tube, translaryngeal catheter, or cricothyrotomy. It is not considered an appropriate procedure for urgent situations such as airway obstruction or cardiac arrest.

Oxygen-Powered, Manually Triggered Devices

Oxygen-powered, manually triggered devices have been used in prehospital care for more than 20 years, despite little scientific evidence supporting their use. Pressure-cycled ventilators and resuscitator-inhalators are obsolete (Class III) and should not be used.

Today most manually triggered (time-cycled) devices (oxygen-powered breathing devices) deliver high instantaneous flow rates by a manual control button. This is inconsistent with the 1986 recommendation to limit their flow to 40 L/min.[79-81] These devices can be used with a mask, an endotracheal tube, an esophageal airway, or a tracheostomy tube. With high flow rates, gastric distention is likely when these devices are used with a mask. Unfortunately the flow rate from these devices as currently manufactured is back-pressure dependent, and they may cease to deliver gas flow prematurely without alerting the rescuer.[81] This is more likely to occur in patients with high airway resistance or poor lung compliance or both, and particularly in those receiving chest compressions. In victims with normal pulmonary mechanics, these devices still deliver high inspiratory flow rates and predispose to gastric insufflation. Even in intubated victims, high flow rates may lead to maldistribution of ventilation and intrapulmonary shunting.

To overcome these problems, manually triggered, oxygen-powered resuscitators should provide

- A constant flow rate of 100% oxygen at less than 40 L/min
- An inspiratory pressure relief valve that opens at approximately 60 cm H_2O and vents any remaining volume to the atmosphere or ceases gas flow; the valve may be set to 80 cm H_2O when used by advanced rescuers but only under expert medical direction
- An audible alarm that sounds whenever the relief valve pressure is exceeded to alert the rescuer that the victim requires high inflation pressures and may not be receiving adequate ventilatory volumes
- Satisfactory operation under common environmental conditions and extremes of temperature
- A demand flow system that does not impose additional work. Many oxygen-powered breathing devices currently available have restricted flow rates of 40 L/min and require unacceptably high triggering pressures in the demand mode and should not be used for spontaneously breathing patients.

Oxygen-powered devices also should have the following minimum design features: (1) a standard 15-mm/22-mm coupling for mask, endotracheal tube, EOA, tracheostomy tubes, and other alternative invasive airways; (2) a rugged, breakage-resistant mechanical design that is compact and easy to hold; and (3) a trigger positioned so that both hands of the rescuer can remain on the mask to hold it in position. These devices must not be used by untrained persons because the potential for complications is high. They should not be used on pediatric patients.

Technique

The unit is checked and an appropriate mask or other airway adjunct is attached. The mask is placed on the victim's face, using both hands to maintain a tight fit and to keep the lower jaw elevated. The valve is opened by activating the level or pushing the button.

The chest is observed for proper expansion. The valve is deactivated as soon as the chest rises. The flow of oxygen then ceases, and the exhaled gases are vented through a one-way valve into the atmosphere.

This type of device can also be used in the spontaneously breathing patient. The valve is opened by the negative pressure generated by the inspiratory effort of the patient; flow ceases when the negative pressure ends.

Complications

In patients who are not intubated, opening of the lower esophageal sphincter and subsequent gastric distention is a frequent complication. Barotrauma to the lungs manifested by pneumothorax or subcutaneous emphysema is also possible with the use of these devices. **Oxygen-powered breathing devices are not designed for use in pediatric patients.**

Automatic Transport Ventilators

Automatic transport ventilators (ATVs) specifically designed for prehospital care have been used in Europe since the early 1980s.[82] Their acceptance in the United States has been slow, partly because of concerns that ventilation cannot be synchronized with external chest compression in cardiac arrest. However, if necessary, the rescuer controlling the airway can indicate to the other rescuer when the device is triggered, and in intubated patients it is unnecessary to synchronize ventilation with compression.

A number of ATVs are available commercially.[83-85] Recent studies comparing ATVs with bag-valve devices during intrahospital transport show that ATVs are superior at maintaining a constant minute ventilation and adequate arterial blood gases.[86,87] Bag-valve devices are effective only when tidal volume and minute ventilation are constantly monitored, an approach that is impractical in prehospital care.[88]

Recent studies have also shown that ATVs are as effective as other devices used in prehospital care in intubated patients.[83,89,90] In addition, studies on mechanical models and in animals demonstrate the superiority of ATVs for ventilating unintubated patients in respiratory arrest.[42] Nevertheless, further studies evaluating the use of these devices are warranted.

ATVs offer many advantages to alternative methods of ventilation:

- In intubated patients they free the rescuer for other tasks.
- In unintubated patients the rescuer has both hands free for mask and airway maintenance.
- Cricoid pressure can be applied with one hand while the other seals the mask on the face.
- They provide a specific tidal volume, respiratory rate, and minute ventilation once set.

Recent studies have shown improved lung inflation with diminished or absent gastric insufflation when ATVs were compared with other devices, including mouth-to-mask, bag-valve–mask, and manually triggered devices, because of the lower inspiratory flow rates and longer inspiratory times provided by ATVs.

Disadvantages of ATVs include the need for an oxygen source and their unsuitability in children less than 5 years of age. Because ATVs require either an oxygen source or, in one instance, electric power, a bag-valve device or a mask should always be available if oxygen is depleted or if oxygen or electric power is unavailable.

ATVs should function as constant inspiratory flow rate generators and should have the following minimum features:

- A lightweight connector with a standard 15-mm/22-mm coupling for a mask, endotracheal tube, or other airway adjunct
- A lightweight (2- to 5-kg), compact, rugged design
- Capability of operating under all common environmental conditions and extremes of temperature
- A peak inspiratory pressure limiting valve set at 60 cm H_2O with the option of an 80 cm H_2O pressure (available for use at the discretion of the medical director) that is easily accessible to the user
- An audible alarm that sounds when the peak inspiratory limiting pressure is generated to alert the rescuer that low compliance or high airway resistance is resulting in a diminished tidal volume delivery
- Minimal gas consumption (eg, at a tidal volume of 1 L and a rate of 10 breaths per minute [10 L/min ventilation], the device should run for a minimum of 45 minutes on an E cylinder)
- Minimal gas compression volume in the breathing circuit
- Ability to deliver an FIO_2 of 1.0
- An inspiratory time of 2 seconds in adults and 1 second in children and maximal inspiratory flow rates of approximately 30 L/min in adults and 15 L/min in children
- At least two rates, 10 breaths per minute for adults and 20 breaths per minute for children

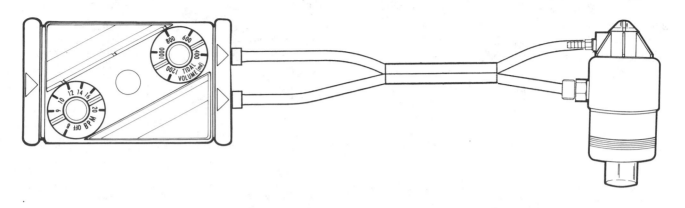

Fig 18. An automatic transport ventilator with adjustable knobs for frequency and tidal volume.

If a demand flow valve is incorporated into the ATV, it should deliver a peak inspiratory flow rate on demand of at least 100 L/min at −2 cm H_2O triggering pressure to minimize the work of breathing.

Some ATVs allow faster breathing rates. Caution should be used in selecting these higher rates since adequate time for exhalation is imperative to prevent air-trapping and a PEEP effect.[12] Additional desirable features include a pressure manometer, provision for continuous positive airway pressure in more sophisticated ventilators, at least two controls (one for rate and one for tidal volume), and low-pressure alarms to indicate depletion of oxygen cylinders and ventilator disconnect. ATVs that meet the recommendations noted above are Class I.

Technique

The unit is checked and attached to an appropriate airway adjunct. Tidal volume and (on some units) rate are set, and, if necessary, the unit is turned on (Fig 18). The chest is observed for proper expansion. The tidal volume knob can be adjusted to provide the desired chest excursion. The device should be checked periodically.

Complications

In the unintubated patient, gastric distention may occur. Since the device is gas powered, loss of gas supply may make it inoperative. In settings where gas supply is limited, a bag-valve device should be kept as a backup.

Suction Devices

The rigid pharyngeal catheter (Yankauer) is used to clear secretions, blood clots, and other foreign material from the mouth and pharynx. The tracheobronchial suction catheter is used to clear secretion through the endotracheal tube or the nasopharynx. High suction pressure is needed for pharyngeal suction (higher than −120 mm Hg). The tracheobronchial suction catheter should have a design that will

- Produce minimal trauma to the mucosa with molded ends and side holes
- Be long enough to pass through the tip of the endotracheal tube
- Have minimal frictional resistance during insertion through the endotracheal tube
- Be sterile and disposable

Technique of Tracheobronchial Suctioning[29]

The equipment is checked, and the suction pressure is set between −80 and −120 mm Hg. The patient is preoxygenated with 100% oxygen for 5 minutes.

Using sterile technique, the catheter is inserted without closing the side opening in the proximal end of the catheter. The catheter is advanced to the desired location, approximately at the level of the carina. Suction is applied intermittently by closing the side opening while the catheter is withdrawn with a rotating motion. The patient's electrocardiographic rhythm should be monitored.

Suction should not be applied for more than 15 seconds. If arrhythmias or bradycardias are present, suctioning is immediately discontinued and the patient is manually ventilated and oxygenated.

Before repeating the procedure, the patient is ventilated with 100% oxygen for about 30 seconds.

Complications [91,92]

The most serious complication of suctioning is the sudden onset of severe hypoxemia secondary to a decrease in lung volume and interrupting ventilation. If severe enough this may lead to cardiac arrest. Suctioning produces stimulation to the airway similar to that produced during endotracheal intubation and may increase arterial pressure and tachycardia. Significant cardiac arrhythmias or bradycardias may occur during suctioning, and this may be due to the decrease in myocardial oxygen supply secondary to hypoxemia or to an increase in oxygen demand due to hypertension or an increase in heart rate. Some patients may manifest bradycardia and hypotension due to vagal stimulation. The stimulation of the catheter in the mucosa may trigger coughing, resulting in increased intracranial pressure and reduced cerebral blood flow. The incidence of mucosal damage is high and includes edema, hemorrhage, and areas of ulceration and loss of integrity, which may result in tracheal infection.

References

1. Melker RJ. Asynchronous and other alternative methods of ventilation during CPR. *Ann Emerg Med.* 1984;13(pt 2):758-761.
2. Safar P, Escarraga LA, Chang F. Upper airway obstruction in the unconscious patient. *J Appl Physiol.* 1959;14:760-764.
3. Morikawa S, Safar P, DeCarlo J. Influence of the head-jaw position upon upper airway patency. *Anesthesiology.* 1961;22:265-270.
4. Ruben HM, Elam JO, Ruben AM, Greene DG. Investigation of upper airway problems in resuscitation: studies of pharyngeal x-rays and performance by laymen. *Anesthesiology.* 1961;22:271-279.
5. Guildner CW. Resuscitation — opening the airway: a comparative study of techniques for opening an airway obstructed by the tongue. *JACEP.* 1976;5:588-590.
6. Boidin MP. Airway patency in the unconscious patient. *Br J Anaesth.* 1985;57:306-310.
7. Lilienfeld SM, Berman RA. Correspondence. *Anesthesiology.* 1950;11:136-137.
8. Spoerel WE. The unprotected airway. In: Spoerel WE, ed. *Problems of the Upper Airway.* Boston, Mass: Little, Brown and Company; 1972;10:1-36. International Anesthesiology Clinics.
9. Pepe PE, Copass MK, Joyce TH. Prehospital endotracheal intubation: rationale for training emergency medical personnel. *Ann Emerg Med.* 1985;14:1085-1092.
10. Sellick BA. Cricoid pressure to control regurgitation of stomach contents during induction of anaesthesia. *Lancet.* 1961;2:404-406.
11. Wraight WJ, Chamney AR, Howells TH. The determination of an effective cricoid pressure. *Anaesthesia.* 1983;38:461-466.
12. Pepe PE, Marini JJ. Occult positive end-expiratory pressure in mechanically ventilated patients with airflow obstruction: the auto-PEEP effect. *Am Rev Respir Dis.* 1982;126:166-170.
13. Falk JL, Rackow EC, Weil MH. End-tidal carbon dioxide concentration during cardiopulmonary resuscitation. *N Engl J Med.* 1988;318:607-611.
14. Sayah AJ, Peacock WF, Overton DT. End-tidal CO_2 measurement in the detection of esophageal intubation during cardiac arrest. *Ann Emerg Med.* 1990;19:857-860.
15. Ornato JP, Garnett AR, Glauser FL. Relationship between cardiac output and the end-tidal carbon dioxide tension. *Ann Emerg Med.* 1990;19:1104-1106.
16. Ornato JP, Shipley JB, Racht EM, et al. Multicenter study of a portable, hand-size, colorimetric end-tidal carbon dioxide detection device. *Ann Emerg Med.* 1992;21:518-523.
17. Blanc VF, Tremblay NA. The complications of tracheal intubation: a new classification with a review of the literature. *Anesth Analg.* 1974;53:202-213.
18. Jones GO, Hale DE, Wasmuth CE, Homi J, Smith ER, Viljoen J. A survey of acute complications associated with endotracheal intubation. *Cleve Clin Q.* 1968;35:23-31.
19. Taryle DA, Chandler JE, Good JT Jr, Potts DE, Sahn SA. Emergency room intubations — complications and survival. *Chest.* 1979;75:541-543.
20. Thompson DS, Read RC. Rupture of the trachea following endotracheal intubation. *JAMA.* 1968;204:995-997.
21. Wolff AP, Kuhn FA, Ogura JH. Pharyngeal-esophageal perforations associated with rapid oral endotracheal intubation. *Ann Otol Rhinol Laryngol.* 1972;81:258-261.
22. Stauffer JL, Petty TL. Accidental intubation of the pyriform sinus: a complication of 'roadside' resuscitation. *JAMA.* 1977;237:2324-2325.
23. Derbyshire DR, Chmielewski A, Fell D, Vater M, Achola K, Smith G. Plasma catecholamine responses to tracheal intubation. *Br J Anaesth.* 1983;55:855-860.
24. Pollard BJ, Junius F. Accidental intubation of the oesophagus. *Anaesth Intensive Care.* 1980;8:183-186.
25. Keith A. The mechanism underlying various methods of artificial respiration. *Lancet.* March 13, 1909:745-749.
26. Salem MR, Wong AY, Mani M, Sellick BA. Efficacy of cricoid pressure in preventing gastric inflation during bag-mask ventilation in pediatric patients. *Anesthesiology.* 1974;40:96-98.
27. Bernhard WN, Cottrell JE, Sivakumaran C, Patel K, Yost L, Turndorf H. Adjustment of intracuff pressure to prevent aspiration. *Anesthesiology.* 1979;50:363-366.
28. Nordin U. The trachea and cuff-induced tracheal injury: an experimental study on causative factors and prevention. *Acta Otolaryngol.* 1977;345(suppl):1-71.
29. Shapiro BA, Harrison RA, Trout CA. *Clinical Application of Respiratory Care.* Chicago, Ill: Year Book Medical Publishers Inc; 1975:130-137.
30. Elam JO, Greene DG. Mission accomplished: successful mouth-to-mouth resuscitation. *Anesth Analg.* 1961;40:578-580.
31. Ruben H. The immediate treatment of respiratory failure. *Br J Anaesth.* 1964;36:542-549.
32. Safar P. Pocket mask for emergency artificial ventilation and oxygen inhalation. *Crit Care Med.* 1974;2:273-276.
33. Harrison RR, Maull KI, Keenan RL, Boyan CP. Mouth-to-mask ventilation: a superior method of rescue breathing. *Ann Emerg Med.* 1982;11:74-76.
34. Lawrence PJ, Sivaneswaran N. Ventilation during cardiopulmonary resuscitation: which method? *Med J Aust.* 1985;143:443-446.
35. Ruben H. A new non-rebreathing valve. *Anesthesiology.* 1955;16:643-645.
36. Carden E, Hughes T. Evaluation of manually operated self-inflating resuscitation bags. *Anesth Analg.* 1975;54:133-138.
37. Elam JO. Bag-valve-mask O_2 ventilation. In: Safar P, Elam JO, eds. *Advances in Cardiopulmonary Resuscitation.* The Wolf Creek Conference on Cardiopulmonary Resuscitation. New York, NY: Springer-Verlag Inc; 1977:73-79.
38. Elling R, Politis J. An evaluation of emergency medical technicians' ability to use manual ventilation devices. *Ann Emerg Med.* 1983;12:765-768.
39. Hess D, Baran C. Ventilatory volumes using mouth-to-mouth, mouth-to-mask, and bag-valve-mask techniques. *Am J Emerg Med.* 1985;3:292-296.
40. Cummins RO, Austin D, Graves JR, Litwin PE, Pierce J. Ventilation skills of emergency medical technicians: a teaching challenge for emergency medicine. *Ann Emerg Med.* 1986;15:1187-1192.
41. Johannigman JA, Branson RD, Davis K Jr, Hurst JM. Techniques of emergency ventilation: a model to evaluate tidal volume, airway pressure, and gastric insufflation. *J Trauma.* 1991;31:93-98.
42. Fuerst RS, Banner MJ, Melker RJ. Gastric inflation in the unintubated patient: a comparison of common ventilating devices. *Ann Emerg Med.* 1992;21:636. Abstract.
43. Don Michael TA, Lambert EH, Mehran A. 'Mouth-to-lung airway' for cardiac resuscitation. *Lancet.* 1968;2:1329. Abstract.
44. Don Michael TA. The esophageal obturator airway: a critique. *JAMA.* 1981;246:1098-1101.
45. Smith JP, Bodai BI, Seifkin A, Palder S, Thomas V. The esophageal obturator airway: a review. *JAMA.* 1983;250:1081-1084.
46. Donen N, Tweed WA, Dashfsky S, Guttormson B. The esophageal obturator airway: an appraisal. *Can Anaesth Soc J.* 1983;30:194-200.
47. Bryson TK, Benumof JL, Ward CF. The esophageal obturator airway: a clinical comparison to ventilation with a mask and oropharyngeal airway. *Chest.* 1978;74:537-539.
48. Pilcher DB, DeMeules JE. Esophageal perforation following use of esophageal airway. *Chest.* 1976;69:377-380.
49. Yancey W, Wears R, Kamajian G, Derovanesian J. Unrecognized tracheal intubation: a complication of the esophageal obturator airway. *Ann Emerg Med.* 1980;9:18-20.
50. Auerbach PS, Geehr EC. Inadequate oxygenation and ventilation using the esophageal gastric tube airway in the prehospital setting. *JAMA.* 1983;250:3067-3071.
51. Pepe PE, Zachariah BS, Chandra NC. Invasive airway techniques in resuscitation. *Ann Emerg Med.* 1993;22:393-403.

52. Gordon AS. Improved esophageal obturator airway (EOA) and new esophageal gastric tube airway (EGTA). In: Safar P, Elam JO, eds. *Advances in Cardiopulmonary Resuscitation*. New York, NY: Springer-Verlag Inc; 1977:58-64.

53. Niemann JT, Rosborough JP, Myers R, Scarberry EN. The pharyngeo-tracheal lumen airway: preliminary investigation of a new adjunct. *Ann Emerg Med*. 1984;13:591-596.

54. Brain AI, McGhee TD, McAteer EJ, Thomas A, Abu-Saad MA, Bushman JA. The laryngeal mask airway: development and preliminary trials of a new type of airway. *Anaesthesia*. 1985;40:356-361.

55. Eisenberg RS. A new airway for tracheal or esophageal insertion: description and field experience. *Ann Emerg Med*. 1980;9:270-272.

56. Berman RA. A method for blind oral intubation of the trachea or esophagus. *Anesth Analg*. 1977;56:866-867.

57. Frass M, Frenzer R, Rauscha F, Weber H, Pacher R, Leithner C. Evaluation of esophageal tracheal Combitube in cardiopulmonary resuscitation. *Crit Care Med*. 1987;15:609-611.

58. Pennant JH, Walker MB. Comparison of the endotracheal tube and laryngeal mask in airway management by paramedical personnel. *Anesth Analg*. 1992;74:531-534.

59. McMahan S, Ornato JP, Racht EM, et al. Multi-agency prehospital evaluation of the pharyngeo-tracheal lumen (PTL) airway. *Prehosp Disaster Med*. 1992;7:13-18.

60. McMahon JM, Bartlett R, Schafermayer RW, et al. Comparison of the pharyngeal-tracheal lumen airway to the endotracheal tube: an EMS field trial. *Prehosp Disaster Med*. 1989;4:77. Abstract.

61. Frass M, Rodler S, Frenzer R, Ilias W, Leithner C, Lackner F. Esophageal tracheal Combitube, endotracheal airway, and mask: comparison of ventilatory pressure curves. *J Trauma*. 1989;29: 1476-1479.

62. Frass M, Frenzer R, Rauscha F, Schuster E, Glogar D. Ventilation with the esophageal tracheal Combitube in cardiopulmonary resuscitation: promptness and effectiveness. *Chest*. 1988;93:781-784.

63. Frass M, Frenzer R, Zdrahal F, Hoflehner G, Porges P, Lackner F. The esophageal tracheal Combitube: preliminary results with a new airway for CPR. *Ann Emerg Med*. 1987;16:768-772.

64. Hammargren Y, Clinton JE, Ruiz E. A standard comparison of esophageal obturator airway and endotracheal tube ventilation in cardiac arrest. *Ann Emerg Med*. 1985;14:953-958.

65. Meislin HW. The esophageal obturator airway: a study of respiratory effectiveness. *Ann Emerg Med*. 1980;9:54-59.

66. Strate RG, Fischer RP. Midesophageal perforations by esophageal obturator airways. *J Trauma*. 1976;16:503-509.

67. Jacoby JJ, Hamelberg W, Ziegler CH, Flory FA, Jones JR. Transtracheal resuscitation. *JAMA*. 1956;162:625-628.

68. Dallen LT, Wine R, Benumof JL. Spontaneous ventilation via transtracheal large-bore intravenous catheters is possible. *Anesthesiology*. 1991;75:531-533.

69. Spoerel WE, Narayanan PS, Singh NP. Transtracheal ventilation. *Br J Anaesth*.1971;43:932-939.

70. Jacobs HB. Emergency percutaneous transtracheal catheter and ventilator. *J Trauma*. 1972;12:50-55.

71. Smith RB, Babinski M, Klain M, Pfaeffle H. Percutaneous transtracheal ventilation. *JACEP*. 1976;5:765-770.

72. Poon YK. Case history number 89: a life-threatening complication of cricothyroid membrane puncture. *Anesth Analg*. 1976;55: 298-301.

73. Brantigan CO, Grow JB Sr. Cricothyroidotomy: elective use in respiratory problems requiring tracheotomy. *J Thorac Cardiovasc Surg*. 1976;71:72-81.

74. McGill J, Clinton JE, Ruiz E. Cricothyrotomy in the emergency department. *Ann Emerg Med*. 1982;11:361-364.

75. Simon RR, Brenner BE. Emergency cricothyroidotomy in the patient with massive neck swelling, part 1: anatomical aspects. *Crit Care Med*. 1983;11:114-118.

76. Simon RR, Brenner BE, Rosen MA. Emergency cricothyroidotomy in the patient with massive neck swelling, part 2: clinical aspects. *Crit Care Med*. 1983;11:119-123.

77. Melker RJ, Banner MJ. Work imposed by breathing through cricothyrotomy tubes. Presented at the Sixth World Congress on Emergency and Disaster Medicine; September 1989; Hong Kong.

78. Florete OG. Airway management. In: Civetta JM, Taylor RW, Kirby RR, eds. *Critical Care*. 2nd ed. Philadelphia, Pa: JB Lippincott Co; 1992:1430-1431.

79. Pearson JW, Redding JS. Evaluation of the Elder demand valve resuscitator for use by first-aid personnel. *Anesthesiology*. 1967;28:623-624.

80. Osborn HH, Kayen D, Horne H, Bray W. Excess ventilation with oxygen-powered resuscitators. *Am J Emerg Med*. 1984;2:408-413.

81. Melker RJ, Banner MJ. Positive pressure and spontaneous ventilation characteristics of demand-flow valves: implications for resuscitation. *Ann Emerg Med*. In press.

82. Harber T, Lucas BG. An evaluation of some mechanical resuscitators for use in the ambulance service. *Ann R Coll Surg Engl*. 1980;62:291-293.

83. Branson RD, McGough EK. Transport ventilators. In: Banner MJ, ed. *Problems in Critical Care*. Philadelphia, Pa: JB Lippincott Co; 1990;4:254-274.

84. Nolan JP, Baskett PJF. Gas-powered and portable ventilators: an evaluation of six models. *Prehosp Disaster Med*. 1992;7:25-34.

85. McGough EK, Banner MJ, Melker RJ. Variations in tidal volume with portable transport ventilators. *Respiratory Care*. 1992;37: 233-239.

86. Braman SS, Dunn SM, Amico CA, Millman RP. Complications of intrahospital transport in critically ill patients. *Ann Intern Med*. 1987;107:469-473.

87. Gervais HW, Eberle B, Konietzke D, Hennes HJ, Dick W. Comparison of blood gases of ventilated patients during transport. *Crit Care Med*. 1987;15:761-763.

88. Weg JG, Haas CF. Safe intrahospital transport of critically ill ventilator-dependent patients. *Chest*. 1989;96:631-635.

89. Melker RJ. A clinical evaluation of the pneuPAC ventilator. Presented at the Fourth World Congress on Intensive and Critical Care Medicine; July 1985; Jerusalem, Israel.

90. Hurst JM, Davis K Jr, Branson RD, Johannigman JA. Comparison of blood gases during transport using two methods of ventilatory support. *J Trauma*. 1989;29:1637-1640.

91. Marx GF, Steen SN, Arkins RE, et al. Endotracheal suction and death. *N Y State J Med*. 1968;68:565-566.

92. Shim C, Fine N, Fernandez R, Williams MH Jr. Cardiac arrhythmias resulting from tracheal suctioning. *Ann Intern Med*. 1969;71: 1149-1153.

Arrhythmias

Chapter 3

This chapter introduces the novice to basic methods of identifying cardiac electrical rhythms and describes the characteristics of various rhythms. An appendix discusses the cellular electrical activity of the heart.

Causes of Cardiac Arrhythmias

Cardiac arrhythmias result from the following three mechanisms:

- *Disturbances in Automaticity.* This may involve a speeding up or slowing down of areas of automaticity such as the sinus node (sinus tachycardia or sinus bradycardia), the atrioventricular (AV) node, or the myocardium. Abnormal beats (more appropriately called *depolarizations* rather than *beats* or *contractions*) may arise through this mechanism from the atria, the AV junction, or the ventricles. Abnormal rhythms, such as atrial or ventricular tachycardia (VT), may also occur.
- *Disturbances in Conduction.* Conduction may be either too rapid (as in Wolff-Parkinson-White syndrome) or too slow (as in atrioventricular [AV] block). The mechanism of reentry depends on the presence of slowed conduction.
- *Combinations of Altered Automaticity and Conduction.* A simple example would be a premature atrial contraction with first-degree AV block or atrial tachycardia with 3:1 or higher grades of AV block.

The Electrocardiogram: Key to Interpreting Arrhythmias

The electrocardiogram (ECG) is a recording of the electrical forces produced by the heart. The body acts as a giant conductor of electrical currents. Any two points on the body may be connected by electrical "leads" to register an ECG or to monitor the rhythm of the heart. The tracing recorded from the electrical activity of the heart forms a series of waves and complexes that have been arbitrarily labeled (in alphabetical order) the P wave, the QRS complex, the T wave, and the U wave (Fig 1). The waves or deflections are separated in most patients by regularly occurring intervals.

Depolarization of the atria produces the P wave; depolarization of the ventricles produces the QRS complex (Fig 2). Repolarization of the ventricles causes the T wave. The significance of the U wave is uncertain, but it may be due to repolarization of the Purkinje system. It appears at a time when many premature ventricular complexes (PVCs) occur and is affected by a variety of factors, such as digitalis and electrolytes.

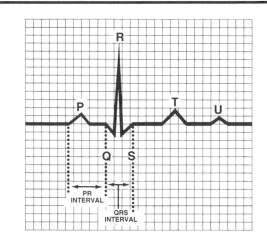

Fig 1. The electrocardiogram.

The PR interval extends from the beginning of the P wave (the beginning of atrial depolarization) to the onset of the QRS complex (the beginning of ventricular depolarization)(Fig 2). It should not exceed 0.20 second as measured on ECG graph paper, where each small square represents 0.04 second. The QRS complex represents the electrical depolarization of the ventricles. The upper limit of normal duration of the QRS is less than 0.12 second. A QRS duration of less than 0.12 second means that the impulse was initiated from the AV node or above (supraventricular). A wide QRS ($\geq$0.12 second) may signify conduction that either arises from the ventricle or comes from supraventricular tissue. Prolonged conduction through the ventricle produces a widened QRS.

The key to arrhythmia interpretation is the analysis of the form and interrelations of the P wave, the PR interval, and the QRS complex. The ECG should be analyzed with respect to its rate, its rhythm, the site of the dominant pacemaker, and the configuration of the P and QRS waves. The relation of the ECG rhythm strip to cardiac anatomy is shown in Fig 2. This is referred to as the normal sinus rhythm. The middle line in the diagram is at the bundle branches of the conduction system. Any malfunction above this point will affect the P wave and PR interval, whereas malfunction below this level will affect the QRS complex.

P Wave. If for some reason the sinus node fails to act as the normal cardiac pacemaker, other atrial foci may take over, and the P wave may have a different configuration. Alternatively, a secondary pacemaker (eg, the AV junction) may provide an "escape rhythm."

PR Interval. When conduction through the atria, the AV node, or bundle of His is slowed, the PR interval becomes longer. Changes in conduction through the AV

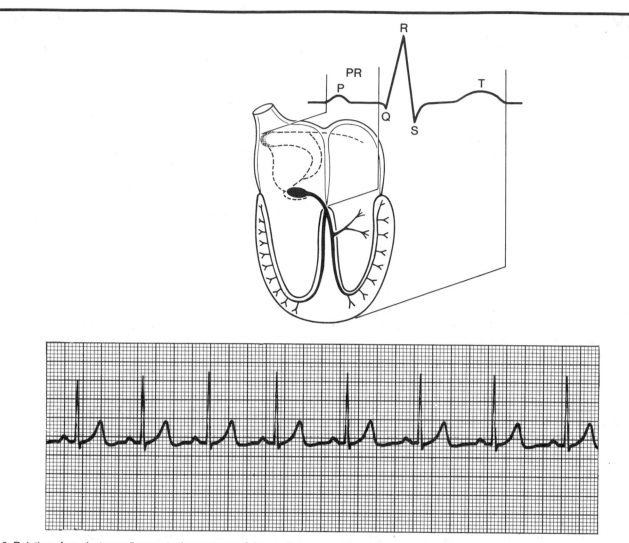

Fig 2. Relation of an electrocardiogram to the anatomy of the cardiac conduction system.

node are the most common cause of changes in the PR interval.

QRS Complex. If there is a delay or interruption in conduction in either bundle branch, the QRS will widen in a manner typical for either right or left bundle branch block. An ectopic focus that initiates an impulse from the ventricle also can alter the shape of the QRS. When an ectopic beat arises above the bundle branches, the ventricles are activated in a normal fashion and the QRS complex will remain the same, assuming that there is no conduction delay in either bundle branch. If the depolarization occurs below the bundle branches, the QRS complex will be widened and notched or slurred because a different sequence of conduction will ensue.

Monitoring Systems

There are many types of cardiac monitoring systems, but they generally consist of a monitor screen (cathode ray oscilloscope) on which the ECG is displayed and a write-out system that directly transcribes the rhythm strip onto paper. The write-out may be automatic or controlled by a switch, and a ratemeter may be set to write out a rhythm strip if the rate goes below a preset figure (eg, 50 beats per minute) or above a certain rate (eg, 120 beats per minute) for at least 6 seconds, and sometimes for as long as 30 seconds. A ratemeter triggered by the QRS complex of the ECG is usually part of the system. Lights and beepers may provide visual and audible signals of the heart rate.

Monitor leads or electrodes may be attached to the patient's chest or extremities. The chest leads must be placed to show clearly the waves and complexes of the ECG strip and to leave the chest clear for defibrillation if necessary.

Conventional locations for the chest electrodes in emergency medicine and intensive care units are illustrated in Fig 3. The arrow indicates the direction of polarity from negative to positive. In lead I the positive electrode is below the left clavicle and the negative below the right (Fig 3A). In lead II the positive electrode is below the left pectoral muscle and the negative below the right clavicle (Fig 3B). Lead III is displayed by attaching the positive electrode beneath the left pectoral muscle and the negative below the left clavicle (Fig 3C). Although these simulate or approximate the I, II, and III leads of the standard ECG, they are not identical.

Another popular monitoring lead is the MCL_1 lead (Fig 3D). To connect this lead, the negative electrode is placed near the left shoulder, usually under the outer third of the left clavicle, and the positive is placed to the right of the sternum in the fourth intercostal space. The ground electrode in all four leads can usually be placed almost anywhere but is commonly located below the right pectoral muscle or under the left clavicle. The electrodes are often color-coded for ease of application, lessening confusion in location. The negative lead is usually white, the positive lead is red, and the ground lead is black, green, or brown. The popular phrase "white-to-right, red-to-ribs, and black left over" helps to recall where the leads for lead II should be placed.

Remember the following points when monitoring patients:

1. A prominent P wave should be displayed if organized atrial activity is present. Leads that show the P wave clearly should be chosen.
2. The QRS amplitude should be sufficient to properly trigger the ratemeter.
3. The patient's precordium must be kept exposed so that defibrillation paddles can be readily used if necessary.
4. Monitoring is for rhythm interpretation only. One should not try to read ST abnormalities or attempt more elaborate ECG interpretation.
5. Artifacts should be noted: a straight line will show if the electrode is loose, or a bizarre, wavy baseline resembling ventricular fibrillation (VF) may appear if an electrode is loose or the patient moves. Sixty-cycle interference also may be present.

Always remember that any ECG findings should be correlated with clinical observation of the patient.

Different electrode placements may be used for telemetry or other special purposes. The positive electrode should be to the left or below the negative electrode. Otherwise the deflections will all be reversed and the rhythm strips can be confusing.

How to Identify Arrhythmias[1-4]

All rhythm interpretation must be correlated with other signs of the condition of the patient for a successful outcome of any resuscitation attempt. Always remember the admonition "treat the patient, not the monitor."

It is necessary that the student develop a method of analysis of ECG strips that allows him or her to consistently identify the rhythm demonstrated. The analysis of ECG records is usually one of two types. One of these is sight reading, the technique used by many experienced ECG interpreters. Sight readers identify ECGs by looking at the whole pattern. This technique often requires little

separation of the individual wave forms of the ECG. Sight reading takes much experience and continued regular viewing of rhythm strips to be successful. It is of little use to the beginner.

Those with less experience evaluating ECGs will need to develop a method that allows them to separate the different wave forms in the ECG and systematically identify rhythm disorders. One such method is discussed below. There are many other techniques. Students will undoubtedly adjust this or any other method for maximum personal comfort as their experience increases. This is perfectly acceptable. There is no magic in any of the systems for ECG identification.

This ECG analysis method is based on three simple questions that allow the student to break down the various parts of the ECG and use those parts to separate rhythms into classes that simplify treatment selections. The system described is tailored to the setting of cardiac arrest.

ECG Analysis: Question 1

The first question is

> • **Is there a normal-looking QRS complex?**

It is important to ask this question first since it will identify most of the immediately life-threatening arrhythmias. If there is no QRS complex, the rhythm must be asystole or VF. A normal QRS complex is shown in Fig 2.

Ventricular Fibrillation

Description

Ventricular fibrillation is the single most important rhythm for the ECC provider to recognize. It is a rhythm in which multiple areas within the ventricles display marked variation in depolarization and repolarization (Fig 4). Since there is no organized ventricular depolarization, the ventricles do not contract as a unit. When observed directly, the ventricular myocardium appears to be quivering.

There is no cardiac output. This is the most common mechanism of cardiac arrest resulting from myocardial ischemia or infarction. The terms *coarse* and *fine* have been used to describe the amplitude of the waveforms in VF (Figs 4 and 5). Coarse VF usually indicates the recent onset of VF, which can be readily corrected by prompt defibrillation. The presence of fine VF that approaches asystole often means there has been a considerable delay since collapse, and successful resuscitation is more difficult.

Treatment: Initial treatment is always defibrillation. Only defibrillation provides definitive therapy. The exact benefit of antifibrillatory agents administered to persistent

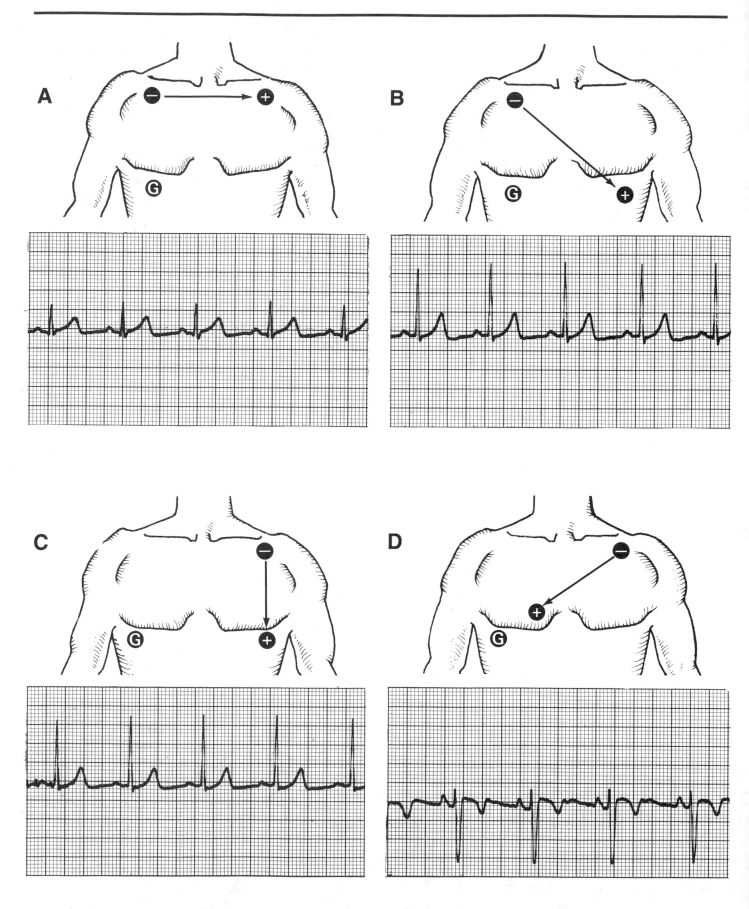

Fig 3. Location for chest electrodes. A, Lead I; B, lead II; C, lead III; D, lead MCL$_1$.

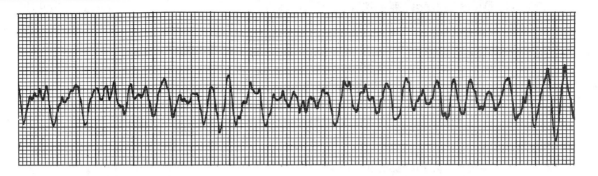

Fig 4. Coarse ventricular fibrillation. Note high amplitude waveforms, which vary in size, shape, and rhythm, representing chaotic ventricular electrical activity. There are no normal-looking QRS complexes.

Fig 5. Fine ventricular fibrillation ("coarse" asystole). In comparison with Fig 4, amplitude of electrical activity is much reduced. Note complete absence of QRS complexes. Slow undulations like this are virtually indistinguishable from asystole.

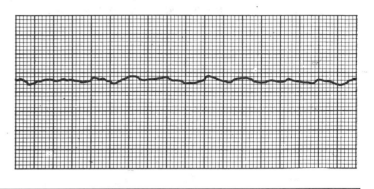

VF independent of defibrillation is unknown. Because their contribution (if any) remains doubtful, never delay defibrillation while waiting for pharmacologic agents to have an effect. See chapter 1, Fig 2, the VF/VT treatment algorithm, for details.

Summary of ECG Criteria

- There are no normal-looking QRS complexes.
- Rate: VF rate is very rapid and usually too disorganized to count.
- Rhythm: The rhythm is irregular. The electrical waveforms vary in size and shape. *There is no QRS complex.* ST segments, P waves, and T waves are absent as well.

Ventricular Asystole (Cardiac Standstill)

Description

Ventricular asystole (Fig 6) represents the total absence of ventricular electrical activity. Since depolarization does not occur, there is no ventricular contraction. This may occur as a primary event in cardiac arrest, or it may follow VF or pulseless electrical activity.

Ventricular asystole can occur also in patients with complete heart block in whom there is no escape pacemaker (see "Third-Degree AV Block" below). VF may masquerade as asystole; it is best always to check two leads perpendicular to each other to make sure that asystole is not VF. In addition, the distinction between

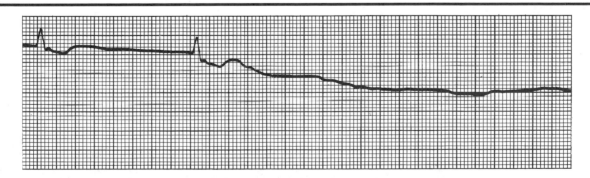

Fig 6. Ventricular asystole. Only two QRS complexes are seen, probably representing ventricular escape beats. They are followed by an absence of electrical activity. These are not normal looking.

very fine VF and asystole without any escape beats (agonal QRS complexes) may be very difficult. If it might be VF, it should be treated, like VF, with defibrillation. However, shocks to asystole are potentially harmful.

Treatment: Use epinephrine and atropine and actively search for reversible causes. See the asystole treatment algorithm (chapter 1, Fig 4) for details.

Summary of ECG Criteria

There is a complete absence of ventricular electrical activity. Sometimes, however, P waves may occur, or rare, erratically occurring ventricular escape beats (agonal beats) may be seen. Patients with these beats will not have a pulse and must be treated immediately if they are to be saved. If no organized QRS complex is seen and the patient has a pulse, then the ECG is improperly connected, turned off, or improperly calibrated.

Ventricular Tachycardia

Description[5]

Ventricular tachycardia is defined as three or more beats of ventricular origin in succession at a rate greater than 100 beats per minute (Fig 7). There are no normal-looking QRS complexes. The rhythm is usually regular, but on occasion it may be modestly irregular. This arrhythmia may be either well tolerated or associated with grave, life-threatening hemodynamic compromise. The hemodynamic consequences of VT depend largely on the presence or absence of myocardial dysfunction (such as might result from ischemia or infarction) and on the rate of VT. Atrioventricular dissociation usually is present. This means that the sinus node is depolarizing the atria in a normal manner at a rate either equal to or slower than the ventricular rate. Thus sinus P waves sometimes can be recognized between QRS complexes. They bear no fixed relation to the QRS complexes unless the atrial and ventricular rates happen to be equal. Conduction from atria to ventricles is usually prevented because the AV node or ventricular conduction system is refractory due to ventricular depolarizations. Sometimes retrograde conduction from ventricles to atria occurs. In this instance there will be a relation between the QRS complex and the retrograde P wave. Thus, it may be difficult to distinguish VT from a supraventricular tachycardia with aberrant ventricular conduction. This is discussed below.

Occasionally an atrial impulse arrives when the AV node and His-Purkinje system are not refractory and AV conduction can occur. This results in a *capture beat*, in which ventricular conduction occurs over the normal pathways, resulting in a normal-appearing (narrow) QRS complex. A capture beat occurs at a shorter RR interval than the RR interval of the VT. AV conduction also may occur simultaneously with depolarization of the ventricular focus. In this instance the ventricle will be depolarized in part over the normal pathway and in part from the ventricular focus. The resulting QRS complex will be intermediate in morphology between a normal QRS and a QRS of ventricular origin. In this instance the RR interval will not change. This is called a *fusion beat*. Ventricular tachycardia may be monomorphic (all QRSs with the same shape) or polymorphic (varying QRS shapes during the tachycardia).

Treatment: Ventricular tachycardia when sustained but hemodynamically stable is initially treated with lidocaine, procainamide, or bretylium. The tachycardia algorithm (chapter 1, Fig 6) presents the recommended pharmacologic agents and sequence of interventions. Ventricular tachycardia that is hemodynamically unstable should be treated the same as VF.

Summary of ECG Criteria

- There are no normal-looking QRS complexes.
- Rate: Greater than 100 beats per minute and usually not faster than 220 beats per minute
- Rhythm: Usually regular but may be irregular
- P waves: In rapid VT the P waves are usually not recognizable. At slower ventricular rates, P waves may be recognized and may represent normal atrial depolarization from the sinus node at a rate slower than VT, but the electrical activities do not affect one another.
- QRS, ST segment, T wave:
  — The PVC is premature; ie, it must occur before the next expected sinus beat unless atrial fibrillation is present since preactivity cannot be assessed.

Fig 7. Ventricular tachycardia. The rhythm is regular at a rate of 158 beats per minute. The QRS is wide. No evidence of atrial depolarization is seen.

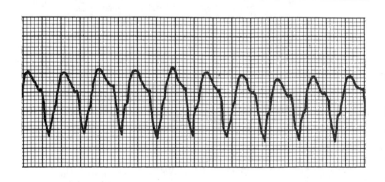

— The width of the QRS is 0.12 second or greater.
— The QRS morphology is often bizarre, with notching.
— The ST segment and T wave are usually opposite in polarity to the QRS.
— When multiformed (or multifocal), the coupling interval and morphology of the QRS vary.

Occasionally a narrow QRS complex may occur with a slightly shorter RR interval (capture beat), or a QRS complex may be seen with morphological features intermediate between a beat of ventricular origin and one of supraventricular origin but with a constant RR interval (fusion beat).

Torsades de Pointes[5]

Torsades de pointes (Fig 8) is a form of VT in which the QRSs appear to be constantly changing. Its name derives from the fact that its electrical activity appears to be twisted into a helix. This form of VT is due to drug toxicity or an idiosyncratic reaction to type IA antiarrhythmic agents, such as quinidine, procainamide, or disopyramide, or other agents that prolong the QT interval. Hypokalemia, hypomagnesemia, and bradycardias can also initiate torsades de pointes. This arrhythmia is usually accompanied by prolongation of the QT interval. The QT interval is measured from the onset of the QRS complex to the end of the T wave of the beat or beats just preceding the onset of torsades de pointes. At most rates the QT interval is 0.40 second or less, though it may be prolonged at slow rates. If the QT is abnormally prolonged in a patient receiving a type IA antiarrhythmic agent, consider the possibility of inducing torsades.

Treatment: Discontinuation of offending agents is crucial. Other treatments include magnesium sulfate and overdrive pacing.

Premature Ventricular Complex

Some patients will have regular QRS complexes interspersed with occasional unusual-looking complexes. These unusual conformations are called PVCs. This aberrant activity can cause more serious ventricular arrhythmias. Clinical deterioration depends on the frequency of the PVCs.

Description

A PVC is a depolarization that arises in either ventricle before the next expected sinus beat, ie, prematurely (Fig 9). It may result from the firing of an automatic focus or reentry.

Since PVCs originate in the ventricle, the normal sequence of ventricular depolarization is altered; ie, instead of the two ventricles depolarizing simultaneously, they depolarize sequentially. In addition, conduction occurs more slowly through the myocardium than through specialized conduction pathways. This results in a wide (0.12 second or greater) and bizarre-appearing QRS. The sequence of repolarization is also altered, usually resulting in an ST segment and T wave in a direction opposite to the QRS complex.

The interval between the previous normal beat and the PVC (the coupling interval) usually remains constant when PVCs are due to reentry from the same focus (uniform PVCs) (Fig 10). When the coupling interval and the QRS morphology vary, the PVCs may be arising from different areas within the ventricles, or if the PVCs are arising from a single focus, ventricular conduction may vary (Fig 11). Such PVCs are referred to as multifocal or, more appropriately, multiformed.

A PVC may occur nearly simultaneously with the firing of the sinus node. The antegrade impulse originating in the sinus node (resulting in normal atrial depolarization) and the retrograde impulse traveling toward the atria from the ventricles may meet in the AV node. Then neither can spread further because of the other's refractory period. Since the rhythm of the sinus node is undisturbed, a fully compensatory pause usually results (ie, the next P wave should occur at the proper time) (Fig 12). However, on occasion retrograde conduction can spread to the atria and reset the SA node.

PVCs may occur as isolated complexes, or they may occur repetitively in pairs (two PVCs in a row) (Fig 13). When three or more PVCs occur in a row, VT is present.

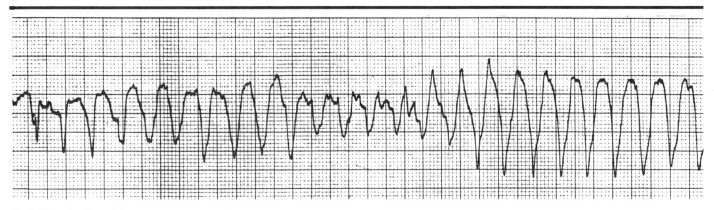

Fig 8. Torsades de pointes.

When VT lasts for more than 30 seconds, it is arbitrarily defined as *sustained ventricular tachycardia.*

If every other beat is a PVC, ventricular bigeminy is present (Fig 14). If every third beat is a PVC, the term *ventricular trigeminy* is used; if every fourth beat is a PVC, *ventricular quadrigeminy* is present; and so forth.

A PVC that falls on the T wave (during the so-called vulnerable period of ventricular repolarization) may precipitate VT or VF (Fig 15). However, PVCs occurring after the T wave may also initiate such VT (Fig 16).

Treatment: Isolated or non–VT PVCs are rarely treated except for needed symptomatic relief. In the setting of an acute myocardial infarction, PVCs indicate the need to aggressively treat the ischemia/infarction with oxygen, nitroglycerin, morphine, and thrombolytic therapy. Simply making the PVCs diminish with lidocaine does little to the underlying pathology and can lure physicians into an invalid clinical security that the problem has been resolved.

Summary of ECG Criteria

- QRS: Not normal looking. Usually broadened to more than 0.12 second.
- Rhythm: Irregular.
- P waves: The sinus P wave is usually obscured by the QRS, ST segment, or T wave of the PVC. It may, however, sometimes be recognized as a notching during the ST segment or T wave. Retrograde P waves may occur. The presence of a sinus P wave (when it cannot be seen) may be inferred by the presence of a fully compensatory pause.

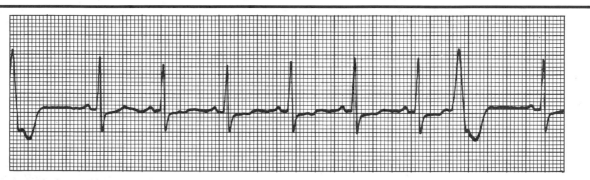

Fig 9. Premature ventricular complex.

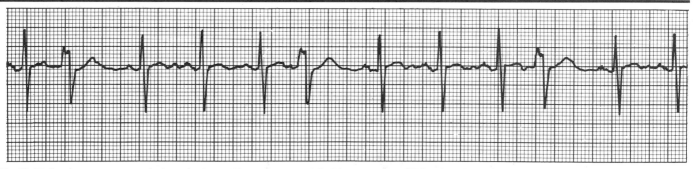

Fig 10. Unifocal premature ventricular complexes. Note occurrence of wide, premature QRS complexes. Interval between preceding normal QRS and PVC (coupling interval) remains constant, and morphology remains the same.

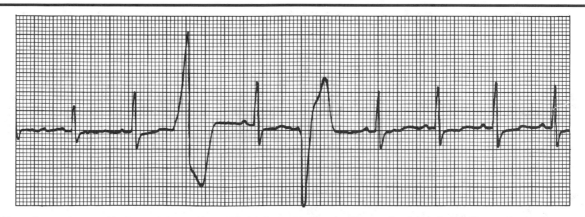

Fig 11. Multiformed premature ventricular complexes. Note variation in morphology and in coupling interval of PVCs.

Again, one simple question will separate the immediately life-threatening arrhythmias as well as help identify PVCs. The first question is

---

• Is there a normal-looking QRS complex?

If the patient has an ECG with a QRS complex with a pulse and a reasonable blood pressure, treatment options can be selected more slowly. If the patient has a normal-looking QRS complex and there is no pulse, the patient is in a form of pulseless electrical activity (PEA) and must be treated immediately.

Pulseless Electrical Activity

Description

PEA is the presence of some type of electrical activity other than VF or VT, but a pulse cannot be detected by palpation of any artery.

Treatment: The one major action that must be taken is to search for reversible causes. Nonspecific therapeutic interventions include epinephrine and (if the rate is slow) atropine, administered as presented in the PEA algorithm (chapter 1, Fig 3). Personnel should provide proper airway management and aggressive hyperventilation

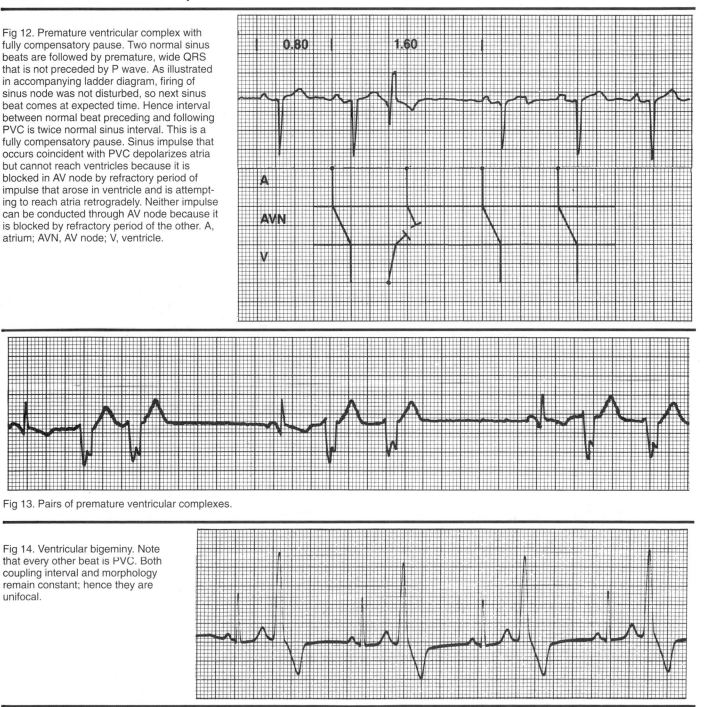

Fig 12. Premature ventricular complex with fully compensatory pause. Two normal sinus beats are followed by premature, wide QRS that is not preceded by P wave. As illustrated in accompanying ladder diagram, firing of sinus node was not disturbed, so next sinus beat comes at expected time. Hence interval between normal beat preceding and following PVC is twice normal sinus interval. This is a fully compensatory pause. Sinus impulse that occurs coincident with PVC depolarizes atria but cannot reach ventricles because it is blocked in AV node by refractory period of impulse that arose in ventricle and is attempting to reach atria retrogradely. Neither impulse can be conducted through AV node because it is blocked by refractory period of the other. A, atrium; AVN, AV node; V, ventricle.

Fig 13. Pairs of premature ventricular complexes.

Fig 14. Ventricular bigeminy. Note that every other beat is PVC. Both coupling interval and morphology remain constant; hence they are unifocal.

because hypoventilation and hypoxemia are frequent causes of PEA. A fluid challenge can be given since PEA may be due to hypovolemia.

Summary of ECG Criteria

Any rhythm or electrical activity that fails to generate a palpable pulse is PEA.

ECG Analysis: Question 2

Once the QRS complex has been identified and analyzed, a second question must be asked:

> • Is there a P wave?

Several arrhythmias are identified by the absence or abnormal appearance of P waves. When there are unorganized, very rapid electrical signals between the QRS complexes and no discernible P wave, the rhythm is atrial fibrillation.

Atrial Fibrillation[4]

Description

Atrial fibrillation (Figs 17 and 18) may result from multiple areas of reentry within the atria or from multiple ectopic foci. Atrial fibrillation may be associated with sick sinus syndrome, hypoxia, increased atrial pressure, pericarditis, and many other conditions. In the setting of acute ischemic heart disease, increased left atrial pressure secondary to congestive heart failure is the most common cause. The atrial electrical activity is very rapid (approximately 400 to 700 per minute), but each electrical impulse results in the depolarization of only a small islet of atrial myocardium rather than the whole atrium.

As a result, there is no contraction of the atria as a whole. Since there is no uniform atrial depolarization, there is no P wave. The chaotic electrical activity does produce a deflection on the ECG, referred to as a fibrillatory wave (Figs 17 and 18). Fibrillatory waves vary in size and shape and are irregular in rhythm. Transmission of these multiple atrial impulses into the AV node is thought to occur at random, resulting in an irregular rhythm. Some impulses are conducted into but not through the AV node; ie, they are blocked within the AV node. This is a form of "concealed conduction" and is important since such nonconducted impulses contribute to the overall refractoriness of the AV node. For this reason the ventricular rate of atrial fibrillation is often slower (averaging 160 to 180 per minute) than that seen in atrial tachycardia or atrial flutter. Atrial fibrillation is usually the result of some underlying form of heart disease (usually with congestive heart failure) and may occur intermittently or as a chronic rhythm. It may, however, be seen in a paroxysmal form in which there is no other evidence of heart disease.

Treatment: Rate control is the initial treatment goal, using agents such as diltiazem, verapamil, β blockers, or digoxin. Chemical cardioversion, usually after a period of anticoagulation, can then be attempted with procainamide or quinidine. Electrical cardioversion is the third

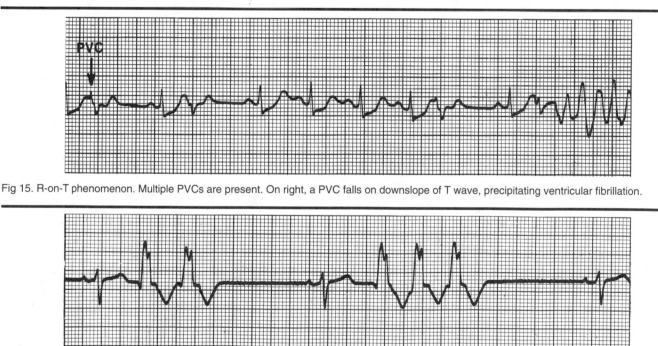

Fig 15. R-on-T phenomenon. Multiple PVCs are present. On right, a PVC falls on downslope of T wave, precipitating ventricular fibrillation.

Fig 16. Precipitation of ventricular tachycardia by late-cycle PVC. Note brief salvo of ventricular tachycardia that is initiated by PVC occurring well beyond T wave.

therapeutic option, after rate control and chemical cardioversion. Place a higher priority on electrical cardioversion in symptomatic patients if the atrial fibrillation is of new onset and is known to be of short duration, eg, 1 to 3 days.

If the patient with atrial fibrillation and a rapid ventricular response is in clinical distress, synchronized cardioversion is the treatment of choice. Hypotension induced by atrial fibrillation is usually seen only in patients with acute myocardial infarction or abnormalities of ventricular filling, eg, idiopathic hypertrophic subaortic stenosis or mitral stenosis. These patients should be immediately cardioverted. The vast majority of patients with atrial fibrillation will have ventricular rates of 120 to 200 beats per minute. If acute ischemic heart disease is present, cardioversion is recommended. Other asymptomatic patients, even those with a modest response (less than 120 beats per minute), can be treated conservatively by controlling their rate initially with digitalis, verapamil, or β-adrenergic blocking agents. In the undigitalized patient, β-adrenergic blocking agents and verapamil may not cause sufficient slowing and may lead to congestive heart failure.

Once the heart rate is controlled or if symptoms occur, a decision about cardioversion should be made. Success in cardioverting and preventing recurrence of atrial fibrillation depends on atrial size and the length of time the patient has been in atrial fibrillation. The larger the atrial size and the longer the patient has been in atrial fibrillation, the lower the likelihood of successful maintenance of sinus rhythm. Before cardioversion is attempted either electrically or pharmacologically with an agent such as quinidine or procainamide, anticoagulation should be considered. Patients with mitral stenosis, cardiomyopathy, and large atria are more likely to have thrombus in the atrium and are thus at higher risk for emboli and stroke. Anticoagulation must be considered.

Summary of ECG Criteria

- Rate: The atrial rate as a rule cannot be counted. In the untreated patient, the ventricular rate is usually 160 to 180 beats per minute.
- Rhythm: The ventricular rhythm is irregularly irregular. Where there are clearly fibrillatory waves indicating the presence of atrial fibrillation but the QRSs are regular, there must be some additional factor present, such as third-degree AV block or accelerated junctional rhythm or both. Both of these are often the result of digitalis intoxication.
- P waves: Organized atrial electrical activity is absent, so there are no P waves. Chaotic electrical activity, or fibrillatory waves, may be seen.
- QRS interval: Ventricular depolarization is normal unless aberrant ventricular conduction occurs.
- R wave amplitude varies irregularly.

Atrial Flutter[4]

If there are P waves but they occur rapidly with a characteristic "sawtooth" appearance, then the rhythm is atrial flutter.

Description

This arrhythmia is the result of a reentry circuit within the atria (Fig 19). Atrial depolarization occurs in a caudad-

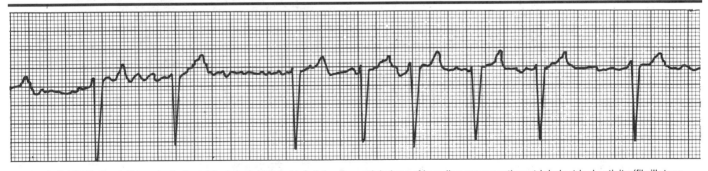

Fig 17. Atrial fibrillation with controlled ventricular response. Note irregular undulations of baseline representing atrial electrical activity (fibrillatory waves). The fibrillatory waves vary in size and shape and are irregular in rhythm. Conduction through the AV node occurs at random; hence ventricular rhythm is irregular.

Fig 18. Atrial fibrillation with rapid ventricular response.

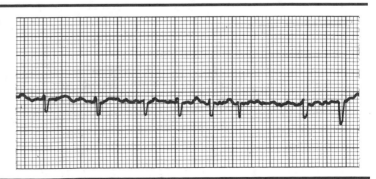

to-cephalad direction and hence is best observed in leads II, III, and aVF. It is often described as resembling a sawtooth or picket fence. Such a wave is called a *flutter wave.*

While it is possible to have 1:1 AV conduction, more commonly there is a physiological block at AV nodal level because the refractory period of the AV node results in 2:1 AV conduction or even higher grades of block.

Since the atrial rate is most commonly about 300 per minute, 2:1 AV block usually is present, and the ventricular rate is usually 150 per minute. The AV conduction ratio may be altered by AV nodal disease, increased vagal tone, and certain drugs (eg, digitalis, propranolol, verapamil) that will induce a higher degree of AV block (eg, 3:1, 4:1) or at times a variable block (Figs 20 and 21). Atrial flutter seldom occurs in the absence of organic heart disease. It is seen in association with mitral or tricuspid valvular heart disease, acute or chronic cor pulmonale, and coronary heart disease. It is rarely a manifestation of digitalis intoxication.

Treatment: If the patient is hypotensive, having ischemic pain, or in severe congestive heart failure, synchronized cardioversion is the treatment of choice. If the patient is only mildly symptomatic, pharmacologic therapy can be tried first. However, many experts recommend that cardioversion should always be the initial therapy. The ventricular rate can be slowed with diltiazem, verapamil, digitalis, or β-blocking agents. Verapamil and β blockers may exacerbate bradycardia and congestive heart failure. If digitalis is used to control the rate, care must be taken to avoid digitalis intoxication. Once the rate is controlled, the patient can be placed on a type I antiarrhythmic agent, such as quinidine or procainamide, to convert flutter. After a reasonable trial of pharmacologic conversion, the patient should be electrically cardioverted.

Summary of ECG Criteria

- Atrial rate: Usually 300 beats per minute, ranging between 220 and 350 beats per minute
- Rhythm: The atrial rhythm is regular. The ventricular rhythm may be regular if a constant degree of AV block is present (such as 2:1 or, less commonly, 1:1) but can be grossly irregular if variable block is present.
- P waves: Flutter waves resemble a sawtooth or picket fence and are best seen in leads II, III, or aVF. In the presence of 2:1 or 1:1 conduction ratios, it may be difficult to identify the flutter waves. In this instance carotid sinus massage (or IV adenosine used diagnostically) may produce a transient delay in AV nodal conduction, resulting in a higher degree of AV block. This will "uncover" the flutter waves, permitting their identification.
- PR interval: Usually the PR interval is regular, but it may vary.

- QRS interval: This pattern is usually normal, but aberrant ventricular conduction, usually with right bundle-branch block, can occur.

ECG Analysis: Question 3

The third question to ask in evaluating ECGs is

> - **What is the relationship between the P waves and the QRS complexes?**

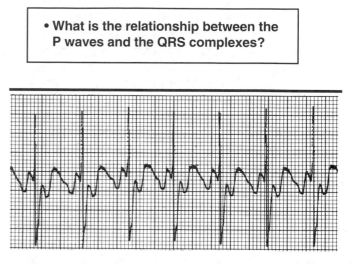

Fig 19. Atrial flutter. The atrial rate is 250 beats per minute, and the rhythm is regular. Every other flutter wave is conducted to ventricles (2:1 block), resulting in regular ventricular rhythm at a rate of 125 beats per minute.

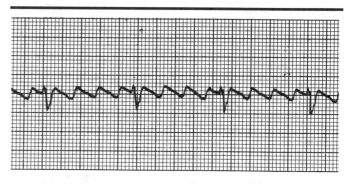

Fig 20. Atrial flutter with high-grade AV block. Atrial rhythm is regular (260 beats per minute), but only every fourth flutter wave is followed by a QRS (4:1 conduction).

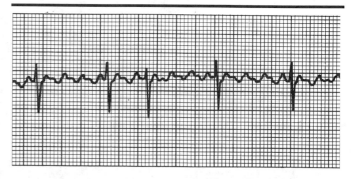

Fig 21. Atrial flutter with variable AV block. Atrial rhythm is regular, but variable AV block is present (2:1, 4:1 conduction ratios), resulting in irregular ventricular rhythm.

Remember that in the normal ECG every QRS complex is preceded by a P wave, and the time between the two forms is less than 0.20 second. Heart blocks are rhythms that are caused by altered conduction through the AV node. As conduction in the AV node slows, the interval between the P wave and the QRS complex lengthens. If slowing in the node becomes pronounced, some P waves will be blocked in the AV node. In the worst case no P waves will pass through the AV node to excite the ventricles.

The heart blocks are divided into three degrees. First-degree heart blocks are characterized by PR intervals longer than 0.20 second and all of the P waves are followed by QRS complexes. Second-degree heart blocks are characterized by some P waves being blocked at the AV node. This results in some P waves occurring without following QRS complexes. Third-degree heart block is characterized by a complete dissociation between P waves and QRS complexes. A hint for separating the heart blocks into degrees is that first- and third-degree blocks usually have regular QRS rates.

Atrioventricular Block

Atrioventricular block is defined as a delay or interruption in conduction between atria and ventricles. It may be due to (1) lesions along the conduction pathway (eg, calcium, fibrosis, necrosis), (2) increases in the refractory period of a portion of the conduction pathway (such as may occur in the AV node when digitalis is administered), or (3) shortening of the supraventricular cycle length, ie, rapid atrial rates, with encroachment on the normal refractory period (as with atrial flutter, in which 2:1 AV block at the level of the AV node occurs because the normal AV node refractory period will not allow conduction at a rate of 300 beats per minute but will allow it at 150 beats per minute).

AV block may be classified in two ways:

1. According to the degree of block:
   - Partial blocks
     — First-degree AV block
     — Second-degree AV block (type I and type II), 2:1, and advanced (3:1 or greater)
   - Third-degree or complete AV block
2. According to the site of block:
   - AV node
   - Infranodal
     — Bundle of His
     — Bundle branches

Each degree of block (first, second, third) may occur either at the level of the AV node or below it. This distinction is not academic since pathogenesis, treatment, and prognosis differ.

First-Degree AV Block

Description

First-degree AV block (Fig 22) is simply a delay in passage of the impulse from atria to ventricles. This delay usually occurs at the level of the AV node but may be infranodal.

Treatment: Treatment for first-degree heart block is usually unnecessary when it occurs without symptoms.

Summary of ECG Criteria

- There is a normal-looking QRS.
- Rhythm: Regular.
- P waves: Each P wave is followed by a QRS complex.
- PR interval: This interval is prolonged beyond 0.20 second. It usually remains constant but may vary.

Second-Degree AV Block

In second-degree AV block, some impulses are conducted and others are blocked. This type of block is subdivided into two additional types.

Type I Second-Degree AV Block (Wenckebach)

Description. This form of block almost always occurs at the level of the AV node (rarely at His bundle or bundle branch level) and is often due to increased parasympathetic tone or to drug effect (eg, digitalis, propranolol, or verapamil). It is usually transient and prognosis is good. *Second-degree type I AV block is characterized by a progressive prolongation of the PR interval.* Decreasing conduction velocity through the AV node occurs until an impulse is completely blocked (Fig 23). Usually only a single impulse is blocked, and the pattern is repeated.

The repetition of this pattern results in "group beating," eg, three conducted sinus beats with progressively lengthening PR intervals and a fourth sinus beat that is not followed by a QRS. Such a "group" is referred to as *4:3 conduction.* Although the conduction ratio may remain constant, it is usual for it to change, eg, 4:3, 3:2, 2:1. The ventricular rhythm is irregular except in the presence of 2:1 block.

Treatment: Specific treatment is rarely needed unless severe signs and symptoms are present. Clinicians should place a high priority on identifying underlying causes. See the bradycardia treatment algorithm (chapter 1, Fig 5).

Summary of ECG Criteria:

- There is a normal-looking QRS.
- Rate: The atrial rate is unaffected, but the ventricular rate will be less than the atrial rate because of the nonconducted beats.

- Rhythm: The atrial rhythm is usually regular. The ventricular rhythm is usually irregular with progressive shortening of the RR interval before the blocked impulse. The RR interval that brackets the non-conducted P wave is less than twice the normal cycle length.
- P waves: The P waves will appear normal, and each P wave will be followed by a QRS complex except for the blocked P wave.
- PR interval: There is a progressive increase in PR interval until one P wave is blocked.

Type II Second-Degree AV Block

Description. This form of second-degree AV block (Fig 24) occurs below the level of the AV node either at the bundle of His (uncommon) or the bundle branches (common). It is usually associated with an organic lesion in the conduction pathway, and unlike type I second-degree AV block, it is rarely the result of increased parasympathetic tone or drug effect. It is thus associated with a poorer prognosis, and complete heart block may develop. A hallmark of this type of second-degree AV block is that the PR interval does not lengthen before a dropped beat. More than one nonconducted beat may occur in succession. This type of block most often occurs at the level of the bundle branches.

For a dropped beat to occur, there must be complete block in one bundle branch (ie, right or left bundle-branch block) with intermittent interruption in conduction in the contralateral bundle as well. Thus, type II second-degree AV block is often associated with a wide QRS complex (Fig 24). When block occurs at the His bundle, the QRS may be narrow since ventricular conduction is not disturbed in beats that are not blocked. The rhythm may be irregular when block is intermittent or when the conduction ratio is variable. With a constant conduction ratio (eg, 2:1) the ventricular rhythm is regular.

Treatment: See the bradycardia algorithm (chapter 1, Fig 5) for the recommended intervention sequence. Again note that there should be clinical indications for treatment.

Summary of ECG Criteria:

- QRS: The QRS will be normal when the block is at the bundle of His. However, the QRS will be widened with the features of bundle-branch block if the block is at the bundle branches.
- Rate: The atrial rate is unaffected, but the ventricular rate will be less than the atrial rate.
- Rhythm: The atrial rhythm is usually regular, whereas the ventricular rhythm is most often irregular, with pauses corresponding to the nonconducted beats.

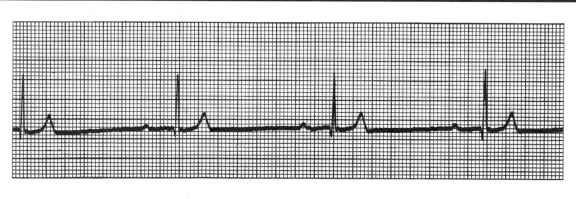

Fig 22. First-degree AV block. The PR interval is prolonged to 0.31 second.

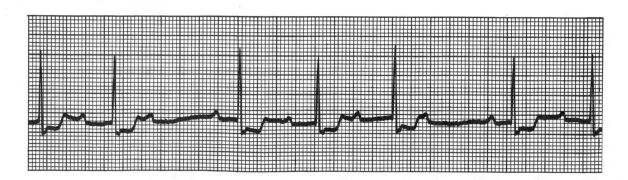

Fig 23. Second-degree AV block type I. Atrial rhythm is nearly regular, but there are pauses in ventricular rhythm because every fourth P wave does not conduct into ventricles. Note progressive prolongation of PR interval, indicating increasing conduction delay in AV node before non-conducted beat. There are four P waves and three QRS complexes in this example, representing a 4:3 cycle. The QRS complexes are normal.

- P waves: The P waves will appear normal, and each will be followed by a QRS except for the blocked P wave.
- PR interval: This interval may be normal or prolonged, but it will remain constant. There may be shortening of the PR interval after a pause.

Third-Degree AV Block

Description

Third-degree AV block indicates complete absence of conduction between atria and ventricles. The atrial rate is always equal to or faster than the ventricular rate in complete heart block. It may occur at the level of the AV node (Fig 25), the bundle of His, or the bundle branches. As in second-degree AV block, this distinction is not merely academic since pathogenesis, treatment, and prognosis may vary considerably, depending on the anatomic level of block. When third-degree AV block occurs at the AV node, a junctional escape pacemaker frequently will initiate ventricular depolarization. This is usually a stable pacemaker with a rate of 40 to 60 beats per minute. Since it is located above the bifurcation of the bundle of His, the sequence of ventricular depolarization usually is normal, resulting in a normal QRS. This type of third-degree AV block can result from increased parasympathetic tone associated with inferior infarction, from toxic drug effects (eg, digitalis, propranolol), or from damage to the AV node. Third-degree AV block with a junctional escape rhythm is usually transient and is associated with a favorable prognosis.

When third-degree AV block occurs at the infranodal level, it is most often due to block involving both bundle branches. This indicates the presence of extensive infranodal conduction system disease. When it results from coronary atherosclerosis, it is usually associated with extensive anterior myocardial infarction. It usually does not result from increases in parasympathetic tone or from drug effects. The only escape mechanism available is in the ventricle distal to the site of block. Such a ventricular escape pacemaker has an intrinsic rate that is slow, less than 40 beats per minute. Like any depolarization origi-nating in a ventricle, the QRS complex will be wide (Fig 26). It is not a stable pacemaker, and episodes of ventricular asystole are common (Fig 27).

Treatment: See the bradycardia algorithm (chapter 1, Fig 5). The major interventions are atropine, transcutaneous pacing, catecholamine infusions (dopamine or epinephrine), and transvenous pacemaker. Isoproterenol is rarely indicated.

Summary of ECG Criteria

- QRS: Generally normal looking. When block occurs at the AV node or bundle of His, the QRS complex will appear normal. When block occurs at bundle branch level, the QRS complex will be widened.
- P waves: Normal.
- Rate: The atrial rate will be unaffected by third-degree AV block. The ventricular rate will be slower than the atrial rate. With intranodal third-degree AV block, the ventricular rate is usually 40 to 60 beats per minute; with infranodal third-degree AV block, the ventricular rate is usually less than 40 beats per minute.
- Rhythm: The atrial rhythm is usually regular, although sinus arrhythmia may be present. The ventricular rhythm will be regular.
- PR interval: Since the atria and ventricles are depolarized from different pacemakers, they are independent of each other, and the PR interval will vary.

The major characteristics for heart blocks are summarized in the Table.

Junctional Complexes

In some patients conducting tissue near the AV node has taken over the pacemaker function of the heart. These patients will have slow heart rates (40 to 60 beats per minute) and inverted but narrow QRS complexes, and often one can see retrograde P waves in leads II and III.

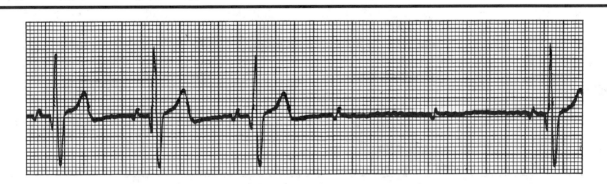

Fig 24. Second-degree AV block type II. In this example three conducted sinus beats are followed by two nonconducted P waves. The PR interval of conducted beats remains constant, and QRS is wide.

Summary of ECG Features of AV Block

ECG feature		First-degree	Second-degree	Third-degree (complete)
Rate	A	Unaffected	Unaffected	Unaffected
	V	Same as A	Slower than A	Slower than A
Ventricular rhythm		Same as A	Type I: Irregular Type II: Irregular or regular	Regular
P-QRS relationship		Consistent 1:1	Type I: Variable (recurring pattern) Type II: Fixed	Absent
QRS duration		Unaffected	Type I: Narrow Type II: Usually wide	Depends on site of escape rhythm
Site of block		Anywhere from AV node to bundle branches	Type I: AV node Type II: His or below	Anywhere from AV node to bundle branches

Premature Junctional Complexes

Description

A premature junctional complex is an electrical impulse that originates in the AV junction and occurs before the next expected sinus impulse. This often results in retrograde atrial depolarization (hence the P wave in leads II, III, and aVF will be negative) (Fig 28). The retrograde P wave may precede, coincide with, or follow the QRS. The relation of a retrograde P wave to QRS complex depends on the relative conduction times from the site of origin within the junction to the atria and ventricles. It is therefore likely that an impulse arising in the higher portion of the junction, above the AV node, would result in a P wave occurring before or during the QRS complex, whereas

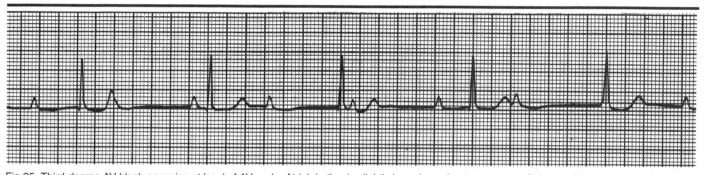

Fig 25. Third-degree AV block occurring at level of AV node. Atrial rhythm is slightly irregular owing to presence of sinus arrhythmia. Ventricular rhythm is regular at slower rate (44 beats per minute). There is no constant PR interval. The QRS complexes are narrow, indicating they are of supraventricular origin but below level of block.

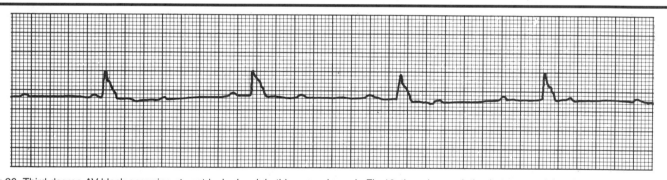

Fig 26. Third-degree AV block occurring at ventricular level. In this example, as in Fig 10, there is no relation between atrial and ventricular rhythm. Ventricular rhythm is regular at very slow rate (38 beats per minute). The QRS is wide because block is at bundle branch level, and ventricular pacemaker is distal to that level.

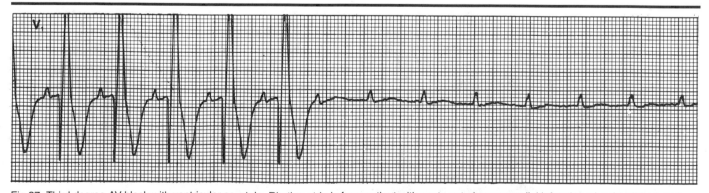

Fig 27. Third-degree AV block with ventricular asystole. Rhythm strip is from patient with acute anterior myocardial infarction who developed right bundle-branch block as indicated by wide QRS complex with terminal R wave (left half of rhythm strip). Complete heart block abruptly developed. On right side of rhythm strip, only P waves are seen. There is absence of ventricular escape, resulting in ventricular asystole.

one arising at a lower level would result in a P wave that occurs after the QRS complex. Conduction from the junction to the ventricles usually occurs along normal pathways. Thus the QRS complex is usually normal, although it can be wide owing to either a bundle-branch block or aberrant conduction. The pause following a premature junctional complex may be noncompensatory (if the sinus node is depolarized by the premature beat) or fully compensatory if the sinus node has discharged before it is reached by the premature beat.

Treatment: Specific suppressive treatment is rarely needed.

Summary of ECG Criteria

- QRS: Usually normal. The interval may sometimes be widened (aberrant ventricular conduction), usually indicating right bundle-branch block.
- Rhythm: Irregular.
- P waves: Because atrial depolarization is usually retrograde, P waves are generally negative in leads II, III, and aVF. P waves can precede, coincide with, or follow the QRS. Either a noncompensatory or a fully compensatory pause may occur.
- PR interval: If the P wave precedes the QRS, the PR interval is usually less than 0.12 second. However, the PR interval may be prolonged. Complete AV block may occur.

Junctional Escape Complexes and Rhythms

Description

The AV junction can function as a pacemaker. It initiates impulses at a rate of 40 to 60 beats per minute, equivalent to an RR interval between 1.0 and 1.5 seconds. Under normal circumstances, the sinus node pacemaker, which is faster, predominates. If the AV node is not depolarized by the arrival of a sinus impulse within approximately 1.0 to 1.5 seconds, it will initiate an impulse. This is called a *junctional escape complex*. It occurs because of failure of the sinus node to initiate an appropriately timed impulse or because of a conduction problem between the sinus node and the AV junction (Fig 29). A repeated series of such impulses is referred to as a *junctional escape rhythm*.

Treatment: Most commonly, junctional escape complexes and rhythms are events of automaticity. They may also be due to digitalis intoxication. In nonparoxysmal junctional tachycardia due to digitalis intoxication, digitalis should be withheld. The serum potassium level should be checked, and if low, potassium should be given to raise the serum potassium to the normal range. If the patient is severely compromised, antibodies to digitalis may be used.

Summary of ECG Criteria

- There is a normal-looking QRS.
- Rate: A junctional escape rhythm has a rate of 40 to 60 beats per minute.

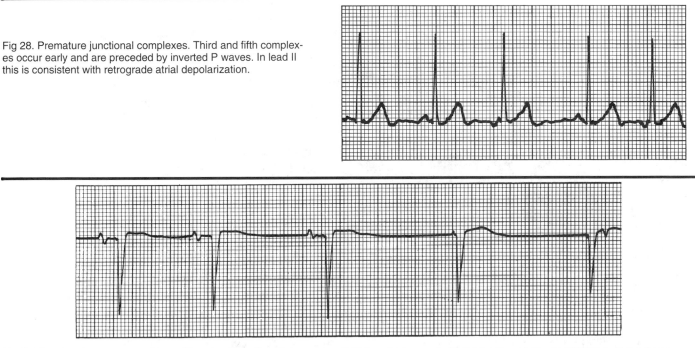

Fig 28. Premature junctional complexes. Third and fifth complexes occur early and are preceded by inverted P waves. In lead II this is consistent with retrograde atrial depolarization.

Fig 29. Junctional escape complexes. Sinus bradycardia with increasing PP interval (sinus arrhythmia) is present. Second PP interval is 1.2 seconds. Third PP interval is 1.5 seconds, but before it can be conducted to ventricles, a junctional escape complex occurs. Morphology is similar to sinus beats, consistent with site of origin in AV junction. Fourth and fifth QRSs also represent junctional escape complexes.

- Rhythm: The presence of some junctional escape complexes may lead to an irregular rhythm. Junctional escape complexes occur approximately 1.0 second or more following the last depolarization. A junctional escape rhythm is usually regular.
- P waves: Retrograde P waves (negative) may be seen in leads II, III, and aVF. P waves may precede, coincide with, or follow the QRS. Sinus P waves, at a rate equal to or slower than the junctional rhythm, may occur. This may result in AV dissociation (discussed in more detail in "Ventricular Tachycardia").
- PR interval: This interval is variable but is usually less than the PR interval of the normally conducted beat from the sinus node.
- QRS interval: Ventricular conduction is usually normal unless a ventricular conduction problem is present or aberrant conduction occurs (see "The Electrocardiogram").

A final group of rhythms needs to be identified on the basis of rate. These include sinus bradycardia, sinus tachycardia, and supraventricular tachycardia.

Sinus Tachycardia

Description

Sinus tachycardia (Fig 30) is characterized by an increase in the rate of discharge of the sinus node. Perhaps secondary to multiple factors (eg, exercise, fever, anxiety, hypovolemia), it is a physiological response to a demand for a higher cardiac output. Never "treat" sinus tachycardia; treat the cause of sinus tachycardia.

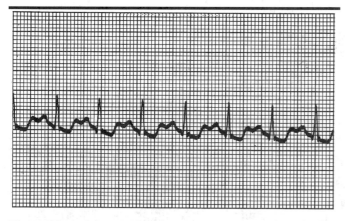

Fig 30. Sinus tachycardia. Note regular rhythm at the rate of 121 beats per minute. Each QRS is preceded by upright P wave in lead II.

Summary of ECG Criteria

- Normal-looking QRS
- Rate: Greater than 100 beats per minute
- Rhythm: Regular
- P waves: Upright in leads I, II, and aVF

Sinus Bradycardia

Description

Sinus bradycardia (Fig 31) is characterized by a decrease in the rate of atrial depolarization due to slowing of the sinus node. It may be secondary to sinus node disease, increased parasympathetic tone, or drug effects (eg, digitalis, propranolol, or verapamil).

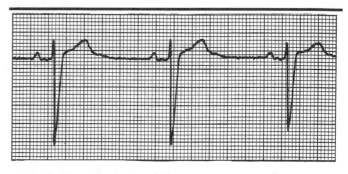

Fig 31. Sinus bradycardia. Sinus rate is 46 beats per minute and rhythm is regular.

Summary of ECG Criteria

- Normal-looking QRS
- Rate: Less than 60 beats per minute
- Rhythm: Regular
- P waves: Upright in leads I, II, and aVF

Supraventricular Tachycardia

Description

Supraventricular tachycardias may be either uniform or multifocal. Multifocal atrial tachycardia occurs most often in patients with respiratory failure. Supraventricular tachycardias include the following:

Paroxysmal supraventricular tachycardia (PSVT)
Nonparoxysmal atrial tachycardia
Multifocal atrial tachycardia
Junctional tachycardia (accelerated or nonparoxysmal)
Atrial flutter
Atrial fibrillation

This section presents only two of the multiple clinical forms of uniform supraventricular tachycardias.

Paroxysmal Supraventricular Tachycardia (PSVT). This is a distinct clinical syndrome characterized by repeated episodes (ie, paroxysms) of tachycardia with an abrupt onset lasting from a few seconds to many hours. These episodes usually end abruptly and often can be terminated by vagal maneuvers. Such paroxysms may recur for many years.

PSVT is due to a reentry mechanism, most often involving the AV node alone or the AV node and an extra—AV nodal bypass tract. Infrequently the sinoatrial node is involved. The QRS complexes are narrow unless preexistent or rate-dependent bundle-branch block is present or unless antegrade conduction to the ventricles occurs over an extra—AV nodal pathway, such as a Kent bundle in Wolff-Parkinson-White syndrome. Atrial depolarization is retrograde, resulting in inverted P waves in ECG leads II, III, and aVF. The P waves may occur just before, during, or after the QRS complexes; they are not discerned if they occur during the QRS complexes (Fig 32). Episodes of paroxysmal tachycardia are usually well tolerated in the young in the absence of other coexisting forms of heart disease. In the elderly and in those with other forms of heart disease (especially coronary atherosclerosis or stenosis of the mitral or aortic valves), serious problems such as myocardial ischemia, infarction, or pulmonary edema can be precipitated by the rapid heart rate.

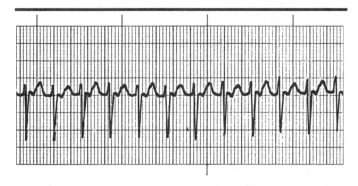

Fig 32. Paroxysmal supraventricular tachycardia (PSVT).

Treatment: The most common treatment includes vagal maneuvers, adenosine, verapamil, or β blockers, as described in the tachycardia algorithm (chapter 1, Fig 6). If the QRS complexes are broad and VT cannot be ruled out, IV lidocaine can be administered. Ablation procedures that destroy a part of the reentrant path are increasing in use. Such procedures can result in a long-term cure in appropriate patients.

Nonparoxysmal Atrial Tachycardia. This arrhythmia is secondary to some other primary event. The most common cause is digitalis intoxication. When the primary event is corrected, the atrial tachycardia may be terminated. Its mechanism of production involves the rapid firing of an automatic focus within either atrium due to enhanced automaticity. Although the paroxysmal and nonparoxysmal forms of atrial tachycardia may be indistinguishable on the ECG (hence the importance of an accurate history), certain important ECG clues may be present. In the undigitalized patient, paroxysmal atrial tachycardia is usually associated with 1:1 AV conduction. Nonparoxysmal atrial tachycardia is usually characterized by AV block (Fig 33). The ventricular rate may be irregular or regular, depending on the constancy of the AV block.

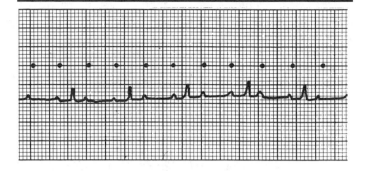

Fig 33. Atrial tachycardia with block. The atrial rate is 200 beats per minute, and the rhythm is regular. Every other P wave is conducted to ventricles (2:1 conduction ratio). P waves are indicated by dots.

Summary of ECG Criteria

- Rate: The atrial rate is usually 140 to 220 beats per minute.
- Rhythm: The atrial rhythm is regular. The ventricular rhythm is most often regular with 1:1 AV conduction when the atrial rate is under 200. Especially with the nonparoxysmal variety, 2:1 AV block is common. Higher grades of block may also occur.
- P waves: P waves may be difficult to identify because they can be buried in the preceding T wave. They usually differ morphologically from sinus P waves when the comparison can be made. However, especially in the nonparoxysmal variety, the P waves may be quite similar to P waves of sinus origin.
- PR interval: This interval may be normal or prolonged.
- QRS interval: The QRS interval may be normal or prolonged because of bundle-branch block or aberrant conduction.

Supraventricular and Ventricular Complexes and Rhythms

Clinicians can find it difficult to differentiate ventricular ectopic beats or VT from supraventricular ectopic beats or supraventricular tachycardia with aberrant ventricular conduction. The problem is complex, and sometimes differentiation is virtually impossible, even by experienced electrocardiographers. Usually such distinctions are beyond the core knowledge of ACLS.

The clinical significance of the distinction, however, is considerable. Ventricular tachycardia is a potentially life-threatening arrhythmia, usually requiring immediate treatment, whereas supraventricular arrhythmias usually are less dangerous.[6]

An extremely important point to remember is that the treatment of rapid, wide, regular QRS tachycardias with such agents as verapamil in the belief that they may represent a supraventricular tachycardia with aberrant conduction can have disastrous consequences when these tachycardias turn out to be VT, which is more common.[6]

Wide-QRS tachycardias of uncertain origin should be considered VT and treated as such until proven otherwise. For example, in the presence of deteriorating hemodynamics, electrocardioversion should be pursued emergently. If the patient is stable in the presence of rapid, wide-QRS tachycardia, **do not treat with verapamil** but consider such agents as procainamide.

In summary, emergency care providers should remember:

> *Rule No. 1:* Wide-QRS tachycardia is VT until proven otherwise.
>
> *Rule No. 2:* Always remember rule No. 1.

These treatment points are presented in the tachycardia algorithm (chapter 1, Fig 6). This algorithm was constructed to prohibit inappropriate use of verapamil and to ensure that clinicians treat unknown wide-complex tachycardia as VT.

Summary of ECG Analysis

Three questions assist in the orderly evaluation of the ECG:

---

1. **Are there normal-looking QRS complexes?**
2. **Are there normal-looking P waves?**
3. **What is the relationship between the P waves and the QRS complexes?**

These three questions will allow the student to discriminate among most of the heart rhythms important to ECC. It is important to recognize what such a scheme can and cannot do. First, this scheme is designed to triage patients into those groups that need immediate attention and those that can be dealt with more leisurely. Second, this system is not designed to identify all aberrations of the ECG, and it will not prepare the student to interpret subtle alterations in heart rhythm. Finally, the student will likely develop refinements on this basic scheme as he or she gains experience.

References

1. Dunn MI, Lipman BS. *Lipman-Massie Clinical Electrocardiography.* 8th ed. Chicago, Ill: Year Book Medical Publishers Inc; 1989.
2. Marriott HJL. *Practical Electrocardiography.* 8th ed. Baltimore, Md: Williams & Wilkins Co; 1988.
3. Marriott HJL, Myerburg RJ. Recognition of cardiac arrhythmias and conduction disturbances. In: Hurst JW, ed. *The Heart, Arteries and Veins.* 7th ed. New York, NY: McGraw-Hill Information Services Co, Health Professions Division; 1990:489-534.
4. Zipes DP. Specific arrhythmias: diagnosis and treatment. In: Braunwald E, ed. *Heart Disease: A Textbook of Cardiovascular Medicine.* 4th ed. Philadelphia, Pa: WB Saunders Co; 1992:667-725.
5. Akhtar M. Clinical spectrum of ventricular tachycardia. *Circulation.* 1990; 82:1561-1573.
6. Stewart RB, Bardy GH, Greene HL. Wide complex tachycardia: misdiagnosis and outcome after emergent therapy. *Ann Intern Med.* 1986;104:766-771.

Appendix: Electrical Activity of the Heart[1,2]

Myocardial Cell Types

Two groups of cells within the myocardium are important to cardiac function:

1. *The Working Myocardial Cells*

These cells possess *contractility,* the ability to shorten and then return to their original length. For a working cell to contract, the cell membrane must be electrically discharged (a process called *depolarization*). This discharge changes the electrical charge across the cell membrane as certain ions (especially sodium) increase their ability to move across the cell membrane. The process of depolarization also allows calcium to enter the cell, where it activates the attraction between the actin and myosin filaments of the sarcomere (the basic contractile unit of the myocardial fiber), resulting in contraction.

2. *The Electrical System*

Cells belonging to the electrical system of the heart are responsible for the formation of an electrical current and for conduction of this impulse to the working cells of the myocardium. Certain cells of the electrical system can generate an electrical impulse (a property referred to as *automaticity* or *spontaneous depolarization*). These cells are known as *pacemaker cells.* They are found in the sinus (or sinoatrial [SA]) node, the atrial conduction pathways, the area above the AV node, the lower portion of the AV node, the bundle of His, the bundle branches, and in the ventricular Purkinje system. The AV node, the bundle of His, and an area immediately above the AV node are called the *AV junction.* The electrical impulse is conducted over specialized myocardial (not neural) pathways.

Basic Electrophysiology

For a cell to do work by contracting or to conduct an impulse, it must be electrically charged. This charge arises from the concentration gradient of ions across the cell membrane. There are different concentrations of potassium, sodium, and calcium inside and outside the cell. This normal gradient causes a -80 to -90 mV electrical charge to occur across the membrane. When the cell is activated, this charge heads toward $+35$ mV, causing either conduction or contraction to be initiated.

The process of depolarization results in a momentary change in the physical properties of the cell membrane. Positively charged ions can enter the cell, causing the inside of the cell to become electrically positive. Ions enter the cell through two channels. The fast channel operates when membrane potentials are more negative than –60 mV, permitting the rapid entry of sodium ions. This is the *normal channel* for nonpacemaker myocardial cells. The slow channel operates at membrane potentials that are less negative than –50 mV. This channel permits the entry of calcium ions (and possibly sodium ions). Slow channel depolarization, as well as potassium flux, is responsible for the pacemaker activity of the sinus node and the AV junction. Slow channel depolarization may be responsible for abnormal types of depolarization such as might exist in an area of myocardium bordering an infarct. In this situation, local extracellular hyperkalemia may occur and result in a reduction in the resting membrane potential (eg, from a normal of –90 mV to –40 mV).

In the action potential of a typical ventricular myocardial (working) cell, the resting membrane potential (the electrical potential across the cell membrane before depolarization) is approximately –80 to –90 mV (Fig 34). The inside of the cell membrane is electrically negative compared with the outside of the cell membrane. This is due to the distribution of ions across the complex cell membrane. Sodium is found in high concentration outside the cell and in low concentration inside the cell. Because of this concentration gradient, sodium ions attempt to enter the cell. Energy is expended to develop this gradient. However, during this phase of the action potential, the cell membrane is relatively impermeable to sodium. Potassium is found in high concentration inside the cell and in low concentration outside the cell. This ion, in small amounts, is able to cross the cell membrane. Therefore, during phase 4, potassium is able to traverse the cell membrane from inside to outside. Because of this direction of potassium flux or movement, the interior of the cell becomes electrically negative while the exterior is positive. The resting membrane potential, then, depends primarily on the potassium gradient across the cell membrane.

At the onset of depolarization (Fig 34), a complex gating mechanism (the fast channel) in the cell membrane opens momentarily (the duration is approximately 1 ms), permitting the rapid entry of sodium into the cell with its concentration gradient. Since there is now a flow of positively charged ions from outside to inside the cell, the interior of the cell becomes electrically positive (about +20 mV) while the outside of the cell membrane is negative. This portion of the action potential is called *phase 0*. When phase 0 occurs in the ventricular muscle cells at the same time, the QRS complex of the ECG is generated. The P wave is generated by phase 0 in the atrial muscle mass. As the gating mechanism closes and the entry of sodium slows down, the electrical charge inside the cell becomes less positive, initiating the repolarization process (*phase 1*). During *phase 2* the action potential is approximately isoelectric and the cell remains depolarized. Significant amounts of sodium are no longer entering the cell through the fast channel, whereas calcium and possibly sodium are entering the cell through the slow channel. Phase 2 of the ventricular muscle occurs at

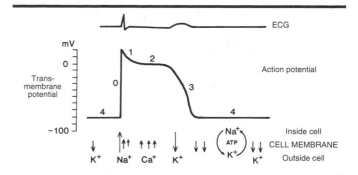

Fig 34. Schematic representation of ventricular myocardial working cell action potential. Arrows indicate times of major ionic movement across cell membrane.

the time of the ST segment of the ECG. *Phase 3* represents rapid repolarization, during which the inside of the cell again becomes negative. This is caused by an increased efflux or movement of potassium ions from inside to outside the cell. Phase 3 in the ventricular muscle occurs during the T wave.

Repolarization is completed at the end of phase 3. The interior of the cell is again approximately –90 mV. However, the ionic distribution across the cell membrane is different from that immediately before onset of depolarization. Because of the entry of sodium into the cell and the loss of potassium from the cell, there is a higher concentration of intracellular sodium and a lower concentration of intracellular potassium. This would not prevent the cell from being depolarized a second time, but repeated depolarizations without an appropriate redistribution of sodium and potassium ions would lead to a serious impairment of cell function. Hence, during *phase 4* a special pumping mechanism in the cell membrane is activated. It transports sodium ions from inside to outside the cell and brings potassium ions into the cell. This pumping mechanism depends on adenosine triphosphate (ATP) as its energy source.

The level of resting membrane potential (phase 4) at the onset of depolarization is an important determinant of the conductivity (ability to cause an adjoining cell to depolarize and the speed by which the adjoining cell is depolarized) of that electrical impulse to other cells. The less negative the resting membrane potential at the onset of phase 0 (eg, –60 mV as opposed to –90 mV), the slower the rate of rise of phase 0. Conductivity is directly related to the rate of rise of phase 0 of the action potential. Among the factors that determine the rate of rise of phase 0 (and hence conductivity) are the sodium gradient across the cell membrane at the onset of phase 0 and potassium gradient during phase 4. For example, an increase in extracellular potassium will result in a decrease in the potassium gradient and a decrease in the resting membrane potential.

The action potential of a pacemaker cell differs significantly from that of a working myocardial cell (Fig 35). Pacemaker cells possess the property of automaticity; ie,

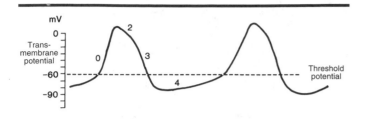

Fig 35. Schematic representation of pacemaker cell action potential.

they are able to depolarize spontaneously. An important feature of the pacemaker cell action potential is that phase 4 does not remain at a constant level. During this phase there is a gradual lessening of the resting membrane potential. This occurs because of the entry of small amounts of calcium as well as sodium and a decrease in the outward flow of potassium ions during phase 4. Hence, the resting membrane potential becomes less negative (a process called *spontaneous diastolic depolarization*).

When the resting membrane potential reaches a certain critical voltage (threshold), phase 0 begins. Since phase 0 begins at a less negative resting membrane potential, the rate of rise of phase 0 is slower than is seen in a normal myocardial working cell. The slow rate of rise of the action potential (phase 0) in cells of the sinus node and AV junction depends on the accelerated entry of calcium and, possibly, sodium ions through the slow channel.

The slope of phase 4 is important in the rate of impulse formation. The steeper the slope, the more rapid the rate of the pacemaker cell; the more gradual the slope, the slower the rate. Activation of the sympathetic nervous system (or administration of a catecholamine) makes the slope steeper and thereby enhances automaticity. Stimulation of the parasympathetic nervous system (ie, vagal stimulation) produces the opposite effect. Commonly used antiarrhythmic drugs (lidocaine, procainamide, quinidine, disopyramide, flecainide, amiodarone, tocainide, mexiletine, diphenylhydantoin) may decrease the rate of spontaneous depolarization.

Clinically the most important groups of pacemaker cells are found in the sinus node, the AV junction, and the ventricular conduction system. The rate of spontaneous depolarization (the "firing rate") differs in these several locations. The sinus node is the primary pacemaker of the heart and has a firing rate of 60 to 100 beats per minute. The firing rate of the AV junction is 40 to 60 per minute, and that of the ventricle (Purkinje fibers) is less than 40 per minute. This decrement in the firing rate has important physiological implications. The lower pacemakers (AV junction and ventricle) fail to reach threshold potential (ie, they are prevented from spontaneously depolarizing) before being depolarized in phase 4 by a sinus node impulse. Thus, the pacemakers in the AV junction and ventricle are "escape pacemakers"; ie, they do not spontaneously produce an electrical impulse unless the faster

pacemaker (eg, the sinus node) fails. Hence, if the sinus rate falls significantly below 60 per minute, a junctional escape beat should occur. Likewise, if a supraventricular impulse does not reach the ventricles within approximately 1.5 seconds (equivalent to a rate of 40 per minute), a ventricular escape beat should occur. However, the rates of these escape pacemakers can be increased or decreased in various disease states, with drugs, or with sympathetic or parasympathetic stimulation.

Another important concept is that of the refractory period (Fig 36). The refractory period of the ventricle begins with the onset of phase 0 (the onset of the QRS complex) and terminates at the end of phase 3 (the end of the T wave). It can most conveniently be divided into two portions: the absolute refractory period and the relative refractory period. During the absolute refractory period, the cell cannot propagate or conduct an action potential. During the relative refractory period, a strong stimulus may result in a propagated but not necessarily normal action potential. The absolute refractory period begins with the onset of phase 0 and ends midway through phase 3 (at about the apex of the T wave); the relative refractory period extends through the remainder of phase 3 (to the end of the T wave).

Mechanisms of Impulse Formation

There are two basic mechanisms whereby an electrical impulse may arise in the myocardium: automaticity and reentry.

Automaticity. An impulse may arise through the mechanism of automaticity described above. Other, "abnormal" forms of automaticity may also be responsible for impulse formation and have been related to abnormalities in slow channel activity:

1. An afterpotential is a transient decrease in the resting membrane potential following the action potential (ie, during phase 4). If such an afterpotential is able to reach threshold, spontaneous depolarization will occur.
2. Multiple afterpotentials may occur (these are referred to as *oscillations*).
3. Differences in potential between nearby groups of cells may result when incomplete repolarization occurs in one group of cells (eg, in cells adjacent to an infarct), whereas normal repolarization occurs elsewhere. Current may then flow between these groups of cells, causing the normal cells to depolarize.
4. Triggered automaticity describes the induction of an automatic focus dependent on an initiating premature beat, which because of an abnormal repolarization causes a second depolarization or a series of depolarizations.

Reentry. The second mechanism for impulse formation is reentry, which may occur in the sinus node, the atrium, the AV junction, or the ventricular conduction sys-

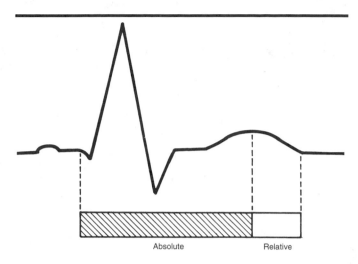

Fig 36. Relation of refractory period to electrocardiogram.

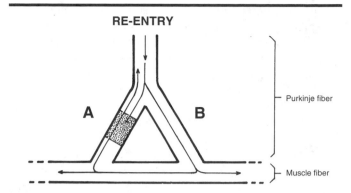

Fig 37. Diagrammatic representation of mechanism of reentry. Branches of Purkinje fiber that join muscle fiber are represented by A and B. Shaded area in A represents area of unidirectional block.

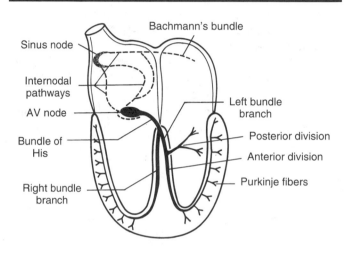

Fig 38. Diagrammatic representation of cardiac conduction system.

tem. It may be responsible for isolated beats, such as PVCs, or abnormal rhythms, such as ventricular tachycardia. As an example of this mechanism (Fig 37), consider an electrical impulse traveling down a ventricular Purkinje fiber that divides into two branches, A and B, and joins a muscle fiber. If conduction in both Purkinje branches is normal, the electrical impulse will travel down both branches to the muscle fiber. If, however, unidirectional (antegrade) block is present in one Purkinje branch (A) and conduction down the other branch (B) is slow, the electrical impulse will reach the muscle fiber through branch B. It will then travel down the muscle fiber. When it reaches branch A, the electrical impulse can be conducted back through A (since only antegrade block was present) to the original Purkinje fiber. From that point, this electrical impulse can travel through the remainder of the Purkinje system, giving rise to an ectopic impulse (eg, a PVC). The same result would occur if the refractory period of branch A was longer than that of branch B. When an electrical impulse reached the point of division, it would find A refractory and would travel down B and then down the muscle fiber. It could then be conducted retrogradely through A if A had recovered from its refractory period.

The basic components of the reentry mechanism include dual conduction pathways, one of which has unidirectional block (or a longer refractory period); the other has slow conduction so that transit time around the circuit is long enough that the refractory period of the Purkinje conduction tissue at the site of and proximal to the block is no longer absolute. Many of these changes from the normal pattern are caused by diseases, such as coronary artery disease and cardiomyopathy.

Conduction of the Cardiac Impulse

The normal cardiac impulse originates in the sinus node, a structure located in the superior portion of the right atrium at its juncture with the superior vena cava (Fig 38).

Conduction from the sinus node is thought to occur over internodal pathways. Three internodal pathways have been described. The anterior pathway arises at the cranial end of the sinus node. It divides into branches, one to the left atrium (Bachmann's bundle) and the other along the right side of the interatrial septum to the AV node. The middle internodal pathway arises along the endocardial surface of the sinus node and descends through the interatrial septum to the AV node. The posterior pathway arises from the caudal end of the sinus node and approaches the AV node at its posterior aspect. The speed of conduction through the atria is approximately 1000 mm/s.

The AV node is located inferiorly in the right atrium, anterior to the ostium of the coronary sinus, and above the tricuspid valve. The speed of conduction is slowed (about 200 mm/s) through the AV node. The AV node is anatomically a complicated network of fibers. These fibers converge at its lower margin to form a discrete bundle of fibers, the bundle of His (or AV bundle). This structure penetrates the anulus fibrosis and arrives at the upper margin of the muscular interventricular septum, where it gives origin to the bundle branches.

The left bundle branch arises as a series of radiations at right angles to the bundle of His. Although the anatomy of these radiations is complex and variable, two groups can be considered. The superior, anterior radiation courses down the anterior aspect of the interventricular septum to the anterolateral papillary muscle, where it breaks up into a Purkinje network. The inferior, posterior radiation is shorter and thicker, passing posteriorly to the base of the posteromedial papillary muscle, where it branches into the Purkinje network. Purkinje fibers to the interventricular septum may arise as a separate radiation or as fibers from either the anterior or posterior radiation.

The right bundle branch courses down the interventricular septum on the right side. It contributes Purkinje fibers to the septum only near the apex of the right ventricle. At the lower end of the septum, it passes into the right ventricular wall, where it branches into a Purkinje network.

As the electrical impulse leaves the AV node, it passes into the bundle of His and then down the bundle branches simultaneously. The first section of the ventricle to begin depolarization is the midportion of the interventricular septum from the left side. The free walls of the ventricles are depolarized simultaneously. The speed of conduction through the ventricular Purkinje network is rapid, about 4000 mm/s.

References

1. Smith WM. Mechanisms of cardiac arrhythmias and conduction disturbances. In: Hurst JW, ed. *The Heart, Arteries and Veins.* 7th ed. New York, NY: McGraw-Hill Information Services Co, Health Professions Division; 1990:473-489.
2. Zipes DP. Genesis of cardiac arrhythmias: electrophysiological considerations. In: Braunwald E, ed. *Heart Disease: A Textbook of Cardiovascular Medicine.* 4th ed. Philadelphia, Pa: WB Saunders Co; 1992:588-627.

Defibrillation

Defibrillation is the therapeutic use of electric current delivered in large amounts over very brief periods of time. The defibrillation shock temporarily depolarizes ("stuns") an irregularly beating heart and thus allows more coordinated contractile activity to resume. Physiologically the shock depolarizes the myocardium, terminating ventricular fibrillation (VF) or other arrhythmias and allowing normal electrical activity to occur.

Importance of Defibrillation

Rationale for Early Defibrillation

A simple rationale supports defibrillation as early as possible:
- The most frequent initial rhythm in sudden cardiac arrest is VF.
- The only effective treatment for VF is electrical defibrillation.
- The probability of successful defibrillation diminishes rapidly over time.
- VF tends to convert to asystole within a few minutes.

Many adult patients in VF can survive neurologically intact even if defibrillation is performed as late as 6 to 10 minutes after the arrest.[1-5] CPR performed while waiting for the defibrillator appears to prolong VF and to contribute to preservation of heart and brain function.[4-6] Basic CPR alone, however, cannot convert hearts in VF to a normal rhythm.

The speed with which defibrillation is performed is the major determinant of the success of resuscitative attempts. Nearly all neurologically intact survivors, who in some studies number more than 90%, had a ventricular tachyarrhythmia that was treated by early defibrillation.[1-5] It appears from studies in which Holter monitors were used that ventricular tachycardia (VT) is the initial rhythm disturbance[4] in up to 85% of persons with sudden, out-of-hospital, nontraumatic cardiac arrest. These studies, however, are somewhat biased, in that they represent patients who were on a Holter monitor. Most of these patients had underlying heart disease, and the majority were taking antiarrhythmic drugs at the time of the study. Ventricular tachycardia, however, is frequently short lived and converts rapidly to VF, from which the only hope for successful resuscitation lies in early defibrillation. Furthermore, the proportion of patients with VF also declines with each passing minute as more and more of these patients deteriorate into asystole, from which successful resuscitation is extremely unlikely. The remaining non–VF patients have a low probability of survival with current resuscitation techniques. Four to eight minutes after collapse, approximately 50% of patients are still in VF (Fig 1).[2,7-10]

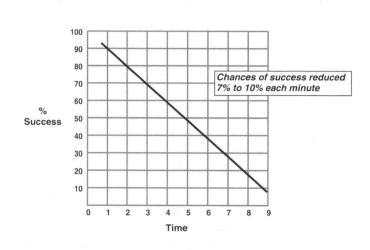

Fig 1. Resuscitation success versus time. From Cummins.[11]

Survival rates from cardiac arrest can be remarkably high if the event is witnessed. For example, when people in supervised cardiac rehabilitation programs suffer a witnessed cardiac arrest, defibrillation is usually performed within minutes. In four studies of cardiac arrest in this setting, 90 of 101 victims (89%) were resuscitated.[12-15] This is the highest survival rate for a defined out-of-hospital population.

Improved survival rates for patients with cardiac arrest have been reported from communities that had no prehospital ACLS services but added early defibrillation programs. The most impressive results were reported from King County, Wash, where the survival rate for patients with VF improved from 7% to 26%,[16] and from rural Iowa, where the survival rate for VF rose from 3% to 19%.[17] More modest results have been observed in rural communities of southeastern Minnesota,[18] northeastern Minnesota,[19] and Wisconsin[20] (Table 1).

Table 1. Effectiveness of Early Defibrillation Programs[11]

Location	Before Early Defibrillation		After Early Defibrillation		Odds Ratio for Improved Survival
King County, Wash	7		26	(10/38)	3.7
Iowa	3	(1/31)	19	(12/64)	6.3
Southeast Minnesota	4	(1/27)	17	(6/36)	4.3
Northeast Minnesota	2	(3/118)	10	(8/81)	5.0
Wisconsin	4	(32/893)	11	(33/304)	2.8

Values are percent surviving and, in parentheses, how many patients had ventricular fibrillation.

A major determinant in these studies was time. It is clear that the earlier defibrillation occurs, the better the prognosis. Emergency personnel have only a few minutes after the collapse of a victim to reestablish a sustained perfusing rhythm (Fig 2). CPR can sustain a patient for a short period but cannot directly restore an organized rhythm. Restoration of an adequate perfusing rhythm requires defibrillation and advanced cardiac care, which must be administered within a few minutes of the initial arrest. Table 2 compares the differences in survival observed in different types of EMS systems. These systems differ in the strength of their chain of survival, especially in terms of early access (percentage of witnessed arrest), early CPR (percentage of witnessed arrest with citizen CPR), and early defibrillation (percentage with defibrillation by first responders). Automated external defibrillators (AEDs) increase the range of personnel who can use a defibrillator and thus shorten the time between collapse and defibrillation. This exciting prospect accounts for addition of this material to the ACLS training curriculum.

Successful defibrillation depends on the metabolic state of the myocardium: longer duration of VF leads to greater myocardial deterioration. Consequently, shocks are less likely to convert VF to a spontaneous rhythm. If VF is of short duration, as in patients with VF occurring in a coronary care unit or with a witnessed cardiac arrest, VF is very likely to respond to a shock. Because speed of defibrillation is the major determinant of survival from both in-hospital and out-of-hospital cardiac arrest, recent efforts have attempted to shorten the time between cardiac arrest and defibrillation. This can be done by training experienced emergency responders both in-hospital and out-of-hospital to use AEDs.[5,14,16,17,23]

Table 2. Range of Survival Rate to Hospital Discharge for All Cardiac Arrests and Ventricular Fibrillation by System Type: Data From 29 Locations[21]

System Type	Survival: All Rhythms (%)	Weighted Average (%)	Survival: Ventricular Fibrillation (%)	Weighted Average (%)
EMT only	2-9	5	3-20	12
EMT-D	4-19	10	6-26	16
Paramedics	7-18	10	13-30	17
EMT/paramedic	4-26	17	23-33	26
EMT-D/paramedic	13-18	17	27-29	29

EMT indicates emergency medical technician; EMT-D, emergency medical technician-defibrillation.

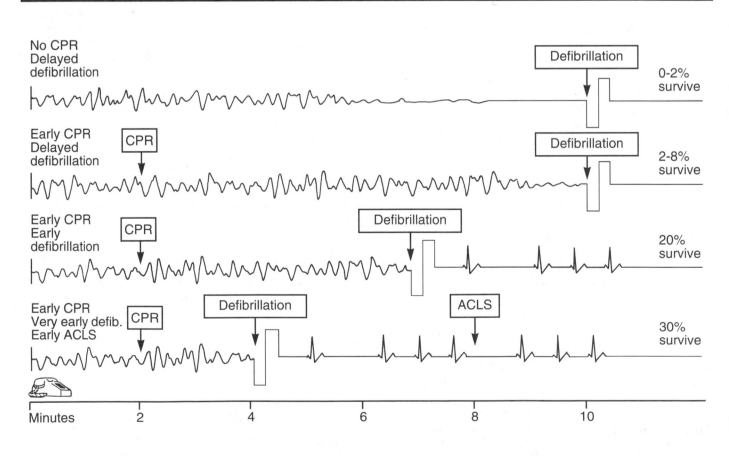

Fig 2. Survival rates are estimates of probability of survival to hospital discharge for patients with witnessed collapse and with ventricular fibrillation as initial rhythm. Estimates are based on a large number of published studies, which are collectively reviewed in References 21 and 22.

The AHA strongly endorses the position that all ambulances that may transport cardiac patients should carry either a manual or an automatic defibrillator and that the emergency personnel should be trained in its use.[24] The AHA recommends that these principles be applied to in-hospital resuscitation as well, where AED placement is clearly underused.

Principle of Early Defibrillation

The principle of early defibrillation states that all BLS personnel must be trained to operate, be equipped with, and be permitted to operate a defibrillator if in their professional activities they are expected to respond to people in cardiac arrest. This concept is now widely accepted.[7,8,20,25-29] BLS personnel include all first-responding emergency personnel, whether in-hospital or out-of-hospital (eg, emergency medical technicians, non–EMT first responders, firefighters, volunteer emergency personnel, physicians, nurses, and paramedics). Early defibrillation has become the standard of care for patients with either prehospital or in-hospital cardiac arrest,[30] except in sparsely populated and remote prehospital settings where the frequency of cardiac arrest is low and rescuer response times are very long.[31-33] Early defibrillation should be available in geographically isolated parts of the hospital where code team response times are greater than 1 minute. Early defibrillation should be available in geographically separate facilities where patients with potential for cardiac instabilities may be seen, such as drug and alcohol detoxification centers, or wherever sedation, anesthetics, or electroshock therapies are needed. Early defibrillation should be considered in free-standing settings where employees or the public are likely to seek first assistance from healthcare personnel. Conceptually and practically, defibrillation should be considered part of BLS. In the mid-1990s use of AEDs will probably become a core part of all BLS training, with nearly all intermediate-level BLS providers using AEDs and not manual defibrillators.

Overview of Defibrillators

A defibrillator is a device that administers a controlled electrical shock to patients to terminate a cardiac arrhythmia. The technique of administering the electrical shock is usually referred to as *defibrillation* if it is used to terminate VF, or *cardioversion* if it is administered for other arrhythmias — typically atrial fibrillation, atrial flutter, or ventricular tachycardia (VT).

A direct-current defibrillator consists of a variable transformer allowing the operator to select a variable voltage potential, an AC to DC converter that includes a capacitor to store the energy, a charge switch that allows the capacitor to charge, and discharge switches to complete the circuit from the capacitor to the electrodes. Most commercially available defibrillators use a half sinusoidal waveform for external defibrillation. For technical rea-

sons, implantable automatic defibrillators often use trapezoidal waveforms. Bidirectional or multipathway waveforms have been shown to be effective for automatic internal defibrillation (electrodes applied directly to the heart).[34] The effectiveness of such waveforms for transthoracic defibrillation is under investigation.

Automated external defibrillators (Fig 3) also deliver electrical shocks to patients but have several distinguishing characteristics. First, they are attached to the patient through adhesive sternal-apex pads on flexible cables. This allows "hands-free" defibrillation, a feature available with conventional defibrillation as well. Second, AEDs have internal microprocessor-based detection systems that analyze the rhythm for the characteristics of VF/VT. If VF/VT is present, the AEDs "advise" the operator to deliver a shock. AEDs are "automated" in the sense that the device, and not the operator, analyzes the rhythm and determines the presence of VF/VT.

Energy, Current, and Voltage

A few terms in basic electricity help with understanding defibrillation. A defibrillation shock passes a large flow of electrons through the heart over a brief period. This flow of electrons is called *current,* which is measured in *amperes.* The *pressure* pushing this flow of electrons is referred to as the electrical *potential,* and potential is measured in *volts.* There is always a *resistance* to this flow of electrons, which is called *impedance,* measured in *ohms.* In short, electrons flow with a certain pressure for a certain period of time (usually milliseconds) through a substance that has resistance.

A series of formulas defines these relationships. The electrical potential (measured in volts) multiplied by current (measured in amperes) equals the *power* (measured in *watts*). One watt is the power produced by one ampere of current flowing with a pressure of one volt. This power sustained over a duration of time (seconds) determines the total *energy* (joules).

Formula 1: Power (watts) = potential (volts) × current (amperes)

Formula 2: Energy (joules) = power (watts) × duration (seconds)

Formula 3: Energy (joules) = potential (volts) × current (amperes) × duration (seconds)

Although the operator selects the shock energy (in joules), it is the current flow (in amperes) that actually defibrillates. With a constant amount of energy stored in the capacitor, the delivered current depends on the impedance (resistance) present between the defibrillator electrodes. Fig 4 illustrates the effect of increasing resistance on delivered current. Notice the important point that the resistance (impedance) cuts down the electron flow (amperes) dramatically, as demonstrated in Formula 4:

Formula 4: Current (amperes) = potential (volts)/impedance (ohms)

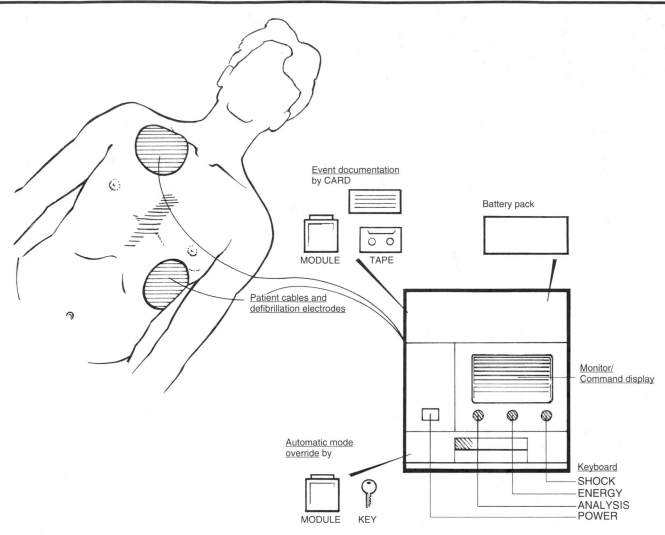

Fig 3. Schematic drawing of automated external defibrillator and its attachments to patient.

Transthoracic Impedance

Defibrillation is accomplished by passage of sufficient electrical current (amperes) through the heart for a brief period of time. Current flow is determined by the energy chosen (joules) and the transthoracic impedance (ohms), or resistance to current flow. Many factors determine transthoracic impedance. These include energy selected, electrode size, electrode-skin coupling material, number and time interval of previous shocks, phase of ventilation, distance between electrodes (size of the chest), and electrode-to-chest contact pressure.[35-44] Human transthoracic impedance has been reported to range from 15 to 150 ohms, with the average adult human impedance about 70 to 80 ohms.[37,43,45-48] If transthoracic impedance is high, a low-energy shock may fail to pass enough current through the heart to achieve defibrillation. Clinicians should not expect a sudden "jump" of the patient with every defibrillation attempt. Defibrillation "failures" are sometimes reported by mistake because the operator failed to see dramatic muscular jerks by the patient. Skeletal muscle response can be affected by sedation, anesthesia, drug overdoses, the patient's muscle mass and general condition, body temperature, and the interval without spontaneous circulation.[45,46,49]

To reduce impedance when using hand-held defibrillation paddles, the defibrillator operator should always apply a defibrillation electrode gel or paste made specifically for defibrillation. Adhesive defibrillation electrodes connected directly to the defibrillator ("remote" or "hands-off" defibrillation) as well as gelled pads permeated with electrode paste are also acceptable. Use of bare paddles without a coupling material between the electrodes and the chest wall results in very high transthoracic impedance.[43] Although the phase of respiration influences impedance,[41,43] most arrested patients will be in end-expiration, especially those with firm paddle-to-chest contact pressure, and this will give a lower impedance. It is important to use an appropriate conductive material between the paddles and the chest to maximize current flow. Use of improper gels or pastes can cause burns or sparks and can pose a serious risk of fire in an oxygen-enriched environment.[50]

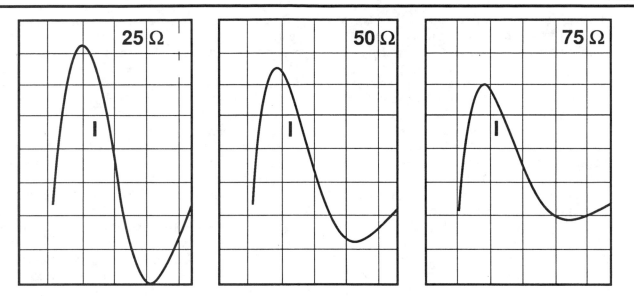

Fig 4. Relationship between transthoracic current (I) and impedance (ohms) in defibrillation. As transthoracic impedance increases, current flow decreases. At high impedance, current flow may be inadequate to achieve defibrillation.

Electrode Size

In general, the larger the electrode, the less the impedance, but too large an electrode can result in inadequate contact with the chest or a large portion of the current traversing extracardiac pathways and missing the heart.[51] For adults most defibrillation electrodes range from 8.5 to 12 cm in diameter, and these are effective.[37,39,48,52]

Infants and children require smaller electrodes. However, high transthoracic impedance in children is found when small "pediatric" paddles are used.[53] Thus, larger "adult" paddles should be used as soon as the paddles will fit completely on the child's chest. This transition occurs at approximately 10 kg, the average weight of a 1-year-old child.[53] Recent research has demonstrated lower impedance and improved current flow with the largest defibrillation pad that can fit on the pediatric chest.[54] Accordingly, children older than 1 year can be defibrillated with adult paddles unless the child is unusually small.

Electrode Position

Electrode placement for defibrillation and cardioversion is important. The electrodes should be placed in a position that will maximize current flow through the myocardium. The recommended placement is anterior-apex (sternal). The anterior electrode is placed to the right of the upper part of the sternum below the clavicle and the apex electrode to the left of the nipple with the center of the electrode in the midaxillary line (Fig 5).[55] An acceptable alternative approach is to place one paddle anteriorly over the left *precordium* and the other posteriorly behind the heart, in the left infrascapular location. Another approach would be to place the anterior paddle over the left apex with the posterior paddle placed in the left infrascapular location.[48,55-57] All of these pathways will

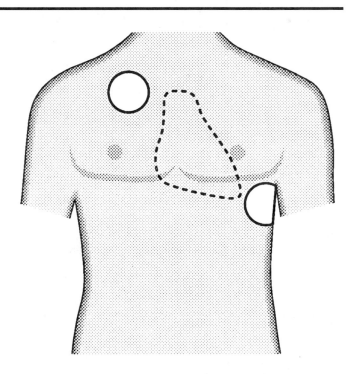

Fig 5. Recommended anterior-apex position for defibrillation. The anterior electrode should be to the right of the upper sternum below the clavicle. The apex electrode should be placed to the left of the nipple with the center of the electrode in the midaxillary line.

maximize current flow through the cardiac chambers. If hand-held paddles are used, the paddles should be applied to the chest wall firmly. Care should be taken that the electrodes are well separated and that paste or gel is not smeared between the electrodes on the chest. Otherwise, current may flow preferentially along the chest wall, "missing" the heart, or arc into the air between electrodes, causing an electrical hazard to bystanders and the device operator.

Self-adhesive monitor/defibrillator electrode pads are as effective as rigid metal paddles, are probably safer and more convenient, and can be used in any of these locations.[48]

When cardioversion or defibrillation is performed in patients with permanent pacemakers, care should be taken to avoid placing the electrodes near the pacemaker generator since direct defibrillation can rarely cause temporary or permanent pacemaker malfunction. In addition, the pacemaker generator box can absorb much of the current of defibrillation directly from the pads or paddles and reduce the chances of success. Patients with permanent pacemakers who have been defibrillated or cardioverted should have the pacing and sensing thresholds checked after the shock and should be examined for integrity of programming.[58] Nevertheless, never withhold defibrillation or cardioversion from pacemaker patients if either is indicated.

Energy Requirements for Defibrillation and Cardioversion

Adult Requirements

If energy and current are too low, the shock will not terminate the arrhythmia; if energy and current are too high, functional and morphological damage may result.[49,59-62] There is no clear relation between body size and energy requirements for defibrillation in adults. Transthoracic impedance plays an important role (see below).[45,49]

In a prospective, out-of-hospital study, defibrillation rates and the proportion of patients resuscitated and later discharged from the hospital were virtually identical in patients receiving shocks of 175 J and 320 J.[63] Since most commercially available defibrillators have a 200-J energy setting, the recommended first shock energy for defibrillation is 200 J.

The appropriate energy level for second shocks should be 200 to 300 J. Transthoracic impedance declines with repeated shocks. Therefore, higher current flow will occur with subsequent shocks, even at the same energy.[37,43,44] These arguments would favor repeating the second shock at the same energy level as the first if the first shock fails to terminate VF. On the other hand, only modest reductions in transthoracic impedance occur in humans after repeated shocks.[37] A greater and more predictable increase in current will occur if the shock energy is raised, and this favors giving the second shock at a higher energy than the first. To reconcile these positions, a range of energies, from 200 to 300 J, is acceptable for the second shock.

If the first two shocks fail to defibrillate, a third shock, of 360 J, should be delivered immediately. If VF is initially terminated by a shock but then recurs during the arrest sequence, shocks should be reinitiated at the energy level that previously resulted in successful defibrillation. Shock energies should be increased only if a shock fails to terminate VF.

BLS should be performed until the arrival of the defibrillator. However, since the most important determinant of survival in adult out-of-hospital VF is rapid defibrillation and the success of defibrillation is adversely affected by delay, shocks should be given as soon as a defibrillator arrives.[14,16,17,23] If three rapidly administered shocks fail to defibrillate, CPR should be continued, IV access accomplished, epinephrine administered, ventilation established or continued, and then shocks repeated. Interposed CPR between shocks one and two and two and three provides less benefit than rapid shocks.

Cardioversion of ventricular and supraventricular tachycardia, including atrial fibrillation and atrial flutter, requires less energy. The recommended initial energy is 100 J with stepwise increases in energy should initial shocks fail.[49,55] The electrical cardioversion algorithm notes that 50 J can be used for atrial flutter and 200 J for polymorphic VT.

The cardioversion energy required to terminate VT depends on the morphological characteristics and rate of the arrhythmia. Monomorphic VT responds well to cardioversion shocks beginning at an energy of 100 J.[64] Polymorphic VT, a more rapid and disorganized arrhythmia, behaves like VF. The initial shock energy should be 200 J with stepwise increases if the first shock fails to cardiovert.[64]

Pediatric Defibrillation

A critical ventricular mass is necessary to sustain VF.[65] Ventricular fibrillation is uncommon in children and rare in infants. Cardiac arrest in the pediatric age group is most often secondary to respiratory arrest. When an infant or child is found to be without a pulse, therapy should first be directed toward providing adequate ventilation and oxygenation and supporting the circulation by external chest compressions. Bradycardia is secondary to respiratory arrest and is most likely to respond to this approach. If VF is present, a weight-related energy dose of 1 J/ lb (2 J/kg) is recommended.[60] If defibrillation is not successful, the energy dose should be doubled and shocks repeated. Since bone is a poor conductor, position the paddles/pads away from major bony structures such as the spine or clavicles. Allow at least 1 to 2 inches clearance between the pads or paddles. It is possible to defibrillate newborn patients propped on their side using anterior-posterior pad/paddle placement.

Current-Based Defibrillation

Current-based defibrillation is a promising alternative approach to defibrillation. The defibrillator operator selects electric current (amperes) instead of energy (joules). This approach avoids the problem of low energy selection in the face of high impedance (resulting in too low a current flow and failure to defibrillate), or high-energy selection in the face of low impedance (resulting in an excessive current flow, myocardial damage, and failure to defibrillate).[45,49] Recent advances allow instantaneous measurement of transthoracic impedance before delivery of a defibrillating shock.[45] The optimal current for ventricular defibrillation appears to be 30 to 40 A.[46,47,49] An operator could specify the desired current, the transthoracic impedance could be instantly measured, and a "smart" defibrillator could deliver the exact current that the operator had selected. Several clinical studies using this approach have demonstrated that it is feasible and effective.[46,47,66] In patients with average transthoracic impedance, the presently recommended standard energy dose of 200 J will generate an appropriate first shock of 30 A of current. In patients with higher impedance, 200-J shocks may generate inadequate current. For such patients a current-based approach should be beneficial.[45-47,49,66]

Current requirements for VT will vary according to the form of the arrhythmia. Monomorphic VT should convert with as low as 18 A of current, whereas polymorphic VT should receive initial shocks of 30 A, similar to VF.[64]

Synchronized Cardioversion

Synchronization of delivered energy reduces the chances that a shock will induce VF, which can occur when electrical energy impinges on the relative refractory portion of the cardiac electrical activity.[56] Thus, synchronization is recommended for supraventricular tachycardia, atrial fibrillation, and atrial flutter. In some patients synchronization in VT may be difficult and misleading because of the form of the arrhythmia. The VT patient who is pulseless and unconscious should receive immediate unsynchronized defibrillation. It may be difficult to provide synchronized shocks to patients with broad, bizarre, or rapid VT. If delays occur with synchronized shocks, switch at once to unsynchronized shocks. Should any shock cause VF, then a second, unsynchronized defibrillation shock should be delivered immediately to terminate VF.

Asystole

There is no evidence that attempting to "defibrillate" asystole is beneficial. However, in some subjects, coarse VF can be present in some leads while very small undulations are present in others. This may mimic asystole in some leads. Therefore, more than one ECG lead should be viewed before concluding that the patient should not receive a shock because of asystole.[67] Asystole should **not** be routinely shocked under the rationale of "you cannot make asystole worse." Empiric shocks to asystole can inhibit the recovery of natural pacemakers in the heart and completely eliminate any chance of recovery.

Procedure for Defibrillation

Once the decision is made to defibrillate, the following steps should be taken:

1. Place the patient in a safe environment, away from pooled water or a metal surface under either patient or rescuer.
2. Apply appropriate conductive materials to hand-held electrodes or use monitor/defibrillator electrode pads.
3. Turn on the defibrillator.
4. Select the energy level; 200 J is recommended for the initial shock for VF.
5. Charge the capacitor.
6. Ensure proper placement of the electrodes on chest: the apex–high right parasternal position is standard (Fig 5). If hand-held paddle electrodes are used, apply firm pressure on each. Do not lean on the paddles because they may slip. Be sure there is no smearing of coupling material between the paddles, or the current may preferentially follow this low-resistance pathway along the chest wall, "missing" the heart. Remove any transdermal medication patches.
7. Make sure no personnel are directly or indirectly in contact with the patient. If ventilation via a bag-mask device or endotracheal tube is being performed, the rescuer should step back and momentarily release the bag. It is unnecessary to disconnect a bag from an endotracheal tube if the tube is well secured.
8. Deliver the electric shock by depressing both discharge buttons simultaneously.

Special Situations

Defibrillation of Patients With Automatic Implantable Cardioverter-Defibrillators

Patients with implantable cardioverter-defibrillators (ICDs) are at high risk for VF. When caring for a patient with an ICD who has experienced cardiac arrest, rescuers should know the following:

1. If the ICD discharges while the rescuer is touching the victim, the rescuer may feel the shock, but it will not be dangerous. Personnel shocked by ICDs report sensations similar to contact with an electrical outlet.
2. ICDs are protected against damage from conventional transchest defibrillator shocks, but they require an ICD readiness check after external defibrillation occurs.
3. If VF or VT is present despite an ICD, an external shock should be given immediately because it is likely that the ICD failed to defibrillate the heart. After an initial series of shocks, the ICD will become operative again only if a period of nonfibrillatory rhythm occurs to reset the unit.[68]

4. ICD units generally use patch electrodes that cover a portion of the epicardial surface, and these may reduce transcardiac current from transthoracic shocks.[69] Thus, if transthoracic shocks of up to 360 J fail to defibrillate an ICD patient, the chest electrode positions should be immediately changed (eg, anterior-apex to anteroposterior) and the transthoracic shocks repeated. The different electrode positions could increase transcardiac current flow and facilitate defibrillation.

Defibrillation of Patients With Hypothermia

See chapter 10, "Special Resuscitation Situations," on treatment of patients with hypothermia.

Precordial Thump

Ventricular tachycardia has been converted to sinus rhythm by a precordial thump. Reports of the efficacy of this maneuver have varied, from 11% to 25% of VT cases.[70,71] VF has also been terminated by a thump but only in a very small number of cases.[70] A thump is generally ineffective for termination of prehospital VF.[71] Moreover, a precordial thump may be deleterious, converting VT to more malignant rhythms, such as faster VT, VF, asystole, and electromechanical dissociation.[71-73]

Since a single thump can be delivered quickly and easily, it may be considered an optional technique (Class IIb) in a witnessed cardiac arrest where the patient is pulseless and a defibrillator is not immediately available.[70] Because a precordial thump is only occasionally effective for termination of VF,[71-73] it should never be allowed to delay electrical defibrillation. Because it may cause VT to deteriorate to VF, asystole, or electromechanical dissociation, precordial thump should never be used in the patient with VT who has a pulse unless a defibrillator and pacemaker are available immediately.[70] It is a technique that should be taught only to allied health professionals, not to lay rescuers.

Importance of Automated External Defibrillation

Every person trained in ACLS must also be familiar with AEDs and know how to interact with emergency personnel equipped with these devices.[7,8,25,26,74-80] Defibrillation was once a skill reserved for emergency care providers trained in all aspects of ACLS, but it is now performed by BLS personnel who have less training.[25,78,79] The availability of AEDs has sparked this extension of defibrillation capability and permitted wider achievement of earlier defibrillation.[2] AEDs eliminate the need for training in rhythm recognition and make early defibrillation by minimally trained personnel practical and achievable.[7,8,25,26,74-80] AEDs were originally for use by emergency personnel

and for family members and associates of people at high risk for sudden cardiac death.[81] Now the range of personnel who may be trained in the use of these devices is much broader.[82] ACLS and BLS providers, both in-hospital and prehospital, should be able to use AEDs and know the protocols for their use. They will be called on with increasing frequency to interact with medical personnel or community members who also can use these devices.

Overview of Automated External Defibrillators

Types of Automated External Defibrillators

The generic term *automated external defibrillators* refers to external defibrillators that incorporate a rhythm analysis system. Some devices are considered "fully" automated, whereas others are semiautomated or shock-advisory defibrillators.[83] All AEDs are attached to the patient by two adhesive pads and connecting cables,[52] as shown in Fig 3. These adhesive pads have two functions — to record the rhythm and to deliver the electric shock. A fully automated defibrillator requires only that the operator attach the defibrillatory pads and turn on the device. If VF (or VT above a preset rate) is present, the device will charge its capacitors and deliver a shock.

Semiautomated or shock-advisory devices require additional operator steps, including pressing an "analyze" control to initiate rhythm analysis and pressing a "shock" control to deliver the shock. The shock control is pressed only when the device identifies VF and "advises" the operator to press the shock control.

Fully automated defibrillators were developed with simple requirements for use by operators with limited training. In general, this user group has comprised family members of high-risk patients and emergency personnel who are rarely called on to treat patients in cardiac arrest.

Shock-advisory AEDs may be safer because they never enter the analysis mode unless activated by the operator and they leave the final decision of whether to deliver the shock to the operator. This increase in safety is more theoretical than real because clinical experience suggests that the devices are equally safe with or without the operator pushing the final shock button.[83]

Automated Analysis of Cardiac Rhythms

Unlike many other devices and approaches in emergency medicine, AEDs have been extensively tested, both in vitro against libraries of recorded cardiac rhythms[84] and clinically in numerous field trials.[18,85-92] The accuracy of the devices in rhythm analysis has been high. The rare errors noted with AEDs in field trials have

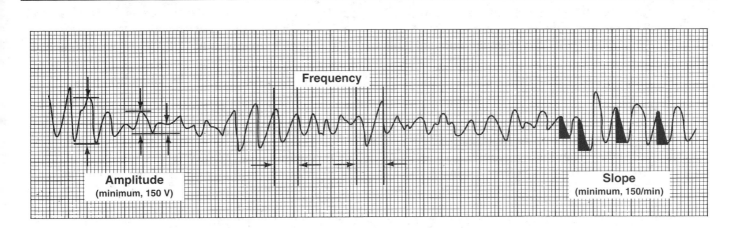

Fig 6. Features of surface electrocardiogram analyzed by automated external defibrillators.

been almost solely errors of omission where the device failed to recognize certain varieties of VF or VT or where operators failed to follow recommended operating procedures, such as avoidance of patient movement.[93,94]

The available AEDs are highly sophisticated, microprocessor-based devices that analyze multiple features of the surface ECG signal, including frequency, amplitude, and some integration of frequency and amplitude such as slope or wave morphology (Fig 6). A variety of filters check for QRS-like signals, radio transmission, or 60-cycle interference as well as for loose electrodes and poor electrode contact. Some intermittent radio transmissions can produce ECG artifact if a transmitter or receiver is used within 6 feet of a patient during rhythm analysis. Some devices are programmed to detect spontaneous patient movements or movement of the patient by others.

AEDs take multiple "looks" at the patient's rhythm, each look lasting a few seconds. If several of these analyses confirm the presence of a rhythm for which a shock is indicated and the other checks are consistent with a nonperfusing cardiac status, the fully automated defibrillator will charge and deliver a shock to the patient. The semiautomated device will signal the operator that a shock is advised. It does this after charging the capacitors, which does not occur until appropriate VF or VT has been identified. Once the capacitors are charged, a shock is advised. The operator can then clear the patient, push a shock button, and the shock is delivered.

Inappropriate Shocks or Failure to Shock

Extensive clinical experience has revealed that AEDs are rarely misled by patient movements (eg, seizures and agonal respirations), by repositioning of the patient by others, or by artifactual signals,[85-92] although some rare difficulties have been reported.[93-95] Failure to follow the manufacturer's instructions in the use of a fully automatic AED has in rare instances (less than one tenth of one

percent) resulted in the delivery of inappropriate electrical countershocks.[93] AEDs should be placed in the analysis mode *only* when full cardiac arrest has been confirmed and *only* when all movement, particularly the movement of patient transport, has ceased. Agonal respiration poses a problem because some devices may not be able to complete analysis cycles if the patient continues to display gasping respirations. Avoid using radio receivers and transmitters during rhythm analysis. The major errors reported in clinical trials have been occasional failures to deliver shocks to rhythms that may benefit from electrical therapy, such as extremely fine or coarse VF.

Ventricular Tachycardia

Although not designed to deliver synchronized shocks, most AEDs will shock monomorphic and polymorphic VT if the rate exceeds preset values. All rescuers who operate AEDs are trained to attach the device only to unconscious patients who are pulseless and without normal respirations. With this approach the operator serves as a second verification system to confirm that the patient has suffered a cardiac arrest. In an apneic, pulseless patient, electric shocks are indicated whether the rhythm is supraventricular tachycardia, VT, or VF. There have been rare case reports of shocks delivered to conscious patients with perfusing ventricular or supraventricular arrhythmias. These are operator errors, not device errors, and are preventable with good training of rescuers and good patient-assessment skills.[92]

Interruption of CPR

Emergency personnel must ensure that no one is touching the patient while the AED analyzes the rhythm, charges the capacitors, and delivers the shocks. Chest compression and ventilation must cease while the device is operating; this permits accurate analysis of the cardiac rhythm and prevents accidental shocks to the rescuers.

Movements induced by CPR can cause the AED to stop its analysis. The time between activating the rhythm analysis system, which is when CPR must stop, and the delivery of a shock averages 10 to 15 seconds.

This time without CPR that occurs when AEDs are used is a recognized exception to the AHA guidelines, which recommend that CPR not be stopped for more than 5 seconds. With the use of AEDs, the negative effects of temporarily stopping CPR are outweighed by the positive effects of delivering an early defibrillatory shock. For patients in refractory VF after the first shock, CPR may have to be interrupted for even longer periods to deliver the recommended three sequential shocks. Consequently, the guidelines for CPR and ECC recommend a maximum period of 90 seconds for diagnosing VF and delivering three shocks.[30,p2942]

Advantages and Disadvantages of Automated External Defibrillators

The major distinction between an automated and a conventional defibrillator is that a person must interpret the cardiac rhythm when a conventional defibrillator is used, but an electronic device interprets the rhythm when an AED is used.

Initial Training and Continuing Education

Conventional defibrillators require regular training and continuing education in rhythm recognition and device operation. The only psychomotor skills required by an AED user are recognition of a cardiac arrest, proper attachment of the device, and adherence to the memorized treatment sequence. Learning to use and operate an AED is easier than learning to perform CPR.[96] Many of the advantages of AEDs stem from brief, convenient training sessions and minimal continuing education.[97] In systems in which compensation must be provided for the initial training time and skills-review classes, the use of AEDs offers considerable financial savings.[98] In systems in which the anticipated number of cardiac arrests is low, skills maintenance is a major concern.[31,32] AEDs offer considerable advantages in these situations because little continuing education is needed.

Speed of Operation

In clinical trials, emergency personnel using an AED deliver the first shock an average of 1 minute sooner than personnel using conventional defibrillators.[88,89]

Rhythm Detection

Field studies have compared the rhythm detection ability of AEDs with that of emergency personnel.[88,89] Although AEDs have not achieved 100% accuracy in rhythm detection, they perform as well as EMTs who use conventional defibrillators.[88,89] The errors of correctly used AEDs have been limited to identification of very fine or very coarse VF. Available AEDs have responded appropriately to almost all perfusing rhythms and to cardiac arrest rhythms for which shocks are not indicated.

Remote Defibrillation Through Adhesive Pads

Another advantage of AEDs stems from the use of the adhesive defibrillatory pads attached to the patient by connecting cables.[48] This approach permits remote "hands-off" defibrillation, which is a safer method from the operator's perspective, particularly in the close confines of aeromedical and ground transport vehicles. Adhesive defibrillatory pads may also offer consistently better paddle placement during a lengthy resuscitation attempt. Some conventional defibrillators have adapters that permit operation through remote adhesive pads. These are becoming more widely used. All AEDs, however, have adhesive monitor/defibrillator electrode pads. With adhesive pads the operator cannot bear down with the heavy pressure used with conventional defibrillator paddles. This pressure lowers the transthoracic resistance by improving contact between the electrodes and the skin and bringing the paddles closer to each other by pressing the air from the lungs. The adhesive pads offer comparable low impedance, however, because of their larger pad surface area.[99]

Rhythm Monitoring

In clinical settings that require frequent rhythm monitoring, the liquid crystal rhythm displays of some AEDs are not yet fully comparable to the bright cathode-ray displays of conventional defibrillators.

Use of Automated External Defibrillators During Resuscitation Attempts

Operational Steps

All AEDs can be operated by following four simple steps:

1. Turn on the power.
2. Attach the device.
3. Initiate analysis of the rhythm.
4. Deliver the shock, if indicated and safe.

Brands and models of AEDs have a variety of features and controls and may differ in characteristics such as paper strip recorders, rhythm display methods, energy levels, and messages to the operator. Operators should understand how each brand and model approaches the four steps.

Standard Operational Procedures

Compared with the Megacode resuscitation procedures for ACLS, resuscitation attempts in which AEDs are used are relatively simple because there are fewer therapeutic options. Only automated defibrillation and basic CPR can be implemented.

Most response teams, including those in hospital, in medical clinics, or out of hospital, consist of at least two people. One team member operates the defibrillator, and another begins BLS. No other activities, including setting up oxygen delivery systems, suction equipment, intravenous lines, or mechanical CPR devices, should take precedence over or delay rhythm analysis and defibrillation. These interventions should proceed simultaneously if possible. The rescuer responsible for defibrillation concentrates on operating the defibrillator, while other rescuers attend to airway management, ventilations, and chest compressions.

The rescuer places the AED close to the supine patient's left ear and performs the defibrillation protocols from the patient's left side. This position provides better access to the defibrillator controls and easier placement of the defibrillatory pads and allows the other rescuer room to perform CPR. However, this position may not be possible in all clinical settings. Some EMS systems have adopted different operator roles and positions with equal success.

Depending on the manufacturer, the AED is turned on by pressing a power switch or by lifting the monitor screen to the "up" position. This activates the voice-ECG tape recorder and permits environmental sounds and operator statements to be recorded along with the patient's cardiac rhythm. Most AEDs can also be operated as a conventional defibrillator, though this may require special steps.

The adhesive defibrillator pads are opened quickly and attached first to the defibrillator cables and then to the patient's chest. The pads are placed in a modified lead II position (upper-right sternal border and lower-left ribs over the apex of the heart). When the pads are attached, CPR and other patient motion should be stopped and the analysis control should be pressed. All movement affecting the patient during analysis must be avoided, and radio transmitters and receivers should not be in operation. Assessment of the rhythms takes from 5 to 15 seconds, depending on the brand of AED. If VF is present, the device will announce that a shock is indicated by a printed message, a visual alarm, or often a voice-synthesized statement.

Safe Automated Defibrillation

The rescuer must always state loudly a "clear-the-patient" message, such as "I'm clear," "You're clear," "Everybody clear," before pressing the shock control. In most devices, pressing the "analyze" button initiates charging of the capacitors if a treatable rhythm is detected. The device shows that charging has started with a tone, a voice-synthesized message, or a light indicator. Shock delivery usually produces some contraction of the patient's musculature like that seen with the use of a conventional defibrillator. After the first shock is delivered, CPR is not restarted. Instead, the analyze control is pressed immediately to start another rhythm analysis cycle. If VF persists, the device will indicate this, and the "charging" and "shock-indicated" sequence is repeated for the second and third shocks. The goal is to analyze quickly for any persisting rhythm treatable by electric shocks (Fig 7).

Pediatric Guidelines

Cardiac arrest in the pediatric age group is seldom caused by VF. Defibrillation, therefore, is of rare importance in pediatric resuscitation and certainly should not take priority over airway clearance and maintenance. It is recommended that currently available AEDs not be used in infant cardiac arrest because they are not capable of the lower energy settings required for pediatric defibrillation and the algorithms were not designed for pediatric rhythms. For children older than 8 years, follow the standard operating procedures. This recommendation reflects the sense that the opportunity to defibrillate a child in VF should not be missed, despite the fact that AED experience in pediatric resuscitation is severely limited. Evidence suggests that VF does occur in young people in association with congenital heart problems, drug overdoses, and illicit drug use (eg, glue sniffing), and these patients merit assessment for the presence of VF/VT.

Hypothermia Associated With Cardiac Arrest

People in VF with extremely low temperatures (core temperatures less than 85°F) do not respond well to defibrillation. First rescuers are often not equipped to detect body core temperatures. Defibrillation should not be withheld from the cold patient in VF. Analyze the rhythm and shock up to three times if advised by the defibrillator. If hypothermic patients do not respond to three shocks, stop defibrillation attempts, resume CPR and rewarming efforts, and transport the patient to a more advanced treatment facility.

Cardiac Arrest Associated With Trauma

People whose cardiac arrest occurred as a direct result of major trauma seldom respond to defibrillation. In trauma patients, begin CPR, assess the rhythm, initiate BLS interventions (including airway, oxygenation, and control of hemorrhage and spine), then defibrillate if VF is present. This benefits the patients in whom VF cardiac arrest may have precipitated the trauma.

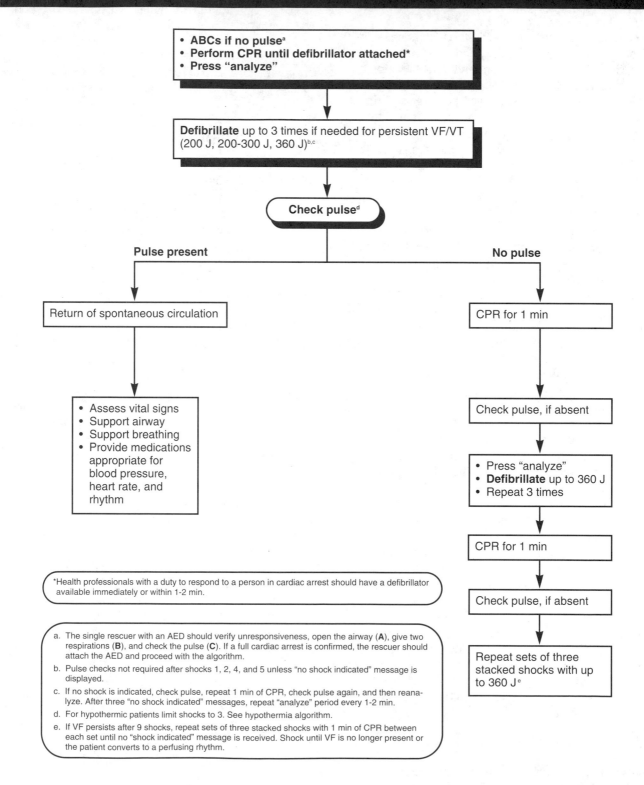

Automated External Defibrillation (AED) Treatment Algorithm
Emergency cardiac care pending arrival of ACLS personnel

- **ABCs if no pulse**[a]
- **Perform CPR until defibrillator attached***
- **Press "analyze"**

↓

Defibrillate up to 3 times if needed for persistent VF/VT
(200 J, 200-300 J, 360 J)[b,c]

↓

Check pulse[d]

Pulse present — **No pulse**

Pulse present:

Return of spontaneous circulation

↓

- Assess vital signs
- Support airway
- Support breathing
- Provide medications appropriate for blood pressure, heart rate, and rhythm

No pulse:

CPR for 1 min

↓

Check pulse, if absent

↓

- Press "analyze"
- **Defibrillate** up to 360 J
- Repeat 3 times

↓

CPR for 1 min

↓

Check pulse, if absent

↓

Repeat sets of three stacked shocks with up to 360 J[e]

*Health professionals with a duty to respond to a person in cardiac arrest should have a defibrillator available immediately or within 1-2 min.

a. The single rescuer with an AED should verify unresponsiveness, open the airway (**A**), give two respirations (**B**), and check the pulse (**C**). If a full cardiac arrest is confirmed, the rescuer should attach the AED and proceed with the algorithm.

b. Pulse checks not required after shocks 1, 2, 4, and 5 unless "no shock indicated" message is displayed.

c. If no shock is indicated, check pulse, repeat 1 min of CPR, check pulse again, and then reanalyze. After three "no shock indicated" messages, repeat "analyze" period every 1-2 min.

d. For hypothermic patients limit shocks to 3. See hypothermia algorithm.

e. If VF persists after 9 shocks, repeat sets of three stacked shocks with 1 min of CPR between each set until no "shock indicated" message is received. Shock until VF is no longer present or the patient converts to a perfusing rhythm.

Fig 7. Recommended treatment algorithm for ventricular fibrillation and pulseless ventricular tachycardia when ACLS support is not immediately available and an automated external defibrillator and a trained provider are present.

Automated Internal (Implanted) Defibrillators and Automated External Defibrillators

Some people with a history of malignant arrhythmias have implanted defibrillators that deliver a limited number of low-energy shocks directly to the myocardium. For patients with known ICDs, attach the AED and follow standard operating procedures. If the ICD is in the process of shocking a patient, however, allow the ICD 30 to 60 seconds to complete its treatment cycle.

Persistent Ventricular Fibrillation and No Available ACLS

The energy levels of the second and third shocks can range from 200 to 360 J. The guidelines for CPR and ECC recommend the use of 200 to 300 J for the second shock and an energy level "not to exceed 360 J" for a third shock if the first two shocks fail to defibrillate. Some AEDs are programmed to automatically increase the energy level to 360 J on the third shock. Others allow the operator either to remain at 200 J or to increase the energy level for subsequent shocks. Both approaches are acceptable. Some evidence suggests that lower-energy shocks have a greater likelihood of leaving the patient in persistent VF, whereas higher-energy shocks may more frequently leave the patient in asystole.[63]

If no pulse returns after these three shocks, rescuers with AEDs but without immediate ACLS backup should not press the analysis button but should resume CPR for 60 seconds. They should then analyze the rhythm, check for a pulse, and deliver additional rounds of three "stacked" defibrillatory shocks if VF continues. Most currently available AEDs will return to a sequence of 200-, 200-, and 360-J shocks at this point, although programmable modules allow a variety of protocols, depending on local practice. If the patient must be transported by the AED response team, then standing orders and guidelines will vary depending on local protocols.

AEDs can be left attached to the patient during transport in moving vehicles. However, AEDs should never be placed in the analysis mode in such circumstances because the movement of the transport vehicle can interfere with rhythm assessment. If a patient requires rhythm analysis and treatment during transport, the vehicle must be brought to a complete stop. CPR should be administered during transport when indicated.

Recurrent Ventricular Fibrillation — Refibrillation With No Available ACLS

The patient may regain a perfusing rhythm after receiving shocks and at some later time refibrillate. In such cases the rescuer using an AED should restart the treatment sequence at the level of the last successful defibrillation shock.[96] Whenever the "no shock indicated"

message is received, the rescuer should check for a pulse and if there is none, resume CPR. Three "no shock indicated" messages indicate that there is a low probability that the rhythm present can be successfully shocked. Therefore, the rhythm analysis time periods should be repeated only at 1- to 3-minute intervals.

Single Rescuer With an Automated External Defibrillator

In some situations a single rescuer equipped with, or with immediate access to, an AED may have to respond to a person in cardiac arrest. The rescue sequence is *verify unresponsiveness, open the airway, give two respirations, and check the pulse.* If no pulse, attach the AED and proceed with the algorithm for VF and pulseless VT (Fig 7). Activation of the EMS system should occur whenever the "no shock indicated" message is displayed or when someone else arrives on the scene.

No Pulse Checks Between Shocks

The ACLS Subcommittee recommends that there be no pulse check between the stacked shocks, ie, after shocks 1, 2, 4, and 5. In the past, ACLS VF protocols required a pulse check after these shocks because the leads may have become dislodged, an artifact may be producing "false" VF, or an unrecognized perfusing rhythm may have returned. These sources of error do not occur with AEDs, which have sensors to detect loose electrodes, artifactual rhythms, and regular rhythms associated with return of palpable pulse. Mandating a pulse check between shocks for AEDs will delay rapid identification of persistent VF, interfere with the assessment capabilities of the devices, and increase the possibility of operator errors.

Summary of Standard Operational Procedures

The rescuer using an AED in the absence of ACLS can memorize an easy treatment sequence:

1. Use AEDs only in situations of apparent cardiac arrest.
2. Always shock in sets of three.
3. Every time the chest is touched after the first assessment, it should be to perform CPR for 1 minute.
4. Continue to shock until the "no shock indicated" message is received.

Coordination of ACLS-Trained Provider With Personnel Using Automated External Defibrillators

With the increasing availability of AEDs, ACLS-trained emergency personnel will interact frequently with

AED-trained personnel. The following guidelines are suggested for this interface between ACLS personnel and personnel using AEDs:

1. ACLS-trained (and authorized) providers always have authority over the scene.

2. On arrival, ACLS-trained providers should ask for a quick report from the automated defibrillation providers and direct them to proceed with their protocols. This is particularly applicable when ACLS-trained providers are unfamiliar with the operation of the AED.

3. ACLS-trained providers should use the AED for additional shocks and rhythm monitoring. They can direct the providers to operate the AED. To save time, avoid disorganization, and allow a coordinated transfer of care, ACLS providers should not remove the AED and attach a separate conventional defibrillator unless the AED in use lacks a rhythm display screen. Most AEDs have the capacity for manual override by ACLS-trained providers, should that be necessary. The method and ease of manual override will vary among models.

4. ACLS-trained providers should consider the shocks delivered by the AED operators as part of their ACLS protocols. For example, if the patient remains in VF after three shocks by the AED, then ACLS personnel should enter the ACLS VF treatment sequence at the point at which the first three shocks have been delivered. Consequently, ACLS providers should move immediately to perform endotracheal intubation, establish IV line access, and administer epinephrine.

5. In most circumstances, the AED should be removed and a conventional defibrillator attached only when the patient has regained a spontaneous rhythm or is ready for transport to another location. Some models of AEDs lack a rhythm display monitor; thus, ACLS personnel will want to attach a conventional defibrillator when clinically convenient.

In-hospital Use of AEDs: Delays in Defibrillation

A number of US and British medical centers have begun to use AEDs for in-hospital resuscitation attempts.[100,101] Nursing leaders in British hospitals first established in-hospital early defibrillation programs in which ward nurses were trained to use AEDs placed in convenient locations.[100,101] This work has documented a disturbing performance problem that exists in many medical facilities — long delays (5 to 10 minutes) can occur before in-hospital response teams deliver the first defibrillation.[101-103]

Delayed defibrillation occurs infrequently in monitored beds and critical care units, but it occurs in non–critical care hospital beds and in outpatient and diagnostic facilities, where hundreds of patients enter and leave each day. In such areas centralized response teams can take many minutes to arrive with a defibrillator, attach it, and deliver the shocks.[101-102] "Code 911" committees inappropriately may place more emphasis on arrival of the code team than on delivery of the first defibrillation shock.

In-hospital practice, like out-of-hospital care, must shift from a focus on CPR as the sole form of BLS. Basic life support includes CPR *and* defibrillation. Many medical centers have purchased AEDs for placement in non–critical care areas. Trained health personnel working in these areas know to retrieve an AED from a designated location, attach it to the patient, and deliver appropriate shocks if the rhythm is VF. Most general floor and outpatient clinic nurses know from previous code experiences that many minutes can pass between the unexpected collapse of one of their patients and the arrival of the code team with all their equipment. For these reasons ACLS courses now teach providers the skill of automated external defibrillation.[104] Allied health personnel, however, must want to use the skill, and medical centers must agree to provide the equipment and training. Leadership and support for this innovative approach to achieve early defibrillation must come from the allied health personnel themselves.[100,101]

At the very least, medical center resuscitation teams should review their data on the time interval from recognition of the emergency to notification of the team and to delivery of the first shock, as recommended by the Utstein Style.[105] They may be surprised to learn that their response intervals are much longer than assumed.[101] If the teams are averaging more than 2 minutes in specific hospital locations, then a nurse – early defibrillation program merits careful consideration. Part of the rationale for requiring more training in the use of AEDs in the ACLS course originated in the need to support this movement toward in-hospital automated external defibrillation.

Postresuscitation Care

Once an AED provider team completes its protocol, several things may happen: (1) patients may display a maximal response to resuscitation and be awake, responsive, and breathing spontaneously; (2) a palpable pulse may be restored with a variety of hemodynamic profiles and thus a variety of neurological and respiratory responses; (3) cardiac arrest may persist without a rhythm that will respond to shocks; or (4) a pulseless VT or VF may remain. In each event patient care remains paramount. If the patient regains a pulse, the resuscitation team will continue to provide supportive care with one or a combination of the following:

- Proper airway control and ventilatory management
- Supplemental oxygen as soon as it is available
- Appropriate airway clearance if vomiting occurs
- Continued monitoring of vital signs
- Physical stabilization and transport
- Continued support while awaiting arrival of the ACLS team

Maintaining Defibrillators in a State of Readiness

After documentation by the US Food and Drug Administration (FDA) that apparent defibrillator malfunction was occurring with unacceptable frequency, the agency launched an educational effort to reduce both the magnitude and the frequency of such problems. The development of user checklists evolved from this effort.[106] The principle of checklists is not new. Aircraft pilots have used them for years as mandatory components of assessment of the preparedness of an aircraft for flight. Likewise, FDA-developed checklists for anesthesiologists have been evaluated as part of an assessment of the operational state of anesthesia machines. Thus, checklists were considered likely to be applicable to users of defibrillators as well, with the assumption that a commitment to their use on a regular basis would be the most successful means of reducing problems encountered by defibrillator users. In fact, the majority of reported malfunctions are traceable to the operator error of improper maintenance of the defibrillator and its batteries.[107,108] The checklists are designed to identify and prevent such deficiencies, not only by providing a means for uniform device testing but also by increasing user familiarity with available equipment.

Some points need to be emphasized in the use of these checklists:

1. Users must be trained in the proper use of checklists if the lists are to fulfill their intended function.
2. The actual users of the defibrillators must perform the check to maintain their familiarity with all aspects of specific device function and operation.
3. The checklists should be used frequently, perhaps as often as every shift. The intent of this recommendation is to make certain that all personnel responsible for operation of the device will have a rotating opportunity to assess its (and their own) state of preparedness for operation. A maintenance schedule should be developed for volunteer services to ensure a daily defibrillator check. Such a schedule should provide a rotation so that all personnel use the checklists.
4. Use of the checklists is intended to be supplementary to, and not in any way a replacement for, regularly scheduled, more detailed maintenance checks recommended by the manufacturer.
5. Nickel-cadmium (Ni-Cad) batteries in particular require specific maintenance procedures that should be carried out at room temperature (68°F to 72°F). Batteries should undergo reconditioning (usually deep discharge-charge cycling three times) every 90 days, and their capacity should be determined after the discharge-charge cycle. If battery capacity is less than 80%, the battery should be replaced. Shelf-life tests performed at least semiannually determine the ability of the battery to hold its charge. Manufacturer's guidelines should be followed in the performance of a shelf-life test and batteries removed from service if they do not hold a charge to manufacturer's specifications. Battery maintenance logs should document the dates and results of both reconditioning and shelf-life tests for each battery. Batteries not put into service should be kept at room temperature in a battery support system. Alternatively, fully charged batteries can be stored at temperatures between 40°F and 80°F but should be recharged before returning to active service. Properly maintained nickel-cadmium batteries have a useful service life of about 2 years. After this time batteries should either be replaced or their performance observed closely for evidence of deterioration.

    Lead-acid batteries should be kept fully charged and recharged after use. It is recommended that lead-acid batteries be connected to a charger when not in a defibrillator. If lead-acid batteries are left discharged for long periods, battery damage can result. Batteries should be charged at temperatures in the range of 32°F to 100°F to avoid incomplete or slow charging at below 32°F and battery damage above 100°F. Unlike nickel-cadmium batteries, lead-acid batteries do not require periodic reconditioning. The status of lead-acid batteries can be assessed by testing in the defibrillator. At 1- to 3-month intervals, a fully charged battery should be placed in the defibrillator and repeated test shocks delivered into a test load, following manufacturer's specifications. If a low battery message is conveyed before the manufacturer's suggested limit (eg, fewer than 20 360-J shocks), the battery should be replaced. As with nickel-cadmium batteries, lead-acid batteries should also be replaced after 2 years of service life unless testing indicates no evidence of deteriorating performance. Manufacturer's periodic maintenance recommendations need to be followed to maintain both defibrillator and batteries in optimum condition. It is imperative that those who operate and maintain defibrillators understand and comply with the specific recommendations for periodic maintenance as stated in defibrillator operator's manuals.
6. With manual defibrillators for which the remote defibrillation option with adhesive pads is used instead of paddles, a charge-discharge cycle with a simulator can be used.
7. Using these checklists as a format, some manufacturers have developed checklists specific for their devices. Provided all of these assessments are included in such device-specific checklists, they are suitable for this purpose.

Revised reporting requirements for adverse incidents related to use of defibrillators and other medical devices are now mandated by the Safe Medical Devices Act of

1990. The new regulation, known as MEDWATCH,* requires healthcare facilities to report deaths and serious injuries or illnesses in which devices such as defibrillators were considered contributing factors. Deaths must be reported to both the FDA and the device manufacturer. Serious injuries or illnesses must be reported to the manufacturer or forwarded to the FDA if the manufacturer is unknown. The reports must be submitted within 10 working days of the incident. Others are requested to voluntarily report such incidents. Manufacturers will still be required to report injuries and deaths to the FDA. Thus, the defibrillator checklists are being made available for use at a time when reporting requirements are being intensified. Adherence to regular use of these checklists is critical and timely.

A commitment to use of checklists will reduce the incidence of the types of problems being reported by defibrillator users. The nationwide implementation of early defibrillation in a wide variety of settings and with diverse frequencies of device use would seem to confer a compelling impetus and even urgency for the need for preventive maintenance wherever defibrillators are placed.

*Contact FDA MEDWATCH Program, 5600 Fishers Lane, Rockville, MD 20852-9787. Telephone 1-800-FDA-0178.

Manual Defibrillators: Operator's Shift Checklist

Date _____   Shift _____   Location _____

Mfr/Model No. _____   Serial No. or Facility ID No. _____

At the beginning of each shift, inspect the unit. Indicate whether all requirements have been met. Note any corrective actions taken. Sign the form.

	OK as Found	Corrective Action/ Remarks
1. Defibrillator Unit Clean, no spills, clear of objects on top, casing intact		
2. Paddles (including pediatric adapters)* a. Clean, not pitted b. Release from housing easily c. If internal paddles are included, verify their availability in a sterile package. Periodically inspect as with external paddles.		
3. Cables/Connectors a. Inspect for cracks, broken wire, or damage b. Connectors engage securely and are not damaged		
4. Supplies a. Two sets of pads in sealed packages, within expiration date* f. Razor b. Monitoring electrodes g. Spare ECG paper c. Alcohol wipes h. Spare charged battery available* d. Hand towel i. Cassette tape* e. Scissors j. Gel or other conductive medium present and stored properly*		

5. Power Supply
a. Battery-powered units
  (1) Verify fully charged battery in place
  (2) Spare charged battery available
  (3) Follow appropriate battery rotation schedule per manufacturer's recommendations
b. AC/battery backup units
  (1) Plugged into live outlet to maintain battery
  (2) Test on battery power and reconnect to line power		

6. Indicators/ECG Display a. Power-on display b. Self-test OK* c. Monitor display functional d. "Service" message display off e. Battery charging; low battery light off* f. Correct time displayed; set with dispatch center*		
7. ECG Recorder a. Adequate ECG paper b. Recorder prints		
8. Charge-Display Cycle for Paddle or Adhesive Pad Defibrillation a. Disconnect AC plug – battery backup units b. Charge to manufacturer's recommended test energy level c. Charge indicators working d. Discharge per manufacturer's instructions e. Reconnect line power		
9. Pacemaker* a. Pacer output cable intact b. Pacer pads present (set of two) c. Inspect per manufacturer's operational guidelines		
Major Problem(s) Identified (Out of Service)		

*Applicable only if the unit has this supply or capability

Signature _____

Automated Defibrillators: Operator's Shift Checklist

Date _____ Shift _____ Location _____

Mfr/Model No. _____ Serial No. or Facility ID No. _____

At the beginning of each shift, inspect the unit. Indicate whether all requirements have been met. Note any corrective actions taken. Sign the form.

	OK as Found	Corrective Action/ Remarks
1. Defibrillator Unit Clean, no spills, clear of objects on top, casing intact		
2. Cables/Connectors a. Inspect for cracks, broken wire, or damage b. Connectors engage securely and are not damaged*		
3. Supplies a. Two sets of pads in sealed packages, within expiration date* b. Hand towel c. Scissors d. Razor e. Alcohol wipes* f. Monitoring electrodes* g. Spare charged battery* h. Adequate ECG paper* i. Manual override module, key, or card* j. Cassette tape, memory module, and/or event card plus spares*		
4. Power Supply a. Battery-powered units (1) Verify fully charged battery in place (2) Spare charged battery available (3) Follow appropriate battery rotation schedule per manufacturer's recommendations b. AC/battery backup units (1) Plugged into live outlet to maintain battery charge (2) Test on battery power and reconnect to line power		
5. Indicators*/ECG Display a. Remove cassette tape, memory module, and/or event card* b. Power-on display c. Self-test OK d. Monitor display functional* e. "Service" message display off* f. Battery charging; low battery light off* g. Correct time displayed; set with dispatch center		
6. ECG Recorder* a. Adequate ECG paper b. Recorder prints		
7. Charge/Display Cycle a. Disconnect AC plug – battery backup units* b. Attach to simulator c. Detects, charges, and delivers shock for VF d. Responds correctly to nonshockable rhythms e. Manual override functional* f. Detach from simulator g. Replace cassette tape, module, and/or memory card *		
8. Pacemaker* a. Pacer output cable intact b. Pacer pads present (set of two) c. Inspect per manufacturer's operational guidelines		
Major Problem(s) Identified (Out of Service)		

*Applicable only if the unit has this supply or capability

Signature _____

Training

Sources of Information

AHA training materials on AEDs are provided in *Automated External Defibrillation*. This publication also includes information for the electrical therapy lecture and the electrical therapy teaching station in the ACLS provider's course.

The publication includes a detailed instructor's curriculum and instructor's guidelines for a separate provider's course on AEDs. The AHA does not intend to approve, control, or directly supervise such courses because EMS agencies in most states already provide these functions. Instead, this material is intended to provide a standardized, national curriculum and course content that can be adapted for local use. It is hoped that the AHA-approved algorithms and recommendations for the proper use of AEDs will lead to greater national uniformity in the use of these devices.

General Points About Training

Because of the intrinsic simplicity of AEDs, a markedly expanded range of persons can now be trained to provide early defibrillation. Persons who may want training in the use of AEDs include general hospital floor nurses, general office nurses, oral surgeons, dentists, physician assistants, nurse practitioners, security and law enforcement personnel, ship and airplane crews, supervisory personnel at senior citizen centers and exercise facilities, and the entire range of professional prehospital providers, including first responders, firefighters, and EMTs. In addition, physicians who are not involved in daily emergency care but nevertheless perceive themselves at risk of encountering a patient in cardiac arrest may be interested in learning to use AEDs.

Maintenance of Skills

Survey results and experience in rural communities have demonstrated that, depending on the rate of cardiac arrest in a community, an emergency responder may go several years without treating a patient in cardiac arrest.[31,33] Therefore, every program director must determine how to ensure correct performance when such an event occurs. Principles of adult education suggest that frequent practice of a psychomotor skill such as operating an AED in a simulated cardiac arrest offers the best skill maintenance.

Frequency of Practice

The frequency and content of these practice sessions have been established by several successful programs.[16,25,31] Currently most systems permit a maximum of 90 days between practice drills and have found this to be satisfactory. Note that this is a **maximum** interval between drills. Many emergency personnel and systems drill as often as once a month. The most successful long-term skill maintenance occurs when individual rescuers voluntarily take a few minutes to perform a quick check of the equipment on a frequent and regular basis. This check includes a visual inspection of the defibrillator components and controls and a mental review of the steps to be followed and the controls to be operated in the event of a cardiac arrest.

Session Content

The practice sessions can be as elaborate as interest and time allow and can include more advanced discussions of ECC. The following is recommended as a minimum content of a 30- to 60-minute practice session that should occur at least once every 90 days:

- Performance review of the care of recent patients
- Review of equipment operation and maintenance
- Review of standing orders
- Discussion of treatment possibilities
- Scenario practice of field protocols with a training manikin, a defibrillator, and a rhythm simulator; this practice should simulate actual cardiac arrests and include entrance to the scene, two-person response teams, ongoing CPR, a variety of initial rhythms, and a variety of postshock responses
- An objective skills test, with a skills checklist (see the supplement to the instructor's manual)

Medical Control

In emergencies, critical medical procedures must be performed by the first trained personnel who respond. Within the constraints of governing laws and regulations, healthcare providers can perform some medical procedures in emergencies but only with the medical authorization of a physician. The authorizing physician assumes medical control and takes legal responsibility for the performance of the emergency care providers. The authorizing physician issues standing orders, which are in effect direct orders to perform specified tasks for a patient. The emergency rescuer must always operate under the authority of the medical license of the medical director and the enabling administrative codes of the state or other governing body.

Successful Completion of Course

The AHA does **not** provide medical control for interventions taught in BLS or ACLS classes. Successful completion of an AHA course, including any automated external defibrillation provider's course that follows AHA recommendations, means only that a certain level of cognitive and performance standards has been met. Successful completion does not warrant performance, nor does it qualify or authorize a person to perform any procedure on a patient. Licensure and certification is a function of the appropriate state legislative or local health or EMS authority. Such licensure and certification may or may not be related to successful completion of a course following ACLS guidelines. The primary objectives of any automated defibrillation provider's course that follows AHA recommendations are educational.

Case-by-Case Review

Every event in which an AED is used (or could have been used) must be reviewed by the medical director or designated representative. This means that every incident in which CPR is performed must have a medical review to establish whether the patient was treated in accordance with professional standards and local standing orders. In each review, whether VF and other rhythms were treated appropriately with shocks and with BLS must be considered. Other dimensions of performance that can be evaluated include command of the scene, safety, efficiency, speed, professionalism, ability to troubleshoot, completeness of patient care, and interactions with other professionals and bystanders.[109]

Methods of Case-by-Case Review

The three ways in which the case-by-case review is performed are by a written report, by review of the recordings made by the voice-ECG tape recorders attached to AEDs, and by solid-state memory modules and magnetic tape recordings that store information about each use of the device. The latter two methods are innovative approaches to event documentation, recordkeeping, and data management that have been recently developed and incorporated into AEDs.[109] Case reviews that use all three approaches appear to offer the most complete information. Particular requirements or constraints in some systems, however, may dictate various combinations of these approaches rather than all three. Future innovations in event documentation, such as digital voice recordings, annotated rhythm strips, and other microprocessor-based approaches, offer even more options. Concern that close documentation of events would lead to an increased risk of liability has thus far proved unfounded.

Quality Assurance

Quality assurance refers to both microperformance, which is the performance of personnel involved in the treatment of individual patients, and macroperformance, which is the overall effectiveness of a system that uses AEDs. Quality assurance requires establishment of a system's performance goals, a review to determine whether those goals are being met, and feedback to move the system closer to unmet goals.[97] Review of the treatment of an individual patient in cardiac arrest can lead to identification of a problem in a system's training program.

Organized collection and review of patient data can identify systemwide problems and allow assessment of each link in the chain of survival for the adult victim of sudden cardiac death. Such data represent quality assurance activities, and as such should not expose clinical providers or organizations to increased risk of liability allegations. Adult victims of witnessed cardiac arrest caused by VF appear to be the best group on which to focus. The lower-than-expected hospital discharge rates of this group may be explained by long ambulance response times, delayed EMS activation, infrequent witnessed arrests, rare bystander CPR, or slow on-scene performance. Each of these problems can be addressed with a specific programwide effort. Continued systematic and uniform data collection will determine whether the new efforts succeed.

References

1. Eisenberg MS, Bergner L, Hallstrom A. Paramedic programs and out-of-hospital cardiac arrest, I: factors associated with successful resuscitation. *Am J Public Health.* 1979;69:30-38.
2. Eisenberg MS, Hallstrom AP, Copass MK, Bergner L, Short F, Pierce J. Treatment of ventricular fibrillation: emergency medical technician defibrillation and paramedic services. *JAMA.* 1984;251:1723-1726.
3. Weaver WD, Copass MK, Bufi D, Ray R, Hallstrom AP, Cobb LA. Improved neurologic recovery and survival after early defibrillation. *Circulation.* 1984;69:943-948.
4. Cobb LA, Werner JA, Trobaugh GB. Sudden cardiac death, I: a decade's experience with out-of-hospital resuscitation. *Mod Concepts Cardiovasc Dis.* 1980;49:31-36.
5. Cobb LA, Hallstrom AP. Community-based cardiopulmonary resuscitation: what have we learned? *Ann N Y Acad Sci.* 1982;382:330-342.
6. Bayes de Luna A, Coumel P, Leclercq JF. Ambulatory sudden cardiac death mechanisms of production of fatal arrhythmia on the basis of data from 157 cases. *Am Heart J.* 1989;117:151-159.
7. Newman MM. National EMT-D study. *J Emerg Med Serv.* 1986;11:70-72.
8. Newman MM. The survival advantage: early defibrillation programs in the fire service. *J Emerg Med Serv.* 1987;12:40-46.
9. Eisenberg M, Bergner L, Hallstrom A. Paramedic programs and out-of-hospital cardiac arrest, II: impact on community mortality. *Am J Public Health.* 1979;69:39-42.
10. Eisenberg MS, Copass MK, Hallstrom A, Cobb LA, Bergner L. Management of out-of-hospital cardiac arrest: failure of basic emergency medical technician services. *JAMA.* 1980;243:1049-1051.
11. Cummins RO. From concept to standard-of-care? review of the clinical experience with automated external defibrillators. *Ann Emerg Med.* 1989;18:1269-1275.
12. Fletcher GF, Cantwell JD. Ventricular fibrillation in a medically supervised cardiac exercise program: clinical, angiographic, and surgical correlations. *JAMA.* 1977;238:2627-2629.
13. Haskell WL. Cardiovascular complications during exercise training of cardiac patients. *Circulation.* 1978;57:920-924.
14. Hossack KF, Hartwig R. Cardiac arrest associated with supervised cardiac rehabilitation. *J Cardiac Rehab.* 1982;2:402-408.
15. Van Camp SP, Peterson RA. Cardiovascular complications of outpatient cardiac rehabilitation programs. *JAMA.* 1986;256:1160-1163.
16. Eisenberg MS, Copass MK, Hallstrom AP, et al. Treatment of out-of-hospital cardiac arrests with rapid defibrillation by emergency medical technicians. *N Engl J Med.* 1980;302:1379-1383.
17. Stults KR, Brown DD, Schug VL, Bean JA. Prehospital defibrillation performed by emergency medical technicians in rural communities. *N Engl J Med.* 1984;310:219-223.
18. Vukov LF, White RD, Bachman JW, O'Brien PC. New perspectives on rural EMT defibrillation. *Ann Emerg Med.* 1988;17:318-321.

19. Bachman JW, McDonald GS, O'Brien PC. A study of out-of-hospital cardiac arrests in northeastern Minnesota. *JAMA.* 1986; 256:477-483.

20. Olson DW, LaRochelle J, Fark D, Aprahamian C, Aufderheide TP, Mateer JR, Hargarten KM, Stueven HA. EMT-defibrillation: the Wisconsin experience. *Ann Emerg Med.* 1989;18:806-811.

21. Eisenberg MS, Horwood BT, Cummins RO, Reynolds-Haertle R, Hearne TR. Cardiac arrest and resuscitation: a tale of 29 cities. *Ann Emerg Med.* 1990;19:179-186.

22. Eisenberg MS, Cummins RO, Damon S, Larsen MP, Hearne TR. Survival rates from out-of-hospital cardiac arrest: recommendations for uniform definitions and data to report. *Ann Emerg Med.* 1990; 19:1249-1259.

23. Eisenberg MS, Bergner L, Hallstrom A. Cardiac resuscitation in the community: importance of rapid provision and implications for program planning. *JAMA.* 1979;241:1905-1907.

24. Kerber RE. Statement on early defibrillation from the Emergency Cardiac Care Committee, American Heart Association. *Circulation.* 1991;83:2233.

25. Cummins RO. EMT-defibrillation: national guidelines for implementation. *Am J Emerg Med.* 1987;5:254-257.

26. Cummins RO, Eisenberg MS. EMT defibrillation: a proven concept. *ECC National Faculty Newsletter.* 1984;1:1-3.

27. ACT (Advanced Coronary Treatment Foundation). EMT defibrillation: ACT Foundation issues policy statement. *J Emerg Med Serv.* 1983;8:37.

28. Prehospital defibrillation by basic-level emergency medical technicians. *Ann Emerg Med.* 1984;13:974.

29. Paris PM. EMT-defibrillation: a recipe for saving lives. *Am J Emerg Med.* 1988;6:282-287.

30. Standards and guidelines for cardiopulmonary resuscitation (CPR) and emergency cardiac care (ECC). *JAMA.* 1986;255:2905-2984.

31. Stults KR, Brown DD. Special considerations for defibrillation performed by emergency medical technicians in small communities. *Circulation.* 1986;74(pt 2):IV-13-IV-17.

32. Ornato JP, McNeill SE, Craren EJ, Nelson NM. Limitation on effectiveness of rapid defibrillation by emergency medical technicians in a rural setting. *Ann Emerg Med.* 1984;13:1096-1099.

33. Cummins RO, Eisenberg MS, Graves JR, Damon SK. EMT-defibrillation: is it right for you? *J Emerg Med Serv.* 1985;10:60-64.

34. Jones DL, Klein GJ, Guiraudon GM, Sharma AD, Kallok MJ, Bourland JD, Tacker WA. Internal cardiac defibrillation in man: pronounced improvement with sequential pulse delivery to two different lead orientations. *Circulation.* 1986;73:484-491.

35. Geddes LA, Tacker WA, Cabler P, Chapman R, Rivera R, Kidder H. Decrease in transthoracic impedance during successive ventricular defibrillation trials. *Med Instrum.* 1975;9:179-180.

36. Dahl CF, Ewy GA, Ewy MD, Thomas ED. Transthoracic impedance to direct current discharge: effect of repeated countershocks. *Med Instrum.* 1976;10;151-154.

37. Kerber RE, Grayzel J, Hoyt R, Marcus M, Kennedy J. Transthoracic resistance in human defibrillation: influence of body weight, chest size, serial shocks, paddle size and paddle contact pressure. *Circulation.* 1981;63:676-682.

38. Ewy GA, Ewy MD, Nuttall AJ, Nuttall AW. Canine transthoracic resistance. *J Appl Physiol.* 1972;32:91-94.

39. Thomas ED, Ewy GA, Dahl CF, Ewy MD. Effectiveness of direct current defibrillation: role of paddle electrode size. *Am Heart J.* 1977;93:463-467.

40. Connell PN, Ewy GA, Dahl CF, Ewy MD. Transthoracic impedance to defibrillator discharge: effect of electrode size and electrode-chest wall interface. *J Electrocardiol.* 1973;6:313-M.

41. Ewy GA, Hellman DA, McClung S, Tarren D. Influence of ventilation phase on transthoracic impedance and defibrillation effectiveness. *Crit Care Med.* 1980;8:164-166.

42. Ewy GA, Ewy MD, Silverman J. Determinants for human transthoracic resistance to direct current discharge. *Circulation.* 1972; 46(suppl II):II-150. Abstract.

43. Sirna SJ, Ferguson DW, Charbonnier F, Kerber RE. Factors affecting transthoracic impedance during electrical cardioversion. *Am J Cardiol.* 1988;62:1048-1052.

44. Sirna SJ, Kieso RA, Fox-Eastham KJ, Seabold J, Charbonnier F, Kerber RE. Mechanisms responsible for the decline in transthoracic impedance after DC shocks. *Am J Physiol.* 1989;257(pt 2): H1180-H1183.

45. Kerber RE, Kouba C, Martins J, Kelly K, Low R, Hoyt R, Ferguson D, Bailey L, Bennett P, Charbonnier F. Advance prediction of transthoracic impedance in human defibrillation and cardioversion: importance of impedance in determining the success of low-energy shocks. *Circulation.* 1984;70:303-308.

46. Lerman BB, DiMarco JP, Haines DE. Current-based versus energy-based ventricular defibrillation: a prospective study. *J Am Coll Cardiol.* 1988;12:1259-1264.

47. Dalzell GW, Cunningham SR, Anderson J, Adgey AA. Initial experience with a microprocessor controlled current-based defibrillator. *Br Heart J.* 1989;61:502-505.

48. Kerber RE, Martins JB, Kelly KJ, Ferguson DW, Kouba C, Jensen SR, Newman B, Parke JD, Kieso R, Melton J. Self-adhesive pre-applied electrode pads for defibrillation and cardioversion. *J Am Coll Cardiol.* 1984;3:815-820.

49. Kerber RE, Martins JB, Kienzle MG, Constantin L, Olshansky B, Hopson R, Charbonnier F. Energy, current, and success in defibrillation and cardioversion: clinical studies using an automated impedance-based method of energy adjustment. *Circulation.* 1988;77:1038-1046.

50. Hummell RS, Ornato JP, Wienberg SM, Clarke AM. Spark-generating properties of electrode gels used during defibrillation: a potential fire hazard. *JAMA.* 1988;260:3021-3024.

51. Hoyt R, Grayzel J, Kerber RE. Determinants of intracardiac current in defibrillation: experimental studies in dogs. *Circulation.* 1981;64: 818-823.

52. Stults KR, Brown DD, Cooley F, Kerber RE. Self-adhesive monitor/defibrillation pads improve prehospital defibrillation success. *Ann Emerg Med.* 1987;16:872-877.

53. Atkins DL, Sirna S, Kieso R, Charbonnier F, Kerber RE. Pediatric defibrillation: importance of paddle size in determining transthoracic impedance. *Pediatrics.* 1988;82:914-918.

54. Samson RA, Atkins DL, Kerber RE. Pediatric defibrillation: what is the optimal size of self-adhesive preapplied electrode pads? *Circulation.* 1993;88(suppl):I-194. Abstract.

55. Guidelines for cardiopulmonary resuscitation and emergency cardiac care. *JAMA.* 1992;268:2171-2298.

56. Lown B. Electrical reversion of cardiac arrhythmias. *Br Heart J.* 1967;29:469-489.

57. Kerber RE, Jensen SR, Grayzel J, Kennedy J, Hoyt R. Elective cardioversion: influence of paddle-electrode location and size on success rates and energy requirements. *N Engl J Med.* 1981;305: 658-662.

58. Levine PA, Barold SS, Fletcher RD, Talbot P. Adverse acute and chronic effects of electrical defibrillation and cardioversion on implanted unipolar cardiac pacing systems. *J Am Coll Cardiol.* 1983;1:1413-1422.

59. Geddes LA, Tacker WA, Rosborough JP, Moore AG, Cabler PS. Electrical dose for ventricular defibrillation of large and small animals using precordial electrodes. *J Clin Invest.* 1974;53:310-319.

60. Gutgesell HP, Tacker HA, Geddes LA, Davis JS, Lie JT, McNamara DG. Energy dose for ventricular defibrillation of children. *Pediatrics.* 1976;58:898-901.

61. Dahl CF, Ewy GA, Warner ED, Thomas ED. Myocardial necrosis from direct current countershock. *Circulation.* 1974;50:956-961.

62. Pantridge JF, Adgey AA, Webb SW, Anderson J. Electrical requirements for ventricular defibrillation. *Br Med J.* 1975;2:313-315.

63. Weaver WD, Cobb LA, Copass MK, Hallstrom AP. Ventricular defibrillation: a comparative trial using 175-J and 320-J shocks. *N Engl J Med.* 1982;307:1101-1106.

64. Kerber RE, Kienzle MG, Olshansky B, Waldo AL, Wilber D, Carlson MD, Aschoff AM, Birger S, Fugatt L, Walsh S, Rockwell M, Charbonnier F. Ventricular tachycardia rate and morphology determine energy and current requirements for transthoracic cardioversion. *Circulation.* 1992;85:150-163.

65. Zipes DP, Fischer J, King RM, Nicoll A, Jolly WW. Termination of ventricular fibrillation in dogs by depolarizing a critical amount of myocardium. *Am J Cardiol.* 1975;36:37-44.

66. Kerber RE, Kienzle MG, Olshansky B, Carlson MD, Waldo AL, Wilber D, Aschoff AM, Birger S, Walsh S, Fox-Eastham K, Rockwell M, Charbonnier F. Current-based transthoracic defibrillation is superior to energy-based defibrillation in patients with high transthoracic impedance. *Circulation.* 1991;84(suppl II):II-612. Abstract.

67. Ewy GA, Dahl CF, Zimmerman M, Otto C. Ventricular fibrillation masquerading as ventricular standstill. *Crit Care Med.* 1981;9: 841-844.

68. Mirowski M, Reid PR, Mower MM, Watkins L, Gott VL, Schauble JF, Langer A, Heilman MS, Kolenik SA, Fischell RE, Weisfeldt ML. Termination of malignant ventricular arrhythmias with an implanted automatic defibrillator in human beings. *N Engl J Med.* 1980;303: 322-324.

69. Walls JT, Schuder JC, Curtis JJ, Stephenson HE Jr, McDaniel WC, Flaker GC. Adverse effects of permanent cardiac internal defibrilla-tor patches on external defibrillation. *Am J Cardiol.* 1989;64:1144-1147.

70. Caldwell G, Millar G, Quinn E, Vincent R, Chamberlain DA. Simple mechanical methods for cardioversion: defense of the precordial thump and cough version. *Br Med J Clin Res.* 1985;291: 627-630.

71. Miller J, Tresch D, Horwitz L, Thompson BM, Aprahamian C, Darin JC. The precordial thump. *Ann Emerg Med.* 1984;13:791-794.

72. Yakaitis RW, Redding JS. Precordial thumping during cardiac resuscitation. *Crit Care Med.* 1973;1:22-26.

73. Gertsch M, Hottinger S, Hess T. Serial chest thumps for the treat-ment of ventricular tachycardia in patients with coronary artery dis-ease. *Clin Cardiol.* 1992;15:181-188.

74. Atkins JM. Emergency medical service systems in acute cardiac care: state of the art. *Circulation.* 1986;74(pt 2):IV-4-IV-8.

75. Cummins RO, Eisenberg MS, Stults KR. Automatic external defib-rillators: clinical issues for cardiology. *Circulation.* 1986;73:381-385.

76. White RD. EMT-defibrillation: time for controlled implementation of effective treatment. *ECC National Faculty Newsletter.* 1986;8:1-2.

77. Atkins JM, Murphy D, Allison EJ Jr, Graves JR. Toward earlier defibrillation. *J Emerg Med Serv.* 1986;11:70.

78. Eisenberg MS, Cummins RO. Defibrillation performed by the emer-gency medical technician. *Circulation.* 1986;74(pt 2):IV-9-IV-12.

79. Ruskin JN. Automatic external defibrillators and sudden cardiac death. *N Engl J Med.* 1988;319:713-715. Editorial.

80. Cummins RO, Eisenberg MS, Moore JE, Hearne TR, Andresen E, Wendt R, Litwin PE, Graves JR, Hallstrom AP, Pierce J. Automatic external defibrillators: clinical, training, psychological, and public health issues. *Ann Emerg Med.* 1985;14:755-760.

81. Cummins RO, Eisenberg MS, Bergner L, Hallstrom A, Hearne T, Murray JA. Automatic external defibrillation: evaluations of its role in the home and in emergency medical services. *Ann Emerg Med.* 1984;13:798-801.

82. Jacobs L. Medical, legal, and social implications of automatic exter-nal defibrillators. *Ann Emerg Med.* 1986;15:863-864. Editorial.

83. Stults KR, Cummins RO. Fully automatic vs shock advisory defibril-lators: what are the issues? *J Emerg Med Serv.* 1987;12:71-73.

84. Cummins RO, Stults KR, Haggar B, Kerber RE, Schaeffer S, Brown DD. A new rhythm library for testing automatic external defibrillators: performance of three devices. *J Am Coll Cardiol.* 1988;11:597-602.

85. Diack AW, Welborn WS, Rullman RG, Walter CW, Wayne MA. An automatic cardiac resuscitator for emergency treatment of cardiac arrest. *Med Instrum.* 1979;13:78-83.

86. Jaggarao NS, Heber M, Grainger R, Vincent R, Chamberlain DA. Use of an automated external defibrillator-pacemaker by ambu-lance staff. *Lancet.* 1982;2:73-75.

87. Cummins RO, Eisenberg M, Bergner L, Murray JA. Sensitivity, accuracy, and safety of an automatic external defibrillator. *Lancet.* 1984;2:318-320.

88. Stults KR, Brown DD, Kerber RE. Efficacy of an automated exter-nal defibrillator in the management of out-of-hospital cardiac arrest: validation of the diagnostic algorithm and initial clinical experience in a rural environment. *Circulation.* 1986;73:701-709.

89. Cummins RO, Eisenberg MS, Litwin PE, Graves JR, Hearne TR, Hallstrom AP. Automatic external defibrillators used by emergency medical technicians: a controlled clinical trial. *JAMA.* 1987;257: 1605-1610.

90. Gray AJ, Redmond AD, Martin MA. Use of the automatic external defibrillator-pacemaker by ambulance personnel: the Stockport experience. *Br Med J Clin Res.* 1987;294:1133-1135.

91. Weaver WD, Hill D, Fahrenbruch CE, et al. Use of the automatic external defibrillator in the management of out-of-hospital cardiac arrest. *N Engl J Med.* 1988;319:661-666.

92. Jakobsson J, Nyquist O, Rehnqvist N. Effects of early defibrillation of out-of-hospital cardiac arrest patients by ambulance personnel. *Eur Heart J.* 1987;8:1189-1194.

93. Sedgwick ML, Watson J, Dalziel K, Carrington DJ, Cobbe SM. Efficacy of out-of-hospital defibrillation by ambulance technicians using automated external defibrillators: the Heartstart Scotland Project. *Resuscitation.* 1992;24:73-87.

94. Dickey W, Dalzell GW, Anderson JM, Adgey AA. The accuracy of decision-making of a semi-automatic defibrillator during cardiac arrest. *Eur Heart J.* 1992;13:608-615.

95. Ornato JP, Shipley J, Powell RG, Racht EM. Inappropriate electri-cal countershocks by an automated external defibrillator. *Ann Emerg Med.* 1992;21:1278-1281.

96. Stults KR, Brown DD. Refibrillation managed by EMT-Ds: inci-dence and outcome without paramedic back-up. *Am J Emerg Med.* 1986;4:491-495.

97. Bradley K, Sokolow AE, Wright KJ, McCullough WJ. A compari-son of an innovative four-hour EMT-D course with a "standard" ten-hour course. *Ann Emerg Med.* 1988;17:613-619.

98. Ornato JP, Craren EJ, Gonzalez ER, Garnett AR, McClung BK, Newman MM. Cost-effectiveness of defibrillation by emergency medical technicians. *Am J Emerg Med.* 1988;6:108-112.

99. Wilson RF, Sirna S, White CW, Kerber RE. Defibrillation of high-risk patients during coronary angiography using self-adhesive, preapplied electrode pads. *Am J Cardiol.* 1987;60:380-382.

100. Walters G, Glucksman EE, Evans TR. A two-hour training in defib-rillation for first-aiders. *Resuscitation.* 1992;24:181A.

101. Kaye W, Mancini ME, Giuliano KK, et al. Early defibrillation in the hospital by staff nurses (RN-Ds) using automated external defibril-lators: training and retention issues. *Resuscitation.* 1992;24:186A.

102. Lazzam C, McCans JL. Predictors of survival of in-hospital car-diac arrest. *Can J Cardiol.* 1991;7:113-116.

103. Dickey W, Adgey AA. Mortality within hospital after resuscitation from ventricular fibrillation outside hospital. *Br Heart J.* 1992;67: 334-338.

104. Cummins RO, Thies WH. Automated external defibrillators and the Advanced Cardiac Life Support Program: a new initiative from the American Heart Association. *Am J Emerg Med.* 1991;9:91-93.

105. Cummins RO, Chamberlain DA, Abramson NS, Allen M, Baskett PJ, Becker L, Bossaert L, Delooz HH, Dick WF, Eisenberg MS, et al. Recommended guidelines for uniform reporting of data from out-of-hospital cardiac arrest: the Utstein Style. *Circulation.* 1991; 84:960-975.

106. White RD, Chesemore KF, and the Defibrillator Checklist Task Force. Charge! FDA recommendations for maintaining defibrilla-tor readiness. *J Emerg Med Serv.* 1992;17:70-82.

107. Emergency Care Research Institute. Hazard: user error and defib-rillator discharge failures. *Health Devices.* 1986;15:340-343.

108. Cummins RO, Chesemore K, White RD, Defibrillator Working Group. Defibrillator failures: causes and problems and recommen-dations for improvement. *JAMA.* 1990;264:1019-1025.

109. Cummins RO, Austin D Jr, Graves JR, Hambly C. An innovative approach to medical control: semiautomatic defibrillators with solid-state memory modules for recording cardiac arrest events. *Ann Emerg Med.* 1988;17:818-824.

Emergency Cardiac Pacing

Chapter 5

A variety of devices for pacing the heart have been developed since the first successful cardiac pacing during the 19th century. All cardiac pacemakers deliver an electrical stimulus through electrodes to the heart, causing electrical depolarization and subsequent cardiac contraction. Pacemaker systems are usually named according to the location of the electrodes and the pathway the electrical stimulus travels to the heart. For example, a transcutaneous pacing system delivers pacing impulses to the heart through the skin using cutaneous electrodes. Transvenous pacemakers use electrodes that have been passed via large central veins to the right chambers of the heart. In addition to electrodes, every pacing system requires a pulse generator. The pulse generator can be outside the patient's body (external pacemakers) or surgically implanted inside the body (internal or permanent pacemakers). Types of pacemakers are summarized in Table 1. The introduction of new transcutaneous pacing systems during the 1980s has led to more widespread use of pacing in emergency cardiac care (ECC).[1]

Indications for Pacing

There are numerous indications for elective placement of a permanent pacemaker, and specific recommendations vary among different authors and institutions.[2] Standby pacing capability is required for persons who are stable clinically yet may decompensate or become unstable in the near future from heart block or other causes of bradycardia. A transcutaneous pacemaker can serve as a standby pacemaker in these potentially unstable patients[3] and can act as a therapeutic bridge until placement of a transvenous pacemaker under more controlled circumstances.

Emergency pacing is often required in patients with hemodynamically unstable bradycardia, particularly if the rhythm is unresponsive to pharmacologic therapy. Symptoms of hemodynamic instability include hypotension (systolic blood pressure less than 80 mm Hg), change in mental status, angina, and pulmonary edema. Such patients cannot always tolerate a delay in pacing until arrival at the hospital or until a transvenous pacing catheter is placed.[4,5] Drug treatment may increase the heart rate and improve hemodynamics before pacing. Pacing should not be delayed in such patients if drug therapy is not immediately available. It may be appropriate to initiate pharmacologic therapy and pacing simultaneously to stabilize the patient as rapidly as possible.[5]

Another indication for emergency pacing is bradycardia so slow that it leads to pause-dependent or bradycardia-dependent ventricular rhythms. These ventricular rhythms may be unresponsive to pharmacologic therapy. Some patients with severe bradycardia may develop wide-complex ventricular beats that may repetitively precipitate ventricular tachycardia (VT) or ventricular fibrillation (VF).[4] Increasing the intrinsic heart rhythm with pacing may eliminate the pause- or bradycardia-dependent ventricular rhythms.

Pacing also can be used to terminate malignant supraventricular and ventricular tachycardias.[6] This technique is termed *overdrive* pacing and is performed by pacing the heart for a few seconds at a rate faster than the tachycardia rate, then stopping the pacemaker to allow the heart's intrinsic rhythm to return. Although this technique has shown promise in the treatment of all supraventricular tachycardias,[6-9] drug therapy remains the preferred treatment for stable patients and electrical cardioversion for those who are unstable. Overdrive pacing is limited by the maximum pacing rate of the device, usually 170 to 180 beats per minute.

Pacing has been studied extensively in the treatment of pulseless patients with bradycardia or asystole.[10]

Table 1. Types of Cardiac Pacemakers

Name	Electrode Location	Pulse Generator Location	Synonyms
Transcutaneous	Skin (anterior chest wall and back)	External	External Noninvasive
Transvenous	Venous (venous catheter with tip in right ventricle or right atrium or both)	External	Temporary transvenous Permanent transvenous
Transthoracic	Through the anterior chest wall into the heart	External	Transmyocardial
Transesophageal	Esophagus	External	
Epicardial	Epicardium (electrodes placed on the surface of the heart during surgery)	External or internal	
"Permanent"	Venous or epicardial	Internal	Implanted Internal

Although some studies have shown encouraging results in such patients when pacing was initiated within 10 minutes of cardiac arrest,[3,11] most studies have documented no improvement in survival with pacing.[12-22] Prehospital studies of transcutaneous pacing for *asystolic arrest* have shown no benefit from pacing.[13-16,19]

In particular, pacing should be considered for all patients in cardiac arrest due to drug overdose, especially if the rhythm is profound bradycardia or pulseless electrical activity. The same technique is useful in pulseless electrical activity due to acidosis or electrolyte abnormalities. These patients may have a normal myocardium with a disturbed conduction system. After correction of electrolyte abnormalities or acidosis, rapid pacing can stimulate effective myocardial contractions until the conduction system can recover.

Indications for emergency and prophylactic pacing are summarized in Table 2.

Contraindications to Cardiac Pacing

Severe hypothermia is one of the few relative contraindications to cardiac pacing in the patient with bradycardia. Bradycardia may be physiological in these patients, owing to the decreased metabolic rate associated with hypothermia.[23] More important, the ventricles are more prone to fibrillation and more resistant to defibrillation as core temperature drops.[24]

Pacing is relatively contraindicated in the patient with bradyasystolic cardiac arrest of more than 20 minutes' duration because of the well-documented poor resuscitation rate of these patients. Most bradycardia in children results from hypoxia or hypoventilation and will respond to adequate airway intervention with or without drug therapy. Thus, pacing is rarely required in pediatric arrests but should be considered for children with primary bradycardia from congenital defects or bradycardia following open heart surgery.

Transcutaneous Pacing

In transcutaneous pacing the heart is stimulated with externally applied cutaneous electrodes that deliver an electrical impulse. This impulse is conducted across the intact chest wall to activate the myocardium.[24,25] This technique is also referred to in the literature as *external pacing*, *noninvasive pacing*, *external transthoracic pacing*, and *transchest pacing*. *Transcutaneous pacing* is the preferred term since it best conveys the concept of pacing the heart through skin electrodes and distinguishes the technique from other emergent pacing techniques (transmyocardial or transthoracic, transvenous, transesophageal). It should be noted that transcutaneous pacing is not truly "noninvasive," because current with the potential to cause cardiac and tissue damage is introduced into the body.[26,27] The term *external* also is used in pacemaker terminology to refer to any pulse generator that is not implanted in the body and therefore may refer to transvenous, transthoracic, or transesophageal pacing, as well as to transcutaneous pacing.

Transcutaneous pacing is the initial pacing method of choice in ECC because of the speed with which it can be instituted and because it is the least invasive pacing tech-

Table 2. Indications for Emergency Pacing and Pacing Readiness

Emergent Pacing

Hemodynamically compromising bradycardias* (Class I)

  (Blood pressure <80 mm Hg systolic, change in mental status, angina, pulmonary edema)

Bradycardia with escape rhythms (Class IIa)

  (Unresponsive to pharmacologic therapy)

Overdrive pacing of refractory tachycardia (Class IIb)

   Supraventricular or ventricular

   (Currently indicated only in special situations refractory to pharmacologic therapy or electrical cardioversion)

Bradyasystolic cardiac arrest (Class IIb)

   Pacing not routinely recommended in such patients. If used at all, pacing should be used as early as possible after onset of arrest.

Pacing Readiness

Anticipatory pacing readiness in setting of acute myocardial infarction (Class I)

   • Symptomatic sinus node dysfunction
   • Mobitz type II second-degree heart block†
   • Third-degree heart block†
   • Newly acquired left, right, or alternating bundle branch block or bifascicular block

*Including complete heart block, symptomatic second-degree heart block, symptomatic sick sinus syndrome, drug-induced bradycardias (ie, digoxin, β blockers, calcium channel blockers, procainamide), permanent pacemaker failure, idioventricular bradycardias, symptomatic atrial fibrillation with slow ventricular response, refractory bradycardia during resuscitation of hypovolemic shock, and bradyarrhythmias with malignant ventricular escape mechanisms.

†In patients with an inferior myocardial infarction, relatively asymptomatic second- or third-degree heart block can occur. Pacing in such patients should be based on symptoms or deteriorating bradycardia.

nique available. Since no vascular puncture is required for electrode placement, this technique is preferred in patients who have received or who may require thrombolytic therapy. Most manufacturers now produce defibrillators with a built-in transcutaneous pacemaker offering the rapid availability of pacing. Multifunctional electrodes allow "hands-off" defibrillation, pacing, and electrocardiographic (ECG) monitoring through a single pair of anterior-posterior or sternal-apex chest wall electrodes. Pediatric electrodes are also available and are useful in pediatric patients with bradycardia of a nonrespiratory origin.[28] Limited experience suggests that transcutaneous pacing also may be useful in treating refractory tachyarrhythmias by overdrive pacing,[6-9] but overdrive pacing may also accelerate the tachycardia.

Energy, Current, and Impulse Duration for Transcutaneous Pacing

The modern age of cardiac pacing in humans began in 1952 with the report by Paul Zoll[29] of a successful resuscitation using the transcutaneous technique. This technique was largely abandoned by the 1960s because it was extremely painful and produced marked muscle contraction and cutaneous burns, especially with prolonged use.[29]

Recent refinements in electrode size and pulse characteristics led to the reintroduction of transcutaneous pacing into clinical practice.[25,30] Increasing the pulse duration from 2 to 20 milliseconds or longer was found to decrease the current output required for cardiac capture.[31] Longer impulse durations also make the induction of VF less likely.[31] The "safety factor" (ratio of fibrillation current to pacing current) for transcutaneous pacing is 12 to 15 in animal studies.[32] Larger surface area electrodes (8 cm in diameter) decrease the current density at the skin and therefore decrease pain and tissue burns. Trials of transcutaneous pacemakers using the newer impulse and electrode characteristics have demonstrated the success of these modifications in overcoming the limitations of earlier transcutaneous pacemakers.[33,34] The mean current required for electrical capture is usually 50 to 100 milliamperes (mA).[33] Some patients can tolerate pacing at their capture threshold, but intravenous analgesia and sedation are needed frequently for currents of approximately 50 mA or more.[35]

There is no risk of electric injury to healthcare providers during transcutaneous pacing. Power delivered during each impulse is less than 1/1000 of that delivered during defibrillation. Chest compressions (CPR) can be administered directly over the insulated electrodes while pacing. Inadvertent contact with the active pacing surface during chest compressions results in only a mild shock if any. Grasping a pacing electrode that is "on" would be more painful. Some pacers shut off when an electrode falls off the chest, but only certain brands have this feature.

Equipment for Transcutaneous Pacing

Transcutaneous pacemakers should be standard equipment in all emergency departments and many in-hospital and out-of-hospital care settings. The pacemakers introduced in the early 1980s were largely asynchronous devices with a limited selection of rate and output options. More recent units have demand-mode pacing with more output options and are often combined with a defibrillator in a single unit.

All transcutaneous pacemakers have similar basic features. Most allow operation in either a fixed-rate (non-demand or asynchronous) or a demand mode. Most allow rate selection in a range from 30 to 180 beats per minute. Current output is usually adjustable from 0 to 200 mA. If an ECG monitor is not an integral part of the unit, *an output adapter to a separate monitor is required* to "blank" the large electrical spike from the pacemaker impulse and allow interpretation of the much smaller ECG complex. Without blanking protection, the standard ECG and monitor devices are overwhelmed by the pacemaker spike and the rhythm is uninterpretable. This could be disastrous because the large pacing artifacts *can mask treatable VF* (Fig 1). The majority of pacing units currently manufactured are part of integrated monitor/defibrillator/pacing devices that automatically blank the pacing complex and thereby avoid this problem. Even with blanking protection large pacing artifacts can occur and cause confusion.

Pulse durations on available units vary from 20 to 40 milliseconds and are not adjustable by the operator. Rectangular pulse markers of 20 to 40 milliseconds are visible on the recorder.

Indications for Transcutaneous Pacing

Transcutaneous pacing is indicated for the treatment of hemodynamically significant bradycardias that have not responded to atropine therapy or when atropine therapy is not immediately available. Transcutaneous pacing is used for short intervals as a bridge until transvenous pacing can be initiated or until the underlying cause of the bradyarrhythmia (eg, hyperkalemia, drug overdose) can be reversed.[37]

In conscious patients with hemodynamically stable bradycardia, transcutaneous pacing may not be necessary. It is reasonable to attach electrodes to such patients and leave the pacemaker in the standby mode against the possibility of hemodynamic deterioration while further efforts at treatment of the patient's underlying disorder are being made. This approach has been used successfully in patients with new type II second-degree and third-degree heart block in the setting of cardiac ischemia and infarction.[38] However, if the device is to be used in the standby mode, a preliminary trial of transcutaneous pacing should be undertaken to ensure that capture can be achieved and is tolerated by the patient. If the patient is having difficulty tolerating transcutaneous pacing, administer medications such as diazepam (for treatment of anxiety and muscle contractions) and morphine (for analgesia).

Technique of Transcutaneous Pacing

The two pacing electrodes are attached to the patient's thorax. The anterior electrode is placed to the left of the sternum and centered as close as possible to the point of maximal cardiac impulse. The posterior electrode is placed directly behind the anterior electrode to the left of the thoracic spinal column. Each 8-cm electrode has an adhesive rim and a large surface area for electrode contact. In patients with excessive body hair, shaving may be required to ensure good contact, or alternative pacing electrode positions may be needed. In conscious patients clip rather than shave excessive hair to avoid tiny nicks in the skin that can increase pain and skin irritation.

To initiate transcutaneous pacing, apply the electrodes and activate the device (usually at a rate of 80 beats per minute). In the setting of bradyasystolic arrest, it is reasonable to turn the stimulating current to maximal output,

then decrease the output if capture is achieved. In the setting of a patient with a hemodynamically compromising bradycardia (but not in cardiac arrest), the operator should slowly increase the output from the minimal setting until capture is achieved. Electrical capture is usually characterized by a widening of the QRS complex and especially by a broad T wave. Sometimes only a change in the intrinsic morphology indicates pacing.

Assess electrical capture by monitoring the ECG on the filtered monitor of the pacing unit (Fig 2). It is easy to mistake the wide, slurred afterpotential following an external pacing spike for electrical capture. The only sure sign of electrical capture is the presence of a consistent ST segment and T wave after each pacer spike. The hemodynamic response to pacing also must be assessed, either by pulse, blood pressure cuff, or arterial catheter. The pulse should be taken at the right carotid or right femoral artery to avoid confusion between the jerking muscle contractions caused by the pacer and a pulse. Continue pacing at an output level slightly higher (10%) than the threshold of initial electrical capture.

Failure to capture with transcutaneous pacing may be related to electrode placement or patient size and body habitus, though capture thresholds do not appear to be

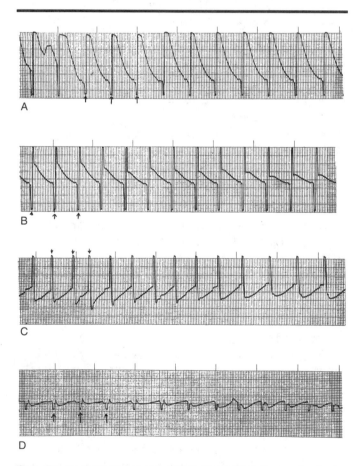

A

B

C

D

Fig 1. The top three rhythm strips (A, B, C) are taken from a standard wall-mounted electrocardiograph monitor. They all demonstrate large pacer spikes without capture. The underlying rhythm cannot be determined and could be treatable ventricular fibrillation. The bottom rhythm strip (D) demonstrates a tracing on the same patient with external pacer monitor (special dampening). Note that the pacing spikes are much smaller, and it is easily seen that the underlying rhythm is asystole, without pacer capture. From Roberts and Hedges.[36]

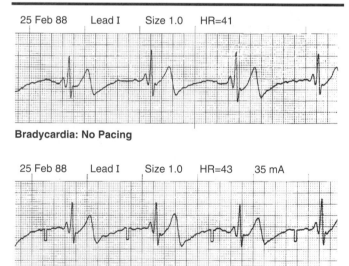

25 Feb 88   Lead I   Size 1.0   HR=41

Bradycardia: No Pacing

25 Feb 88   Lead I   Size 1.0   HR=43   35 mA

Pacing Below Threshold (35 mA): No Capture

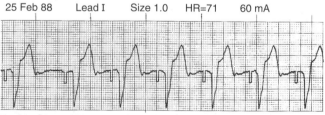

25 Feb 88   Lead I   Size 1.0   HR=71   60 mA

Pacing Above Threshold (60 mA): With Capture (Pacing-Pulse Marker ⊓)

Fig 2. Assessing electrocardiogram capture with transcutaneous pacing. Note that the monitor has been adapted to accommodate the large pacing artifact so as not to obscure the underlying ventricular activity. From Roberts and Hedges.[36]

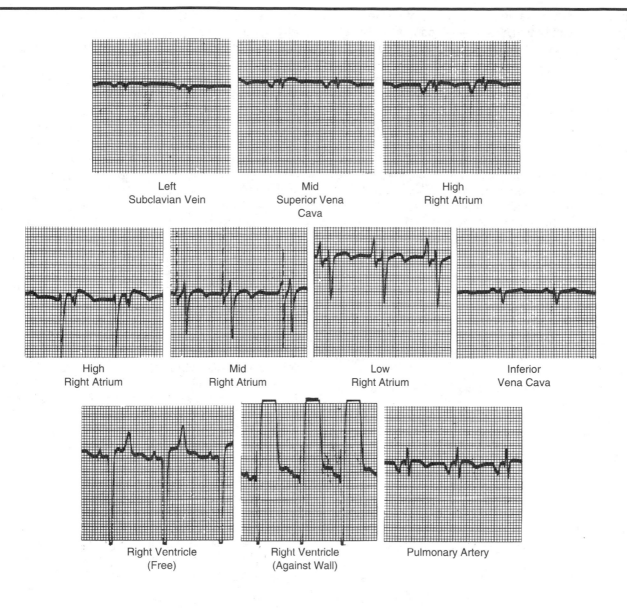

Left
Subclavian Vein

Mid
Superior Vena
Cava

High
Right Atrium

High
Right Atrium

Mid
Right Atrium

Low
Right Atrium

Inferior
Vena Cava

Right Ventricle
(Free)

Right Ventricle
(Against Wall)

Pulmonary Artery

Fig 3. Electrocardiographic monitoring of catheter tip location. Adapted from Bing.[42]

related to body weight or surface area in adults. Patients with barrel-shaped chests and large amounts of intra-thoracic air conduct electricity poorly and may have heart rhythms refractory to capture. A large pericardial effusion, tamponade, and recent thoracic surgery also will increase the output required for capture.[39]

Patients who are conscious or who regain consciousness during transcutaneous pacing will experience discomfort because of muscle contraction.[3,33,34] Analgesia with incremental doses of a narcotic, sedation with a benzodiazepine, or both will make this discomfort tolerable until transvenous pacing can be instituted. When transcutaneous pacing is used as a standby technique, the operator should first document that capture is possible by initiating a brief period of pacing at a rate slightly faster than the patient's intrinsic rate, then return the device to the standby mode.

Pitfalls and Complications of Transcutaneous Pacing

Two major pitfalls with transcutaneous pacing are *failure to recognize the presence of underlying treatable VF* and failure to recognize that the pacemaker is not capturing. This complication is primarily due to the size of the pacing artifact on the ECG screen, a technical problem inherent in systems without dampening circuitry.

Another theoretical complication of transcutaneous pacing is induction of arrhythmias or VF. With cutaneous precordial electrodes, the current required to induce fibrillation is probably greater than the output of external pacers.[32]

Pain from electrical skin and muscle stimulation was a significant complication of earlier transcutaneous pacemakers.[24] Recent studies with the newer units in conscious patients have shown that the technique is often well tolerated and that most patients rate the discomfort as "mild or moderate and easily tolerable,"[3,33,34] but up to one third of patients rate the pain as severe or intolerable.[35,40] The degree of pain varies with the device used and with the output required for capture.

Tissue damage can occur with prolonged transcutaneous pacing, but following manufacturers' recommendations can markedly reduce these problems.[26,27] This potential has been minimized by recent changes in pacemaker and electrode designs. Nonetheless, third-degree burns have been reported in pediatric patients where improper or prolonged pacing has been used.[28] With prolonged pacing there can be changes in pacing thresholds, leading to capture failure. Frequent skin inspection and repositioning the electrodes can remedy this problem.

Transvenous Pacing

Transvenous pacing consists of endocardial stimulation of the right atrium or ventricle or both via an electrode introduced into a central vein. Originally developed in the late 1950s, transvenous pacing was the technique of choice for initial emergency pacing until the reintroduction of transcutaneous pacing in the 1980s.[41] The major difficulties of transvenous pacing are venous access and proper placement of the stimulating electrode.[42-45] Venous access routes most commonly used include the subclavian, internal jugular, femoral, and brachial veins. Transvenous pacing catheters can be inserted through a variety of venous introducers. A soft, flexible, semifloating bipolar catheter is preferred. This type of pacing catheter is safest to use and takes advantage of any forward blood flow that is present.

Transvenous pacing is best suited for use in urgent situations in which there is adequate time for fluoroscopy. In ECC, transcutaneous pacing should be used first as a bridge to stabilize the patient until a transvenous pacer can be placed in a more controlled hospital environment.

Technique for Transvenous Lead Placement

Placement of the catheter tip into the apex of the right ventricle is key to successful transvenous pacing.[45] Several techniques can aid successful placement. Fluoroscopic guidance is the surest method of right ventricular placement. This technique requires familiarity with the fluoroscopic anatomy of the chest.

When fluoroscopy is unavailable, ECG guidance is useful in patients with narrow QRS complexes or P waves.[42] When this technique is used, the standard limb leads of an ECG machine are placed on the patient. The V lead is connected with a standard connector supplied with the pacing catheter, or with an alligator clip to the distal lead of the pacing catheter. The tip of the pacing catheter, as it is being inserted, thus becomes the sensing V lead of the ECG machine. With the ECG machine in the "V" position, the ECG complexes mirror the position of the tip of the pacing catheter. As the catheter approaches and enters the right atrium, the P wave and QRS complex sensed through this lead will become larger. When the tip of the catheter reaches the ventricle, the P wave will diminish in size and disappear at the apex, and the QRS complex will become very large. ST segment elevation signifies placement of the tip against the wall of the ventricle (the position desired for pacing). When this is achieved, the alligator clip is disconnected. The pacing catheter leads are then connected to the pulse generator box to initiate pacing. If QRS deflection becomes smaller during insertion, the tip is moving away from the heart, usually down the inferior vena cava or up a great vein in the neck[42] (Fig 3). Modern ECG devices are usually multichannel, allowing a multilead monitoring technique.

Balloon-tipped "floating" catheters may aid placement when used in conjunction with ECG and fluoroscopic guidance or when used alone. The balloon is inflated after catheter insertion into a central vein. Forward blood flow will then direct the catheter tip toward the ventricle as the operator slowly advances the catheter. As with all balloon-tipped catheters, the balloon should always be deflated before the catheter is pulled back or withdrawn.[44]

Positioning of the pacer tip within the right ventricle is difficult when patients have decreased or no forward blood flow, including most circumstances in which emergency pacing is indicated. Often fluoroscopy is not immediately available, and ECG guidance will aid placement in only the patient with narrow QRS complexes or a discernible P wave.[42] If available, transesophageal or transthoracic echocardiography can be used to position the pacing wire.[46] Balloon-tipped catheters offer little aid in placement during low- or no-flow states. Transcutaneous pacing is preferred in this setting. If transcutaneous pacing is unavailable or ineffective, transvenous pacing may be attempted. In a true emergency, the transvenous electrodes are connected to the pulse generator and the catheter advanced blindly in the hope that the tip will encounter the endocardium of the right ventricle and that capture will result.[47] In this setting, a right internal jugular venous access route should be used.[45] From this approach the catheter traverses a straight line into the right ventricle and rarely curls in the atrium or deflects into the inferior vena cava.

Transvenous Pacemaker Use

Transvenous pacer settings vary with the clinical situation. An initial rate of 80 to 100 beats per minute is appropriate for most patients. Asynchronous mode should be used initially in pulseless (asystolic) patients. In this setting, output should initially be set at maximum (usually 20 mA) then decreased after capture is achieved.

When a transvenous pacer is placed prophylactically in stable patients or when the patient has already been stabilized with transcutaneous pacing, the transvenous catheter tip should be correctly positioned before activating the pulse generator. A pacing rate should be selected; this turns the sensing "on." Output should initially be at a minimum setting and gradually increased until capture is achieved. With optimal tip position, capture should occur at less than 2 mA. If the pacing threshold is less than 0.5 mA, the pacing tip should be slightly withdrawn, since very low thresholds may suggest that the catheter tip is deeply embedded in myocardium. In such situations myocardial perforation may occur. Pacing should be continued at 1.5 to 2 times the threshold output required for capture. Subsequent rate and sensitivity settings should be adjusted as clinically indicated by the patient's hemodynamic status and underlying rhythm disturbance.[47]

Chest radiographs (anteroposterior and lateral) should be obtained after patient stabilization to ensure proper pacing lead tip placement and to evaluate the possibility of pneumothorax from the preceding central venous line placement.[43] Finally, care should be taken to affix the pacing catheter firmly to the insertion site before patient transfer.[47]

Other Pacing Techniques

Transmyocardial Transthoracic Pacing

Transthoracic pacing involves the percutaneous placement of a bipolar pacing wire directly into the right ventricular cavity through a trocar needle. The technique was developed during the 1960s as a faster alternative to transvenous pacer insertion for emergent cardiac pacing.[48,49] Although this technique has been lifesaving in patients with hemodynamically significant bradycardia,[50] it has been replaced in emergency practice by the transcutaneous technique. As with other pacing techniques, clinical series have shown transthoracic pacing to be of little benefit for the patient in prolonged bradyasystolic cardiac arrest.[20,21] Because of a significant incidence of serious complications associated with the procedure (pericardial tamponade, major vessel injury, pneumothorax) and because placement within the right ventricle is frequently unsuccessful, this technique should never be used unless it is the only possible alternative.[20,51,52]

Transesophageal Pacing

Atrial pacing via esophageal electrodes has been used in emergent and diagnostic situations since the 1960s.[53] The technique requires passage of an electrode-bearing esophageal "pill" electrode followed by positioning of the electrode behind the heart.[54] The proximity of the atria to the esophagus allows atrial capture at relatively low currents, producing minimal pain. Ventricular capture requires higher outputs (10 to 80 mA) that may produce pain. In many cases it may not be possible to achieve ventricular capture using the transesophageal route. The transesophageal approach thus is useful only for atrial pacing, a condition that has rare application during resuscitation.[55] However, it is useful for overdrive pacing of atrial arrhythmias.

Epicardial Pacing

Epicardial pacing refers to placement of pacing leads directly onto or through the epicardium under direct visualization. In the emergent situation this is used almost exclusively during open thoracotomy for resuscitation of the patient with penetrating trauma.[56] These patients may develop refractory bradyarrhythmias after initial fluid resuscitation. Dramatic improvement has been reported following epicardial pacing in this situation.[57] Epicardial leads are more commonly placed electively in patients undergoing cardiac surgery for postoperative use in the event of bradycardia.

References

1. Hedges JR, Syverud SA, Dalsey WC. Development in transcutaneous and transthoracic pacing during bradyasystolic arrest. *Ann Emerg Med.* 1984;13:822-827.
2. ACC/AHA guidelines for the early management of patients with acute myocardial infarction. *Circulation.* 1990;82:664-707.
3. Zoll PM, Zoll RH, Falk RH, Clinton JE, Eitel DR, Antman EM. External noninvasive temporary cardiac pacing: clinical trials. *Circulation.* 1985;71:937-944.
4. Roberts JR, Syverud SA. Emergency pacemaker insertion and malfunction. In: Callaham ML, ed. *Current Therapy in Emergency Medicine.* Philadelphia, Pa: BC Decker; 1987:465-471.
5. Hedges JR, Feero S, Shultz B, Easter R, Syverud SA, Dalsey WC. Prehospital transcutaneous cardiac pacing for symptomatic bradycardia. *PACE Pacing Clin Electrophysiol.* 1991;14:1473-1478.
6. Estes NA III, Deering TF, Manolis AS, Salem D, Zoll PM. External cardiac programmed stimulation for noninvasive termination of sustained supraventricular and ventricular tachycardia. *Am J Cardiol.* 1989;63:177-183.
7. Rosenthal ME, Stamato NJ, Marchlinski FE, Josephson ME. Noninvasive cardiac pacing for termination of sustained, uniform ventricular tachycardia. *Am J Cardiol.* 1986;58:561-562.
8. Sharkey SW, Chaffee V, Kapsner S. Prophylactic external pacing during cardioversion of atrial tachyarrhythmias. *Am J Cardiol.* 1985;55:1632-1634.
9. Altamura G, Bianconi L, Boccadamo R, Pistolese M. Treatment of ventricular and supraventricular tachyarrhythmias by transcutaneous cardiac pacing. *PACE Pacing Clin Electrophysiol.* 1989; 12:331-338.
10. Syverud SA. Cardiac pacing. *Emerg Med Clin North Am.* 1988; 6:197-215.
11. Syverud SA, Dalsey WC, Hedges JR. Transcutaneous and transvenous cardiac pacing for early bradyasystolic cardiac arrest. *Ann Emerg Med.* 1986;15:121-124.
12. Dalsey WC, Syverud SA, Hedges JR. Emergency department use of transcutaneous pacing for cardiac arrests. *Crit Care Med.* 1985; 13:399-401.
13. Eitel DR, Guzzardi LJ, Stein SE, Drawbaugh RE, Hess DR, Walton SL. Noninvasive transcutaneous cardiac pacing in prehospital cardiac arrest. *Ann Emerg Med.* 1987;16:531-534.
14. Barthell E, Troiano P, Olson D, Stueven HA, Hendley G. Prehospital external cardiac pacing: a prospective, controlled clinical trial. *Ann Emerg Med.* 1988;17:1221-1226.
15. Hedges JR, Syverud SA, Dalsey WC, Feero S, Easter R, Schultz B. Prehospital trial of emergency transcutaneous cardiac pacing. *Circulation.* 1987;76:1337-1343.
16. Cummins RO, Graves JR, Halstrom A, Larsen MP, Hearne TR,

Ciliberti J, Nicola RM, Horan S. Out-of-hospital transcutaneous pacing by emergency medical technicians in patients with asystolic cardiac arrest. *N Engl J Med.* 1993;328:1377-1382.

17. Hazard PB, Benton C, Milnor P. Transvenous cardiac pacing in cardiopulmonary resuscitation. *Crit Care Med.* 1981;9:666-668.

18. Ornato JP, Carveth WL, Windle JR. Pacemaker insertion for prehospital bradyasystolic cardiac arrest. *Ann Emerg Med.* 1984; 13:101-103.

19. Paris PM, Stewart RD, Kaplan RM, Whipkey R. Transcutaneous pacing for bradyasystolic cardiac arrests in prehospital care. *Ann Emerg Med.* 1985;14:320-323.

20. Tintinalli JE, White BC. Transthoracic pacing during CPR. *Ann Emerg Med.* 1981;10:113-116.

21. White JD. Transthoracic pacing in cardiac asystole. *Am J Emerg Med.* 1983;1:264-266.

22. White JD, Brown CG. Immediate transthoracic pacing for cardiac asystole in an emergency department setting. *Am J Emerg Med.* 1985;3:125-128.

23. Best R, Syverud SA, Nowak RM. Trauma and hypothermia. *Am J Emerg Med.* 1985;3:48-55.

24. Zoll PM, Zoll RH, Belgard AH. External noninvasive electric stimulation of the heart. *Crit Care Med.* 1981;9:393-394.

25. Syverud SA, Hedges JR, Dalsey WC, Gabel M, Thomson DP, Engel PJ. Hemodynamics of transcutaneous cardiac pacing. *Am J Emerg Med.* 1986;4:17-20.

26. Kicklighter EJ, Syverud SA, Dalsey WC, Hedges JR, van der Bel-Kahn JM. Pathological aspects of transcutaneous cardiac pacing. *Am J Emerg Med.* 1985;3:108-113.

27. Pride HB, McKinley DF. Third-degree burns from the use of an external cardiac pacing device. *Crit Care Med.* 1990;18:572-573.

28. Beland MJ, Hesslein PS, Finlay CD, Faerron-Angel JE, Williams WG, Rowe RD. Noninvasive transcutaneous cardiac pacing in children. *PACE Pacing Clin Electrophysiol.* 1987;10:1262-1270.

29. Zoll PM, Linenthal AJ, Norman LR. Treatment of unexpected cardiac arrest by external electric stimulation of the heart. *N Engl J Med.* 1956;254:541-546.

30. Dalsey WC, Syverud SA, Trott A. Transcutaneous cardiac pacing. *J Emerg Med.* 1984;1:201-205.

31. Jones M, Geddes LA. Strength-duration curves for cardiac pacemaking and ventricular fibrillation. *Cardiovasc Res Cent Bull.* 1977;15:101-112.

32. Voorhees WD III, Foster KS, Geddes LA, Babbs CF. Safety factor for precordial pacing: minimum current thresholds for pacing and for ventricular fibrillation by vulnerable-period stimulation. *PACE Pacing Clin Electrophysiol.* 1984;7:356-360.

33. Falk RH, Zoll PM, Zoll RH. Safety and efficacy of noninvasive cardiac pacing: a preliminary report. *N Engl J Med.* 1983;309:1166-1168.

34. Heller MB, Peterson J, Ilkhanipour K, et al. A comparative study of five transcutaneous pacing devices in unanesthetized human volunteers. *Prehosp Disaster Med.* 1989;4:15-20.

35. Madsen JK, Meibom J, Videbak R, Pedersen F, Grande P. Transcutaneous pacing: experience with the Zoll noninvasive temporary pacemaker. *Am Heart J.* 1988;116:7-10.

36. Roberts JR, Hedges JR, eds. *Clinical Procedures in Emergency Medicine.* Philadelphia, Pa: WB Saunders Co; 1985:206,208.

37. Cummins RO, Haulman J, Quan L, Graves JR, Peterson D, Horan S. Near-fatal yew berry intoxication treated with external cardiac pacing and digoxin-specific FAB antibody fragments. *Ann Emerg Med.* 1990;19:38-43.

38. Gessman LJ, Wertheimer JH, Davison J, Watson J, Weintraub W. A new device and method for rapid emergency pacing: clinical use in 10 patients. *PACE Pacing Clin Electrophysiol.* 1982;5:929-933.

39. Hedges JR, Syverud SA, Dalsey WC, Simko LA, van der Bel-Kahn J, Gabel M, Thomson DP. Threshold, enzymatic, and pathologic changes associated with prolonged transcutaneous pacing in a chronic heart block model. *J Emerg Med.* 1989;7:1-4.

40. Dunn DL, Gregory JJ. Noninvasive temporary pacing: experience in a community hospital. *Heart Lung.* 1989;18:23-28.

41. Bartecchi CE. Emergency transvenous cardiac pacing. *Henry Ford Hosp Med J.* 1978;26:13-18.

42. Bing OH, McDowell JW, Hantman J, Messer JV. Pacemaker placement by electrocardiographic monitoring. *N Engl J Med.* 1972; 287:651.

43. Kaul TK, Bain WH. Radiographic appearances of implanted transvenous endocardial pacing electrodes. *Chest.* 1977;72:323-326.

44. Lang R, David D, Klein HO, Di Segni E, Libhaber C, Sareli P, Kaplinsky E. The use of the balloon-tipped floating catheter in temporary transvenous cardiac pacing. *PACE Pacing Clin Electrophysiol.* 1981;4:491-496.

45. Syverud SA, Dalsey WC, Hedges JR, Hanslits ML. Radiologic assessment of transvenous pacemaker placement during CPR. *Ann Emerg Med.* 1986;15:131-137.

46. Porter TR, Ornato JP, Guard CS, Roy VG, Burns CA, Nixon JV. Transesophageal echocardiography to assess mitral valve function and flow during cardiopulmonary resuscitation. *Am J Cardiol.* 1992; 70:1056-1060.

47. Benjamin GC. Emergency transvenous cardiac pacing. In: Roberts JR, Hedges JR, eds. *Clinical Procedures in Emergency Medicine.* Philadelphia, Pa: WB Saunders Co; 1985:170-207.

48. Roe BB, Katz HJ. Complete heart block with intractable asystole and recurrent ventricular fibrillation with survival. *Am J Cardiol.* 1965;15:401-403.

49. Roe BB. Intractable Stokes-Adams disease: a method of emergency management. *Am Heart J.* 1965;69:470-472.

50. Roberts JR, Greenberg MI, Crisanti JW, Gayle SW. Successful use of emergency transthoracic pacing in bradyasystolic cardiac arrest. *Ann Emerg Med.* 1984;13:277-283.

51. Brown CG, Gurley HT, Hutchins GM, MacKenzie EJ, White JD. Injuries associated with percutaneous placement of transthoracic pacemakers. *Ann Emerg Med.* 1985;14:223-228.

52. Roberts JR, Greenberg MI. Emergency transthoracic pacemaker. *Ann Emerg Med.* 1981;10:600-612.

53. Burack B, Furman S. Transesophageal cardiac pacing. *Am J Cardiol.* 1969;23:469-472.

54. Rowe GG, Terry W, Neblett I. Cardiac pacing with an esophageal electrode. *Am J Cardiol.* 1969;24:548-550.

55. Pattison CZ, Atlee JL III, Krebs LH, Madireddi L, Kettler RE. Transesophageal indirect atrial pacing for drug-resistant sinus bradycardia. *Anesthesiology.* 1991;74:1141-1144.

56. Millikan JS, Moore EE, Dunn EL, Van Way CW III, Hopeman AR. Temporary cardiac pacing in traumatic arrest victims. *Ann Emerg Med.* 1980;9:591-593.

57. Lick S, Rappaport WD, McIntyre KE. Successful epicardial pacing in blunt trauma resuscitation. *Ann Emerg Med.* 1991;20:908-909.

Intravenous (IV) cannulation is a means to gain direct access to the venous circulation, either peripheral or central. The purposes of IV cannulation are

- To administer drugs and fluids
- To obtain venous blood for laboratory determinations
- To insert catheters into the central circulation, including the right heart and pulmonary artery, for physiological monitoring and electrical pacing

Personnel who provide advanced life support must be proficient in gaining direct access to the venous circulation as early as possible. An IV lifeline is essential for administering drugs and fluids and ensuring their immediate uptake and distribution.[1] Persons who place IV lines must take appropriate universal precautions to protect the patient and themselves from infectious disease. They must use protective barriers and take care in hand washing and the use and disposal of needles and other sharp instruments.[2]

Many drugs can be administered intramuscularly or subcutaneously, but absorption of drugs from these tissues into the capillary blood depends on blood flow. In low cardiac output states, blood is shunted away from skin and muscle, which markedly impairs uptake and distribution of the drug. If the drug is given IV, access to the circulation is ensured.

The following percutaneous IV techniques are commonly used:

- Peripheral venipuncture
  — Arm vein
  — Leg vein
  — External jugular vein
- Central venipuncture
  — Femoral vein
  — Internal jugular vein
  — Subclavian vein

ACLS providers should know the general guidelines for choice of access route; the available needles, cannulas, and catheters; the general principles of IV therapy; and the specific anatomy, indications, performance criteria, and complications for each of these techniques.

Guidelines for Vascular Access: Choice of a Particular Approach

Peripheral Lines

Cannulation of a peripheral venous access site is the procedure of choice even during CPR because of the speed, ease, and safety with which it can usually be performed. During an emergency, personnel should cannulate the large, easily accessible peripheral veins, such as the cephalic, femoral, or external jugular. Minimal training is required, and several members of the resuscitation team often have the necessary skill. Peripheral sites are easily compressible, which is particularly important in patients who may require thrombolytic therapy.

A disadvantage of peripheral venous cannulation is that these vessels may collapse during low-flow states, making access both difficult and time-consuming. Blind cannulation of the femoral vein during CPR poses special problems because of patient movements and limited space around the patient. In addition, researchers have recently observed prolonged intervals for the entrance of peripherally administered drugs into the central circulation during cardiac arrest. When using peripheral sites during a cardiac arrest, use upper extremity veins, keep the access site elevated, and follow drug administration with a flush of IV fluid.

Central Lines

Cannulate central veins when peripheral sites are not readily available or when access to the central circulation is required to place central venous pressure lines, right heart catheters, or transvenous pacemaker electrodes. The predictable anatomic location of the central vessels permits rapid venous access in emergencies when valuable time might be lost searching for a peripheral site. The large size of the central vessels permits passage of large-bore catheters when rapid volume replacement is needed. The greater flow through the central vessels permits infusion of concentrated solutions that would irritate peripheral vessels.

The primary disadvantage of central venous cannulation is an increased complication rate. The subclavian and internal jugular veins lie close to the carotid and subclavian arteries, the apical pleura of the lungs, the trachea, and various nerves. These structures are frequently damaged, most often when inexperienced operators perform the procedures. In addition, central cannulation carries the risks of air embolus, catheter embolus, and hemorrhage from noncompressible sites. The last may be a particular problem in patients receiving thrombolytic therapy.

While there are advantages and disadvantages to central catheterization techniques, the primary determinant should be the experience of the operator. Complication rates are inversely related to the operator's experience, so it is important to choose the technique with which the operator is most familiar. The supraclavicular subclavian and central internal jugular approaches are both relatively easy to perform, and they are associated with a low incidence of pneumothorax. Furthermore, the rate of catheter tip malposition is much lower when the catheter is inserted from above rather than below the clavicle. The supraclavicular subclavian approach has additional advantages during cardiac arrest in that it can be performed with minimal interruption of chest compression (unlike the infraclavicular approach) and it permits the operator to stand to the side of the patient's head during insertion. In this position there is less interference with airway management than occurs with internal jugular cannulation.

Intravenous Cannulas

There are three types of cannulas: (1) hollow needles, including those attached to a syringe and the butterfly type, (2) indwelling plastic catheters inserted over a hollow needle, and (3) indwelling plastic catheters inserted through a hollow needle or over a guidewire that was previously introduced through a needle.

Plastic catheters, rather than hollow needles, should be used for emergency IV therapy because they can be better anchored and they permit the patient to move more freely. When volume expansion is needed, the catheter should be short and the gauge as large as possible. The flow rate through a 14-gauge catheter 5 cm long averages approximately 125 mL/min. This may be twice the flow through a 16-gauge catheter 20 cm long and three times the flow through a 20-gauge catheter 5 cm long.[3]

The length of the needle and catheter depends on the site of insertion. For cannulation of a peripheral vein, a needle and catheter length of 5 cm is adequate. If a central vein such as the internal jugular or the subclavian is to be cannulated, a needle length of at least 6 or 7 cm is required because the vein may lie up to 5 cm from the point of entry of the needle. The necessary catheter length can be determined by measuring from the point of planned insertion to the appropriate location on the anterior chest that overlies the desired position of the tip in the central circulation. For an internal jugular or subclavian vein insertion, a catheter should be at least 15 to 20 cm long.

If a catheter-over-needle device is used (Fig 1), the venipuncture is made and the catheter is introduced into the vein as the needle is removed. The end of the IV tubing is then connected directly to the end of the plastic catheter. The length of the catheter is limited by the length of the needle required, but the puncture in the vein is exactly the size of the external plastic catheter. This reduces the possibility of blood leaking around the venipuncture site. Over-the-needle devices are not suitable for central venous cannulation because of their limited length.

If a catheter-inside-needle unit is used (Fig 2), the catheter is pushed into the vein through the needle after venipuncture. The needle is retracted to the external end of the catheter, where it remains, and the IV tubing is

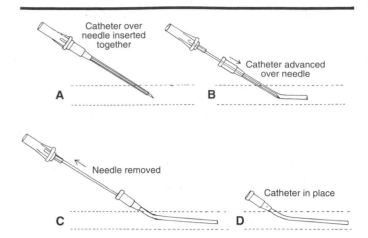

Fig 1. Insertion of catheter over needle.

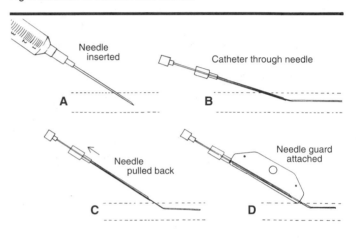

Fig 2. Insertion of catheter through needle.

attached to it. Great caution must be exercised not to retract the catheter through the needle since the sharp tip of the needle may shear off the end of the catheter and could produce a catheter-fragment embolus.

A third alternative is to use a guidewire (Seldinger technique) (Fig 3).[4] This valuable technique is becoming the procedure of choice as guidewire kits become easier to use and as more physicians are properly trained in the technique. Modern guidewire devices use thin-wall 18-gauge needles that theoretically have less potential for damaging structures in their path than do the 14-gauge needles commonly used with through-the-needle devices.

As with other cannulation techniques, personnel should be trained in the proper use of a guidewire before they use it. The guidewire must be several centimeters longer than the catheter to be placed, and the diameter of the wire must be small enough to allow it to pass through both the needle and the catheter. At all times during insertion of a catheter over a guidewire, the end of the guidewire must extend beyond the end of the catheter that remains outside the patient. This prevents the wire from sliding all the way into the catheter and being lost within the circulation. The tip of the guidewire must be

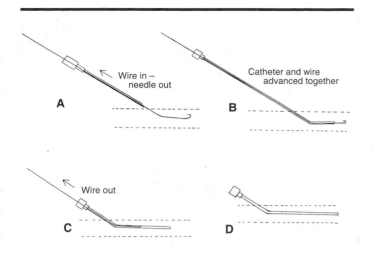

Fig 3. Insertion of catheter over guidewire (Seldinger technique).

flexible. A J-tip facilitates passage of the wire through the tortuous vessels. After the venipuncture is made with the needle, the flexible-tipped or J-tipped guidewire is inserted through the needle. If the guidewire does not pass easily into the vein, it should be removed, a syringe re-attached to the needle, and the needle advanced or withdrawn until it is within the lumen of the vein.

Once the guidewire is successfully placed through the needle into the vein, the needle is removed and a venous dilator/catheter unit is passed over the wire, through the skin, and into the vessel. The dilator device consists of a semirigid thick-wall catheter over which a thin-wall flexible plastic venous catheter is passed. The dilator provides the rigidity necessary to pass the catheter into the vessel. It is frequently necessary to nick the skin at the puncture site with a No. 11 scalpel to facilitate passage of the dilator. A slight twisting motion of the dilator will also make advancement easier. It is important to make sure that the proximal end of the guidewire remains visible during passage of the dilator.

Once the dilator has been advanced far enough to guarantee placement of its tip well within the vessel lumen, the flexible catheter is advanced over the dilator and guidewire into the vessel. The guidewire and dilator can then be removed and the catheter connected to IV tubing.

General Principles of IV Therapy

In an emergency, where speed is essential (especially outside the hospital), strict aseptic technique may be impossible. After the patient is stabilized, the cannula should be removed and replaced under sterile conditions.

If the patient is awake, it is preferable that the overlying skin be anesthetized, using 1% lidocaine without epinephrine, before inserting a large-bore cannula. A scalpel can also be used to make a small skin incision through which larger cannulas will pass more easily. After

the catheter is inserted, sterile infusion tubing with injection sites near the tip of the tubing is attached. The other end of the tubing is connected to a container of sterile normal saline. Ideally this container should be a non-breakable plastic bottle or bag. If a plastic bag is used, it can be placed under the patient's shoulders during transportation, and the weight of the patient will maintain the infusion at the preset rate. The plastic bag should be squeezed before use to detect punctures that may lead to contamination of the contents. No drug that may be absorbed by the plastic should be added to the solution.[5] To keep the IV line open, the rate of infusion should be set at 10 mL/h.

An alternative to the fluid infusion systems commonly used is insertion of a saline lock catheter system. This system is particularly useful for patients who require drug injections but not IV volume infusion. If fluid infusion is needed, the saline lock can be readily removed and standard IV tubing attached to the catheter. Advantages of the saline lock are simplicity and reduced cost because there is no IV tubing or bag. Its disadvantage is that flushing the catheter is more complicated, requiring use of a separate needle and syringe. Newer systems use needleless locks to permit drug and flush infusions without inadvertent needle sticks. During cardiac arrest all peripherally administered drugs should be followed by bolus administration of at least 20 mL of IV flush solution to ensure entry into the central circulation.[6] This may be cumbersome when many drugs are administered with a saline lock system.

Complications Common to All IV Techniques

The risk of certain complications is common to all IV techniques. Local complications include hematoma formation, cellulitis, thrombosis, and phlebitis. Systemic complications include sepsis, pulmonary thrombo-embolism, air embolism, and catheter-fragment embolism.

Peripheral Veins

The most common areas for IV therapy are in the hands and arms. Favored sites are the dorsum of the hands, the wrists, and the antecubital fossae. In the legs the long saphenous veins are the preferred sites for IV therapy. Ideally only the antecubital veins should be used for drug administration during CPR.[1]

Anatomy: Upper Extremities[7, 8] (Fig 4)

On the dorsum of the hand, a series of veins arises from the digital veins that run parallel to the long axis of the hand, interconnected by a series of arches that form the dorsal plexus. At the radial side of the dorsal plexus, a thick vein, the superficial radial vein, runs laterally up to the antecubital fossa and joins the median cephalic vein

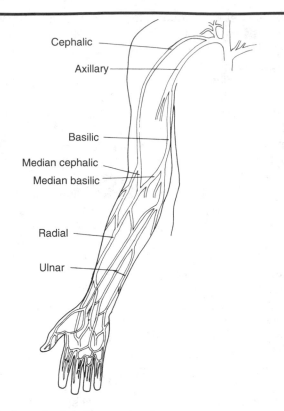

Fig 4. Anatomy of veins of upper extremity.

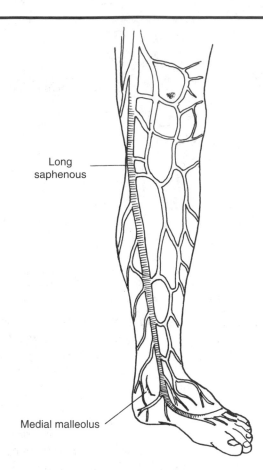

Fig 5. Anatomy of long saphenous vein of leg.

to form the cephalic vein. Other superficial veins on the ulnar aspect of the forearm run to the elbow and join the medial basilic vein to form the basilic vein. The median vein of the forearm bifurcates into a Y in the antecubital fossa, laterally becoming the medial cephalic and medially becoming the median basilic.

The basilic vein passes up the inner side of the arm, becoming deep at the lower third of the arm. As it continues cephalad, it joins the brachial vein to become the axillary vein. The cephalic vein continues laterally up the arm, crosses anteriorly, and becomes deep in the interval between the pectoralis major and deltoid muscles. After a sharp angulation, it joins the axillary vein at a 90° angle, an anatomic detail that makes the cephalic vein unsuitable for insertion of central venous pulmonary artery catheters.

Anatomy: Lower Extremities[7,8] (Fig 5)

The long saphenous vein begins on the inner side of the foot, receiving branches from the dorsal venous arch of the foot. It travels upward in front of the medial malleolus of the tibia to the groove between the upper medial end of the tibia and the calf muscle and passes backward behind the medial condyle of the femur. It then runs somewhat outward and upward on the inner side of the front of the thigh to 1½ inches (3.8 cm) below the inguinal ligament, where it pierces the saphenous opening to end in the femoral vein.

Anatomy: External Jugular Vein[7,8] (Fig 6)

The external jugular vein is formed below the ear and behind the angle of the mandible where a branch of the posterior facial vein joins the posterior auricular vein. The

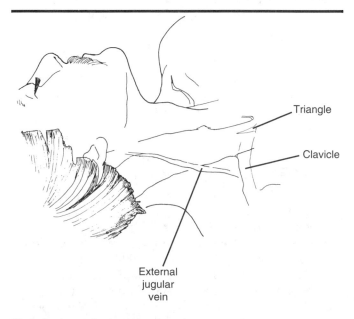

Fig 6. Anatomy of external jugular vein.

external jugular vein then passes downward and obliquely backward across the surface of the sternomastoid muscle, pierces the deep fascia of the neck just above the middle of the clavicle, and ends in the subclavian vein lateral to the anterior scalene muscle. Valves and other veins enter the external jugular vein at the entrance to the subclavian vein. There are also valves in the external jugular vein about 4 cm above the clavicle.

Technique: Arm or Leg Vein

Since the largest of the superficial veins of the arm are in the antecubital fossa, select these initially if the patient is in circulatory collapse or cardiac arrest (Fig 7). In the stable patient, however, the more distal veins of the arm may be selected first, if accessible (Fig 8). Similarly, the long saphenous vein at the medial malleolus may be

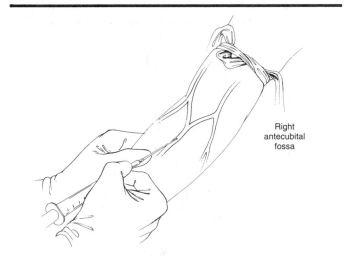

Right antecubital fossa

Fig 7. Antecubital venipuncture.

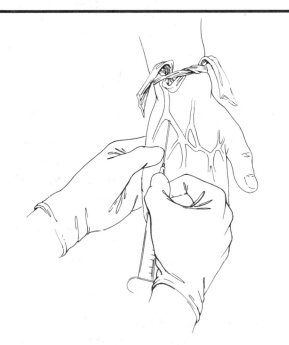

Fig 8. Venipuncture of dorsal hand vein.

used first, but it can be entered at any point along its course. Usually a point between the junction of two veins is chosen for entry, because the vein is more stable here and venipuncture is more easily accomplished. The steps for initiating IV therapy using the arm or leg vein follow:

1. Apply tourniquet proximally.
2. Locate vein and cleanse the overlying skin with alcohol or povidone-iodine.
3. Anesthetize the skin if a large-bore cannula is to be inserted in a conscious patient.
4. Hold vein in place by applying traction on vein distal to the point of entry.
5. Puncture the skin with bevel of needle upward about 0.5 to 1.0 cm from the vein. Enter the vein either from the side or from above.
6. Note blood return and advance the catheter either over or through the needle, depending on the type of catheter-needle device being used. Remove tourniquet.
7. Withdraw and remove needle and attach infusion tubing.
8. Cover the puncture site with povidone-iodine ointment and a sterile dressing. Tape dressing in place.

Technique: External Jugular Vein[9] (Fig 9)

The steps for initiating IV therapy using the external jugular vein are

1. Place the patient in a supine, head-down (Trendelenburg) position to fill the external jugular vein. Turn the patient's head to the opposite side.
2. Cleanse and anesthetize the skin as previously described.
3. Align the cannula in the direction of the vein with the point aimed toward the ipsilateral shoulder.
4. Make venipuncture midway between the angle of the jaw and the midclavicular line, "tourniqueting" the vein lightly with one finger above the clavicle.
5. Proceed as described in the section on technique for arm and leg veins.

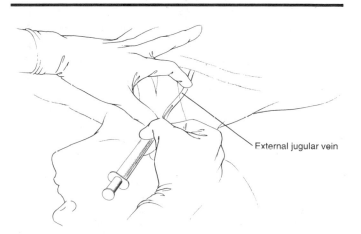

External jugular vein

Fig 9. External jugular venipuncture.

Using Peripheral Veins for IV Therapy

Advantages

The technique is easy to master. Antecubital vein cannulation usually provides an effective route for the administration of drugs during cardiac arrest so that central cannulation or intracardiac injection may be unnecessary. If basic life support measures are under way, antecubital vein catheterization does not interfere with continuing ventilation and chest compression.

After administration of a drug during CPR, raise the arm and give at least a 20-mL bolus of IV fluid to facilitate delivery of the drug into the central circulation. Allow 1 to 2 minutes for agents to reach the central circulation.

Disadvantages

In circulatory collapse it may be difficult or impossible to establish access from a peripheral vein. Recent studies have demonstrated a significant delay in the arrival of a drug at the heart when peripheral IV sites are used for injection even during effective chest compression.[10,11] Compared with drugs given via a central vein, drugs administered via peripheral veins reach a lower peak concentration and take longer to reach the central circulation.[10,12] Hypertonic or irritating solutions should not be administered through a peripheral vein because pain and phlebitis will result. Even if isotonic solutions are used, the incidence of phlebitis is high if the long saphenous vein is used.

Femoral Veins[7,8]

The femoral vein lies in the femoral sheath, medial to the femoral artery immediately below the inguinal ligament. If a line is drawn between the anterior superior iliac spine and the symphysis pubis, the femoral artery runs directly across the midpoint; medial to that point is the femoral vein. If the femoral artery pulse is palpable, the artery can be located with a finger and the femoral vein will lie immediately medial to the pulsation (Fig 10). During CPR palpable pulsations may represent femoral venous pulsations. Hence, if the vein cannot be located medial to the pulsations, aspiration at the area of the pulsations should be attempted. (If a pulse cannot be felt with cardiac compression, the CPR team should be informed.)

The femoral vein is formed from both the deep and superficial (saphenous) veins of the legs. It extends above the inguinal ligament as the external iliac and becomes the common iliac after being joined by the internal iliac. Both common iliacs join to become the inferior vena cava (Fig 11).

Technique

The steps for initiating IV therapy using the femoral vein follow. Although not described in this section, the Seldinger technique is commonly used in this approach.

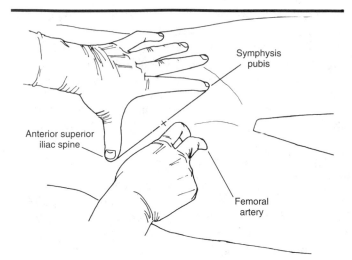

Fig 10. Femoral artery runs directly across the midpoint of line drawn between anterior superior iliac spine and symphysis pubis.

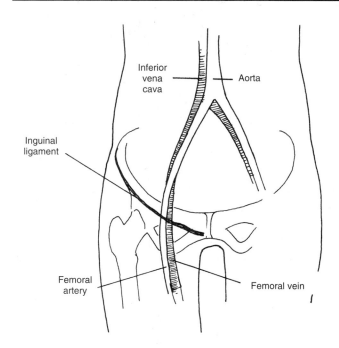

Fig 11. Anatomy of femoral vein. Femoral vein lies medial to femoral artery below inguinal ligament.

1. Cleanse the overlying skin with povidone-iodine *when time permits*. When the procedure is elective, clip (do not shave) pubic hair and sterilely prep and drape the area.
2. Locate the femoral artery by its pulsation or Doppler flowmeter tones or by finding the midpoint of a line drawn between the anterior superior iliac spine and the symphysis pubis.
3. Infiltrate the skin with lidocaine if the patient is awake.
4. Make the puncture with the needle attached to a 5- or 10-mL syringe the breadth of two fingers below the inguinal ligament, medial to the artery, directing the needle cephalad at a 45° angle with the skin or

frontal plane (some prefer to enter at a 90° angle) until the needle will go no farther (Fig 12).

5. Maintain suction on the syringe and pull the needle back slowly until blood appears in the syringe.

6. Lower the needle more parallel to the frontal plane and confirm placement and advance the catheter (if an over-the-needle device) or remove the syringe and insert the catheter (if a through-the-needle device).

7. The catheter is best secured with suture ligature.

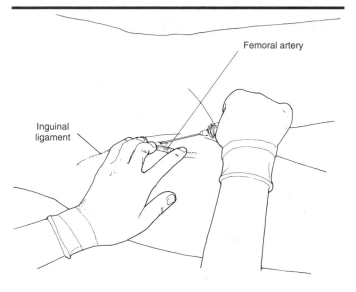

Fig 12. Femoral venipuncture.

Using the Femoral Vein for IV Therapy

Advantages

Interruption of basic life support is unnecessary for femoral cannulation. The femoral vein can be entered when more peripheral veins are collapsed. Once the femoral vein is cannulated, a long catheter can be passed above the diaphragm into the central circulation. Do not use the femoral vein for drug administration during cardiac arrest unless a long catheter that passes above the diaphragm is used.

Disadvantages

Easy location of the vein depends on the presence of the femoral artery pulse; in the absence of an arterial pulse, successful cannulation during CPR is difficult.[13,14] During CPR, venous backflow causes femoral vein pulsations; unsuccessful attempts to cannulate the vein medial to the pulsations should lead to a more lateral approach. Venous return from below the diaphragm is diminished during CPR, and drug delivery times to the central circulation are similar for femoral and peripheral routes.[12,15] For this reason long catheters advanced into the thoracic cavity and large quantities of flush solution are recommended if this technique is used during CPR.

Specific Complications

Hematoma may occur, either from the vein itself or from the adjacent femoral artery. Thrombosis and phlebitis may extend not only to the deep veins but also proximally to the iliac veins or the inferior vena cava. When this occurs, use of the femoral vein may preclude the later use of the saphenous vein.

Inadvertent cannulation of the femoral artery during cardiac arrest may not be recognized since femoral arterial pressure and oxygen tension may be so low that the aspirated blood resembles venous blood. Infusion of a potent vasopressor such as epinephrine into the femoral artery may cause ischemic injury to the involved limb.

Internal Jugular and Subclavian Veins

Anatomy: Internal Jugular Vein[7,8] (Fig 13)

The internal jugular vein emerges from the base of the skull, enters the carotid sheath posterior to the internal carotid artery, and runs posteriorly and laterally to the internal and common carotid artery. Finally, near its termination, the internal jugular vein is lateral and slightly anterior to the common carotid artery.

The internal jugular vein runs medial to the sternomastoid muscle in its upper part, posterior to it in the triangle between the two inferior heads of the sternomastoid in its middle part, and behind the anterior portion of the clavicular head of the muscle in its lower part, ending just above the medial end of the clavicle, where it joins the subclavian vein.

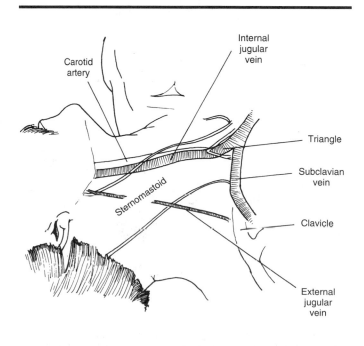

Fig 13. Anatomy of internal jugular vein.

Anatomy: Subclavian Vein[7,8] (Fig 14)

The subclavian vein, which in the adult is approximately 3 to 4 cm long and 1 to 2 cm in diameter, begins as a continuation of the axillary vein at the lateral border of the first rib, crosses over the first rib, and passes in front of the anterior scalene muscle. The anterior scalene muscle is approximately 10 to 15 mm thick and separates the subclavian vein from the subclavian artery, which runs behind the anterior scalene muscle. The vein continues behind the medial third of the clavicle, where it is immobilized by small attachments to the rib and clavicle. At the medial border of the anterior scalene muscle and behind the sternocostoclavicular joint, the subclavian unites with the internal jugular to form the innominate (brachiocephalic) vein. The large thoracic duct on the left and the smaller lymphatic duct on the right enter the superior margin of the subclavian vein near the internal jugular junction. On the right, the brachiocephalic vein descends behind the right lateral edge of the manubrium, where it is joined by the left brachiocephalic vein, which crosses over behind the manubrium. On the right side, near the

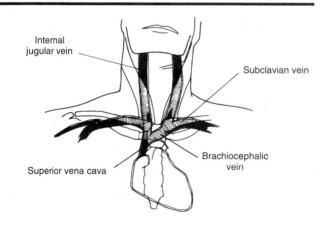

Fig 14. Anatomy of the subclavian vein.

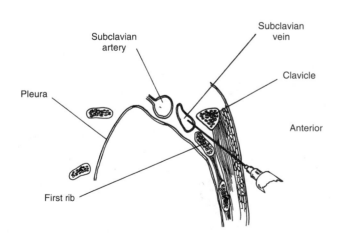

Fig 15. In sagittal section through medial third of clavicle, both apical pleura and subclavian artery can be seen immediately posterior to subclavian vein. Adapted from Davidson et al.[16]

sternal-manubrial joint, the two veins join together to form the superior vena cava. Medial to the anterior scalene muscle, the phrenic nerve, the internal mammary artery, and the apical pleura are in contact with the postero-inferior side of the subclavian vein and the jugulosubclavian junction. In a sagittal section through the medial third of the clavicle, both the apical pleura and the subclavian artery can be seen immediately posterior to the subclavian vein (Fig 15).[16]

Indications for Internal Jugular and Subclavian Venipuncture

The internal jugular and subclavian veins usually remain patent when peripheral veins are collapsed. Their cannulation therefore allows emergency access to the venous circulation when IV therapy is urgently required. Cannulation of these veins is also used to gain access to the central circulation for measurement of central venous pressure, for administration of hypertonic or irritating solutions, and for passing catheters into the heart and pulmonary circulation.

Technique: General Principles[17,18]

The steps for initiating therapy using the internal jugular and subclavian veins follow:

1. Select a 14-gauge needle at least 6 cm long with an inner 16-gauge catheter at least 15 to 20 cm long. If the Seldinger technique is used, select a thin-wall 18-gauge needle to accept a standard guidewire.
2. Determine the depth of catheter placement by measuring from the planned point of insertion to the following surface markers on the chest wall (Fig 16):

   • Sternoclavicular joint — subclavian vein
   • Midmanubrial area — brachiocephalic vein
   • Manubriosternal junction — superior vena cava
   • Five centimeters below the manubriosternal junction — right atrium of the heart
   The tip of a correctly positioned catheter is in the superior vena cava, not the right atrium. Placement in the atrium increases the risk of arrhythmias and myocardial perforation.[19]
3. Place the patient in a supine, head-down position (Trendelenburg) of at least 15° to reduce the chance of air embolism. The Trendelenburg position does not distend the subclavian vein in the euvolemic patient.[20,21] Turn the patient's head away from the side of the venipuncture just enough to provide sufficient access to the puncture site. Rotation beyond 45° should be avoided because this maneuver may increase the incidence of catheter malposition.[21,22] It is not helpful to place a towel between the shoulders to extend the head and make the clavicles more prominent because this decreases the space between the clavicle and first rib, making the subclavian vein less accessible.[21]

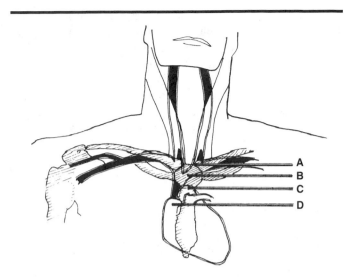

Fig 16. Surface markers on chest wall to determine depth of catheter placement. (A) Sternoclavicular joint — subclavian vein, (B) mid-manubrial area — brachiocephalic vein, (C) manubriosternal junction — superior vena cava, and (D) 5 cm below manubriosternal junction — right atrium.

4. Cleanse the area around the site of puncture with povidone-iodine and drape as for any surgical procedure. Wear sterile gloves. Ideally a face mask should be worn.

5. If the patient is awake, infiltrate the skin with lidocaine.

6. Mount the needle on a 5- or 10-mL syringe containing 0.5 to 1.0 mL saline solution or lidocaine. After the skin has been punctured with the bevel of the needle upward, flush the needle to remove a possible skin plug.

7. As the needle is slowly advanced, maintain negative pressure on the syringe. As soon as the lumen of the vein is entered, blood will appear in the syringe; advance the needle a few millimeters farther to obtain a free flow of blood. Rapid backward movement of the plunger and the appearance of bright red blood indicate that an artery has been entered. Should arterial puncture occur, completely remove the needle and apply pressure, if possible, to the puncture site for at least 10 minutes.

8. Occasionally the vein will not be entered despite the fact that the needle has been inserted to the appropriate depth. Maintain negative pressure on the syringe and slowly withdraw the needle. Blood may suddenly appear in the syringe, indicating that the needle is now in the lumen of the vein. If no blood appears, completely remove the needle and reinsert it, directing it at a slightly different angle, depending on the site of venipuncture.

9. Remove the syringe from the needle, occluding the needle with a finger to prevent air embolism. (A 5-cm water pressure difference across a 14-gauge needle will allow the introduction of approximately 100 mL of air per second.[23]) If the patient is breathing spontaneously, remove the syringe during exhalation. If the patient is being artificially ventilated with either a bag-valve unit or a mechanical ventilator, remove the syringe during the inspiratory (positive-pressure) cycle. Quickly insert the catheter or guidewire through the needle to a predetermined point and remove the needle.

10. If the catheter is inserted through the needle, never pull the catheter backward through the needle, because the sharp end may shear off the tip of the catheter and produce a catheter-fragment embolus.

11. It is occasionally impossible to advance the plastic catheter even though the needle tip is within the vein. Since the catheter must not be withdrawn through the needle, the needle and the catheter must be removed together and the venipuncture attempted again. The use of the flexible straight or J-tipped guidewire should eliminate this problem. Insert the catheter through the needle into the vein, remove the guidewire, attach the syringe, and while maintaining negative pressure on the syringe, reposition the needle until it is in the vein. Remove the syringe and insert the guidewire once again. If the guidewire passes freely into the vein, remove the needle and then pass the catheter over the guidewire into the vein.

12. Where feasible, affix the catheter to the skin with a suture, making certain that the catheter is not compressed by the suture.

13. Attach the IV tubing to the catheter.

14. Apply povidone-iodine ointment to the puncture site and tape the catheter in place.

Technique: Internal Jugular[17]

The right side of the neck is preferred for venipuncture because

- The dome of the right lung and pleura is lower than the left
- There is a relatively straight line to the superior vena cava
- The large thoracic duct is not endangered

In this chapter two approaches are described: posterior and central. In trained hands, each is an effective means of cannulating the internal jugular vein. Some texts also describe an anterior approach, which is more difficult and more often associated with common carotid puncture. In general, the central approach is the easiest to learn and perform successfully. The central and posterior approaches are performed with the patient in the supine, head-down (Trendelenburg) position as described above. In a stable patient, use of a hand-held Doppler probe is helpful for locating the internal jugular vein and nearby carotid artery.

Posterior Approach

The steps for initiating the posterior approach to internal jugular cannulation follow (Fig 17):

1. Introduce the needle under the sternomastoid muscle near the junction of the middle and lower thirds of the lateral (posterior) border (5 cm above the clavicle or just above the point where the external jugular vein crosses the sternomastoid muscle).
2. Aim the needle caudally and ventrally (anteriorly) toward the suprasternal notch at an angle of 45° to the sagittal and horizontal planes and with 15° forward angulation in the frontal plane.
3. The vein should be entered within 5 to 7 cm.

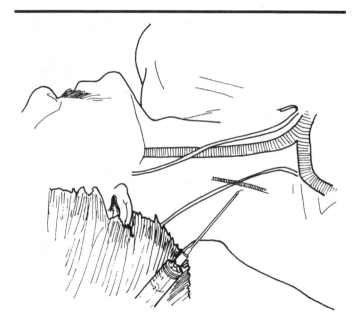

Fig 17. Posterior approach for internal jugular venipuncture.

Central Approach

The steps for initiating the central approach to internal jugular cannulation follow (Fig 18):

1. Locate by observation and palpation the triangle formed by the two heads (sternal and clavicular) of the sternomastoid muscle and the clavicle. It may be helpful to have the conscious patient lift his or her head slightly off the bed to make the triangle more visible. In patients with large or obese necks, the triangle may be difficult to identify. Palpate the suprasternal notch and slowly move laterally, locating first the sternal head of the sternomastoid muscle, then the clavicle, the triangle itself, and finally the clavicular head of the sternomastoid muscle.
2. If the patient is not in cardiac arrest, the carotid pulse is usually palpable within the triangle. If three fingers are used to trace the course of the carotid artery, the vein can be expected to run just lateral

to this position. The relative position of the carotid artery and vein may be confirmed by use of a hand-held Doppler flowmeter if time permits. Alternatively, the vein may be found through use of a small-gauge locator needle inserted as described below. Use of this technique allows the operator to determine the vessel location while minimizing the risk of tissue injury associated with multiple punctures by a large-gauge needle.

3. Insert the needle at the apex of the triangle formed by the two heads of the sternomastoid muscle and the clavicle.
4. Direct the needle caudally at an angle of 45° to the frontal plane. If the carotid artery is palpable, the needle should be directed parallel and just lateral to the course of the artery. If the artery is not palpable, direct the needle parallel to the medial border of the clavicular head of the sternocleidomastoid muscle.
5. The vessel is normally entered at a depth of no more than 2 cm. If the vessel has not been entered at a depth of 4 cm, slowly withdraw the needle, maintaining negative pressure on the syringe. If the vein is still not entered, the needle should be withdrawn to just below the skin surface and redirected a few degrees medially. However, do not direct the needle medially across the sagittal plane, since the carotid artery will be punctured.

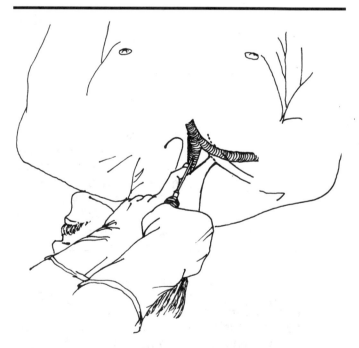

Fig 18. Central approach for internal jugular venipuncture.

Technique: Subclavian Vein[17]

Three approaches for cannulation of the subclavian vein will be described: the direct infraclavicular and supraclavicular approaches and indirect cannulation of the subclavian via the external jugular vein.

Infraclavicular Subclavian Approach

The steps for initiating the direct infraclavicular subclavian puncture follow (Fig 19):

1. The patient must be in a supine, head-down (Trendelenburg) position of at least 15°.
2. Introduce the needle 1 cm below the junction of the middle and medial thirds of the clavicle.
3. Establish a good point of reference by firmly pressing the fingertip into the suprasternal notch. Direct the needle tip toward a point immediately above (cephalad) and behind (posterior to) the fingertip.
4. If possible, hold the syringe and needle parallel to the frontal plane. In larger patients or those with well-developed pectoral muscles, it is often necessary to direct the needle 10° to 20° posterior to the frontal plane.
5. Orient the needle bevel caudally, facilitating the downward turn the catheter must negotiate into the brachiocephalic vein.
6. Vessel puncture generally occurs at a depth of 3 to 4 cm. If vessel entry has not occurred at a depth of 5 cm, slowly withdraw the needle, maintaining negative pressure on the syringe. If the vein is still not entered, the needle should be withdrawn to just below the skin surface and redirected a few degrees cephalad.

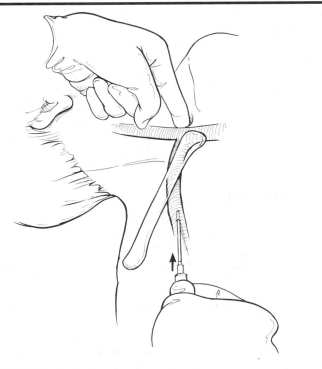

Fig 19. Infraclavicular subclavian venipuncture.

Supraclavicular Approach[24]

The goal of the supraclavicular approach is to puncture the subclavian vein in its superior aspect just as it joins the internal jugular vein.

1. Identify the junction of the clavicle and the clavicular head of the sternocleidomastoid muscle.
2. Introduce the needle 1 cm lateral to the lateral border of the clavicular head and 1 cm posterior to the clavicle.
3. The axis of the syringe should be oriented so that the needle tip is directed 10° above the frontal plane. The axis should also bisect the angle formed by the clavicle and the clavicular head of the sternocleidomastoid muscle with the needle tip directed just cephalad to the contralateral nipple.
4. The needle bevel should be directed medially, facilitating passage of the catheter or guidewire down the brachiocephalic vein.
5. Vessel puncture generally occurs at a depth of 1 to 2 cm. If vessel entry has not occurred at a depth of 3 cm, slowly withdraw the needle, maintaining negative pressure on the syringe. If the vein is still not entered, the needle should be withdrawn to just below the skin surface and redirected a few degrees cephalad.

Cannulation of Subclavian Vein via the External Jugular Vein With a J-Wire[17,25]

Indirect cannulation of the subclavian vein via the external jugular vein is an option when other access routes are unavailable or contraindicated, but it can be a difficult and time-consuming procedure. The steps are as follows:

1. Prepare the patient and make the venipuncture into the external jugular vein as described previously. Use a needle through which the J-wire will pass.
2. Insert a flexible J-tipped wire that fits through both the needle and the catheter (this should be tested before the venipuncture is done) and advance the J-wire into the external jugular and subclavian veins. Gentle manipulation may be necessary to pass the device through venous valves and tortuous vessels. At no time should the wire be forced.
3. With several centimeters of wire still protruding from the distal end of the needle, remove the needle from the vein. As soon as the wire appears, hold it near the skin insertion site to prevent the wire from being inadvertently pulled out of the vein.
4. Make a small incision in the skin with a scalpel to facilitate insertion of the catheter through the skin.
5. Slide the catheter over the wire up to the point of insertion. Make certain that several centimeters of wire are protruding from the other end of the catheter. Slowly advance the catheter and the wire into the vein. As soon as the catheter is in place, remove the wire.
6. Affix the catheter and dress the insertion site as previously described.

Using Internal Jugular and Subclavian Venipuncture

Advantages

Since puncture does not depend on visualization of these veins, rapid access to the circulation is possible even if peripheral veins are collapsed. These approaches also allow direct access to the central circulation.

The internal jugular approach may be preferred to subclavian puncture because there is less risk of pleural puncture and because the hematomas that may form in the neck are visible and compressible. Internal jugular venipuncture may be easier to perform during CPR. It also may be easier to insert a balloon-tipped flow-directed pulmonary artery catheter via the right internal jugular vein since it is in a straight line from the insertion site to the right atrium.

The subclavian route may be preferred, however, because with prolonged subclavian cannulation more neck movement may be possible than with the internal jugular approach.

Disadvantages

Because of the proximity of the veins to the carotid and subclavian arteries, apical pleura, lymphatic ducts, and various nerves, these structures can be damaged by inexperienced operators. Techniques for internal jugular and subclavian venipuncture also require more training than for peripheral venipuncture, and the complication rate is much higher. This may be of particular importance in patients receiving treatment with thrombolytic agents.

If basic life support is being performed, the presence of an additional operator at the patient's head or chest may crowd those performing ventilation and chest compression and either make CPR more difficult to perform or require that it be interrupted altogether to cannulate the veins.

Using Subclavian Cannulation via the External Jugular Vein

Advantages

The technique is easy to learn and perform. The venipuncture is similar to the other peripheral venipunctures, but training and practice are required to use guidewires and insert central catheters safely.

Disadvantages

The complication rate of external jugular puncture is similar to that of any other peripheral venipuncture. However, the wire or the catheter may perforate any of the veins along the course of the insertion. During CPR this technique has the same disadvantages as internal jugular and subclavian venipuncture. In addition, the wire or catheter may not pass into the subclavian vein.

Specific Complications[17,18,26-30]

Local

Bleeding and hematomas may occur from perforating either the vein itself or an adjacent artery. If a hematoma appears on one side of the neck, it is hazardous to attempt puncture on the opposite side because a bilateral hematoma in the neck can severely compromise the airway. Any adjacent structure may be damaged, including the artery, nerve, or lymphatic duct. If the patient has an endotracheal tube with an inflated cuff in place, it is possible to perforate the trachea with the needle and deflate the cuff. Thrombosis of the vein around the catheter may occur, especially with prolonged catheterization. Thrombosis may extend to the superior vena cava and lead to vena caval obstruction and pulmonary thromboembolism.

Systemic

Pneumothorax is a common complication; a follow-up chest x-ray film must be obtained as soon as possible. The position of the catheter tip must be verified by x-ray before infusing hyperalimentation fluids and other hypertonic preparations. Fluid may infiltrate the mediastinum or pleural cavity from an extruded catheter. Bleeding from an injured vein or adjacent artery may lead to hemothorax. Air embolism may occur during insertion or when the IV administration set is disconnected from the catheter hub. The use of three-way stopcocks or extension tubes increases the risk of disconnection. If the catheter tip is in the right atrium or the right ventricle, it may induce cardiac arrhythmias; during manipulation of the patient, perforation of the right atrium or the right ventricle may occur, producing cardiac tamponade. To avoid these complications, the catheter tip should be outside the right atrium in the superior vena cava. Catheters that remain in place longer than 3 days may cause local and systemic infection (bacteremia).

References

1. American Heart Association. Guidelines for cardiopulmonary resuscitation and emergency cardiac care, III: adult advanced cardiac life support. *JAMA.* 1992;268:2199-2241.
2. Centers for Disease Control. Recommendations for preventing transmission of human immunodeficiency virus, hepatitis B virus to patients during exposure-prone invasive procedures. *JAMA.* 1991;266:771-776.
3. Dutky PA, Stevens SL, Maull KI. Factors affecting rapid fluid resuscitation with large-bore introducer catheters. *J Trauma.* 1989;29:856-860.
4. Seldinger SI. Catheter replacement of the needle in percutaneous arteriography; a new technique. *Acta Radiol.* 1953;39:368-376.
5. Plastic containers for intravenous solutions. *Med Lett Drugs Ther.* 1975;17:43-44.
6. Emerman CL, Pinchak AC, Hancock D, Hagen JF. The effect of bolus injection on circulation times during cardiac arrest. *Am J Emerg Med.* 1990;8:190-193.
7. Hamilton WJ, ed. *Textbook of Human Anatomy.* London, England: MacMillan & Co Ltd; 1957.
8. Gray H; Goss CM, eds. *Anatomy of the Human Body.* 28th ed. Philadelphia, Pa: Lea & Febiger; 1966.

9. Engle WA, Rescorla FJ. Vascular access and blood sampling techniques in infants and children. In: Roberts JR, Hedges JR, eds. *Clinical Procedures in Emergency Medicine.* 2nd ed. Philadelphia, Pa: WB Saunders Co; 1991:268-287.

10. Kuhn GJ, White BC, Swetnam RE, et al. Peripheral vs central circulation times during CPR: a pilot study. *Ann Emerg Med.* 1981; 10:417-419.

11. Hedges JR, Barsan WB, Doan LA, et al. Central versus peripheral intravenous routes in cardiopulmonary resuscitation. *Am J Emerg Med.* 1984;2:385-390.

12. Emerman CL, Pinchak AC, Hancock D, Hagen JF. Effect of injection site on circulation times during cardiac arrest. *Crit Care Med.* 1988;16:1138-1141.

13. Emerman CL, Bellon EM, Lukens TW, May TE, Effron D. A prospective study of femoral versus subclavian vein catheterization during cardiac arrest. *Ann Emerg Med.* 1990;19:26-30.

14. Jastremski MS, Matthias HD, Randell PA. Femoral venous catheterization during cardiopulmonary resuscitation: a critical appraisal. *J Emerg Med.* 1984;1:387-391.

15. Dalsey WC, Barsan WG, Joyce SM, Hedges JR, Lukes SJ, Doan LA. Comparison of superior vena caval and inferior vena caval access using a radioisotope technique during normal perfusion and cardiopulmonary resuscitation. *Ann Emerg Med.* 1984; 13:881-884.

16. Davidson JT, Ben-Hur N, Nathen H. Subclavian venipuncture. *Lancet.* 1963;2:1140.

17. Barker WJ. Central venous catheterization: internal jugular approach and alternatives. In: Roberts JR, Hedges JR, eds. *Clinical Procedures in Emergency Medicine.* 2nd ed. Philadelphia, Pa: WB Saunders Co; 1991:340-351.

18. Dronen SC. Central venous catheterization: subclavian vein approach. In: Roberts JR, Hedges JR, eds. *Clinical Procedures in Emergency Medicine.* 2nd ed. Philadelphia, Pa: WB Saunders Co; 1991:325-340.

19. Sheep RE, Guiney WB Jr. Fatal cardiac tamponade: occurrence with other complications after left internal jugular vein catheterization. *JAMA.* 1982;248:1632-1635.

20. Land RE. Anatomic relationships of the right subclavian vein: a radiologic study pertinent to percutaneous subclavian venous catheterization. *Arch Surg.* 1971;102:178-180.

21. Jesseph JM, Conces DJ Jr, Augustyn GT. Patient positioning for subclavian vein catheterization. *Arch Surg.* 1987;122:1207-1209.

22. Bazaral M, Harlan S. Ultrasonographic anatomy of the internal jugular vein relevant to percutaneous cannulation. *Crit Care Med.* 1981;9:307-310.

23. Flanagan JP, Grandisar IA, Gross RJ, Kelly TR. Air embolus: a lethal complication of subclavian venipuncture. *N Engl J Med.* 1969;281:488-489.

24. Dronen S, Thompson B, Nowak R, Tomlanovich M. Subclavian vein catheterization during cardiopulmonary resuscitation: a prospective comparison of the supraclavicular and infraclavicular percutaneous approaches. *JAMA.* 1982;247:3227-3230.

25. Blitt CD, Wright WA, Petty WC, Webster TA. Central venous catheterization via the external jugular vein: a technique employing the J-wire. *JAMA.* 1974;229:817-818.

26. Defalque RJ. Percutaneous catheterization of the internal jugular vein. *Anesth Analg.* 1974;53:116-121.

27. McConnell RY, Fox RT. Experience with percutaneous internal jugular-innominate vein catheterization. *Calif Med.* 1972;117:1-6.

28. Marshall JP, Chadwick SJ, Meyers DS. Catheter perforation of the right ventricle: a complication of endoscopy. *N Engl J Med.* 1974;290:890-891.

29. Peters JL, Armstrong R. Air embolism occurring as a complication of central venous catheterization. *Ann Surg.* 1978;187:375-378.

30. Gibson RN, Hennessy OF, Collier N, Hemingway AP. Major complications of central venous catheterisation: a report of five cases and a brief review of the literature. *Clin Radiol.* 1985;36:205-208.

Cardiovascular Pharmacology I

Chapter 7

Pharmacology I
- Oxygen*
- Epinephrine*
- Atropine*

Antiarrhythmic agents
- Lidocaine*
- Procainamide*
- Bretylium*
- Verapamil and diltiazem
- Adenosine

Miscellaneous
- Magnesium*
- Sodium bicarbonate*
- Morphine
- Calcium chloride

*Agents in the three cardiac arrest algorithms

Pharmacology II
Inotropic vasoactive agents
- Epinephrine
- Norepinephrine
- Dopamine
- Dobutamine
- Isoproterenol
- Amrinone
- Digitalis

Vasodilators/antihypertensives
- Sodium nitroprusside
- Nitroglycerin

β-Adrenergic blockers
- Propranolol
- Metoprolol
- Atenolol
- Esmolol

Diuretics
- Furosemide

Thrombolytic agents
- Anisoylated plasminogen activator complex
- Streptokinase
- Tissue plasminogen activator

Overview: ACLS Pharmacology

Rote Memorization vs Full Understanding

ACLS pharmacology challenges every person who treats cardiac emergencies. Cardiac emergencies require many agents with complex actions and overlapping indications. Personnel must make decisions in a few seconds. In these situations quick mental associations between "rhythm-drug-and-dose" are helpful and at times lifesaving. On the other hand, each order for a medication should be supported by a thorough understanding of the mechanism of action, indications and contraindications, dosages, and precautions. Such understanding requires years of clinical experience supported by conscientious continued education.

Pharmacology Chapters and the ACLS Algorithm and Drugs Handbook

This text tries to meet the needs of both the ACLS provider with minimal clinical background and the more experienced practitioner. Each of these providers must make quick decisions appropriately and accurately.

The AHA pocket booklet *Algorithms and Drugs: A 1993 Handbook for Adult and Pediatric Providers* reproduces the core ACLS clinical algorithms. It summarizes how each drug is supplied, indications and precautions for its use, and recommendations for dosing.

The pocket booklet is supported by the ACLS pharmacology chapters in this textbook. These group the agents, in general, by their class of action: antiarrhythmics, adrenergic agents, thrombolytics, and others. The chapters follow the classic pharmacologic format: mechanism of action, indications, dose, and precautions.

The student of ACLS must understand and master the details of ACLS pharmacology. The summaries in the appendix and the booklet are convenient and helpful, but they are no substitute for in-depth understanding.

Organization of Pharmacology I and II

In general, "Cardiovascular Pharmacology I" presents agents used in the algorithms for full cardiac arrest, including the antiarrhythmics. "Cardiovascular Pharmacology II" presents agents used to treat acute myocardial infarction and its complications, including the inotropic vasoactive agents and the antihypertensive vasodilators.

Objectives of ACLS

ACLS providers should think about ACLS pharmacology in terms of both indications and class of action and should always remember the major objectives of ACLS:

- To correct hypoxemia
- To establish spontaneous circulation at an adequate blood pressure
- To promote optimal cardiac function
- To prevent or suppress significant arrhythmias
- To relieve pain
- To correct acidosis
- To treat congestive heart failure

Oxygen

Oxygen therapy is an essential component of cardiac resuscitation and emergency cardiac care.

Mechanism of Action

Even under ideal conditions expired air contains only 16% to 17% oxygen. Mouth-to-mouth resuscitation produces an alveolar oxygen tension of no more than 80 mm Hg. This tension cannot completely oxygenate mixed venous blood that is severely desaturated, because the victim of cardiac arrest undergoing CPR has low cardiac output (25% to 30% of normal), ventilation perfusion abnormalities, and right-to-left shunts.[1] Similar abnormalities have been described in patients with pulmonary edema and gastric aspiration.[2] Accordingly, personnel must give supplemental oxygen (FIO_2 = 100%) during resuscitation. Modest changes in oxygen tension produce large hemoglobin saturation changes in patients who are on the steep portion of the oxyhemoglobin saturation curve (Fig 1). In hypoxemic patients, oxygen administration elevates arterial oxygen tension, increases arterial oxygen content, and improves tissue oxygenation.[3]

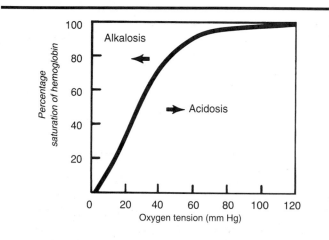

Fig 1. Oxyhemoglobin dissociation curve. On the steep part of the curve small changes in oxygen tension produce large changes in hemoglobin saturation. Acidosis shifts the curve to the right so that for a given oxygen tension hemoglobin saturation falls. Alkalosis shifts the curve to the left so that for a given oxygen tension hemoglobin saturation increases.

Indications

Oxygen should be given to all patients with acute chest pain that may be due to cardiac ischemia,[4] suspected hypoxemia of any cause, and cardiopulmonary arrest. Oxygen should not be withheld from COPD patients with possible myocardial infarction or severe dyspnea out of fear that they have CO_2 retention. These patients need oxygen and careful observation. Prompt treatment of hypoxemia may prevent cardiac arrest.

Dosage

Several devices, including masks and nasal cannulas, can be used to administer oxygen to patients who are breathing spontaneously. Oxygen can also be delivered by positive-pressure ventilation devices, eg, demand valve. Oxygen can be adequately delivered by volume-regulated ventilators even during resuscitation of intubated patients. Use 100% FIO_2 during resuscitation. For further details of oxygen administration see chapters 1 and 2.

Precautions

The major precaution with oxygen is to make sure that high-flow oxygen is being delivered adequately. Oxygen toxicity may occur after prolonged (more than 3 to 5 days) ventilatory support with a high oxygen concentration. However, even 100% oxygen is not hazardous to the patient during the minutes required for clinical resuscitation. It should never be withheld or diluted during resuscitation in the mistaken belief that it will be harmful. In treating patients with chronic pulmonary disease (eg, pulmonary emphysema), it may be necessary to assist ventilation during the administration of oxygen if correction of hypoxemia reduces respiratory drive in a patient who retains CO_2. The respiratory drive is seldom depressed enough to require ventilatory support. (See chapter 2, "Venturi Mask.")

A variety of commercial devices measure end-tidal CO_2 either colorimetrically or quantitatively. Similarly pulse oximetry devices are now incorporated into many automated blood pressure devices and other monitors.

The adequacy of ventilation and oxygenation should be monitored by end-tidal CO_2 measurement and by pulse oximeter rather than by arterial blood gas analysis. Avoid arterial blood gas analysis because of the incidence of complications associated with the aggressive use of anticoagulants and fibrinolytic agents, which are often needed in patients with ischemic heart disease.

Epinephrine

Mechanism of Action

Epinephrine is a natural catecholamine with both α- and β-adrenergic agonist activity. Epinephrine plays a critical role in cardiac arrest.[5] The pharmacologic actions of epinephrine are complex because they are modulated in part by reflex circulatory adjustments. Epinephrine can produce the following cardiovascular responses:

- Increased systemic vascular resistance
- Increased systolic and diastolic blood pressures
- Increased electrical activity in the myocardium
- Increased coronary and cerebral blood flow
- Increased strength of myocardial contraction
- Increased myocardial oxygen requirements
- Increased automaticity

The primary beneficial effect of epinephrine in cardiac arrest is peripheral vasoconstriction, which leads to improved coronary and cerebral perfusion pressure (Figs 2 and 3).[6-8] Epinephrine's potent α_1- and α_2-postsynaptic adrenergic agonist effects improve cerebral and coronary blood flow by preventing arterial collapse and increasing peripheral vasoconstriction.[6-8] Recent studies in animals indicate that epinephrine's α-adrenergic effect (not its β-adrenergic effect) makes ventricular fibrillation (VF) more susceptible to direct current countershock.[5] Pure α-adrenergic agonists appear to be as effective as epinephrine in restoring spontaneous circulation without producing β-adrenergic–mediated myocardial ischemia.[9-12] Although the β-adrenergic effects of epinephrine may increase myocardial lactate production, these effects also appear to improve blood flow to the central nervous system. Epinephrine produces a greater improvement in cerebral blood flow than other adrenergic agents like methoxamine.[13-16]

Epinephrine produces favorable redistribution of blood flow from peripheral to central circulation during CPR. The elevation of coronary perfusion pressure following the administration of epinephrine is beneficial in all forms of cardiorespiratory arrest.[6-8] Epinephrine is a useful vasoactive, inotropic agent in selected patients with refractory circulatory shock, eg, after cardiopulmonary bypass.[17,18]

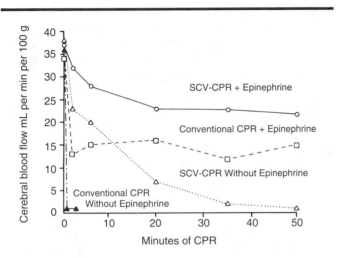

Fig 2. Cerebral blood flow measurement by radiolabeled microsphere technique in dogs during conventional CPR with and without epinephrine. Without epinephrine there is essentially no measureable flow, whereas flow is substantially increased by the drug, correlating with higher perfusion pressures. SCV indicates simultaneous compression ventilation. Adapted from Michael et al.[6]

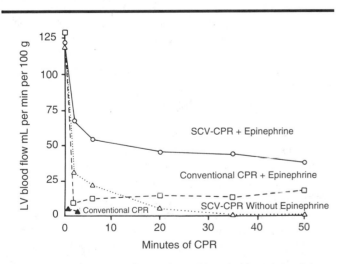

Fig 3. Left ventricular blood flow in dogs with and without epinephrine. As with cerebral blood flow, myocardial blood flow is increased by epinephrine as perfusion pressure is increased. LV indicates left ventricular; SCV, simultaneous compression ventilation. Adapted from Michael et al.[6]

Indications

The indications for epinephrine are cardiac arrest from ventricular fibrillation or pulseless ventricular tachycardia unresponsive to initial countershocks, asystole, or pulseless electrical activity. Also epinephrine infusion can be used to treat patients with profoundly symptomatic bradycardia.

Dosage

Researchers and clinicians have questioned the optimal dose of epinephrine because the "standard" dose of epinephrine (1 mg) is not based on body weight.[19] The standard dose of epinephrine originated from the practice of administering 1-mg intracardiac injections of epinephrine in the operating room.[20] Anecdotal reports stated that 1 to 3 mg of intracardiac epinephrine restarted the arrested heart.[21,22] The original assumption was that 1 mg of intravenous (IV) epinephrine would produce the same pharmacologic response as 1 mg of intracardiac epinephrine. Although patients vary greatly in weight, cardiac size does not. Therefore a 1-mg dose of epinephrine has been recommended for all patients.

The dose-response curve of IV epinephrine was investigated in a series of experiments with animals during the 1980s. This work demonstrated that epinephrine produced its optimal response in animals in the range of 0.045 to 0.20 mg/kg.[23-27] These experimental studies suggested that higher doses of epinephrine might be required in humans to improve hemodynamics and to achieve successful resuscitation. Optimistic case series and retrospective studies published in the late 1980s and early 1990s[19,28-30] set the stage for prospective, randomized trials in humans.[31-34]

Participants at the 1992 National Conference on CPR and ECC reviewed preliminary results from four clinical trials.[31-34] Nine cities provided the out-of-hospital setting for these trials, which involved more than 2400 adult patients. One trial also included in-hospital cardiac arrests.[32] These trials demonstrated increased rates of return of spontaneous circulation with higher doses of epinephrine[31,33] but no statistically significant improvement in survival rates to hospital discharge when compared with standard epinephrine doses (Table). One trial showed a threefold increase in hospital discharge rates

Standard-Dose vs High-Dose Epinephrine: Human Survival Data

Author	HDE Regimen		% Hospital Discharge HDE/SDE	P Value
Lindner et al[31]	5	mg	14/5	NS
Stiell et al[32]	7	mg	3/5	NS
Callaham et al[33]	15	mg	1.7/1.2	NS
Brown et al[34]	0.2	mg/kg	5/4	NS

HDE indicates high dose epinephrine; SDE, standard dose epinephrine; NS, not significant.

in patients with pulseless electrical activity and asystole when treated with 5 mg versus 1 mg epinephrine as the initial dose, but this difference did not reach statistical significance.[31] Another study suggested that patients older than 65 years and those in VF did better with standard doses of epinephrine.[32] Three important conclusions can be derived from these clinical trials.[31-34] First, survival rates are low regardless of the dose of epinephrine. Second, most patients who survived responded to early defibrillation and therefore did not receive epinephrine.[33] Third, these trials failed to detect substantial harm from administration of higher doses of epinephrine. These data strongly reaffirm the value of the "standard" interventions of CPR, airway management, and rapid defibrillation. Furthermore, they indicate that epinephrine, as well as other late interventions, represent a last desperate effort to resuscitate people with a very poor chance of survival.

Based on available clinical data, there is little reason to alter the initial IV dose of 1 mg epinephrine (10 mL of a 1:10 000 solution) during resuscitation. A higher dose of epinephrine (5 mg or approximately 0.1 mg/kg) is considered Class IIb (not specifically recommended; acceptable, possibly helpful) for use after the initial dose. Therefore, the use of higher doses of epinephrine can neither be recommended nor discouraged. Regardless of which subsequent dose of epinephrine is chosen during resuscitation, epinephrine should be administered at intervals that do not exceed 3 to 5 minutes.[35] If the dose is given by peripheral injection, it should be followed by a 20-mL flush of IV fluid to ensure delivery of the drug into the central compartment.[36]

Epinephrine has good bioavailability after proper endotracheal administration.[37] Although the optimal dose of epinephrine for endotracheal delivery is unknown, a dose that is at least 2 to 2.5 times the peripheral IV dose may be needed.[38] Intracardiac administration should be used only during open cardiac massage or when other routes of administration are unavailable.[38,39] Intracardiac injections increase the risk of coronary artery laceration, cardiac tamponade, and pneumothorax and cause interruption of external chest compression and ventilation.

During cardiac arrest and symptomatic bradycardia with profound hypotension, epinephrine may be administered by continuous infusion. In cardiac arrest, the dose should be comparable to the standard IV dose of epinephrine (1 mg every 3 to 5 minutes). This is accomplished by adding 30 mg epinephrine hydrochloride (30 mL of a 1:1000 solution) to 250 mL of normal saline of D_5W to run at 100 mL/h and titrating to desired hemodynamic end point. Continuous infusions of epinephrine should be administered by central venous access to reduce the risk of extravasation and to ensure good bioavailability.

Epinephrine can also be used as a pressor and a chronotropic agent (to raise the blood pressure and the heart rate) for patients who are not in cardiac arrest (eg, in septic shock or symptomatic bradycardia), although it is not the first agent to use. Epinephrine hydrochloride, 1 mg (1 mL of a 1:1000 solution), is added to 500 mL of normal saline or D_5W and administered by continuous infusion. The initial dose for adults is 1 μg/min titrated to desired hemodynamic response (2 to 10 μg/min).

Precautions

Auto-oxidation of catecholamines and related sympathomimetic compounds is pH dependent. Contact of epinephrine with other drugs that have an alkaline pH (such as sodium bicarbonate) can cause auto-oxidation, but the reaction rate is too slow to be clinically important when epinephrine is given by bolus injection or is infused rapidly.[40] Epinephrine should not be added to infusion bags or bottles that contain alkaline solutions.

Even at low doses, epinephrine's positive inotropic and chronotropic effects can precipitate or exacerbate myocardial ischemia. Doses greater than 20 μg/min or 0.3 μg/kg per minute frequently produce hypertension in patients who are not in cardiac arrest.[41] Epinephrine may induce or exacerbate ventricular ectopy, especially in patients who are receiving digitalis.[42]

Atropine

Mechanism of Action

Atropine sulfate is a parasympatholytic drug that enhances both sinus node automaticity and atrioventricular (AV) conduction via its direct vagolytic action.

Indications

In diseased myocardium, heightened parasympathetic tone may precipitate conduction disturbances or asystole.[43] Atropine is indicated as initial therapy for patients with symptomatic bradycardia, including those with heart rates in the "physiological" range but for whom a sinus tachycardia would be more appropriate (eg, a patient who has acute myocardial infarction, symptomatic hypotension, and a heart rate of 70 beats per minute).[44] This condition is referred to as relative bradycardia. In the absence of symptoms or signs of hemodynamic compromise, ischemia, or frequent ventricular ectopy atropine is not needed and may produce adverse consequences.[45]

Atropine can restore normal AV nodal conduction and electrical activity in patients with first-degree AV block or Mobitz type I AV block, and in some patients with bradyasystolic cardiac arrest.[43] Atropine has been reported to be harmful in some patients with AV block at the His-Purkinje level (type II AV block and third-degree AV block with a new wide-QRS complex).[46] Atropine can be used in these situations, but watch closely for paradoxical slowing. Treatment with atropine may improve outcome in patients with bradyasystolic cardiac arrest due to excessive vagal stimulation. Atropine is less effective when asystole or pulseless electrical activity are the result of prolonged ischemia or mechanical injury in the myocardium.[43,47-51]

Several authors have reported on asystolic patients who responded to atropine, though most of these are uncontrolled anecdotes. Brown and coworkers[43] reported that three of eight patients survived after administration of atropine for asystole. All survivors experienced cardiac arrest in the hospital (two in the catheterization laboratory and one in intensive care) and received ACLS within 2 minutes. Stueven and coworkers[48] reported a significant (P<.04) increase in the number of patients who survived until arrival at the emergency department after out-of-hospital arrest with asystole in response to atropine (14% compared with 0% in those who received only epinephrine and bicarbonate); none of the short-term survivors was discharged from the hospital. Iseri et al[50] observed no response in 10 asystolic patients. Coon and coworkers[51] found that 10 of 11 patients who did not receive atropine and 8 of 10 who did receive atropine developed rhythms other than asystole, yet only one patient (who did not receive atropine) was discharged alive. Unfortunately, asystolic cardiac arrest is nearly always fatal regardless of therapy.[51] Although there is no definitive proof of its value, there is little evidence that atropine is harmful in this setting. A well-designed prospective, controlled trial would help determine the utility of atropine in treating asystole.

Dosage

For patients without cardiac arrest, atropine is administered IV in doses of 0.5 to 1.0 mg. The dose may be repeated at 5-minute intervals until the desired response is achieved (ie, an increased heart rate, usually to 60 beats per minute or greater, or abatement of signs and symptoms). Repeated doses of atropine should be avoided when possible, especially in patients with ischemic heart disease. In patients with recurrent episodes of bradycardia, especially those with acute ischemic heart disease, the heart rate can be maintained with an electric pacemaker. When the recurrent use of atropine is essential in patients with coronary artery disease, the total dose should be restricted to 2 to 3 mg (maximum of 0.03 to 0.04 mg/kg) if possible, to avoid the detrimental effects of atropine-induced tachycardia on myocardial oxygen demand.

For patients with bradyasystolic cardiac arrest, a 1-mg dose of atropine is administered IV and is repeated every 3 to 5 minutes if asystole persists. Three milligrams (0.04 mg/kg) given IV is a fully vagolytic dose in most patients.[52] The administration of this dose of atropine should be reserved for patients with bradyasystolic cardiac arrest.

Administration of atropine in doses of less than 0.5 mg can produce a paradoxical bradycardia owing to the central or peripheral parasympathomimetic effects of low doses in adults. This effect can precipitate VF.[44,53]

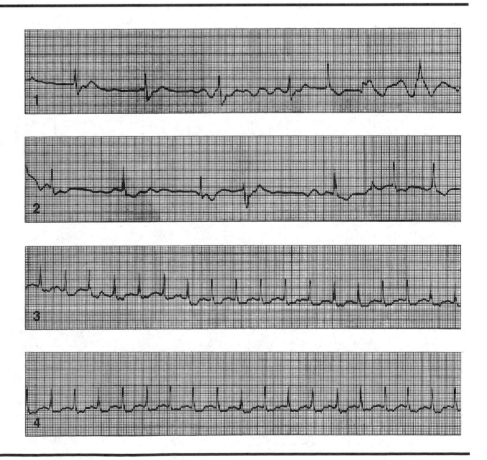

Fig 4. Changes in cardiac rate and rhythm following endotracheal administration of atropine. Measurement of atropine blood levels confirmed absorption of the drug. (1) Initial cardiac rhythm strip, supraventricular mechanism, 30 to 40 beats per minute. (2) Cardiac rhythm strip 75 seconds after endotracheal intubation. Atropine sulfate 1 mg, administered endotracheally. (3) Thirty seconds after endotracheal atropine. (4) Ninety seconds after endotracheal atropine. From Greenberg et al.[55]

Endotracheal administration of atropine can be used in patients without IV access (Fig 4).[39,54] Endotracheally administered atropine produces a rapid onset of action similar to that observed with IV injection.[54,55] The recommended adult dose of atropine for endotracheal administration is 1.0 to 2.0 mg diluted to a total not to exceed 10 mL of sterile water or normal saline.[39,55]

Precautions

Atropine may induce tachycardia, which may be deleterious in patients with coronary artery disease or patients with ongoing myocardial ischemia or infarction. Atropine should always be administered with caution in the setting of myocardial ischemia.[56,57] Ventricular fibrillation and tachycardia have occurred after IV administration of atropine, especially in patients with coronary artery disease.[58-60] Excessive doses of atropine can cause an anticholinergic syndrome of delirium, tachycardia, coma, flushed and hot skin, ataxia, and blurred vision.[61]

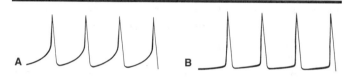

Fig 5. Effect of lidocaine on phase 4 depolarization in canine Purkinje fiber action potentials. A, Before lidocaine administration, there is spontaneous depolarization (automaticity). B, After lidocaine, slope of phase 4 depolarization has been depressed.

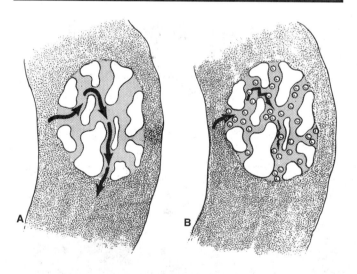

Fig 6. Schematic depiction of conduction through ischemic/ infarcted intramural zone of ventricular muscle. White areas are islands of inexcitable, severely depressed tissue. Dotted areas within ischemic zone are still excitable, though also depressed, and conduct wave front at reduced conduction velocities. Ischemic zone is surrounded by normal muscle. A, Wave front propagates through depressed area at reduced conduction velocity but is able to sustain itself and emerge to reenter surrounding normal myocardium. B, After lidocaine administration, lidocaine-induced further depression of conduction velocity impairs advance of wave front to extent that it is blocked, unable to reenter normal surrounding muscle. Reentrant arrhythmias sustained via such pathways of depressed conduction would then be terminated.

Antiarrhythmic Agents

Arrhythmias result from altered impulse formation (automaticity), abnormal impulse conduction (reentry), triggered rhythms, or a combination of these mechanisms. During myocardial ischemia, any or all mechanisms may exist. In animal studies ischemia also decreases the threshold for VF (the energy necessary to induce VF). Antiarrhythmic drugs comprise a heterogenous group of agents.

Lidocaine

Mechanism of Action

Lidocaine suppresses ventricular arrhythmias by decreasing automaticity (ie, it reduces the slope of phase 4 diastolic depolarization, Fig 5).[62] In addition, its local anesthetic properties help to suppress ventricular ectopy after myocardial infarction by reducing the slope of phase 0 of the action potential.[63] Lidocaine may terminate reentrant ventricular arrhythmias by affecting conduction

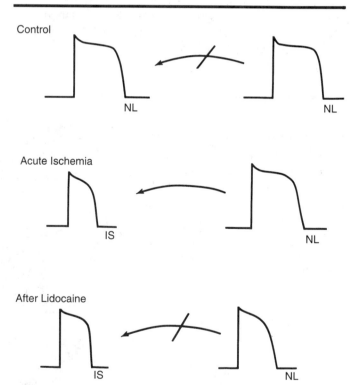

Fig 7. Boundary current in a canine model during acute ischemia and after lidocaine administration. Top, There is no boundary current flow between normal zones (NL) of heart because action potentials are of essentially equal duration. Middle, In acute ischemia of 15-minute duration, current flows from normal zone into acutely ischemic zone (IS). This is because acute ischemia shortens action potential duration in ischemic tissue, which therefore recovers excitability earlier than surrounding normal tissue. This current can pass through ischemic tissue slowly and emerge to reexcite the heart as a premature ventricular complex. Bottom, Lidocaine acts on normal tissue to make action potentials more uniform, thus preventing current flow.

velocity in reentrant pathways (Fig 6).[64] This prevents the emergence of wave fronts from zones of ischemic myocardium. Lidocaine has also been shown to reduce the disparity in action potential duration between ischemic and normal zones and to prolong conduction and refractoriness in ischemic tissue[65] (Fig 7).

During acute myocardial ischemia, the threshold for the induction of VF is reduced (less energy is required, and thus fibrillation is more likely to occur). In some studies lidocaine has been shown to elevate the fibrillation threshold, ie, to reduce the propensity to develop VF.[66] Other experimental studies show that lidocaine may either increase or fail to change the energy needed to reverse VF, ie, the ventricular defibrillation threshold.[67,68] These conflicting results may be due to interactions between lidocaine and the anesthetic agents used in the studies and also to the extent of acidosis in the circulation at the time of the study.

Clinical studies fail to support a major antifibrillatory effect for lidocaine in prehospital VF refractory to direct current countershock.[69] The comparable efficacy of lidocaine when compared with agents that do have primary antifibrillatory effects suggests that some episodes of refractory VF represent recurrent rather than resistant episodes and that lidocaine is capable of preventing these recurrences.[70,71] Studies in laboratory animals suggest that combination antiarrhythmic therapy with lidocaine and bretylium may provide a synergistic effect on the defibrillation threshold.[72]

Elevation of the fibrillation threshold correlates closely with blood levels of lidocaine.[66] Higher plasma lidocaine concentrations (ie, 6 µg/mL) are required to achieve an antifibrillatory effect, whereas lidocaine concentrations of 2 to 5 µg/mL are needed to control ventricular ectopy.[72,73]

Lidocaine usually does not affect myocardial contractility, arterial blood pressure, atrial arrhythmogenesis, or intraventricular conduction, and can facilitate AV conduction.[62] However, several reports show that lidocaine may depress myocardial conduction and/or contractility in patients receiving concurrent antiarrhythmic therapy and those with sick sinus syndrome or left ventricular dysfunction.[74-76]

Indications

Lidocaine is the first antiarrhythmic to use for treatment of ventricular tachycardia (VT) and VF. In controlled trials, lidocaine is as effective as agents with primary antifibrillatory activity.[70,71] It is recommended for patients with pulseless VT and VF that is refractory to electrical countershocks and epinephrine. After VT or VF has been terminated, lidocaine should be given to patients with significant risk factors for malignant ventricular arrhythmias (hypokalemia, myocardial ischemia, or significant left ventricular dysfunction) to prevent recurrent VF. Other causes that can contribute to the development of ventricular ectopy (eg, persistent acidosis, hypoxemia, hypo-magnesemia, hypocalcemia, or drugs) should be sought and corrected.

Lidocaine reduces the incidence of primary VF in patients with acute myocardial infarction but may not necessarily alter mortality.[77-82] A meta-analysis of 14 randomized control trials of lidocaine prophylaxis during acute myocardial infarction showed that mortality was not reduced during the prehospital phase of acute myocardial infarction and suggested that mortality may increase in patients who receive prophylactic lidocaine during the hospital phase of monitored, uncomplicated acute myocardial infarction.[82] This reflects both the abolition of escape rhythms by lidocaine in patients with a propensity to conduction disturbances and a decrease in the overall incidence of VF in acute myocardial infarction patients treated with thrombolytics, β blockers, and aspirin.[46,81,83] Prophylactic lidocaine therapy in patients with either non–Q-wave infarction or minimal risk factors for VF diminishes the potential benefits of treatment and does not change the risk for adverse reactions to lidocaine.[80,82,83] *Routine prophylactic lidocaine therapy in patients with acute myocardial infarction can no longer be recommended.*[46,84,85]

Lidocaine is the drug of choice for the suppression of ventricular ectopy, including VT and VF. Given the propensity of lidocaine to inhibit the development of escape rhythms, its use should be reserved for symptomatic ventricular arrhythmias, sustained VT, or VF. Based on the assumption that most wide-complex tachycardias are ventricular rather than supraventricular in origin, lidocaine is the drug of choice for wide-complex tachycardias of unknown origin.[86]

Dosage

There is extensive literature on the proper way to load and maintain blood levels of lidocaine in an effective suppressive range of 1.5 to 6 µg/mL.[87-89] For refractory VF and pulseless VT, an initial dose of 1.0 to 1.5 mg/kg is suggested for all patients. Cardiac arrest victims may require only a single bolus of lidocaine. Plasma lidocaine concentrations should persist within the therapeutic range for a protracted period because of reduced drug clearance from poor blood flow during CPR.[90] Laboratory animal models show an alteration in the pharmacokinetics of lidocaine because of reduced liver blood flow during cardiac arrest.[90,91] Studies during CPR in humans show that lidocaine may produce a therapeutic effect at doses considered suboptimal in animal models.[69-72]

Because of poor blood flow and prolonged circulatory times observed during CPR, only bolus administration of lidocaine should be used in treating patients in cardiac arrest. After restoration of spontaneous circulation, lidocaine should be administered by continuous IV infusion at a rate of 30 to 50 µg/kg per minute (2 to 4 mg/min).[88] The need for additional bolus doses of lidocaine should be guided by clinical response or plasma lidocaine concentrations.

In cardiac arrest lidocaine can be administered via an endotracheal tube. Use 2 to 2.5 times the IV dose to obtain equivalent blood levels compared with IV administration.

In noncardiac arrest an initial bolus of 1 to 1.5 mg/kg followed by a maintenance infusion at a rate of 30 to 50 µg/kg per minute (2 to 4 mg/min) is required to achieve therapeutic lidocaine levels rapidly.[88] To prevent subtherapeutic lidocaine levels after the initial bolus, a second bolus of 0.5 mg/kg is recommended after 10 minutes. If ventricular ectopy persists, additional bolus injections of 0.5 to 0.75 mg/kg can be given every 5 to 10 minutes to a total dose of 3 mg/kg.[88] The maintenance infusion should be titrated according to clinical needs and plasma lidocaine concentrations.

Lidocaine undergoes blood-flow–dependent hepatic metabolism. Although the loading dose of lidocaine does not need to be reduced, the maintenance dose should be decreased by 50% in the presence of impaired hepatic blood flow (acute myocardial infarction, congestive heart failure, or circulatory shock) because total body clearance of lidocaine is reduced.[92-94] The maintenance dose should also be reduced by 50% in patients older than 70 years, because they have a reduced volume of distribution.[88,95] Since the half-life of lidocaine is increased after 24 to 48 hours of continuous infusion therapy, observe carefully for toxicity. Maintenance doses after 12 to 24 hours should be based on ideal (not actual) body weight and on serum lidocaine levels. Monitoring the concentration of lidocaine in the blood may help avoid toxicity.[94] In patients with renal failure, there is no need to adjust the dose of lidocaine because its clearance and volume of distribution are unchanged. However, renal failure leads to the accumulation of monoethylglycinexylidide (MEGX) and glycinexylidide (GX), lidocaine's metabolites, which have little pharmacologic activity but can produce significant neurotoxicity.[92]

Precautions

Excessive doses of lidocaine can produce neurological changes, myocardial depression, and circulatory depression. Clinical indicators of lidocaine-induced neurological toxicity include drowsiness, disorientation, decreased hearing ability, paresthesia, and muscle twitching.[87] Some patients may become very agitated. More serious toxic effects include focal and grand mal seizures.[62] Treatment consists of withdrawal of lidocaine and, if necessary, administration of anticonvulsants (eg, benzodiazepines, barbiturates, or phenytoin) to control seizures.

Patients with an elevated serum lidocaine concentration and left ventricular dysfunction may experience significant myocardial depression. These patients are prone to proportionally higher serum lidocaine concentrations than are healthy persons (Fig 8).

Although therapeutic doses of lidocaine can be used safely in patients with conduction disturbances, large doses of lidocaine may induce heart block, depress spon-

taneous discharge from the sinus node, or alter AV conduction.[62,76] Lidocaine should not change the AH and HV intervals measured by a bundle of His recording, but use caution in patients with documented conduction system disorder.[96]

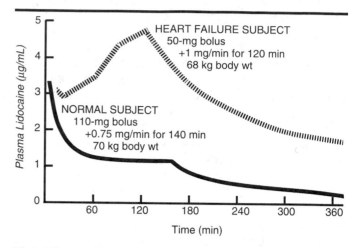

Fig 8. Differences in plasma level response to infused lidocaine in normal subject and heart failure subject of similar size. Within 2 hours concentrations of lidocaine approached toxic levels in patient with advanced heart failure even though infusion rate was near minimum recommended dose.

Procainamide

Mechanism of Action

Procainamide suppresses ventricular ectopy and may be effective when lidocaine has not suppressed life-threatening ventricular arrhythmias.[97] In normal ventricular muscle and Purkinje fibers, procainamide suppresses phase 4 diastolic depolarization, reducing the automaticity of all pacemakers. Procainamide also slows intraventricular conduction. If conduction is already slowed, eg, in ischemic tissue, further slowing may produce bidirectional block and may terminate reentrant arrhythmias.[98,99]

Indications

Procainamide is acceptable and probably helpful in persistent cardiac arrest due to VF. Procainamide is rarely used to treat VF, however, because of the prolonged time required to administer effective doses. Rapid administration of procainamide (faster than 30 mg/min) exacerbates hypotension. Procainamide may be useful in suppressing premature ventricular complexes and recurrent VT that cannot be controlled with lidocaine. Procainamide may also be used to convert supraventricular arrhythmias or prevent their recurrence.[100]

Dosage

The IV dose of procainamide for suppressing premature ventricular complexes and VT is 20 to 30 mg/min until the arrhythmia is suppressed or hypotension ensues or the QRS complex is widened by 50% of its original width or 17 mg/kg of drug has been administered.[97] The loading regimen is followed by a maintenance IV infusion rate of 1 to 4 mg/min.

An alternative approach to the administration of procainamide uses a loading dose of 17 mg/kg infused over 1 hour, followed by a maintenance infusion of 2.8 mg/kg per hour.[101] In patients with cardiac or renal dysfunction, the loading dose is reduced to 12 mg/kg, and the maintenance dose is decreased to 1.4 mg/kg per hour.[102]

Therapeutic concentrations in plasma are achieved in about 15 minutes and are sustained by the maintenance infusion.[102] The reference range for procainamide in blood is 4 to 10 μg/mL.[102] The plasma procainamide concentration should be monitored and kept within the laboratory's therapeutic range for patients with renal failure, for patients who are on a constant infusion of 3 mg/min or more for 24 hours or longer, and for patients who are receiving chronic oral therapy.

Precautions

Procainamide is a ganglionic blocker with potent vasodilatory and modest negative inotropic effects, especially in patients with left ventricular dysfunction.[97,102,103] Procainamide-induced hypotension is most pronounced after rapid IV injection or when high plasma procainamide concentrations are present.[103] Arterial blood pressure and ECG monitoring are essential during IV administration. Effects observed on the ECG include widening of the QRS complex and lengthening of the baseline PR or QT interval. Atrioventricular conduction disturbances, including heart block, or cardiac arrest may follow. QRS widening by 50% of the original QRS length or lengthening of the PR or QT interval by 50% or more of the baseline interval indicates the need to stop procainamide administration. Intravenous procainamide must be administered cautiously to patients with acute myocardial infarction. Procainamide can induce or exacerbate malignant ventricular arrhythmias. This tendency to produce arrhythmias may be somewhat greater when hypokalemia and hypomagnesemia are present.

Bretylium

Bretylium tosylate is an adrenergic neuronal blocking drug introduced in 1950 as an antihypertensive agent. Tolerance for its antihypertensive action and undesirable side effects limited its oral use in the treatment of hypertension.[104-106] Interest in bretylium was revived in the mid 1960s when it was found to possess antifibrillatory activity.[107] Results of studies differ on whether bretylium improves either fibrillation or defibrillation threshold.[67,104,105] Both bretylium and lidocaine increase the fibrillation threshold.[67,73] Lidocaine, however, also increases defibrillation threshold whereas bretylium does not.[67,68] Laboratory animal models of VF during closed-chest CPR

show a synergistic response when bretylium and lidocaine are administered in combination.[72]

No difference in clinical outcome or survival is observed in studies comparing lidocaine and bretylium in patients with out-of-hospital VF.[70,71] Because of a greater potential for adverse hemodynamic effects with bretylium, lidocaine is the drug of first choice for all ventricular ectopy. Bretylium should be considered in patients with refractory malignant ventricular arrhythmias. Combination therapy with bretylium and lidocaine during cardiac arrest has not been studied.

Mechanism of Action

Bretylium is a quaternary ammonium compound with both adrenergic and direct myocardial effects.[108-110] Bretylium's adrenergic effects are biphasic. Initially bretylium releases norepinephrine from adrenergic nerve endings in direct relation to its concentration at the adrenergic terminal.[109] In the non–cardiac arrest setting, these sympathomimetic effects last approximately 20 minutes[109,110] and consist of transient hypertension, tachycardia, and (in some people) increases in cardiac output.[110] Subsequently inhibition of norepinephrine release from peripheral adrenergic terminals results in adrenergic blockade, which generally begins 15 to 20 minutes after injection and peaks 45 to 60 minutes later.[111] At this time clinically significant hypotension may develop, especially with changes in position.[112] In addition, since bretylium blocks the uptake of norepinephrine into adrenergic nerve terminals, it will potentiate the action of exogenous catecholamines.[108]

The antiarrhythmic action of bretylium is poorly understood. It elevates VF threshold, as does lidocaine.[73,108] This effect is observed in both normal and infarcted myocardium and appears independent of bretylium's adrenergic effects.[111] Bretylium also increases the action potential duration and the effective refractory period in normal ventricular muscle and Purkinje fibers without lengthening the effective refractory period relative to action potential duration (Fig 9).[113]

Bretylium's electrophysiological actions are different from those of other antiarrhythmic agents. In general, bretylium does not suppress phase 4 depolarization or the spontaneous firing of Purkinje fibers.[113] Thus, its actions may be more dependent on its adrenergic effects than originally thought.[104]

In infarcted canine hearts, bretylium prolongs action potential duration throughout the normal conduction system but produces very little increase in action potential duration in infarcted regions where action potential duration is already prolonged. Bretylium reduces the disparity in action potential duration and refractory period between normal and infarcted regions and prevents reentry (Fig 10).[114] Bretylium transiently improves conduction velocity in Purkinje fibers in infarcted regions.[114] This effect is related to the initial release of catecholamines.[106,110] Since VF

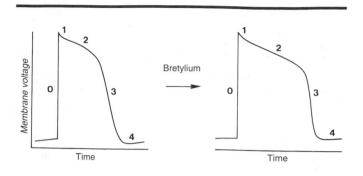

Fig 9. Schematic illustration of normal Purkinje fiber action potential before and after bretylium administration. Drug prolongs duration of action potential and refractory period to greater degree in normal tissue than in ischemic and infarcting tissue. By prolonging refractory period, bretylium may prevent reentry from ischemic zone.

Action Potential Characteristics of Purkinje Cells

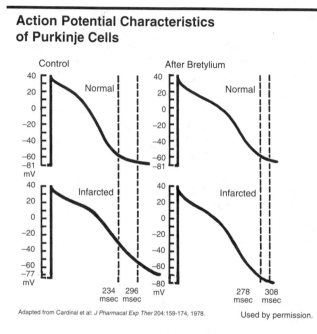

Adapted from Cardinal et al: *J Pharmacal Exp Ther* 204:159-174, 1978.

Used by permission.

Fig 10. Effects of infarction and bretylium on Purkinje fibers from canine hearts 1 to 2 days after coronary artery occlusion. Action potentials in infarcted zones (control, lower left) have lower resting potentials and prolonged durations. This disparity may permit reentrant excitation. Bretylium prolongs duration of action potential and refractory period, primarily in surrounding normal tissue and, to a lesser extent, in the infarcted area. This results in a reduction in disparity in action potential duration and refractory period between infarcted and normal tissue. Reentrant excitation is less likely to occur with more equalized recovery times.

may result from competing wave fronts,[115] improved conduction could conceivably prevent this competition and thus reduce the propensity for VF to develop. Some investigators believe that it is only during this phase of catecholamine release that bretylium is beneficial and that thereafter the negative adrenergic effects result in adverse hemodynamic and electrophysiological effects.[116-118]

Indications

Bretylium is indicated for the treatment of VF and VT refractory to other therapy, including electrical counter-

shock, epinephrine, and lidocaine.[70,116] Bretylium is not considered first-line therapy for either VT or VF because it is no more effective than lidocaine and is more likely to produce adverse hemodynamic effects during CPR (Fig 11).[70] Bretylium should be considered when (1) lidocaine and electrical countershock fail to convert VF; (2) VF recurs despite therapy with lidocaine; or (3) lidocaine and procainamide have been unable to prevent recurrent VT.

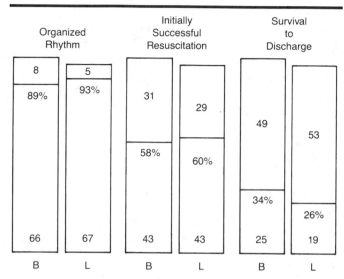

Fig 11. Outcome in a randomized clinical trial comparing bretylium (B, 74 patients) and lidocaine (L, 72 patients) in out-of-hospital VF. Percentages indicate restoration of organized rhythm, initially successful resuscitation, and survival to discharge. There were no significant differences between the two groups. Adapted from Haynes et al.[70]

Dosage

In patients with VF, 5 mg/kg of bretylium is given IV undiluted by rapid injection. The dose should be flushed with 20 mL of IV fluid if it is administered from a peripheral site. After 30 to 60 seconds defibrillation is attempted again. If VF persists, the dose can be increased to 10 mg/kg and given 5 minutes later. After that, 10 mg/kg of bretylium can be repeated twice at 5- to 30-minute intervals to a maximum dose of 35 mg/kg.[108]

In refractory or recurrent VT without a pulse, 500 mg of bretylium (10 mL) can be diluted to 50 mL, and 5 to 10 mg/kg can be injected IV over a period of 8 to 10 minutes. In the conscious patient, hypotension, nausea, and vomiting may follow more rapid injection. If VT persists, a second dose of 5 to 10 mg/kg can be given in 10 to 30 minutes and, if necessary, every 6 to 8 hours thereafter.[118] Alternatively, bretylium can be administered as a continuous infusion at a rate of 2 mg/min. The onset of action of bretylium in VF seems to be within a few minutes; in VT it may be delayed for 20 minutes or more.

Precautions

Postural hypotension is the most common adverse reaction in the non–cardiac arrest patient. It is observed in as many as 60% of patients, although the mean arterial pressure infrequently falls more than 20 mm Hg.[106,118] Treatment includes IV fluids and assumption of a supine or, if necessary, Trendelenberg position. In some cases a vasopressor such as norepinephrine may be required. Hypotension may be refractory to epinephrine.[117] Hypertension and tachycardia may also occur, but these effects are transient, owing to the initial stimulation of norepinephrine release from adrenergic nerve terminals.[107-110] Nausea and vomiting also may occur after rapid injection in the conscious patient. Bretylium should be used with caution in the treatment of arrhythmias accompanying digitalis toxicity because bretylium-mediated catecholamine release may exacerbate digitalis toxicity.[108-110]

Verapamil and Diltiazem

Slow channel activity in cardiac and vascular smooth muscle can be inhibited by calcium channel blockers. This results in several clinically useful effects that differ substantially from one agent to another.[119-122] Verapamil exerts potent, direct negative chronotropic and negative inotropic effects.[123-125] Diltiazem produces direct, potent negative chronotropic effects with only mild direct, negative inotropic actions.[118,119] Verapamil is highly effective for both acute and preventive treatment of supraventricular tachycardias (Class I).[122-125] Diltiazem has been studied less extensively for treatment and prevention of supraventricular tachycardias, but it may be as effective as verapamil.[126-128] Intravenous diltiazem is highly effective in controlling the ventricular response rate in patients with atrial fibrillation (Class I).[129,130]

Mechanism of Action

The therapeutic value of verapamil and diltiazem is due to their slow channel blocking properties, especially on cardiac and vascular smooth muscle.[125] These agents block the slow inward current of both calcium and sodium flux.[131] Verapamil's negative inotropism and chronotropism reduce myocardial oxygen consumption, making it an effective anti-ischemic agent.[125,132] Its negative inotropic effects are counterbalanced by a reduction in systemic vascular resistance caused by its vasodilation of vascular smooth muscle. Diltiazem produces fewer negative hemodynamic effects than verapamil. Both verapamil and diltiazem cause coronary vasodilation.[122,123]

Verapamil and diltiazem slow conduction and prolong refractoriness in the AV node, making them useful in terminating supraventricular tachycardias that use the AV node as part of their reentrant pathway.[133,134] These drugs slow the ventricular response to atrial flutter and fibrillation.[123,135,136] Verapamil and diltiazem depress the amplitude of action potentials in the upper and middle regions of the AV node.[137] The AH interval and the effective functional refractory periods of the AV node lengthen after administration of these calcium channel blockers.[138] In patients with the typical forms of AV nodal tachycardia,

verapamil terminates the arrhythmia by blocking conduction in the antegrade limb of the reentrant circuit.[138] Because it blocks slow-response action potentials, it is potentially beneficial in treating arrhythmias associated with ischemia.[139]

Indications

In ECC verapamil is used in the treatment of paroxysmal supraventricular tachycardia (PSVT) that does not require cardioversion.[121-125,140] Verapamil was the drug of choice until adenosine became available for clinical use in patients with PSVT. Verapamil terminates PSVT by direct effects on the AV node. The most common form of PSVT is due to sustained reentry within the AV node. The next most common type uses the AV node for at least one limb of its reentrant circuit.[132] When used for the proper indications, verapamil terminates more than 90% of episodes of PSVT in adults[121-124] and infants.[141] It is also useful in slowing ventricular response to atrial flutter and fibrillation.[122-124,136]

Verapamil and diltiazem have minimal, direct effects on the bypass tracts of patients with Wolff-Parkinson-White syndrome.[142] However, because of the reduced AV conduction, the refractory period of the bypass tract during antegrade conduction may be shortened indirectly by these agents because of reduced concealed retrograde conduction into the pathway.[142-144] These agents may also shorten the refractory period of the accessory pathway indirectly as a result of increases in adrenergic tone induced by peripheral vasodilation.[144] Thus, the ventricular response to atrial fibrillation in patients with Wolff-Parkinson-White syndrome may be accelerated in response to verapamil, and VF can occur (Fig 12).[143-148] Accordingly, verapamil and diltiazem should be used cautiously, if at all, in patients with Wolff-Parkinson-White syndrome and atrial fibrillation or flutter (Class III). Because a reciprocating tachycardia can degenerate into atrial fibrillation, patients with Wolff-Parkinson-White syndrome who are being treated with these agents for PSVT should be monitored continuously, and a defibrillator should be immediately available.[145,149]

Verapamil is not effective for the treatment of most types of VT (Class III). It may induce severe hypotension and predispose the patient to the development of VF.[150] Avoid verapamil and diltiazem in patients with wide-QRS tachycardia unless it is known with certainty to be supraventricular in origin.[150,151]

Clinical experience with IV diltiazem is more limited.[129,130] However, IV diltiazem, like verapamil, appears to be effective in terminating and preventing PSVT.[126-128] Intravenous diltiazem is indicated for ventricular rate control in patients with atrial fibrillation or flutter. In this setting a loading dose regimen followed by a maintenance infusion effectively controls ventricular response rate in 90% of patients.[130] Diltiazem offers the advantage of producing less myocardial depression than verapamil in patients with left ventricular dysfunction.

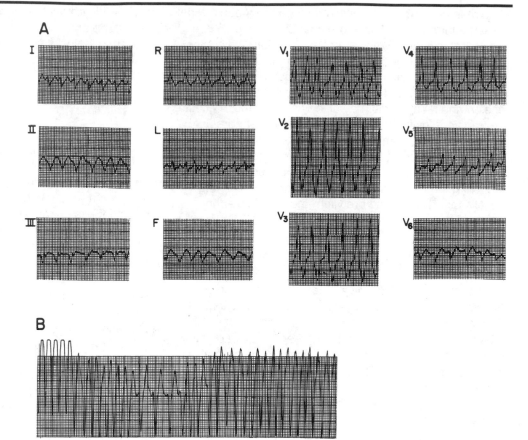

Fig 12. A, Twelve-lead ECG showing atrial fibrillation with ventricular pre-excitation. B, After verapamil injection there is accelerated atrioventricular conduction with an increased ventricular rate. From McGovern et al.[145]

Dosage

Single-Dose Verapamil

As a single dose, give 2.5 to 5.0 mg IV bolus over 1 to 2 minutes. Peak therapeutic effects occur within 3 to 5 minutes of bolus injection.

Repeat Dose

If the initial response is inadequate, the repeat dose is 5 to 10 mg in 15 to 30 minutes after the first dose. Alternatively, a 5-mg bolus injection can be given every 15 minutes until a desired response is achieved or a total dose of 30 mg is administered.

Older Patients

In middle-aged or older patients the IV dose should be administered over at least 3 minutes.

Age 8 to 15 Years

For patients aged 8 to 15 years, 0.1 to 0.3 mg/kg body weight (total single dose range: 2 to 5 mg) is administered as an IV bolus over 1 minute. The repeat dose is 0.1 to 0.2 mg/kg body weight (total single dose range: 2 to 5 mg) 15 to 30 minutes after the first dose if the initial response is inadequate.

Diltiazem

An initial bolus dose of 0.25 mg/kg (20 mg for the average patient) is administered IV over 2 minutes. For control of the ventricular response rate in patients with atrial fibrillation or flutter, the bolus dose is followed by a maintenance infusion at a rate of 5 to 15 mg/h titrated to heart rate. Because diltiazem shows dose-dependent, nonlinear pharmacokinetics, infusion duration exceeding 24 hours and infusion rates above 15 mg/h are not recommended. If satisfactory ventricular rate control is not achieved, a 0.35 mg/kg bolus (25 mg for the average patient) over 2 to 5 minutes may be given 15 minutes after the initial bolus.

For patients with PSVT, a bolus of 0.25 mg/kg is administered IV over 2 minutes. Conversion should occur in approximately 90% of patients. However, a second bolus dose of 0.35 mg/kg may be administered if the PSVT fails to convert to normal sinus rhythm within 15 minutes after the initial bolus.

Precautions

A transient decrease in arterial pressure due to peripheral vasodilation should be expected in response to verapamil or diltiazem.[121] Intravenous calcium injection will restore arterial pressure and has been recommended as pretreatment therapy against hypotension in patients with marginal blood pressure or left ventricular dysfunction.[152] Used in this manner, calcium does not affect the electrophysiological properties of verapamil.[153] Cardiac output usually remains unchanged, reflecting the balance between the intrinsic negative inotropic effects of the drug, its reflex sympathetic response, and vasodilation.[121,154] This is also true in patients with mild to moderate left ventricular dysfunction.[155] However, in patients with severely reduced left ventricular function, IV verapamil may induce hemodynamic compromise.[155] Although diltiazem is less likely to produce this effect, caution should be used in patients with severe left ventricular dysfunction.

Verapamil and diltiazem can be used safely and effectively in patients receiving digitalis, although verapamil will increase serum digitalis concentrations. Unless there is evidence of impaired AV conduction, prior treatment with digitalis is not a contraindication to the use of IV verapamil or diltiazem.[156] Positive synergism between digitalis and verapamil or diltiazem is often observed in patients with atrial tachyarrhythmias.

The use of IV β-adrenergic blocking agents combined with calcium channel blockers is contraindicated because the hemodynamic and electrophysiological effects of these agents will be synergistic. Caution is also recommended when IV calcium channel blockers are given to a patient receiving β blockers orally.

Verapamil and diltiazem should be avoided, or used with caution, in patients with sick sinus syndrome or AV block in the absence of a functioning pacemaker. In patients with acute pump failure, therapy with verapamil or diltiazem is indicated if resolution of the tachycardia will remove the cause of the hemodynamic compromise. Because of its shorter duration of action, adenosine is preferable in PSVT. Severe heart failure is a contraindication to the use of verapamil and a relative contraindication to the use of diltiazem. Bradycardia can occur if cardioversion is done proximate to the administration of verapamil or diltiazem. Diltiazem injection is incompatible with simultaneous furosemide injection.

Adenosine

Mechanism of Action

Adenosine is an endogenous purine nucleoside that slows conduction through the AV node, interrupts AV-nodal reentry pathways, and can restore normal sinus rhythm in patients with PSVT, including PSVT associated with Wolff-Parkinson-White syndrome. Adenosine produces a short-lived pharmacologic response because it is rapidly sequestered by red blood cells. The half-life of free adenosine is less than 10 seconds.

Indications

Since most common forms of PSVT involve a reentry pathway, including the AV node, adenosine is effective in terminating these arrhythmias.[157] If the arrhythmias are not due to reentry involving the AV node or sinus node (eg, atrial flutter, atrial fibrillation, atrial or ventricular tachycardias), adenosine will not terminate the arrhythmia but may produce transient AV or VA block, which may serve to clarify the diagnosis.[158] Thus, adenosine is the initial drug of choice for the diagnosis of supraventricular arrhythmias.

Adenosine is indicated for the conversion of PSVT (including that associated with Wolff-Parkinson-White syndrome) to sinus rhythm. Because of adenosine's short half-life, PSVT may recur. Repeat episodes of PSVT may be treated with additional doses of adenosine, but verapamil or diltiazem may be preferable, if not contraindicated (eg, by Wolff-Parkinson-White syndrome) because of their longer duration of action.

Dosage

The recommended initial dose is a 6-mg rapid bolus over 1 to 3 seconds. The dose should be followed quickly by a 20-mL saline flush. A brief period of asystole (up to 15 seconds) is common after rapid administration. If no response is observed within 1 to 2 minutes, a 12-mg repeat dose should be administered in the same manner. Experience with larger doses is limited, but patients taking theophylline are less sensitive to adenosine and may require larger doses.[159] Conversely, cardiac transplant recipients are more sensitive to adenosine and require only a small dose.[160]

Precautions

Side effects with adenosine are common but transient. Flushing, dyspnea, and chest pain are the most frequently observed.[159] These side effects usually resolve spontaneously within 1 to 2 minutes. Transient periods of sinus bradycardia and ventricular ectopy are common after termination of supraventricular tachycardia with adenosine. Caution is advised in patients with preexisting propensity to bradycardias or conduction defects who do not have a functioning pacemaker because of the risk of prolonged sinus arrest or AV block. Adenosine should be used with caution in patients with denervated, transplanted hearts.[160]

Because of its brief duration of action, adenosine produces few, if any, hemodynamic effects and is less likely to precipitate hypotension if the arrhythmia does not terminate. However, the use of adenosine should be reserved for situations where transient suppression of AV nodal conduction will be of therapeutic or diagnostic value.

Adenosine has several important drug interactions.[159] Therapeutic concentrations of theophylline or related methylxanthines (caffeine and theobromine) block the receptor responsible for adenosine's electrophysiological and hemodynamic effects. Dipyridamole blocks adenosine uptake and potentiates its effects. Alternative therapy should be selected in patients receiving these drugs.

Magnesium

Mechanism of Action

Magnesium is a cofactor in numerous enzymatic reactions. It is essential for the function of the sodium-potassium ATPase pump. It acts as a physiological calcium channel blocker and blocks neuromuscular transmission. The effect of hypomagnesemia in cardiac disease is well known.[161,162] Magnesium deficiency is associated with a high frequency of cardiac arrhythmias, symptoms of cardiac insufficiency, and sudden cardiac death.[161-164] Transient hypomagnesemia not induced by renal magnesium loss has been observed in patients with acute myocardial infarction.[165] Because hypomagnesemia can precipitate refractory VF and can hinder the replenishment of intracellular potassium, it should be corrected if present.

Indications

Magnesium supplementation may reduce the incidence of postinfarction ventricular arrhythmias.[164,165] Magnesium is considered a treatment of choice in patients with torsades de pointes. Evidence that IV magnesium lowers complications associated with acute myocardial infarction continues to accumulate.[164-169] A recent meta-analysis showed that administration of magnesium led to a 58% reduction in cardiac arrest and a 49% reduction in VF and VT.[166] The incidence of supraventricular arrhythmias was also significantly reduced.[166] A recently published prospective, blinded study (LIMIT-2) examined the role of acute IV magnesium therapy (16 mEq over 5 minutes followed by 130 mEq over 24 hours) in 2316 patients with suspected acute myocardial infarction.[168] In this study the 30-day mortality rate was significantly lower (P=.04) in patients receiving magnesium (7.8%) than in those receiving saline placebo (10.3%). The incidence of acute pump failure was reduced by 25% in the magnesium-treated group. The reduction in mortality was not affected by other interventions (thrombolytic therapy, aspirin, β blockers, calcium antagonists, electrical pacing, countershocks, or antiarrhythmic therapy). The side effects of magnesium included transient flushing and an increased incidence of sinus bradycardia.

If the results of the multicenter ISIS-4 trial confirm the beneficial effects of magnesium demonstrated in LIMIT-2, magnesium therapy may soon become routine for patients who are hospitalized for suspected acute myocardial infarction.[169] Preliminary results presented at the AHA 66th Scientific Sessions, November 1993, suggest that the positive effects of magnesium on acute myocardial infarction mortality may not be confirmed in much larger studies.

Dosage

For acute administration during VT, 1 or 2 g of magnesium sulfate (2 to 4 mL of a 50% solution) is diluted in 10 mL of D_5W and administered over 1 to 2 minutes.[170] In VF magnesium should be given IV push. When magnesium is administered, caution should be used to safeguard against clinically significant hypotension or asystole. A 24-hour magnesium infusion (0.5 to 1.0 g [4 to 8 mEq] per hour) may be considered in patients with documented magnesium deficiency on admission to the cardiac care unit. For torsades de pointes even higher doses, up to 5 to 10 g, have been used with success. Clinical research has not yet established the optimum dose.

Precautions

Magnesium toxicity is rare, but side effects from too rapid administration include flushing, sweating, mild bradycardia, and hypotension. Hypermagnesemia may produce depressed reflexes, flaccid paralysis, circulatory collapse, respiratory paralysis, and diarrhea.

Sodium Bicarbonate

Standard CPR generates only 25% to 30% of normal cardiac output, resulting in limited organ perfusion and oxygen delivery.[171] At the tissue level, the accumulation of CO_2 reflects the balance between local production of CO_2, the dissociation of endogenous bicarbonate (buffering the anaerobically generated hydrogen ions), and the reduced clearance of CO_2 due to low blood flow. Continuous CO_2 release from anaerobic metabolism of ischemic tissues, decreased CO_2 transport from the underperfused tissues to the lungs, and reduced pulmonary blood flow, with resultant curtailed alveolar CO_2 elimination, result in the rapid accumulation of CO_2 in the prepulmonary veins and the tissues.[172-174] Decreased expired P_{CO_2} (end-tidal CO_2) and hypercarbic venous acidemia (reflecting tissue acidosis), often with hypocarbic arterial alkalemia, occur during CPR.[172-174] Venous acidemia in the face of arterial alkalemia has been termed the *veno-arterial paradox*.[175]

The degree of acid-base changes observed during CPR depends on the adequacy of blood flow and the duration of ischemia before CPR.[176,177] Acid-base derangements associated with prolonged cardiopulmonary arrest (eg, most out-of-hospital cardiac arrest) are usually found to have a combined metabolic and hypercarbic acidemia. Reduction of the increased tissue CO_2 and associated acidemia found during curtailed organ perfusion is thought to be important. However, laboratory and clinical data fail to conclusively show that low blood pH adversely affects ability to defibrillate, ability to restore spontaneous circulation, or short-term survival.[172,178,179] Response to adrenergic agonists may also be unaffected by tissue acidosis.[180] Furthermore, the three-part acid-base abnormality found during low perfusion — venous hypercarbic acidemia, arterial hypocarbic alkalemia, and metabolic (lactic) acidemia — make the choice of an optimal buffer agent difficult and controversial.

Mechanism of Action

Sodium bicarbonate ($NaHCO_3$) is clinically the most widely used buffer agent. $NaHCO_3$ dissociates to sodium and bicarbonate ions. In the presence of hydrogen ions, these are converted to carbonic acid and hence to CO_2, which is transported to and excreted by the lungs. The formation of the easily excretable CO_2 permits $NaHCO_3$ to function as an efficient buffer, as follows:

$$H^+ + HCO_3^- \Leftrightarrow H_2CO_3 \Leftrightarrow H_2O + CO_2$$

Under conditions of normal ventilation and perfusion, the CO_2 generated by $NaHCO_3$ is eliminated by the lungs, and excesses of hydrogen ions are effectively neutralized. However, since the transport of CO_2 from the tissues to the lungs and removal of CO_2 by the lungs is decreased during CPR, CO_2 generated by the buffering action of $NaHCO_3$ may not be adequately cleared. Because of its free diffusability across cell membranes, CO_2 remaining at the tissue level may induce paradoxical tissue and intracellular hypercarbic acidosis.[181,182] This might result in a decrease in myocardial contractility and resuscitability.[183,184]

Alkalemia[178,185] and plasma hyperosmolality and hypernatremia,[185,186] as well as possible intracerebral hemorrhage, especially in pediatric patients, are potentially deleterious side effects of $NaHCO_3$. $NaHCO_3$ also induces a left shift of the oxyhemoglobin dissociation curve with a decrease in the release of oxygen by hemoglobin.[187] The most important shortcoming of $NaHCO_3$ when used during CPR is its apparent failure to improve defibrillation success[185,188] or increase survival rates after brief cardiac arrest.[178,185,189] This may be related to decreases in coronary perfusion pressure observed when $NaHCO_3$ was administered as the sole resuscitative agent.[190] However, concurrent administration of $NaHCO_3$ and epinephrine improves both coronary perfusion pressure and neurological outcomes in experimental models of cardiac arrest.[191-193]

Indications

Tissue acidosis and resulting acidemia during cardiac arrest and resuscitation are dynamic processes resulting from inadequate ventilation and poor oxygen delivery. These processes depend on the duration of cardiac arrest and the level of blood flow during CPR. Adequate alveolar ventilation and restoration of tissue perfusion, first with chest compressions, then with rapid restoration of spontaneous circulation, are the mainstays of control of acid-base balance during cardiac arrest.

In cardiac arrests of short duration, adequate ventilation and effective chest compressions limit the accumulation of CO_2 during cardiac arrest. The restoration of sufficient blood flow provides oxygen to vital organs and counterbalances the hypercarbic and metabolic acidemia by eliminating CO_2 and metabolizing lactate. Thus, in the early phase of CPR, buffer agents are generally unneces-

sary. In general, the provision of good CPR is the best "buffer therapy."

In certain circumstances, such as preexisting metabolic acidosis, hyperkalemia, or tricyclic or phenobarbital overdose, bicarbonate is beneficial. During CPR bicarbonate therapy should be considered only after the confirmed interventions — such as defibrillation, cardiac compression, intubation, ventilation, and more than one trial of epinephrine — have been used. If buffer therapy is considered necessary, it must be accomplished rapidly. After successful CPR, administration of sodium bicarbonate may help buffer the acid washout seen with the reestablishment of spontaneous circulation.

Dosage

When bicarbonate is used, 1 mEq/kg IV bolus should be given as the initial dose. Give half this dose every 10 minutes thereafter. If blood gas analyses are available soon enough that the results reflect acid-base status at that time, bicarbonate therapy can be guided by calculated base deficit or bicarbonate concentration. To minimize the risk of iatrogenically induced alkalosis, complete correction of the base deficit should be avoided. Ready-to-use injections containing 8.4% sodium bicarbonate (50 mEq/50 mL) are recommended for use during CPR.

Sodium bicarbonate may be administered by continuous infusion when the therapeutic goal is gradual correction of acidosis or alkalinization of blood (eg, in tricyclic antidepressant overdose) or urine (eg, in barbiturate overdose). To administer a sodium bicarbonate infusion, use a 5% sodium bicarbonate solution (297.5 mEq/500 mL). The infusion rate should be guided by arterial blood gas monitoring.

Precautions

In the past much emphasis has been placed on the administration of sodium bicarbonate during cardiac arrest. However, it is the crucial role of P_{CO_2} that must be emphasized. In vitro even partial respiratory compensation of metabolic acidosis can prevent intracellular acidosis.[194] Sodium bicarbonate administration results in the rapid generation of CO_2, a potent negative inotrope.[195,196] The performance of the ischemic heart is closely related to tissue P_{CO_2} and is minimally related to the level of extracellular pH.[196] Cardiac muscle performance is depressed by increases in arterial P_{CO_2}, presumably because of the paradoxical intracellular acidosis that is induced.[194,197] Hydrogen ions liberated during metabolic acidosis also exert a negative inotropic action, but this effect is much slower in onset and may not be fully manifest until 30 minutes have elapsed from onset of an acidosis to a magnitude equivalent to that induced more rapidly by CO_2.[195]

The rapid onset of a carbon dioxide–induced intracellular acidosis is directly related to the rapidity with which CO_2 diffuses intracellularly.[195] Intracellular P_{CO_2} during

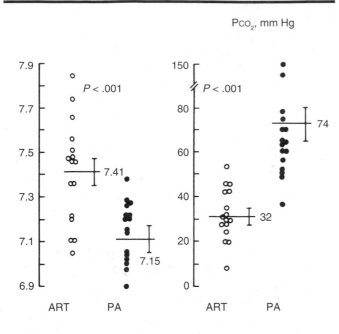

Fig 13. Differences in systemic arterial (ART) and pulmonary artery (PA) pH and Pco_2 in 16 patients during CPR. Measurements were made at a median of 23 minutes after onset of arrest. Average dose of $NaHCO_3$ (+SEM) was 130 + 30 mEq over a median interval of 23 minutes. Numerical mean values for each measurement are indicated on the graph. Mixed venous acidemia from CO_2 retention is evident. $NaHCO_3$ would be expected to worsen this acidosis from CO_2 formation. From Weil et al.[175]

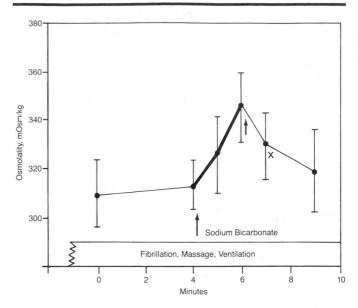

Fig 14. Arterial osmolality in six patients during cardiac resuscitation. Note significant and persistent rise in osmolality after sodium bicarbonate administration (x indicates $P<.05$). From Bishop and Weisfeldt.[185]

experimental acute myocardial ischemia has been shown to rise to more than 300 mm Hg, and corresponding intracellular pH falls to as low as 6.1. Liberation of CO_2 and its rapid intracellular diffusion after sodium bicarbonate administration may produce cerebrospinal fluid acidosis and central venous acidosis during CPR (Fig 13).[175,181]

Other adverse effects from sodium bicarbonate include hypernatremia and hyperosmolality (Fig 14).[185,186] Severe hyperosmolal states during resuscitation may compromise survival.[186] Shift in the oxyhemoglobin saturation curve caused by sodium bicarbonate can inhibit oxygen release to the tissues.

Morphine

Mechanism of Action

Morphine is effective treatment for ischemic chest pain and for acute pulmonary edema.[198] It manifests both analgesic and hemodynamic effects.[199] It increases venous capacitance and reduces systemic vascular resistance, relieving pulmonary congestion.[200] In doing so, it reduces intramyocardial wall tension, which decreases myocardial oxygen requirements.[201] Morphine's hemodynamic effects may be mediated by sympatholytic effects on the central nervous system since they are most pronounced in patients with heightened sympathetic activity.[202]

Indications

Morphine is the traditional drug of choice for the treatment of pain and anxiety associated with acute myocardial infarction. It is also useful for treating patients with acute cardiogenic pulmonary edema.

Dosage

Morphine should be administered IV in small incremental doses of 1 to 3 mg slow IV (over 1 to 5 minutes) until the desired effect is achieved.

Precautions

Like other narcotic analgesics, morphine is a respiratory depressant. Small incremental doses at frequent intervals make serious depression less likely than a single large bolus. Excessive narcosis can be reversed with IV naloxone (0.4 to 0.8 mg). Hypotension is most common and most severe in volume-depleted patients and in patients who are dependent on elevated systemic resistance for maintenance of blood pressure.[203] Hypotension and an inappropriate heart rate response that appears to be vagally mediated also have been described.[203]

Calcium Chloride

Mechanism of Action

Calcium ions increase the force of myocardial contraction.[204] In response to electrical stimulation of muscle, calcium ions enter the sarcoplasm from the extracellular space.[205,206] Calcium ions contained in the sarcoplasmic reticulum are rapidly transferred to the sites of interaction between the actin and myosin filaments of the sarcomere to initiate myofibril shortening.[207] Thus, calcium increases myocardial contractile function. The positive inotropic effects of calcium are modulated by its action on systemic vascular resistance. Calcium may either increase or decrease systemic vascular resistance.[208-210] In normal hearts calcium's positive inotropic and vasoconstricting effects produce a predictable rise in systemic arterial pressure.[208,211]

Indications

Although calcium ions play a critical role in myocardial contractile performance and impulse formation, retrospective and prospective studies in the cardiac arrest setting have not demonstrated benefit from the use of calcium.[212,213] In addition, there is considerable theoretical reason to believe that the high levels induced by calcium administration may be detrimental.[214,215] When hyperkalemia, hypocalcemia (eg, after multiple blood transfusions), or calcium channel blocker toxicity is present, calcium is probably helpful. Otherwise, calcium should not be used. Some clinical experience has observed calcium to be useful to prevent the hypotensive effects of calcium channel blocking agents (IV verapamil and diltiazem).

Dosage

Hyperkalemia and Calcium Channel Overdose

Give 8 to 16 mg/kg of 10% solution. Repeat if necessary.

Prophylaxis of Calcium Channel Blockers

A 10-mL prefilled syringe or ampule of 10% solution of calcium chloride (1 mL = 100 mg) contains 13.6 mEq of calcium. Calcium chloride can be given IV in a dose of 2 to 4 mg/kg of 10% solution (1.36 mEq of calcium per 100 mg of salt per milliliter) and repeated if necessary at 10-minute intervals. Two other calcium salts are available, calcium gluceptate and calcium gluconate. Calcium gluceptate can be given in a dose of 5 to 7 mL; the dose of calcium gluconate is 5 to 8 mL. Calcium chloride is preferable because it produces consistently higher and more predictable levels of ionized calcium in plasma.[216]

Precautions

If the heart is beating, rapid administration of calcium can produce slowing of the cardiac rate. Calcium must be used cautiously in the patient receiving digitalis, because calcium increases ventricular irritability and may precipitate digitalis toxicity. In the presence of sodium bicarbonate, calcium salts will precipitate as carbonates. Thus these drugs cannot be administered together. Calcium may produce vasospasm in coronary and cerebral arteries.

References

1. Ornato JP, Bryson BL, Donovan PJ, Farquharson RR, Jaeger C. Measurement of ventilation during cardiopulmonary resuscitation. *Crit Care Med*. 1983;11:79-82.
2. Wynne JW, Modell JH. Respiratory aspiration of stomach contents. *Ann Intern Med*. 1977;87:466-474.
3. Ayres SM. Mechanisms and consequences of pulmonary edema: cardiac lung, shock lung, and principles of ventilatory therapy in adult respiratory distress syndrome. *Am Heart J*. 1982;103:97-112.
4. Madias JE, Madias NE, Hood WB Jr. Precordial ST-segment mapping, II: effects of oxygen inhalation on ischemic injury in patients with acute myocardial infarction. *Circulation*. 1976;53:411-417.
5. Otto CW, Yakaitis RW. The role of epinephrine in CPR: a reappraisal. *Ann Emerg Med*. 1984;13(pt 2):840-843.
6. Michael JR, Guerci AD, Koehler RC, Shi AY, Tsitlik J, Chandra N, Niedermeyer E, Rogers MC, Traystman RJ, Weisfeldt ML. Mechanisms by which epinephrine augments cerebral and myocardial perfusion during cardiopulmonary resuscitation in dogs. *Circulation*. 1984;69:822-835.
7. Koehler RC, Michael JR, Guerci AD, Chandra N, Schleien CL, Dean JM, Rogers MC, Weisfeldt ML, Traystman RJ. Beneficial effect of epinephrine infusion on cerebral and myocardial blood flows during CPR. *Ann Emerg Med*. 1985;14:744-749.
8. Otto CW, Yakaitis RW, Ewy GA. Spontaneous ischemic ventricular fibrillation in dogs: a new model for the study of cardiopulmonary resuscitation. *Crit Care Med*. 1983;11:883-887.
9. Brillman JA, Sanders AB, Otto CW, Fahmy H, Bragg S, Ewy GA. Outcome of resuscitation from fibrillatory arrest using epinephrine and phenylephrine in dogs. *Crit Care Med*. 1985;13:912-913.
10. Livesay JJ, Follette DM, Fey KH, Nelson RL, DeLand EC, Barnard RJ, Buckberg GD. Optimizing myocardial supply/demand balance with alpha-adrenergic drugs during cardiopulmonary resuscitation. *J Thorac Cardiovasc Surg*. 1978;76:244-251.
11. Ralston SH. Alpha agonist drug usage during CPR. *Ann Emerg Med*. 1984;13(pt 2):786-789.
12. Yakaitis RW, Otto CW, Blitt CD. Relative importance of alpha and beta adrenergic receptors during resuscitation. *Crit Care Med*. 1979;7:293-296.
13. Holmes HR, Babbs CF, Voorhees WD, Tacker WA Jr, de Garavilla B. Influence of adrenergic drugs upon vital organ perfusion during CPR. *Crit Care Med*. 1980;8:137-140.
14. Brown CG, Birinyi F, Werman HA, Davis EA, Hamlin RL. The comparative effects of epinephrine versus phenylephrine on regional cerebral blood flow during cardiopulmonary resuscitation. *Resuscitation*. 1986;14:171-183.
15. Brown CG, Werman HA, Davis EA, Katz S, Hamlin RL. The effect of high-dose phenylephrine versus epinephrine on regional cerebral blood flow during CPR. *Ann Emerg Med*. 1987;16:743-748.
16. Brown CG, Davis EA, Werman HA, Hamlin RL. Methoxamine versus epinephrine on regional cerebral blood flow during cardiopulmonary resuscitation. *Crit Care Med*. 1987;15:682-686.
17. Steen PA, Tinker JH, Pluth JR, Barnhrst DA, Tarhan S. Efficacy of dopamine, dobutamine, and epinephrine during emergence from cardiopulmonary bypass in man. *Circulation*. 1978;57:378-384.
18. Sato Y, Matsuzawa H, Eguchi S. Comparative study of effects of adrenaline, dobutamine, and dopamine on systemic hemodynamics and renal blood flow in patients following open heart surgery. *Jpn Circ J*. 1982;46:1059-1072.
19. Callaham M. Epinephrine doses in cardiac arrest: is it time to outgrow the orthodoxy of ACLS? *Ann Emerg Med*. 1989;18:1011-1012.
20. Beck C, Leighninger D. Reversal of death in good hearts. *J Cardiovasc Surg*. 1962;3:357-375.
21. Beck CS, Rand HJ III. Cardiac arrest during anesthesia and surgery. *JAMA*. 1949;141:1230-1233.
22. Gerbode F. The cardiac emergency. *Ann Surg*. 1952;135:431.
23. Lindner KH, Ahnefeld FW, Bowdler IM. Comparison of different doses of epinephrine on myocardial perfusion and resuscitation success during cardiopulmonary resuscitation in a pig model. *Am J Emerg Med*. 1991;9:27-31.
24. Brown CG, Taylor RB, Werman HA, Luu T, Spittler G, Hamlin RL. Effect of standard doses of epinephrine on myocardial oxygen delivery and utilization during cardiopulmonary resuscitation. *Crit Care Med*. 1988;16:536-539.

25. Brown CG, Werman HA, Davis EA, Hobson J, Hamlin RL. The effects of graded doses of epinephrine on regional myocardial blood flow during cardiopulmonary resuscitation in swine. *Circulation*. 1987;75:491-497.

26. Brown CG, Werman HA, Davis EA, Hamlin R, Hobson J, Ashton JA. Comparative effect of graded doses of epinephrine on regional brain blood flow during CPR in a swine model. *Ann Emerg Med*. 1986;15:1138-1144.

27. Kosnik JW, Jackson RE, Keats S, Tworek RM, Freeman SB. Dose-related response of centrally administered epinephrine on the change in aortic diastolic pressure during closed-chest massage in dogs. *Ann Emerg Med*. 1985;14:204-208.

28. Paradis NA, Koscove EM. Epinephrine in cardiac arrest: a critical review. *Ann Emerg Med*. 1990;19:1288-1301.

29. Gonzalez ER, Ornato JP, Garnett AR, Levine RL, Young DS, Racht EM. Dose-dependent vasopressor response to epinephrine during CPR in human beings. *Ann Emerg Med*. 1989;18:920-926.

30. Gonzalez ER, Ornato JP. The dose of epinephrine during cardiopulmonary resuscitation in humans: what should it be? *DICP*. 1991;25:773-777.

31. Lindner KH, Ahnefeld FW, Prengel AW. Comparison of standard and high-dose adrenaline in the resuscitation of asystole and electromechanical dissociation. *Acta Anesthesiol Scand*. 1991; 35:253-256.

32. Stiell IG, Hebert PC, Weitzman BN, Wells GA, Raman S, Stark RM, Higginson LA, Ahuja J, Dickinson GE. High-dose epinephrine in adult cardiac arrest. *N Engl J Med*. 1992;327:1047-1050.

33. Callaham M, Madsen CD, Barton CW, Saunders CE, Pointer J. A randomized clinical trial of high-dose epinephrine and norepinephrine vs standard-dose epinephrine in prehospital cardiac arrest. *JAMA*. 1992;268:2667-2672.

34. Brown CG, Martin DR, Pepe PE, Stueven H, Cummins RO, Gonzalez E, Jastremski M. A comparison of standard-dose and high-dose epinephrine in cardiac arrest outside the hospital: the Multicenter High-dose Epinephrine Study Group. *N Engl J Med*. 1992;327:1051-1055.

35. Paradis NA, Martin GB, Rivers EP, Goetting MG, Appleton JJ, Feingold M, Nowak RM. Coronary perfusion pressure and return of spontaneous circulation in human cardiopulmonary resuscitation. *JAMA*. 1990;263:1106-1113.

36. Emerman CL, Pinchak AC, Hancock D, Hagen JF. The effect of bolus injection on circulation times during cardiac arrest. *Am J Emerg Med*. 1990;8:190-193.

37. Roberts JR, Greenberg MI, Knaub MA, Kendrick ZV, Baskin SI. Blood levels following intravenous and endotracheal epinephrine administration. *JACEP*. 1979;8:53-56.

38. Aitkenhead AR. Drug administration during CPR: what route? *Resuscitation*. 1991;22:191-195.

39. Hasegawa EA. The endotracheal use of emergency drugs. *Heart Lung*. 1986;15:60-63.

40. Newton DW, Fung EY, Williams DA. Stability of five catecholamines and terbutaline sulfate in 5% dextrose injection in the absence and presence of aminophylline. *Am J Hosp Pharm*. 1981;38:1314-1319.

41. Zaritsky AL, Chernow B. Catecholamines, sympathomimetics. In: Chernow B, Lake CR, eds. *The Pharmacologic Approach to the Critically Ill Patient*. Baltimore, Md: Williams & Wilkins Co; 1983:481-509.

42. Packer M, Gottlieb SS, Kessler PD. Hormone-electrolyte interactions in the pathogenesis of lethal cardiac arrhythmias in patients with congestive heart failure: basis of a new physiologic approach to control of arrhythmia. *Am J Med*. 1986;80(suppl 4A):23-29.

43. Brown DC, Lewis AJ, Criley JM. Asystole and its treatment: the possible role of the parasympathetic nervous system in cardiac arrest. *JACEP*. 1979;8:448-452.

44. Dauchot P, Gravenstein JS. Bradycardia after myocardial ischemia and its treatment with atropine. *Anesthesiology*. 1976;44:501-518.

45. Epstein SE, Goldstein RD, Redwood DR, et al. The early phase of acute myocardial infarction: pharmacologic aspects of therapy (NIH Conference). *Ann Intern Med*. 1973;78:918-936.

46. Gunnar RM, Passamani ER, Bourdillon PD, Pitt B, Dixon DW, Rapaport E, Fuster V, Reeves TJ, Karp RB, Russell RO Jr, et al. Guidelines for the early management of patients with acute myocardial infarction: a report of the American College of Cardiology/American Heart Association Task Force on Assessment of Diagnostic and Therapeutic Cardiovascular Procedures (Subcommittee to Develop Guidelines for the Early Management of Patients with Acute Myocardial Infarction). *J Am Coll Cardiol*. 1990;16:249-292.

47. Myerburg RJ, Estes D, Zaman L, Luceri RM, Kessler KM, Trohman RG, Castellanos A. Outcome of resuscitation from bradyarrhythmic or asystolic prehospital cardiac arrest. *J Am Coll Cardiol*. 1984; 4:1118-1122.

48. Stueven HA, Tonsfeldt DJ, Thompson BM, Whitcomb J, Kastenson E, Aprahamian C. Atropine in asystole: human studies. *Ann Emerg Med*. 1984;13(pt 2):815-817.

49. Ornato JP, Gonzalez ER, Morkunas AR, Coyne MR, Beck CL. Treatment of presumed asystole during pre-hospital cardiac arrest: superiority of electrical countershock. *Am J Emerg Med*. 1985;3:395-399.

50. Iseri LT, Humphrey SB, Siner EJ. Prehospital brady-asystolic cardiac arrest. *Ann Intern Med*. 1978;88:741-745.

51. Coon GA, Clinton JE, Ruiz E. Use of atropine for brady-asystolic prehospital cardiac arrest. *Ann Emerg Med*. 1981;10:462-467.

52. O'Rourke GW, Greene NM. Autonomic blockade and the resting heart rate in man. *Am Heart J*. 1970;80:469-474.

53. Kottmeier CA, Gravenstein JS. The parasympathomimetic activity of atropine and atropine methylbromide. *Anesthesiology*. 1968;29: 1125-1133.

54. Prete MR, Hannan CJ Jr, Burkle FM Jr. Plasma atropine concentrations via intravenous, endotracheal, and intraosseous administration. *Am J Emerg Med*. 1987;5:101-104.

55. Greenberg MI, Mayeda DV, Chrzanowski R, Brumwell D, Baskin SI, Roberts JR. Endotracheal administration of atropine sulfate. *Ann Emerg Med*. 1982;11:546-548.

56. Knoebel SB, McHenry PL, Phillips JF, Widlansky S. Atropine-induced cardioacceleration and myocardial blood flow in subjects with and without coronary artery disease. *Am J Cardiol*. 1974;33:327-332.

57. Richman S. Adverse effect of atropine during myocardial infarction: enhancement of ischemia following intravenously administered atropine. *JAMA*. 1974;228:1414-1416.

58. Massumi RA, Mason DT, Amsterdam EA, DeMaria A, Miller RR, Scheinman MM, Zelis R. Ventricular fibrillation and tachycardia after intravenous atropine for treatment of bradycardias. *N Engl J Med*. 1972;287:336-338.

59. Lunde P. Ventricular fibrillation after intravenous atropine for treatment of sinus bradycardia. *Acta Med Scand*. 1976;199:369-371.

60. Cooper MJ, Abinader EG. Atropine-induced ventricular fibrillation: case report and review of the literature. *Am Heart J*. 1979;97: 225-228.

61. Weiner N. Atropine, scopolamine, and related antimuscarinic drugs. In: Gilman AG, Goodman LS, Gilman A, eds. *The Pharmacological Basis of Therapeutics*. 6th ed. New York, NY: Macmillan Inc; 1980:120-137.

62. Collinsworth KA, Kalman SM, Harrison DC. The clinical pharmacology of lidocaine as an antiarrhythmic drug. *Circulation*. 1974;50: 1217-1230.

63. Kupersmith J, Antman EM, Hoffman BF. In vivo electrophysiological effects of lidocaine in canine acute myocardial infarction. *Circ Res*. 1975;36:84-91.

64. El-Sherif N, Scherlag BJ, Lazzara R, Hope RR. Re-entrant ventricular arrhythmias in the late myocardial infarction period, IV: mechanism of action of lidocaine. *Circulation*. 1977;56:395-402.

65. Kupersmith J. Electrophysiological and antiarrhythmic effects of lidocaine in canine acute myocardial ischemia. *Am Heart J*. 1979; 97:360-366.

66. Spear JF, Moore EN, Gerstenblith G. Effect of lidocaine on the ventricular fibrillation threshold in the dog during acute ischemia and premature ventricular contractions. *Circulation*. 1972;46:65-73.

67. Kerber RE, Pandian NG, Jensen SR, Constantin L, Kieso RA, Melton J, Hunt M. Effect of lidocaine and bretylium on energy requirements for transthoracic defibrillation: experimental studies. *J Am Coll Cardiol*. 1986;7:397-405.

68. Dorian P, Fain ES, Davy JM, Winkle RA. Lidocaine causes a reversible, concentration-dependent increase in defibrillation energy requirements. *J Am Coll Cardiol*. 1986;8:327-332.

69. Harrison EE. Lidocaine in prehospital countershock refractory ventricular fibrillation. *Ann Emerg Med*. 1981;10:420-423.

70. Haynes RE, Chinn TL, Copass MK, Cobb LA. Comparison of bretylium tosylate and lidocaine in management of out-of-hospital ventricular fibrillation: a randomized clinical trial. *Am J Cardiol*. 1981;48:353-356.

71. Olson DW, Thompson BM, Darin JC, Milbrath MH. A randomized comparison study of bretylium tosylate and lidocaine in resuscitation of patients from out-of-hospital ventricular fibrillation in a paramedic system. *Ann Emerg Med*. 1984;13(pt 2):807-810.

72. Chow MS, Kluger J, DiPersio DM, Lawrence R, Fieldman A. Antifibrillatory effects of lidocaine and bretylium immediately post-cardiopulmonary resuscitation. *Am Heart J.* 1985;110:938-943.

73. Anderson JL. Symposium on the management of ventricular dys-rhythmias: antifibrillatory versus antiectopic therapy. *Am J Cardiol.* 1984;54:7A-13A.

74. Gottlieb SS, Packer M. Deleterious hemodynamic effects of lidocaine in severe congestive heart failure. *Am Heart J.* 1989;110:611-612.

75. Applebaum D, Halperin E. Asystole following a conventional thera-peutic dose of lidocaine. *Am J Emerg Med.* 1986;4:143-145.

76. Lown B. Lidocaine to prevent ventricular fibrillation: easy does it. *N Engl J Med.* 1985;313:1154-1156. Editorial.

77. Lie KI, Wellens HJ, van Capelle FJ, Durrer D. Lidocaine in the pre-vention of primary ventricular fibrillation: a double-blind, random-ized study of 212 consecutive patients. *N Engl J Med.* 1974;291:1324-1326.

78. DeSilva RA, Hennekens CH, Lown B, Casscells W. Lignocaine prophylaxis in acute myocardial infarction: an evaluation of ran-domized trials. *Lancet.* 1981;2:855-858.

79. Koster RW, Dunning AJ. Intramuscular lidocaine for prevention of lethal arrhythmias in the prehospitalization phase of acute myocar-dial infarction. *N Engl J Med.* 1985;313:1105-1110.

80. MacMahon S, Collins R, Peto R, Koster RW, Yusuf S. Effects of prophylactic lidocaine in suspected acute myocardial infarction: an overview of results from the randomized, controlled trials. *JAMA.* 1988;260:1910-1916.

81. Kuck KH, Jannasch B, Schluter M, Schafer J, Mathey DG. Ineffective use of lidocaine in preventing reperfusion arrhythmias in patients with acute myocardial infarction. *Z Kardiol.* 1985;74:185-190.

82. Hine LK, Laird N, Hewitt P, Chalmers TC. Meta-analytic evidence against prophylactic use of lidocaine in acute myocardial infarction. *Arch Intern Med.* 1989;149:2694-2698.

83. Antman EM, Berlin JA. Declining incidence of ventricular fibrillation in myocardial infarction: implications for the prophylactic use of lidocaine. *Circulation.* 1992;86:764-773.

84. Carruth JE, Silverman ME. Ventricular fibrillation complicating acute myocardial infarction: reasons against the routine use of lido-caine. *Am Heart J.* 1982;104:545-550.

85. Dunn HM, McComb JM, Kinney CD, Campbell NP, Shanks RG, MacKenzie G, Adgey AA. Prophylactic lidocaine in the early phase of suspected myocardial infarction. *Am Heart J.* 1985;110:353-362.

86. Akhtar M, Shenasa M, Jazayeri M, Caceres J, Tchou PJ. Wide QRS complex tachycardia: reappraisal of a common problem. *Ann Intern Med.* 1988;109:905-912.

87. Benowitz N, Forsyth FP, Melmon KL, Rowland M. Lidocaine dispo-sition kinetics in monkey and man, I: prediction by a perfusion model. *Clin Pharmacol Ther.* 1974;16:87-98.

88. Benowitz NL. Clinical applications of the pharmacokinetics of lido-caine. In: Melmon KL, ed. *Cardiovascular Drug Therapy.* Philadelphia, Pa: FA Davis Co; 1974:77-101.

89. Stargel WW, Shand DG, Routledge PA, Barchowsky A, Wagner GS. Clinical comparison of rapid infusion and multiple injection methods for lidocaine loading. *Am Heart J.* 1981;102:872-876.

90. Barsan WG, Levy RC, Weir H. Lidocaine levels during CPR: differ-ences after peripheral venous, central venous, and intracardiac injection. *Ann Emerg Med.* 1981;10:73-78.

91. Chow MS, Ronfeld RA, Hamilton RA, Helmink R, Fieldman A. Effect of external cardiopulmonary resuscitation on lidocaine phar-macokinetics in dogs. *J Pharmacol Exp Ther.* 1983;224:531-537.

92. Thomson PD, Melmon KL, Richardson JA, Cohn K, Steinbrunn W, Cudihee R, Rowland M. Lidocaine pharmacokinetics in advanced heart failure, liver disease, and renal failure in humans. *Ann Intern Med.* 1973;78:499-508.

93. Thomson PD, Rowland M, Melmon KL. The influence of heart fail-ure, liver disease, and renal failure on the disposition of lidocaine in man. *Am Heart J.* 1971;82:417-421.

94. Davison R, Parker M, Atkinson AJ Jr. Excessive serum lidocaine levels during maintenance infusions: mechanisms and prevention. *Am Heart J.* 1982;104:203-208.

95. Pfeifer HJ, Greenblatt DJ, Koch-Weser J. Clinical use and toxicity of intravenous lidocaine: a report from the Boston Collaborative Drug Surveillance Program. *Am Heart J.* 1976;92:168-173.

96. Kunkel FW, Rowland M, Scheinman MM. Effects of intravenous lidocaine infusion (LI) on atrioventricular (AV) and intraventricular (IV) conduction in patients with bilateral bundle branch block (BBB). *Circulation.* 1973;48(suppl 4):188. Abstract.

97. Giardina EG, Heissenbuttel RH, Bigger JT Jr. Intermittent intra-venous procaine amide to treat ventricular arrhythmias: correlation of plasma concentration with effect on arrhythmia, electrocardio-gram, and blood pressure. *Ann Intern Med.* 1973;78:183-193.

98. Kastor JA, Josephson ME, Guss SB, Horowitz LN. Human ven-tricular refractoriness, II: effects of procainamide. *Circulation.* 1977;56:462-467.

99. Arnsdorf MF. Electrophysiologic properties of antidysrhythmic drugs as a rational basis for therapy. *Med Clin North Am.* 1976;60:213-232.

100. Fenster PE, Comess KA, Marsh R, Katzenberg C, Hager WD. Conversion of atrial fibrillation to sinus rhythm by acute intra-venous procainamide infusion. *Am Heart J.* 1983;106:501-504.

101. Morady F, Kou WH, Schmaltz S, Annesley T, DeBuitleir M, Nelson SD, Kushner JA. Pharmacodynamics of intravenous procainamide as used during acute electropharmacologic testing. *Am J Cardiol.* 1988;61:93-98.

102. Lima JJ, Goldfarb AL, Conti DR, Golden LH, Bascomb BL, Benedetti GM, Jusko WJ. Safety and efficacy of procainamide infusions. *Am J Cardiol.* 1979;43:98-105.

103. Harrison DC, Sprouse JH, Morrow AG. The antiarrhythmic proper-ties of lidocaine and procaine amide: clinical and physiologic studies of their cardiovascular effects in man. *Circulation.* 1963;28:486-491.

104. Euler DE, Scanlon PJ. Mechanism of the effect of bretylium on the ventricular fibrillation threshold in dogs. *Am J Cardiol.* 1985;55:1396-1401.

105. Koo CC, Allen JD, Pantridge JF. Lack of effect of bretylium tosy-late on electrical ventricular defibrillation in a controlled study. *Cardiovasc Res.* 1984;18:762-767.

106. Dollery CT, Emslie-Smith D, McMichael J. Bretylium tosylate in the treatment of hypertension. *Lancet.* 1960;1:296-299.

107. Leveque PE. Anti-arrhythmic action of bretylium. *Nature.* 1965;207:203-204.

108. Koch-Weser J. Drug therapy: bretylium. *N Engl J Med.* 1979;300:473-477.

109. Markis JE, Koch-Weser J. Characteristics and mechanism of ino-tropic and chronotropic actions of bretylium tosylate. *J Pharmacol Exp Ther.* 1971;178:94-102.

110. Heissenbuttel RH, Bigger JT Jr. Bretylium tosylate: a newly avail-able antiarrhythmic drug for ventricular arrhythmias. *Ann Intern Med.* 1979;91:229-238.

111. Sasyniuk BI. Symposium on the management of ventricular dys-rhythmias: concept of reentry versus automaticity. *Am J Cardiol.* 1984;54:1A-6A.

112. Anderson JL. Symposium on the management of ventricular dys-rhythmias: antifibrillatory versus antiectopic therapy. *Am J Cardiol.* 1984;54:7A-13A.

113. Bigger JT Jr, Jaffe CC. The effect of bretylium tosylate on the electrophysiologic properties of ventricular muscle and Purkinje fibers. *Am J Cardiol.* 1971;27:82-92.

114. Cardinal R, Sasyniuk BI. Electrophysiological effects of bretylium tosylate on subendocardial Purkinje fibers from infarcted canine hearts. *J Pharmacol Exp Ther.* 1978;204:159-174.

115. Ideker RE, Klein GJ, Harrison L, et al. Epicardial mapping of the initiation of ventricular fibrillation induced by reperfusion following acute ischemia. *Circulation.* 1978;64(suppl 2):II-57-II-58.

116. Holder DA, Sniderman AD, Fraser G, Fallen EL. Experience with bretylium tosylate by a hospital cardiac arrest team. *Circulation.* 1977;55:541-544.

117. Euler DE, Zeman TW, Wallock ME, Scanlon PJ. Deleterious effects of bretylium on hemodynamic recovery from ventricular fibrillation. *Am Heart J.* 1986;112:25-31.

118. Anderson JL. Bretylium tosylate: profile of the only available class III antiarrhythmic agent. *Clin Ther.* 1985;7:205-224.

119. Ellrodt G, Chew CY, Singh BN. Therapeutic implications of slow-channel blockade in cardiocirculatory disorders. *Circulation.* 1980;62:669-679.

120. Antman EM, Stone PH, Muller JE, Braunwald E. Calcium channel blocking agents in the treatment of cardiovascular disorders, part I: basic and clinical electrophysiologic effects. *Ann Intern Med.* 1980;93:875-885.

121. Singh BN, Collett JT, Chew CY. New perspectives in the pharma-cologic therapy of cardiac arrhythmias. *Prog Cardiovasc Dis.* 1980;22:243-301.

122. Weiss AT, Lewis BS, Halon DA, Hasin Y, Gotsman MS. The use of calcium with verapamil in the management of supraventricular tachyarrhythmias. *Int J Cardiol.* 1983;4:275-284.

123. Waxman HL, Myerburg RJ, Appel R, Sung RJ. Verapamil for control of ventricular rate in paroxysmal supraventricular tachycardia and atrial fibrillation or flutter: a double-blind randomized crossover study. *Ann Intern Med.* 1981;94:1-6.

124. Sung RJ, Elser B, McAllister RG Jr. Intravenous verapamil for termination of re-entrant supraventricular tachycardias: intracardiac studies correlated with plasma verapamil concentrations. *Ann Intern Med.* 1980;93:682-689.

125. McGoon MD, Vlietstra RE, Holmes DR Jr, Osborn JE. The clinical use of verapamil. *Mayo Clin Proc.* 1982;57:495-510.

126. Rozanski JJ, Zaman L, Castellanos A. Electrophysiologic effects of diltiazem hydrochloride on supraventricular tachycardia. *Am J Cardiol.* 1982;49:621-628.

127. Chaffman M, Brogden RN. Diltiazem: a review of its pharmacological properties and therapeutic efficacy. *Drugs.* 1985;29:387-454.

128. Dougherty AH, Jackman WM, Naccarelli GV, Friday KJ, Dias VC. Acute conversion of paroxysmal supraventricular tachycardia with intravenous diltiazem, IV: Diltiazem Study Group. *Am J Cardiol.* 1992;70:587-592.

129. Salerno DM, Dias VC, Kleiger RE, Tschida VH, Sung RJ, Sami M, Giorgi LV. Efficacy and safety of intravenous diltiazem for treatment of atrial fibrillation and atrial flutter: the Diltiazem-Atrial Fibrillation/Flutter Study Group. *Am J Cardiol.* 1989;63:1046-1051.

130. Ellenbogen KA, Dias VC, Plumb VJ, Heywood JT, Mirvis DM. A placebo-controlled trial of continuous intravenous diltiazem infusion for 24-hour heart rate control during atrial fibrillation and atrial flutter: a multicenter study. *J Am Coll Cardiol.* 1991;18:891-897.

131. Shigenobu K, Schneider JA, Sperelakis N. Verapamil blockade of slow Na+ and Ca++ responses in myocardial cells. *J Pharmacol Exp Ther.* 1974;190:280-288.

132. Nayler WG, Szeto J. Effect of verapamil on contractility, oxygen utilization, and calcium exchangeability in mammalian heart muscle. *Cardiovasc Res.* 1972;6:120-128.

133. Haeusler G. Differential effect of verapamil on excitation-contraction coupling in smooth muscle and on excitation-secretion coupling in adrenergic nerve terminals. *J Pharmacol Exp Ther.* 1972;180:672-682.

134. Winbury MM, Howe BB, Hefner MA. Effect of nitrates and other coronary dilators on large and small coronary vessels: a hypothesis for the mechanism of action of nitrates. *J Pharmacol Exp Ther.* 1969;168:70-95.

135. Hwang MH, Danoviz J, Pacold I, Rad N, Loeb HS, Gunnar RM. Double-blind crossover randomized trial of intravenously administered verapamil: its use for atrial fibrillation and flutter following open heart surgery. *Arch Intern Med.* 1984;144:491-494.

136. Plumb VJ, Karp RB, Kouchoukos NT, Zorn GL Jr, James TN, Waldo AL. Verapamil therapy of atrial fibrillation and atrial flutter following cardiac operation. *J Thorac Cardiovasc Surg.* 1982;83:590-596.

137. Wit AL, Cranefield PF. Effect of verapamil on the sinoatrial and atrioventricular nodes of the rabbit and the mechanism by which it arrests reentrant atrioventricular nodal tachycardia. *Circ Res.* 1974;35:413-425.

138. Wellens HJ, Tan SL, Bar FW, Duren DR, Lie KI, Dohmen HM. Effect of verapamil studied by programmed electrical stimulation of the heart in patients with paroxysmal re-entrant supraventricular tachycardia. *Br Heart J.* 1977;39:1058-1066.

139. Spear JF, Horowitz LN, Moore EN, et al. Verapamil-sensitive 'slow-response' activity in infarcted human ventricular myocardium. *Circulation.* 1976;54(suppl 2):II-71-II-75.

140. Josephson ME, Kastor JA. Supraventricular tachycardia: mechanisms and management. *Ann Intern Med.* 1977;87:346-358.

141. Soler-Soler J, Sagrista-Sauleda J, Cabrera A, Sauleda-Pares J, Iglesias-Berengue J, Permanyer-Miralda G, Roca-Llop J. Effect of verapamil in infants with paroxysmal supraventricular tachycardia. *Circulation.* 1979;59:876-879.

142. Spurrell RA, Krikler DM, Sowton E. Effects of verapamil on electrophysiological properties of anomalous atrioventricular connexion in Wolff-Parkinson-White syndrome. *Br Heart J.* 1974;36:256-264.

143. Gulamhusein S, Ko P, Carruthers SG, Klein GJ. Acceleration of the ventricular response during atrial fibrillation in the Wolff-Parkinson-White syndrome after verapamil. *Circulation.* 1982; 65:348-354.

144. Harper RW, Whitford E, Middlebrook K, Federman J, Anderson S, Pitt A. Effects of verapamil on the electrophysiologic properties of the accessory pathway in patients with the Wolff-Parkinson-White syndrome. *Am J Cardiol.* 1982;50:1323-1330.

145. McGovern B, Garan H, Ruskin JN. Precipitation of cardiac arrest by verapamil in patients with Wolff-Parkinson-White syndrome. *Ann Intern Med.* 1986;104:791-794.

146. Gulamhusein S, Ko P, Klein GJ. Ventricular fibrillation following verapamil in the Wolff-Parkinson-White syndrome. *Am Heart J.* 1983;106:145-147.

147. Jacob AS, Nielsen DH, Gianelly RE. Fatal ventricular fibrillation following verapamil in Wolff-Parkinson-White syndrome with atrial fibrillation. *Ann Emerg Med.* 1985;14:159-160.

148. Klein GJ, Bashore TM, Sellers TD, Pritchett EL, Smith WM, Gallagher JJ. Ventricular fibrillation in the Wolff-Parkinson-White syndrome. *N Engl J Med.* 1979;301:1080-1085.

149. Sung RJ, Castellanos A, Mallon SM, Bloom MG, Gelband H, Myerburg RJ. Mechanisms of spontaneous alternation between reciprocating tachycardia and atrial flutter-fibrillation in the Wolff-Parkinson-White syndrome. *Circulation.* 1977;56:409-416.

150. Stewart RB, Bardy GH, Greene HL. Wide complex tachycardia: misdiagnosis and outcome after emergent therapy. *Ann Intern Med.* 1986;104:766-771.

151. Morady F, Baerman JM, DiCarlo LA Jr, DeBuitleir M, Krol RB, Wahr DW. A prevalent misconception regarding wide-complex tachycardias. *JAMA.* 1985;254:2790-2792.

152. Dolan DL. Intravenous calcium before verapamil to prevent hypotension. *Ann Emerg Med.* 1991;20:588-589.

153. Hariman RJ, Mangiardi LM, McAllister RG Jr, Surawicz B, Shabetai R, Kishida H. Reversal of the cardiovascular effects of verapamil by calcium and sodium: differences between electrophysiologic and hemodynamic response. *Circulation.* 1979; 59:797-804.

154. Ferlinz J, Easthope JL, Aronow WS. Effects of verapamil on myocardial peformance in coronary disease. *Circulation.* 1979; 59:313-319.

155. Chew CY, Hecht HS, Collett JT, McAllister RG, Singh BN. Influence of severity of ventricular dysfunction on hemodynamic responses to intravenously administered verapamil in ischemic heart disease. *Am J Cardiol.* 1981;47:917-922.

156. Schamroth L, Krikler DM, Garrett C. Immediate effects of intravenous verapamil in cardiac arrhythmias. *Br Med J.* 1972;1: 660-662.

157. DiMarco JP, Sellers TD, Berne RM, West GA, Belardinelli L. Adenosine: electrophysiologic effects and therapeutic use for terminating paroxysmal supraventricular tachycardia. *Circulation.* 1983;68:1254-1263.

158. DiMarco JP, Sellers TD, Lerman BB, Greenberg ML, Berne RM, Belardinelli L. Diagnostic and therapeutic use of adenosine in patients with supraventricular tachyarrhythmias. *J Am Coll Cardiol.* 1985;6:417-425.

159. Camm AJ, Garratt CJ. Adenosine and supraventricular tachycardia. *N Engl J Med.* 1991;325:1621-1629.

160. Ellenbogen KA, Thames MD, DiMarco JP, Sheehan H, Lerman BB. Electrophysiological effects of adenosine in the transplanted human heart: evidence of supersensitivity. *Circulation.* 1990;81: 821-828.

161. Dyckner T, Wester PO. Magnesium in cardiology. *Acta Med Scand.* 1982;661(suppl):27-31.

162. Ebel H, Gunther T. Role of magnesium in cardiac disease. *J Clin Chem Clin Biochem.* 1983;21:249-265.

163. Hollifield JW. Potassium and magnesium abnormalities: diuretics and arrhythmias in hypertension. *Am J Med.* 1984;77:28-32.

164. Rasmussen HS, McNair P, Norregard P, Backer V, Lindeneg O, Balslev S. Intravenous magnesium in acute myocardial infarction. *Lancet.* 1986;1:234-236.

165. Ceremuzynski L, Jurgiel R, Kulakowski P, Gebalska J. Threatening arrhythmias in acute myocardial infarction are prevented by intravenous magnesium sulfate. *Am Heart J.* 1989;118:1333-1334.

166. Horner SM. Efficacy of intravenous magnesium in acute myocardial infarction in reducing arrhythmias and mortality: meta-analysis of magnesium in acute myocardial infarction. *Circulation.* 1992; 86:774-779.

167. Ott P, Fenster P. Should magnesium be part of the routine therapy for acute myocardial infarction? *Am Heart J.* 1992;124:1113-1118.

168. Woods KL, Fletcher S, Roffe C, Haider Y. Intravenous magnesium sulfate in suspected acute myocardial infarction: results of the second Leicester Intravenous Magnesium Intervention Trial (LIMIT-2). *Lancet*. 1992;339:1553-1558.

169. Seelig MS. Magnesium in acute myocardial infarction (International Study of Infarct Survival 4). *Am J Cardiol*. 1991;68:1221-1222.

170. Ornato JP, Gonzalez ER. Refractory ventricular fibrillation. *Emerg Decisions*. 1986;4:35-41.

171. Ditchey RV, Winkler JV, Rhodes CA. Relative lack of coronary blood flow during closed-chest resuscitation in dogs. *Circulation*. 1982;66:297-302.

172. von Planta M, Weil MH, Gazmuri RJ, Bisera J, Rackow EC. Myocardial acidosis associated with CO_2 production during cardiac arrest and resuscitation. *Circulation*. 1989;80:684-692.

173. Gudipati CV, Weil MH, Gazmuri RJ, Deshmukh HG, Bisera J, Rackow EC. Increases in coronary vein CO_2 during cardiac resuscitation. *J Appl Physiol*. 1990;68:1405-1408.

174. Falk JL, Rackow EC, Weil MH. End-tidal carbon dioxide concentration during cardiopulmonary resuscitation. *N Engl J Med*. 1988;318:607-611.

175. Weil MH, Rackow EC, Trevino R, Grundler W, Falk JL, Griffel MI. Difference in acid-base state between venous and arterial blood during cardiopulmonary resuscitation. *N Engl J Med*. 1986;315:153-156.

176. Adrogue HJ, Rashad MN, Gorin AB, Yacoub J, Madias NE. Assessing acid-base status in circulatory failure: differences between arterial and central venous blood. *N Engl J Med*. 1989;320:1312-1316.

177. Chazan JA, McKay DB. Acid-base abnormalities in cardiopulmonary arrest: varying patterns in different locations in the hospital. *N Engl J Med*. 1989;320:597-598. Letter.

178. Kette F, Weil MH, von Planta M, Gazmuri RJ, Rackow EC. Buffer agents do not reverse intramyocardial acidosis during cardiac resuscitation. *Circulation*. 1990;81:1660-1666.

179. Kerber RE, Pandian NG, Hoyt R, Jensen SR, Koyanagi S, Grayzel J, Kieso R. Effect of ischemia, hypertrophy, hypoxia, acidosis, and alkalosis on canine defibrillation. *Am J Physiol*. 1983;244:H825-H831.

180. Paradis NA, Martin GB, Goetting MG, Rivers EP, Feingold M, Nowak RM. Aortic pressure during human cardiac arrest: identification of pseudo-electromechanical dissociation. *Chest*. 1992;101:123-128.

181. Berenyi KJ, Wolk M, Killip T. Cerebrospinal fluid acidosis complicating therapy of experimental cardiopulmonary arrest. *Circulation*. 1975;52:319-324.

182. Ritter JM, Doktor HS, Benjamin N. Paradoxical effect of bicarbonate on cytoplasmic pH. *Lancet*. 1990;335:1243-1246.

183. Graf H, Leach W, Arieff AI. Evidence for a detrimental effect of bicarbonate therapy in hypoxic lactic acidosis. *Science*. 1985;227:754-756.

184. von Planta I, Weil MH, von Planta M, Gazmuri RJ, Duggal C. Hypercarbic acidosis reduces cardiac resuscitability. *Crit Care Med*. 1991;19:1177-1182.

185. Bishop RL, Weisfeldt ML. Sodium bicarbonate administration during cardiac arrest: effect on arterial pH, Pco_2, and osmolality. *JAMA*. 1976;235:506-509.

186. Mattar JA, Weil MH, Shubin H, Stein L. Cardiac arrest in the critically ill, II: hyperosmolal states following cardiac arrest. *Am J Med*. 1974;56:162-168.

187. Douglas ME, Downs JB, Mantini EL, Ruis BC. Alteration of oxygen tension and oxyhemoglobin saturation: a hazard of sodium bicarbonate administration. *Arch Surg*. 1979;114:326-329.

188. Guerci AD, Chandra N, Johnson E, Rayburn B, Wurmb E, Tsitlik J, Halperin HR, Siu C, Weisfeldt ML. Failure of sodium bicarbonate to improve resuscitation from ventricular fibrillation in dogs. *Circulation*. 1986;74(pt 2):IV-75-IV-79.0

189. von Planta M, Gudipati C, Weil MH, Kraus LJ, Rackow EC. Effects of tromethamine and sodium bicarbonate buffers during cardiac resuscitation. *J Clin Pharmacol*. 1988;28:594-599.

190. Kette F, Weil MH, Gazmuri RJ. Buffer solutions may compromise cardiac resuscitation by reducing coronary perfusion pressure. *JAMA*. 1991;266:2121-2126.

191. Paradis NA, Martin GB, Rosenberg J, Rivers EP, Goetting MG, Appleton TJ, Feingold M, Cryer PE, Wortsman J, Nowak RM. The effect of standard- and high-dose epinephrine on coronary perfusion pressure during prolonged cardiopulmonary resuscitation. *JAMA*. 1991;265:1139-1144.

192. Redding JS, Pearson JW. Resuscitation from ventricular fibrillation: drug therapy. *JAMA*. 1968;203:255-260.

193. Bircher NG. Sodium bicarbonate improves immediate survivorship and 24-hour neurological outcome after ten minutes of cardiac arrest in dogs. *Crit Care Med*. 1991;19:S87. Abstract.

194. Cingolani HE, Mattiazzi AR, Blesa ES, Gonzalez NC. Contractility in isolated mammalian heart muscle after acid-base changes. *Circ Res*. 1970;26:269-278.

195. Minuck M, Sharma GP. Comparison of THAM and sodium bicarbonate in resuscitation of the heart after ventricular fibrillation in dogs. *Anesth Analg*. 1977;56:38-45.

196. Poole-Wilson PA, Langer GA. Effects of acidosis on mechanical function and Ca^{2+} exchange in rabbit myocardium. *Am J Physiol*. 1979;236:H525-H533.

197. Cingolani HE, Faulkner SL, Mattiazzi AR, Bender HW, Graham TP Jr. Depression of human myocardial contractility with 'respiratory' and 'metabolic' acidosis. *Surgery*. 1975;77:427-432.

198. Todres D. The role of morphine in acute myocardial infarction. *Am Heart J*. 1971;81:566-570.

199. Zelis R, Mansour EJ, Capone RJ, Mason DT. The cardiovascular effects of morphine: the peripheral capacitance and resistance vessels in human subjects. *J Clin Invest*. 1974;54:1247-1258.

200. Ward JM, McGrath RL, Weil JV. Effects of morphine on the peripheral vascular response to sympathetic stimulation. *Am J Cardiol*. 1972;29:659-666.

201. Alderman EL. Analgesics in the acute phase of myocardial infarction. *JAMA*. 1974;229:1646-1648.

202. Lee G, DeMaria AN, Amsterdam EA, Realyvasquez F, Angel J, Morrison S, Mason DT. Comparative effects of morphine, meperidine and pentazocine on the cardiocirculatory dynamics in patients with acute myocardial infarction. *Am J Med*. 1976;60:949-955.

203. Semenkovich CF, Jaffe AS. Adverse effects due to morphine sulfate: challenge to previous clinical doctrine. *Am J Med*. 1985;79:325-330.

204. Niedergerke R. The rate of action of calcium ions on the contraction of the heart. *J Physiol*. 1957;138:506-515.

205. Weber A, Herz R, Reiss I. Role of calcium in contraction and relaxation of muscle. *Fed Proc*. 1964;23:896-900.

206. Borle AB. Calcium metabolism at the cellular level. *Fed Proc*. 1973;32:1944-1950.

207. Legato MJ. The myocardial cell: new concepts for the clinical cardiologist. *Circulation*. 1972;45:731-735.

208. Shapira N, Schaff HV, White RD, Pluth JR. Hemodynamic effects of calcium chloride injection following cardiopulmonary bypass: response to bolus injection and continuous infusion. *Ann Thorac Surg*. 1984;37:133-140.

209. Nerothin DD, Kaane PB. Calcium — vasodilator or vasoconstrictor? *Anesth Analg*. 1983;63:175-284.

210. Stanley TH, Isern-Amaral J, Liu WS, Lunn JK, Gentry S. Peripheral vascular versus direct cardiac effects of calcium. *Anesthesiology*. 1976;45:46-58.

211. Eriksen C, Sorensen MB, Bille-Brahe NE, Skovsted P, Lunding M. Haemodynamic effects of calcium chloride administered intravenously to patients with and without cardiac disease during neurolept anaesthesia. *Acta Anaesthesiol Scand*. 1983;27:13-17.

212. Stueven HA, Thompson BM, Aprahamian C, Tonsfeldt DJ. Calcium chloride: reassessment of use in asystole. *Ann Emerg Med*. 1984;13(pt 2):820-822.

213. Harrison EE, Amey BD. Use of calcium in electromechanical dissociation. *Ann Emerg Med*. 1984;13(pt 2):844-845.

214. Dembo DH. Calcium in advanced life support. *Crit Care Med*. 1981;9:358-359.

215. Carlon GC, Howland WS, Kahn RC, Schweizer O. Calcium chloride administration in normocalcemic critically ill patients. *Crit Care Med*. 1980;8:209-212.

216. White RD, Goldsmith RS, Rodriguez R, Moffitt EA, Pluth JR. Plasma ionic calcium levels following injection of chloride, gluconate, and glucepate salts of calcium. *J Thorac Cardiovasc Surg*. 1976;71:609-613.

Cardiovascular Pharmacology II

Chapter 8

This chapter discusses medications used to treat acute myocardial infarction and its complications (eg, congestive heart failure, hypotension, hypertension, and cardiogenic shock). At times these complications can occur with remote myocardial infarction or with other types of myocardial disease (eg, valvular disease). In patients with ischemic heart disease, these complications can exacerbate the imbalance between myocardial oxygen supply and demand. This may increase the likelihood of more severe myocardial ischemia and hemodynamic decompensation. Aggressive treatment with rapid-acting, parenteral agents titrated to desired hemodynamic end points is critical. A detailed understanding of the pharmacology and proper use of these agents is required to attain rapid hemodynamic improvement and to avoid morbidity. The drugs may be classified as follows:

Inotropic vasoactive agents
    Epinephrine
    Norepinephrine (levarterenol, L-norepinephrine)
    Dopamine
    Dobutamine
    Isoproterenol
    Amrinone
    Digitalis

Vasodilators/antihypertensives
    Sodium nitroprusside
    Nitroglycerin

β-Adrenergic blockers
    Propranolol
    Metoprolol
    Atenolol
    Esmolol

Diuretics
    Furosemide

Thrombolytics
    Anisoylated plasminogen activator complex
    Streptokinase
    Tissue plasminogen activator

"Clinical" Pharmacology

Other sections of this book provide a more in-depth discussion of the clinical use of certain agents. For example, thrombolytic therapy is discussed in the chapter on acute myocardial infarction. Inotropic vasoactive agents are presented in more detail and in a clinical context in the "Essentials" chapter.

Cardiovascular Adrenergic Receptors

Adrenergic receptors regulate cardiac, vascular, bronchiolar, and gastrointestinal smooth muscle tone.[1] There are three types of adrenergic receptors: α-adrenergic (α_1 and α_2), β-adrenergic (β_1 and β_2), and dopaminergic.[2-4] Catecholamines differ from one another in their binding affinity for adrenergic receptors (Table 1).

Table 1. Sympathomimetic Amines

Drug	Usual IV Dosage	Adrenergic Effect α	Adrenergic Effect β	Arrhythmogenic Potential
Epinephrine (Adrenalin)	0.5-1.0 mg	+	++	+++
	1-200 µg per min	++	+++	+++
Norepinephrine (Levophed)	2-80 µg per min	+++	++	++
Dopamine (Intropin)	1-2 µg/kg per min	+	+*	+
	2-10 µg/kg per min	++	++*	++
	10-30 µg/kg per min	+++	++	+++
Dobutamine (Dobutrex)	2-30 µg/kg per min	+	+++	++
Isoproterenol (Isuprel)	2-10 µg/min	0	+++	+++
Amrinone† (Inocor)	2-15 µg/kg per min	0	0*	++

*Increases renal and splanchnic blood flow.
†Phosphodiesterase inhibitor.

α_1 Receptors are present in the postsynaptic region of neurons in vascular smooth muscle. The stimulation of the vascular receptor leads to vasoconstriction. α_1 Receptors in myocardium mediate positive inotropic and negative chronotropic effects.[5] The relative potency of clinically available adrenergic agonists, on α_1 receptors, in order of increasing potency, is phenylephrine, norepinephrine, and epinephrine.[6]

Presynaptic α_2 receptors modulate vascular tone in large blood vessels[7] and provide a counter-regulatory mechanism for α_1-receptor activity. When these receptors are stimulated, release of norepinephrine is inhibited, decreasing adrenergic activity by limiting norepinephrine accumulation. In the central nervous system, stimulation of the α_2 receptors inhibits reflex arcs in the locus ceruleus, leading to peripheral vasodilation.[8,9] α_2 Postsynaptic receptors also can mediate arteriolar and venous vasoconstriction.[7]

Stimulation of β_1 receptors increases heart rate and myocardial contractility. Stimulation of β_2 receptors causes vasodilation and leads to relaxation of bronchial, uterine, and gastrointestinal smooth muscle. β_2-Receptor activity also modulates fat metabolism and glycogenolysis and drives potassium intracellularly, inducing hypokalemia.[10] This effect may play an important role in the induction of arrhythmias during ischemia and may explain the beneficial effects of β-adrenergic blockade both acutely and for secondary prevention of cardiac events after myocardial infarction. Stimulation of β_2-adrenergic receptors results in renin release, which is inhibited by high doses of β-blocking agents.

Low doses of dopamine stimulate dopaminergic receptors to produce renal and mesenteric vasodilation, but venous tone is increased by α-adrenergic stimulation.[11] At higher concentrations of dopamine, the α-adrenergic effects of dopamine produce renal and mesenteric vasoconstriction. Coronary arteries possess both α- and β-adrenergic receptors.[12,13]

Histochemical studies suggest that α-adrenergic receptors predominate in the larger epicardial coronary arteries and that β-adrenergic receptors predominate in the smaller arteries.[14] Stimulation of α-receptors (eg, by agents like norepinephrine or dopamine or by stimulation of sympathetic nerves) produces coronary vasoconstriction.[13-16] Coronary vasoconstriction usually is promptly antagonized by local metabolic factors such as adenosine, which are elaborated in response to cardiac work.[17] In patients with coronary artery disease, the coronary vasoconstriction from a given stimulus may be enhanced, and paradoxical responses due to endothelial injury are common.[18] Thus, catecholamines with α-agonist properties must be used with caution, if at all, in patients with acute ischemic disease. α_2-Postsynaptic receptors may be particularly important in mediating coronary vasospasm. Calcium channel blockers blunt α_2-receptor–mediated vasoconstriction, one reason for their efficacy in antagonizing coronary vasoconstriction.[7] Stimulation of β-adrenergic receptors generally results in coronary vasodilation.

Adrenergic tone is in balance with, and is to some extent modulated by, the parasympathetic nervous system, which has effects on electrophysiological function[19] and coronary vasomotion.[20] Other mechanisms that have been postulated for abnormalities in coronary vasomotion other than autonomic influences include (1) an imbalance between vasoactive platelet–mediated products such as thromboxane A_2 and prostacyclin; (2) endothelial dysfunction leading to paradoxical response to normal vasodilating stimuli; and (3) loss of vasodilating substances such as endothelium relaxing factor.[21]

Norepinephrine

Mechanism of Action

Norepinephrine is a naturally occurring catecholamine that differs chemically from epinephrine only by the absence of a methyl group on the terminal amine. Epinephrine and norepinephrine are approximately equipotent in their ability to stimulate β_1-adrenergic (cardiac) receptors, but their relative stimulatory effects on α_1- and β_2-adrenergic receptors are quite different. Norepinephrine is a potent α-receptor agonist with minimal effect on β_2 receptors. Norepinephrine increases myocardial contractility because of its β_1-adrenergic effects, whereas its potent α-adrenergic effects lead to arterial and venous vasoconstriction.[22]

Norepinephrine's positive inotropic and vasopressor effects have been used in the treatment of refractory shock. However, the increased vascular resistance induced by norepinephrine may counteract its inotropic effects. Norepinephrine increases blood pressure predominantly by elevating systemic vascular resistance and may not improve, but may actually diminish, cardiac output. Because norepinephrine increases myocardial oxygen demand, it can exacerbate myocardial ischemia, especially if coronary vasoconstriction is induced by stimulation of coronary α receptors. Norepinephrine should be used as an agent of last resort in the medical treatment of patients with ischemic heart disease.[23]

Indications

Norepinephrine is used for the treatment of hemodynamically significant hypotension refractory to other sympathomimetic amines. Norepinephrine is more likely to be useful when total peripheral resistance is low. Hypotension and low systemic vascular resistance occur rarely in patients with acute myocardial infarction[24] but are more common in patients with septic shock and neurogenic shock. The use of norepinephrine should be considered a temporizing measure. Successful management requires not only support of the blood pressure but also correction of the underlying abnormalities.

Dosage

Norepinephrine bitartrate USP is available in 4-mL ampules containing 1 mg norepinephrine base per milliliter (2 mg norepinephrine bitartrate per milliliter). It should be mixed in 250 mL of either 5% dextrose and water (D_5W) or saline to provide a concentration of 16 µg/mL of the norepinephrine base. Norepinephrine should be infused through a central venous catheter to minimize the risk of extravasation (see "Precautions"). Infusions of 0.5 to 1.0 µg/min are generally used as a starting dose. The infusion rate is then titrated to achieve the desired effect, which usually is the maintenance of an adequate blood pressure (one reasonable criterion is a systolic blood pressure of at least 90 mm Hg) at the lowest possible dose. The average adult dose is 2 to 12 µg/min. Patients with refractory shock may require large doses, up to 30 µg/min of norepinephrine to maintain an adequate blood pressure. Norepinephrine should be administered via a volumetric infusion system that ensures a precise flow rate. The use of this drug should be viewed as a temporizing measure, and the dose should be reduced or the infusion discontinued as soon as possible. Norepinephrine should be tapered slowly to avoid abrupt and severe hypotension.

Precautions

Because peripheral blood pressure measurements are often inaccurate when severe vasoconstriction is present, central intra-arterial pressure monitoring may be necessary for accurate determination of arterial pressure.[25] If the central and peripheral "cuff" pressures are the same, arterial monitoring should be discontinued. When continuous invasive arterial blood pressure monitoring is not used, cuff or Doppler blood pressure should be monitored every 5 minutes during titration and then at frequent intervals, based on the patient's hemodynamic status. In patients requiring vasopressor support with norepinephrine, hemodynamic monitoring should be carried out to assess changes in cardiac output, pulmonary occlusive pressure, and peripheral arterial resistance.

Norepinephrine increases myocardial oxygen requirements without producing a compensatory increase in coronary blood flow. This can be deleterious in patients with myocardial ischemia or infarction. Norepinephrine may precipitate arrhythmias, especially in volume-depleted patients and in patients with limited myocardial reserves. Norepinephrine is contraindicated when hypotension is due to hypovolemia except as a temporizing measure to maintain coronary and cerebral perfusion pressure until volume replacement can be achieved.

Extravasation of norepinephrine produces ischemic necrosis and sloughing of superficial tissues. If extravasation occurs, phentolamine (5 to 10 mg diluted in 10 to 15 mL of saline solution) should be infiltrated into the area to antagonize the norepinephrine-induced vasoconstriction and to minimize necrosis and sloughing.

Dopamine

Mechanism of Action

Dopamine hydrochloride is a chemical precursor of norepinephrine that stimulates dopaminergic, β_1-adrenergic, and α-adrenergic receptors in a dose-dependent fashion.[22] Dopamine also stimulates the release of norepinephrine. Low doses of dopamine (1 to 2 µg/kg per minute) stimulate dopaminergic receptors to produce cerebral, renal, and mesenteric vasodilation, but venous tone is increased owing to α-adrenergic stimulation.[11] Urine output may increase, but heart rate and blood pressure are usually unchanged. In the dosage range of 2 to 10 µg/kg per minute, dopamine stimulates both β_1- and α-adrenergic receptors. β_1-Adrenergic stimulation increases in cardiac output and partially antagonizes the α-adrenergic–mediated vasoconstriction. This results in

enhanced cardiac output and only modest increases in systemic vascular resistance.

At doses above 2.5 µg/kg per minute, dopamine produces substantial increases in venous tone and central venous pressures. At doses greater than 10 µg/kg per minute, the α-adrenergic effects of dopamine predominate. This results in renal, mesenteric, and peripheral arterial, and venous vasoconstriction with marked increases in systemic vascular resistance, pulmonary vascular resistance, and further increases in preload. Doses above 20 µg/kg per minute produce hemodynamic effects similar to those of norepinephrine.

As with all vasoactive agents, there is substantial variability in the response to dopamine. Accordingly, the drug must be titrated to hemodynamic effect. Dopamine increases myocardial work without compensatory increases in coronary blood flow.[26] The imbalance between oxygen supply and demand may result in myocardial ischemia.

Indications

Dopamine is indicated for hemodynamically significant hypotension in the absence of hypovolemia. One reasonable definition for the presence of significant hypotension is a systolic arterial blood pressure of less than 90 mm Hg associated with evidence of poor tissue perfusion, oliguria, or changes in mental status. Dopamine should be used at the lowest dose that produces adequate perfusion of vital organs. The presence of increased vascular resistance, pulmonary congestion, or increased preload is a relative contraindication to the use of dopamine. In these settings, dopamine should be used in low doses (1 to 2 µg/kg per minute) to enhance renal blood flow.

Treatment with dopamine is usually reserved for hypotension that occurs with symptomatic bradycardia or after return of spontaneous circulation. Norepinephrine should be added if more than 20 µg/kg per minute of dopamine is needed to maintain blood pressure. Gonzalez and colleagues[27] studied the vasopressor response to incremental doses of intravenous (IV) epinephrine (1, 3, and 5 mg) with and without dopamine (15 µg/kg per minute) in nine prehospital cardiac arrest victims. Epinephrine alone produced a significant ($P < .05$) dose-dependent vasopressor effect on systolic and diastolic blood pressure. The concomitant administration of epinephrine and dopamine did not produce an additive vasopressor effect. A recent study using a prolonged model of cardiac arrest shows that dopamine is less effective than epinephrine at improving hemodynamics during CPR.[28]

Immediately after resuscitation, higher doses of dopamine may be required to induce the transient hypertension recommended to improve cerebral perfusion. It is important to remember that dopamine's α-adrenergic effects, even at low infusion rates, elevate pulmonary artery occlusive pressure and may induce or exacerbate pulmonary congestion despite a rise in cardiac output (Figure).[11] Vasodilators (eg, nitroglycerin or nitroprusside) can be used to reduce preload and improve cardiac output by antagonizing increases in venous and arterial resistance produced by dopamine. The combination of dopamine and nitroprusside produces hemodynamic effects similar to those of dobutamine.[29]

Dosage

Dopamine is available for IV use only. The contents of one or two ampules (400 mg per ampule) should be mixed in 250 mL of D_5W. This yields a concentration of 1600 or 3200 µg/mL. The initial rate of infusion is 1 to 5 µg/kg per minute. The infusion rate may be increased

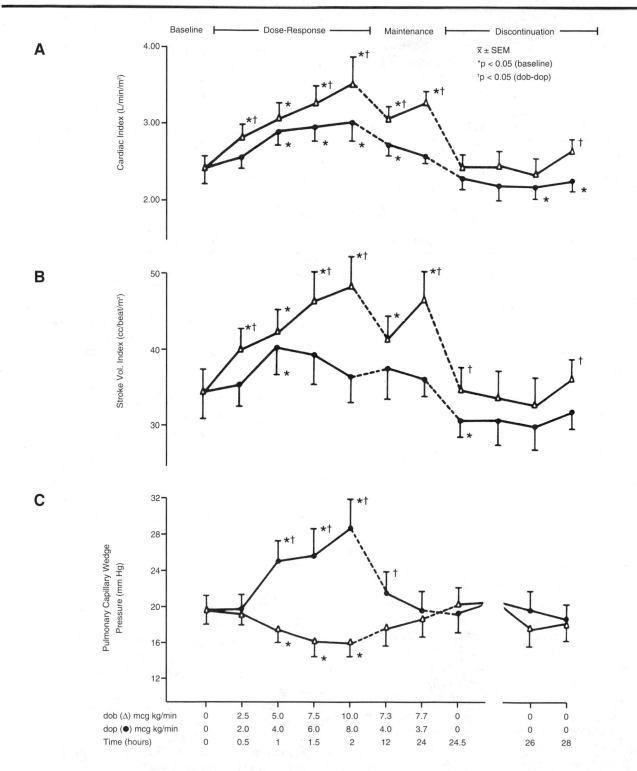

Graphs showing the effects of dopamine (dop) and dobutamine (dob) on cardiac index (A), stroke volume index (B), and the pulmonary capillary wedge pressure (C).

until blood pressure, urine output, and other indicators of end-organ perfusion improve. A final dosage range of 5 to 20 µg/kg per minute is recommended. To minimize side effects, the lowest infusion rate that results in satisfactory hemodynamic performance should be used. Dopamine should be administered via a volumetric infusion pump to ensure precise flow rates. Hemodynamic monitoring is essential for proper use of dopamine in patients who have ischemic heart disease or congestive heart failure. Monitoring should be instituted before, or as soon as possible after, initiation of treatment. Dopamine should be tapered gradually to avoid an acute hypotensive response.

Precautions

Dopamine will increase heart rate and may induce or exacerbate supraventricular and ventricular arrhythmias. Furthermore, even at low doses dopamine's venous and arterial vasoconstricting effects can exacerbate pulmonary congestion and compromise cardiac output. Occasionally these effects may require a reduction in dosage or discontinuation of the infusion. Despite hemodynamic improvements, myocardial oxygen consumption and myocardial lactate production may increase in response to higher doses of dopamine, indicating that coronary blood supply is not sufficiently augmented to compensate for the increased cardiac work. This imbalance between supply and demand would be expected to induce or exacerbate myocardial ischemia.[26] Nausea and vomiting are frequent side effects of dopamine, especially at high doses. Like norepinephrine, dopamine produces cutaneous tissue necrosis and sloughing if interstitial extravasation occurs. Treatment for dopamine-induced extravasation is similar to that for norepinephrine.

Monoamine oxidase inhibitors such as isocarboxazid (Marplan), pargyline hydrochloride (Eutonyl), tranylcypromine sulfate (Parnate), and phenelzine sulfate (Nardil) may potentiate the effects of dopamine. Patients receiving these agents should be treated with one tenth of the usual dose of dopamine. Agents with similar hemodynamic effects (eg, the initial effects of bretylium tosylate) may be synergistic with dopamine.[30] Patients receiving phenytoin may experience hypotension during concomitant administration of dopamine.[31] Like other catecholamines, dopamine may precipitate hypertensive crisis in patients with pheochromocytoma and is contraindicated.

Dopamine should not be added to solutions containing sodium bicarbonate or other alkaline IV solutions since dopamine is slowly inactivated at alkaline pH. The kinetics of this reaction are slow enough that dopamine and alkaline solutions (aminophylline, phenytoin, sodium bicarbonate) that are administered over a short period can be infused through the same venous catheter.[32]

Dobutamine

Mechanism of Action

Dobutamine is a synthetic sympathomimetic amine that exerts its potent inotropic effects by stimulating β_1- and α_1-adrenergic receptors in the myocardium.[33] Dobutamine stimulates peripheral α_1-adrenergic receptors, but this is antagonized by more potent β_2-adrenergic stimulation, leading to a mild vasodilatory response. Dobutamine-mediated increases in cardiac output also lead to a decrease in peripheral vascular resistance. At conventional doses (2 to 20 µg/kg per minute), dobutamine is less apt to induce tachycardia than either isoproterenol or dopamine. However, higher doses of dobutamine produce a tachycardic response. Dobutamine increases renal and mesenteric blood flow by increasing cardiac output. It does not produce direct renal and mesenteric vasodilation via dopaminergic receptors. However, urine volume and flow appear to increase equally with dopamine and dobutamine, suggesting that enhanced renal perfusion secondary to increased cardiac output is the most important determinant of renal function. The net hemodynamic effects of dobutamine are similar to those of dopamine combined with a vasodilator such as nitroprusside.[29] Dobutamine increases cardiac output and reduces pulmonary artery occlusive pressure and peripheral vascular resistance.[34]

The beneficial hemodynamic effects of dobutamine and its lack of induction of endogenous norepinephrine release minimize its effects on myocardial oxygen demand and produce a more favorable balance between oxygen supply and demand than either norepinephrine or dopamine.[33] Dobutamine's positive inotropic effect is also balanced by increased coronary blood flow.[26] For these reasons dobutamine does not increase infarct size or elicit arrhythmias when it is titrated to avoid significant increases in heart rate.[35] Heart rate may decrease as hemodynamics improve, but cardioacceleration should be avoided because this may aggravate myocardial ischemia. Direct measurement of central hemodynamics, including cardiac output, is required to assess the clinical response to dobutamine.

Dopamine and dobutamine have been used together.[36-38] The combination of moderate doses of both drugs (7.5 µg/kg per minute) maintains arterial pressure with less increase in pulmonary occlusive pressure and less pulmonary congestion than dopamine alone.[38] Combination therapy with dopamine and dobutamine produces significant hemodynamic improvements but does not alter survival in patients with cardiogenic shock.[37] Although inotropic and vasoactive agents may not alter mortality rates in some patients with severe cardiogenic shock, these agents can be used to maintain vital organ perfusion while other interventions (eg, myocardial revascularization) that can salvage the myocardium are undertaken.

Indications

Dobutamine is useful in the treatment of patients with pulmonary congestion and low cardiac output and in hypotensive patients with pulmonary congestion and left ventricular dysfunction who cannot tolerate vasodilators. Dobutamine and moderate volume loading are the treatment of choice in patients with hemodynamically significant right ventricular infarction.[39] Dobutamine may also be used to improve left ventricular work in patients with septic shock.

Dosage

Dobutamine may be effective at low doses (eg, 0.5 µg/kg per minute). The usual dosage range is 2 to 20 µg/kg per minute. The smallest effective dose should be used as determined by hemodynamic monitoring. Dobutamine-mediated increases in heart rates of more than 10% from initial values should be avoided in patients with coronary artery disease. Two to four ampules of dobutamine (250 mg per ampule) should be mixed in 250 mL of D_5W or normal saline. Dobutamine should be administered via a volumetric infusion pump to ensure precise flow rates.

Precautions

Dobutamine may cause tachycardia, arrhythmias, and fluctuations in blood pressure. It can provoke myocardial ischemia, especially if tachycardia is induced. Other side effects include headache, nausea, tremor, and hypokalemia.

Isoproterenol

Mechanism of Action

Isoproterenol hydrochloride is a synthetic sympathomimetic amine with nearly pure β-adrenergic-receptor activity.[22] Its potent inotropic and chronotropic properties frequently result in increased cardiac output despite a reduction in mean blood pressure due to peripheral vasodilation and venous pooling. However, isoproterenol markedly increases myocardial oxygen requirements and may induce or exacerbate myocardial ischemia. Newer inotropic agents (dobutamine, amrinone) that are less prone to induce ischemia or arrhythmias have replaced isoproterenol in most clinical settings.

Indications

Isoproterenol can be used for the temporary control of hemodynamically significant bradycardia in the patient with a pulse. The major indication now is for bradycardia in the denervated transplanted heart. Atropine, pacing, dopamine, and epinephrine should be used before isoproterenol for symptomatic bradycardia.

Electronic pacing provides better control than isoproterenol without increasing myocardial oxygen consumption and the risk of tachyarrhythmias. Pacing should be used instead of isoproterenol or as soon as possible after isoproterenol has been given as a temporizing measure. When used for chronotropic support, isoproterenol may exacerbate ischemia or hypotension. Isoproterenol's vasodilatory effects lower coronary perfusion pressure during cardiac arrest and increase the mortality rate in laboratory animal models.[40] Isoproterenol is contraindicated in the routine treatment of cardiac arrest.

Dosage

The dose of isoproterenol needed for chronotropic support is usually small. No more than 10 µg/min should be necessary. The initial starting dose is 2 µg/min, with gradual titration of the dose upward until a heart rate of approximately 60 beats per minute is reached. One milligram of isoproterenol is diluted in 250 mL of D_5W to yield a concentration of 4 µg/mL. Isoproterenol should be administered via a volumetric infusion pump to ensure a precise flow rate.

Precautions

Because isoproterenol increases myocardial oxygen requirements, it should be avoided in patients with ischemic heart disease. Isoproterenol's potent chronotropic properties can induce serious arrhythmias, including ventricular tachycardia (VT) and ventricular fibrillation (VF). Isoproterenol may also exacerbate tachyarrhythmias due to digitalis toxicity and may precipitate hypokalemia.

Amrinone

Mechanism of Action

Amrinone is a rapid-acting inotropic agent available for parenteral use. Amrinone is a phosphodiesterase inhibitor. Its inotropic and vasodilator effects are not reversed by adrenergic-blocking drugs or by norepinephrine depletion.[41] Amrinone has been studied extensively in patients with congestive cardiomyopathy, but its efficacy in patients with ischemic heart disease is not established.[42]

Amrinone's net hemodynamic effects are similar to those of dobutamine. Cardiac output increases and peripheral resistance and preload are diminished at doses between 2.0 and 15 µg/kg per minute. Higher doses produce a tachycardia similar to that observed with dobutamine.[42,43] Amrinone can exacerbate ischemia and should be used with caution, if at all, in patients with ischemic heart disease.[44] Monitoring of central hemodynamics is essential for proper dose titration during initiation of therapy with amrinone.

Indications

Amrinone should be considered for use in patients with severe congestive heart failure refractory to diuretics, vasodilators, and conventional inotropic agents.

Dosage

Since amrinone has a long half-life (4 to 6 hours), a loading dose of 0.75 mg/kg is recommended to promptly achieve therapeutic levels. Because the afterload-reducing effects of amrinone are directly proportional to dosage and rate of administration, the loading dose should usually not exceed 1 mg/kg. Although the loading dose may be given over 2 to 5 minutes, it is better to give it over 10 to 15 minutes to minimize the risk of hypotension in patients with significant left ventricular dysfunction and marginal blood pressures. The bolus dose is followed by a maintenance infusion begun at a rate of 2 to 5 µg/kg per minute and titrated up to a rate of 10 to 15 µg/kg per minute according to hemodynamic response.

Because of the potential for chemical incompatibility, amrinone lactate should not be diluted directly in dextrose-containing solutions before injection. It may be administered directly into a venous-access line flowing with dextrose-containing IV solutions. For continuous IV infusion, amrinone lactate injection should be diluted to a final concentration of 1 to 3 mg/mL in 0.45% or 0.9% sodium chloride. Amrinone infusions should be administered by means of an infusion pump that ensures a precise flow rate.

Precautions

Amrinone can induce or worsen myocardial ischemia. Hemodynamic monitoring is essential since changes in central hemodynamics may occur in the absence of changes in heart rate or blood pressure. To minimize side effects from amrinone, the lowest dose that produces the desired hemodynamic effect should be used.

Amrinone can cause thrombocytopenia in 2% to 3% of patients. This adverse effect is seen within 48 to 72 hours after initiation of therapy. The fall in platelets is rarely associated with significant bleeding and usually resolves when the drug is discontinued. Platelet reduction appears to be dose dependent and is likely due to an amrinone-induced decrease in platelet survival time. Other side effects include gastrointestinal upset, myalgia, fever, hepatic dysfunction, and ventricular irritability. Because amrinone contains metabisulfite, its use is contraindicated in patients allergic to sulfiting agents.

The Tapering of Vasoactive Drugs

Inotropic and vasoactive agents should be tapered gradually under close supervision. These agents affect neurohormonal control of blood pressure and circulatory

volume. Therefore, the infusion rate should be reduced gradually, and intravascular fluid should be repleted if necessary to avoid hypotension.

Digitalis Glycosides

Mechanism of Action

Digitalis glycosides have been used for decades to treat cardiac disorders. Digoxin is the form of digitalis glycoside now used almost exclusively in clinical practice.

Digoxin is used to increase myocardial contractility and to control the ventricular response to atrial flutter and fibrillation. The positive inotropic effect of digitalis is due to the inhibition of membrane-bound sodium potassium ATPase. This effect alters calcium flux and increases the concentration of calcium in the sarcoplasmic reticulum, which in turn increases contractility.[45] The inotropic effects of digitalis do not depend on catecholamine liberation and are unaffected by β-adrenergic receptor blockade.[46] Digitalis evokes vasoconstriction in coronary and mesenteric vascular beds.[47]

Digitalis exerts direct and indirect effects on the sinoatrial and atrioventricular (AV) nodes. It directly and indirectly (by increasing vagal tone) depresses impulse conduction through the AV node but increases the rate of atrial conduction. The proper dose of digitalis depends on the route of administration and the desired effect. Higher doses are often required to control the ventricular response to atrial fibrillation than for inotropic support. Digitalis toxicity is more common when the serum level is high. However, toxicity may be present with low serum levels, and it may be absent despite elevated levels, because it is the amount of digitalis glycoside in the myocardium and not the circulating blood level that determines toxicity.[48]

Indications

Digitalis helps control the ventricular response to atrial fibrillation or atrial flutter and may convert paroxysmal supraventricular tachycardia to normal sinus rhythm. In patients with left ventricular dysfunction, it may also convert atrial flutter to atrial fibrillation. Digoxin may be used for supraventricular rhythm disturbances if the patient is hemodynamically stable and does not require emergent electrical cardioversion. The inotropic effects of digoxin are less potent than those of parenteral inotropes, and it may cause significant toxicity and adverse drug interactions in critically ill patients.[49] Digitalis has little role in the management of acute congestive heart failure.[49] Recent clinical studies have confirmed that digitalis produces sustained hemodynamic benefits during chronic treatment and improves outcome in patients with congestive heart failure.[50,51]

Dosage

Digoxin can be administered either orally or IV. Intravenous digoxin administration avoids the problem of gastrointestinal absorption and produces a more rapid onset of action and peak effect than oral administration. Following IV administration, the negative chronotropic and dromotropic effects of digoxin are seen within 5 to 30 minutes, and peak effects in 1½ to 3 hours. The inotropic effects of digoxin lag slightly behind its electrophysiological response.

In nonemergencies, treatment can be initiated orally. Regardless of route of administration, the relatively long elimination half-time of digoxin (36 hours) necessitates administration of an initial loading dose. Loading doses of digoxin in the range of 10 to 15 µg/kg lean body weight generally provide therapeutic effect with minimum risk of toxicity.[52] The maintenance dose is affected by body size and renal function. Clinical guides to the adequacy of digitalization include control of supraventricular arrhythmias and improvement in congestive heart failure. Uses of the other digitalis preparations have been reviewed elsewhere.[45]

Precautions

Digitalis toxicity is a common and important problem occurring with an incidence varying from 7% to 20%.[53,54] Virtually every rhythm disturbance has been described with digitalis toxicity. The most frequent are atrial and ventricular premature complexes, ventricular bigeminy, and VT. Accelerated junctional rhythm or nonparoxysmal junctional tachycardia, paroxysmal atrial tachycardia with 2:1 AV block, and high levels of AV block are less common but are characteristic, electrocardiographic observations of digitalis excess. Noncardiac manifestations of digitalis toxicity include anorexia, nausea, vomiting, diarrhea, visual disturbances, and changes in mental status, including psychosis, lassitude, and agitation. Toxicity is more frequent in patients with hypokalemia, hypomagnesemia, or hypercalcemia.[54]

When digitalis toxicity is suspected, the drug must be stopped, and the serum digitalis concentrations should be measured. Although normal blood levels do not exclude toxicity, patients with serum digitalis concentrations above 2.5 ng/mL tend to be at greater risk for digitalis toxicity. Correction of coexistent hypokalemia is important. The serum potassium level should be increased until it is normal unless heart block is present. Caution is necessary in patients with heart block since it can be worsened by the administration of potassium. Additional treatment may include lidocaine, phenytoin, or propranolol for control of ventricular or supraventricular arrhythmias.[55,56] A temporary pacemaker may be required to treat high-grade AV block. Catecholamines are relatively contraindicated since they may aggravate the potential for serious ventricular arrhythmias.

Electrical cardioversion can be dangerous in the setting of clinical digitalis toxicity with arrhythmias and can precipitate a fatal ventricular arrhythmia. Cardioversion should be reserved for the treatment of life-threatening, hemodynamically significant arrhythmias. If cardioversion is necessary in a digitalis-intoxicated patient, the lowest possible energy levels (10 to 20 J) should be tried initially.[57] However, cardioversion is usually safely accomplished in patients with serum digoxin concentrations below 2 ng/mL.

Antidigoxin antibodies are the treatment of choice for massive digoxin overdose or refractory digitalis toxicity.[58] Massive overdoses of digitalis may induce hyperkalemia.[59] Because it induces mesenteric and coronary vasoconstriction, digitalis may induce ischemia or mesenteric infarction.[47] Multiple drug interactions with digitalis have been described.[52] Because quinidine, verapamil, and amiodarone reduce the elimination of digoxin from the body, patients receiving concurrent therapy with agents usually require a 50% reduction in the maintenance dose of digoxin to avoid a potentially toxic drug interaction.

Sodium Nitroprusside

Mechanism of Action

Sodium nitroprusside is a potent peripheral vasodilator with effects on both arterial and venous smooth muscle. Its effects are seen almost immediately and cease within minutes after the infusion is stopped. Nitroprusside is metabolized by red blood cells to hydrocyanic acid, which is converted to thiocyanate by the liver and excreted by the kidneys. Hepatic or renal dysfunction can affect the clearance of the drug and its potentially toxic metabolites, cyanide and thiocyanate.[60]

Nitroprusside is used in the emergency treatment of hypertension and heart failure. Nitroprusside reduces blood pressure by reducing peripheral arterial resistance and by increasing venous capacitance and thus preload. Arterial effects are not lost even when preload is markedly diminished, although tachycardia ensues.[61] In the absence of heart failure, cardiac output either falls or remains unchanged.

When heart failure is present, nitroprusside generally increases cardiac output by diminishing vascular impedance and increasing stroke volume.[62] The increase in stroke volume usually is sufficient to maintain the systemic blood pressure at or only slightly below the pretreatment level. In patients with left ventricular failure, nitroprusside-induced tachycardia suggests an inadequate (relative or absolute) left ventricular filling pressure.[63] The hemodynamic improvement induced in the presence of left ventricular failure or hypertension may be of particular significance to patients with ischemic heart disease. Nitroprusside reduces myocardial work and may therefore mitigate ischemia. However, some data suggest that nitroprusside also may reduce coronary perfusion to ischemic myocardium,[64] which may counterbalance some or all of the beneficial effects on myocardial work.

Numerous studies have reported improvement in left ventricular function, tissue perfusion, cardiac output, and clinical status in patients with low cardiac output and high systemic vascular resistance.[65,66] Nitroprusside tends to reduce pulmonary occlusive pressure to a greater extent than dobutamine because of its more potent venodilating effects and its ability to enhance diastolic relaxation of the left ventricle.[67,68]

Indications

Sodium nitroprusside is the parenteral treatment of choice for hypertensive emergencies when immediate reduction of peripheral resistance is necessary because it reduces blood pressure rapidly, it is easily titratable, it is generally well tolerated, and its action can be rapidly reversed if necessary simply by discontinuing the infusion. Nitroprusside is also very useful in the treatment of patients with acute left ventricular failure. Nitroprusside may be used when heart failure and pulmonary congestion are acute or poorly controlled by diuretic therapy. In this setting, combined therapy with dopamine and nitroprusside frequently is more effective than the use of either agent alone. The net hemodynamic effects of this combination are similar to the effects of dobutamine and may be less costly.[29] Since nitroprusside has the potential to induce myocardial ischemia, IV nitroglycerin with or without dobutamine is a preferred choice if diuretics do not adequately control patients with pulmonary edema and coronary artery disease.

Dosage

Continuous infusions of nitroprusside are prepared by adding 50 to 100 mg of nitroprusside (after reconstituting the dry powder in 2 to 3 mL of dextrose in water) to 250 mL of dextrose in water or 0.9% sodium chloride. The solution must be wrapped promptly in aluminum foil or another opaque material to protect it from deterioration upon exposure to light. The freshly prepared solution may have a very faint brownish tint without any change in drug potency. Nitroprusside in aqueous solution will react with a variety of substances to form highly colored reaction products. If this occurs, the infusion should be replaced. Once prepared, the solution should be used immediately.[60] Treatment should begin with an infusion rate of 0.1 µg/kg per minute titrated to the desired end point. Hemodynamic monitoring is essential for proper titration when treating congestive heart failure. The average therapeutic dose of nitroprusside ranges from 0.5 to 8.0 µg/kg per minute. Nitroprusside should be administered by an infusion system that ensures a precise flow rate.

Precautions

When treating congestive heart failure, monitoring of central hemodynamic pressures is essential for safety and proper titration of effect. Systemic arterial pressure must be monitored frequently. Hypotension is the most common adverse reaction seen with nitroprusside. Nitroprusside-induced hypotension may precipitate myocardial ischemia, infarction, or stroke. Hypoxemia and deterioration of the ventilation-perfusion relation can occur.[69,70] Elderly patients and volume-contracted patients may be more sensitive to the drug and should be treated with lower doses. There is controversy about the possibility that nitroprusside can reduce coronary blood flow and exacerbate ischemia despite a lower myocardial work load. In the presence of congestive heart failure, IV nitroglycerin has a similar hemodynamic profile but improves ischemia and is preferred over nitroprusside in patients with coronary artery disease.[71,72]

Nitroprusside is metabolized to thiocyanate by the liver. Thiocyanate intoxication due to nitroprusside is uncommon unless large doses of nitroprusside are given (greater than 3 µg/kg per minute), prolonged infusions are used (greater than 2 to 3 days), or the patient has renal failure. Blood levels of thiocyanate should be monitored when high or prolonged dosage regimens are used or renal failure is present. If blood thiocyanate levels remain below 10 mg/100 mL, continued use of the agent is usually safe. Signs of thiocyanate toxicity include tinnitus, visual blurring, changes in mental status, nausea, abdominal pain, hyperreflexia, and seizures. Cyanide toxicity is a rare complication of nitroprusside therapy in patients with hepatic dysfunction.[60]

Nitroglycerin

Mechanism of Action

Nitroglycerin relaxes vascular smooth muscle by binding to specific vascular receptors and causing the formation of disulfide bonds.[73] Nitrate preparations differ principally in their rate of onset, duration of action, potency, and route of administration. Although nitrates have multiple uses, only the use of sublingual and IV nitroglycerin for the treatment of angina pectoris, acute myocardial infarction, and left ventricular failure will be discussed here.

Nitroglycerin is effective in relieving angina pectoris. Relief usually occurs in 1 to 2 minutes but may take as long as 10 minutes.[74] In the past this response was considered useful as a clinical diagnostic test for angina,[75] but it is often misleading and should not be relied upon since other conditions (eg, esophageal spasm) can respond to nitrates as well. Nitrates relieve angina pectoris in part by dilating the smooth muscle of the venous system, which inhibits venous return and decreases intramyocardial wall tension. The decrease in left ventricular work and wall tension usually improves subendocardial perfusion. Nitroglycerin also dilates large coronary (conduit) arteries, antagonizes vasospasm, and increases coronary collateral blood flow to ischemic myocardium.[76,77] These effects are particularly important when myocardial ischemia is due to abnormal coronary vasomotion.[78] Sublingual nitroglycerin decreases left ventricular filling pressure without significantly lowering systemic vascular resistance. Cardiac output usually falls in response to the decreased preload or remains the same when left ventricular filling pressure is normal or elevated at the time of administration.[79,80]

In patients with congestive heart failure, IV nitroglycerin reduces left ventricular filling pressure and systemic vascular resistance.[81-83] The decline in ventricular volume and systolic wall tension decreases myocardial oxygen requirements and usually reduces myocardial ischemia.[84] The net effect is an increase in cardiac output. Intravenous nitroglycerin produces a slightly greater reduction of preload and a slightly lesser reduction of impedance than does nitroprusside.[85] Nitroglycerin loses its arterial effects when preload is reduced,[86] whereas nitroprusside retains its arterial effects even if preload is reduced.[61] Nitroglycerin does not usually increase heart rate if preload is adequate.

Indications

Sublingual nitroglycerin is the drug of choice for the treatment of an anginal episode. It is effective for exertional as well as rest angina. For angina pectoris one tablet (0.3 to 0.4 mg) should be given sublingually. The dose may be repeated twice at 5-minute intervals as needed. If the pain is not gone after three sublingual tablets, the patient should seek medical attention immediately. For acute relief of angina, nitroglycerin may be sprayed onto the oral mucosa using a lingual aerosol canister that delivers 0.4 mg nitroglycerin per metered spray. Topical nitroglycerin ointment provides an easy route of administration for acute as well as chronic therapy with nitroglycerin. One to two inches of 2% nitroglycerin ointment may be applied over a 2- to 4-inch area of the skin. Unlike the ointment preparation, nitroglycerin patches should not be used for acute therapy.

With unstable angina pectoris or myocardial infarction, IV administration of nitroglycerin is preferred. Although oral nitrates result in a similar reduction in the frequency of anginal pain in patients with unstable angina, oral administration produces variable bioavailability and has a delayed onset of action.[87] Patients with coronary vasospasm (Prinzmetal's variant angina) usually respond promptly to sublingual nitroglycerin.

Nitroglycerin is the parenteral agent of choice for the emergency treatment of congestive heart failure, particularly in patients with ischemic heart disease. In patients with congestive heart failure, IV nitroglycerin and sodium nitroprusside exert similar beneficial hemodynamic

effects.[85] Both lower systemic arterial resistance and increase venous capacitance. Intravenous nitroglycerin has slightly more potent venous effects and nitroprusside slightly more potent arterial effects. Arterial dilation with nitroglycerin is more critically dependent on preload.[61,86] Thus, either agent can be used to improve hemodynamics. Intravenous nitroglycerin is preferred in the setting of acute ischemic heart disease because of its potent antiischemic effects. Intravenous nitroglycerin may reduce infarct size when it is used to treat congestive heart failure[88] associated with infarction and in patients with inferior wall infarction.[89,90] Nitroglycerin also acutely inhibits infarct expansion. However, there are insufficient data to warrant the routine use of nitroglycerin to limit infarct size.[91]

Nitroglycerin is often used in conjunction with thrombolytic therapy and aspirin in patients with acute myocardial infarction.[92-94] It should decrease vasospasm at the site of plaque rupture and exert a synergistic antiplatelet effect with aspirin.[94,95] Recent data suggest that IV nitroglycerin may antagonize the action of heparin and alter the response to tissue plasminogen activator (alteplase). Carefully conducted, prospective, clinical trials have failed to show a consistent adverse interaction between nitroglycerin and heparin,[96] but an occasional patient may have a reduced anticoagulant response to heparin in the presence of IV nitroglycerin.[97] Preliminary studies suggest that there may be pharmacodynamic interaction between nitroglycerin and alteplase.[98] This interaction appears to diminish the thrombolytic potential of alteplase, probably by reducing plasma alteplase concentrations.

Nitroglycerin should be used cautiously in patients with acute myocardial infarction because it may induce hypotension, which can compromise coronary artery perfusion and aggravate myocardial ischemia.[92,93] A reduction in blood pressure of 10% or less has been deemed safe in patients with coronary artery disease.[89,90] Studies evaluating the response of the chest pain of patients with acute infarction have not shown a benefit from IV nitroglycerin.[89,99]

Dosage

When used sublingually, the recommended starting dose of nitroglycerin is 0.3 to 0.4 mg. The drug is less effective orally because of deactivation in the liver. A dose of 0.3 or 0.4 mg can be repeated at 5-minute intervals to a total dose of three tablets if discomfort is unrelieved.

Intravenous nitroglycerin may be administered by bolus or by continuous infusion.[100] A bolus of 12.5 to 25 μg nitroglycerin may be administered before the initiation of a continuous nitroglycerin infusion (200 to 400 μg/mL) at a rate of 10 to 20 μg/min. The infusion should be increased by 5 or 10 μg/min every 5 to 10 minutes until the desired hemodynamic or clinical response is achieved (eg, fall in systemic vascular resistance or left ventricular filling pressure, relief of chest pain). Most patients respond to 50 to 200 µg/min, and the lowest possible dose should be used. An occasional patient may require up to 500 µg/min. The pharmacologic effects of nitroglycerin are primarily dependent on the patient's intravascular volume and to a lesser extent on the dose administered. Hypovolemia blunts the beneficial effects of nitroglycerin and increases the risk of hypotension. Nitroglycerin should be administered by an infusion system that ensures a precise flow rate to minimize the risk of hypotension.

Recent data strongly suggest that the maintenance of sustained plasma nitroglycerin concentrations will rapidly induce tolerance to the hemodynamic effects of nitroglycerin.[101] Increasing the dose of nitroglycerin will temporarily overcome the tolerance that develops and reestablish the response in some but not all patients (so-called pseudotolerance). Intermittent dosing, with nitrate-free periods, and use of the lowest possible effective dose are strongly recommended to reduce the likelihood of nitrate tolerance.[102]

Precautions

Headache is a common consequence of therapy with nitroglycerin. Blood pressure may fall, resulting in nausea, giddiness, faintness, or syncope. Such symptoms are often aggravated by the erect position. Patients should be instructed to sit or lie down when taking nitroglycerin and to use the smallest dose that will relieve angina. Hypotension in a recumbent patient often responds to elevation of the legs. With chronic therapy patients usually accommodate to both the hypotensive effects and the headaches.

Hypotension sufficient to produce hypoperfusion is the most serious side effect of nitroglycerin, particularly in patients where perfusion is impaired because of arterial obstruction. Hypotension is best treated by stopping or reducing the dose of nitrates and then administering fluids. If bradycardia accompanies nitroglycerin-induced hypotension (ie, vasovagal reflex arc), atropine along with discontinuation of nitroglycerin and fluid replacement is the treatment of choice.[103] The rapid titration of IV nitroglycerin in patients with congestive heart failure requires hemodynamic monitoring to ensure efficacy and safety. Nitroglycerin may cause methemoglobinemia and ventilation-perfusion mismatch, which can result in hypoxemia.[104]

β Blockers: Propranolol, Metoprolol, Atenolol, and Esmolol

Mechanism of Action

β-Blocking agents attenuate the effects of circulating catecholamines by blocking their ability to bind to β-adrenergic receptors. Propranolol, metoprolol, atenolol,

and esmolol are available for IV use. Propranolol hydrochloride is a nonselective β blocker (ie, it affects both β₁- and β₂-adrenergic receptors) without intrinsic sympathomimetic activity.[105,106] Because it is nonselective, it has effects on both cardiac systems (negative inotropism and chronotropism) and pulmonary systems (bronchoconstriction). Metoprolol, atenolol, and esmolol are β₁-selective agents. At low doses (less than 200 mg/d for metoprolol and less than 300 µg/kg per minute for esmolol) these agents tend to inhibit mostly β₁ receptors.[106] At higher doses, metoprolol and esmolol lose their β₁ selectivity.[106,107]

β Blockers reduce heart rate, blood pressure, myocardial contractility, and myocardial oxygen consumption. These actions explain their effectiveness in the treatment of angina pectoris and hypertension. β Blockers can help control arrhythmias that are dependent on catecholamine stimulation for their initiation or propagation, perhaps in part by antagonizing β₂-mediated hypokalemia.[10,108] Propranolol has been reported to control recurrent episodes of VT or VF refractory to other antiarrhythmics, especially when these arrhythmias are caused by myocardial ischemia.

β Blockers are also useful in slowing the ventricular response and preventing atrial fibrillation, atrial flutter, and paroxysmal supraventricular tachycardia because they reduce AV nodal conduction. Some β blockers (eg, propranolol) have a quinidine-like effect on myocardial membranes and the cardiac action potential that facilitates their antiarrhythmic effect.[109,110]

β Blockers can reduce creatine kinase–determined infarct size in patients with Q-wave myocardial infarctions and can prevent reinfarction when given concomitantly with thrombolytic agents.[92,94,111] Experimental data suggest that β blockers may protect ischemic myocardium during coronary artery occlusion by reducing myocardial oxygen demand and by inhibiting lipid peroxidation during reperfusion.[94,111-113] The well-documented benefits of β blockers for prevention of sudden death after acute myocardial infarction are likely related to their antiadrenergic effects on ischemic burden and the threshold for malignant arrhythmias.

The effects of competitive inhibition of β-receptor sites by β blockers depends in part on receptor number and the level of circulating catecholamines. Differences in the drug metabolism among patients may also explain the lack of correlation between dose or plasma level and response. Following IV administration, propranolol and metoprolol produce a sustained response that lasts for 6 to 8 hours. Esmolol is rapidly metabolized by esterases in the cytosol of erythrocytes. Its elimination half-life is approximately 9 minutes (range, 5 to 23 minutes), and its duration of action is 15 to 20 minutes. The relative β₁ selectivity of esmolol and its short-lived action provide an extra margin of safety in patients who are critically ill, but the agent is more costly.

Indications

The primary indication for β blockers in emergency cardiac care is for control of recurrent VT, recurrent VF, or rapid supraventricular arrhythmias refractory to other therapies. β Blockers are most effective when these arrhythmias are attributable to excess β-adrenergic stimulation or are precipitated by myocardial ischemia. They are useful in patients with hypertension and tachycardia if left ventricular function is not severely depressed.

The use of β blockers in the setting of acute myocardial infarction is controversial. Some studies suggest a reduction in myocardial infarct size or mortality, or both, when β blockers are administered early after the onset of acute myocardial infarction.[113-117] Atenolol,[92] metoprolol,[118,119] and propranolol[120] significantly reduce the incidence of VF in acute myocardial infarction patients not treated with thrombolytic agents. β Blockers may also produce potential benefits in patients receiving thrombolytic agents.[94,121-124] When used within 4 hours after thrombolytic therapy, β blockade may reduce the rate of nonfatal reinfarction and recurrent ischemia. In thrombolytic-treated patients, β blockers may reduce mortality and recurrent myocardial infarction if administered within 2 hours of the onset of symptoms. However, these effects are observed only in patients at low risk and were not of sufficient magnitude to warrant a recommendation at this time of the routine use of β blockers in patients receiving thrombolytic agents.

There is conclusive evidence that chronic β-blocker therapy reduces mortality after myocardial infarction. The use of β blockers is recommended as prophylaxis for prevention of sudden death after myocardial infarction if there are no strong contraindications to their use.[118] The use of β blockers either acutely or for chronic prevention after acute myocardial infarction requires careful consideration of the patient's left ventricular function and co-existing medical problems.

Dosage

Intravenous β blockers should be administered slowly with frequent and careful monitoring of blood pressure, electrocardiogram, and clinical response. The recommended dose of atenolol is 5 mg IV over 5 minutes. Wait 10 minutes, then give a second dose of 5 mg slow IV (over 5 minutes). In 10 minutes, if the patient tolerates the dose well, an oral dose of 50 mg may be started. Then give an oral dose of 50 mg twice daily.

Metoprolol is given in IV doses of 5 mg over 2 to 5 minutes and repeated at 5-minute intervals to a total of 15 mg. An oral regimen is then initiated at a dose of 50 mg twice a day for at least 24 hours and increased to 100 mg twice a day.

Propranolol can be administered at an IV dose of 1 to 3 mg given over 2 to 5 minutes (not to exceed 1 mg/min). This dose can be repeated after 2 minutes to a total dose of 0.1 mg/kg. The oral maintenance regimen is 180 to 320 mg/d, given in divided doses.

Esmolol has a rapid onset and short duration and is used for brief, initial control of ventricular rate in patients with various supraventricular tachycardias. The agent reaches steady-state blood levels in 30 minutes. Rate control has generally been achieved by this time and the infusion can be titrated and stopped.

Esmolol hydrochloride is available in 10-mL ampules containing 2.5 g. It must be diluted to a final, maximal concentration of 10 mg/mL before administration. In general this is accomplished by placing the 2.5 g of esmolol in 250 mL of solution. The infusion of esmolol is begun with a loading dose of 250 to 500 μg/kg for 1 minute followed by a maintenance dose of 25 to 50 μg/kg per minute for 4 minutes. The maintenance infusion is titrated upwards by 25 to 50 μg/kg per minute at 5- to 10-minute intervals to a maximum of 300 μg/kg per minute.

Precautions

The principal adverse effects of β-blocking agents are precipitation of hypotension, congestive heart failure, and bronchospasm. Exercise caution for critically ill patients who may be dependent on β-adrenergic receptor support. Therapy may be hazardous when cardiac function is depressed, as is the case after cardiac arrest.

Congestive heart failure induced by β blockers can be managed with diuretics and vasodilators, but it often requires inotropic support. In patients with reactive airway disease, β-adrenergic blockers may produce serious and even fatal bronchoconstriction. Should bronchospasm occur, it can be managed by the administration of sympathomimetics and aminophylline. Treatment with β blockers is contraindicated in patients who exhibit significant AV block or bradycardia. Atropine may restore an adequate heart rate when bradycardia is induced by β blockers. If the bradycardia remains resistant to atropine, consider transcutaneous pacemakers, or dopamine or epinephrine infusions. Isoproterenol can be considered as a last resort.

Adverse effects from β blockers may be increased when β blockers are combined with other agents with similar actions (eg, calcium channel blockers, antihypertensive agents, and antiarrhythmic agents). Pharmacokinetic and pharmacodynamic drug interactions are also common with β blockers. For example, reduction in blood flow induced by β blockers may inhibit a drug's metabolism and potentiate its pharmacologic response (eg, lidocaine).[105,106]

Furosemide

Mechanism of Action

Furosemide is a potent, rapidly acting diuretic that inhibits reabsorption of sodium and chloride in the ascending loop of Henle.[125] In patients with pulmonary edema, IV furosemide exerts direct venodilating effects that reduce venous return and thus central venous pressures.[126] This effect is seen before the onset of diuresis. Diuresis begins roughly 10 minutes after treatment, reaches peak effect in about 30 minutes, and lasts for about 6 hours. These reductions in intravascular volume are generally associated with a decline in cardiac output, especially in patients with acute myocardial infarction.[127]

In patients with chronic heart failure and excess extravascular fluid, diuresis may be induced in part by changes in osmolarity. When this occurs, the egress of extravascular fluid into the intravascular space results in no net change in intravascular volume.[128] In addition, a generalized pressor response has been described when large doses of furosemide are administered IV to patients with chronic heart failure.[129]

In patients with acute myocardial infarction and other disease states associated with abnormal left ventricular compliance, diuretics must be used cautiously since small changes in volume may induce large changes in left ventricular pressure.[127] This may reduce cardiac output or induce hypotension, which can reduce coronary perfusion. Because the effects of diuretics on preload are synergistic with those of morphine and nitrates, combination therapy should be used with caution.

Indications

In emergency cardiac care, furosemide is indicated for the emergency treatment of pulmonary congestion associated with left ventricular dysfunction.

Dosage

The initial dose of furosemide is 20 to 40 mg IV (or 0.5 to 1.0 mg/kg as an initial dose and up to 2 mg/kg in toto). It should be injected slowly over at least 1 to 2 minutes. Patients who fail to respond to bolus administration of furosemide may respond to continuous infusions per hour.[130-133] Furosemide infusions at rates of 0.25 to 0.75 mg/kg per hour may produce adequate diuresis even in patients with renal dysfunction.[132] A prospective, randomized, crossover study in patients with severe congestive heart failure showed that furosemide infusions (2.5 to 3.3 mg/h for 48 hours preceded by a loading dose of 30 to 40 mg) produced significantly greater diuresis and natriuresis than an intermittent administration regimen (30 to 40 mg every 8 hours for 48 hours).[134] Total urine output increased by 12% to 26% and total sodium excretion increased by 11% to 33% ($P < .01$) without any difference in side effects.

Precautions

Dehydration and hypotension can result from overzealous diuresis. Sodium, potassium, calcium, and magnesium depletion are common and may pose a serious threat to patients with coronary heart disease as well as those receiving digitalis or antiarrhythmic agents. Hyperosmolality and metabolic alkalosis can occur. Since furosemide is a sulfonamide derivative, it may induce allergic reactions in patients with sensitivity to sulfonamides.

Thrombolytic Agents

Mechanism of Action

Thrombolytic agents activate both soluble plasminogen and surface-bound plasminogen to form plasmin. When generated close to the fibrin clot, plasmin digests fibrin and dissolves the clot. Streptokinase, urokinase, and anisoylated plasminogen streptokinase activator complex (anistreplase) are non–clot-selective thrombolytic agents. These agents stimulate the conversion of circulating plasminogen to plasmin and induce a systemic lytic response. Recombinant tissue plasminogen activator (alteplase) and recombinant single-chain urokinase plasminogen activator are fibrin-selective agents because they activate circulating plasminogen to a lesser extent than surface-bound plasminogen. However, fibrin selectivity is relatively dose dependent, and all agents will activate circulating plasminogen to different degrees. To date, fibrin specificity has not been shown to lower the risk of serious bleeding.

Three thrombolytic agents are currently available for clinical use in the United States: anistreplase, streptokinase, and alteplase. Comparative trials of streptokinase and a standard 3- to 4-hour infusion of alteplase demonstrate no difference in mortality rates between treatment groups in patients with acute myocardial infarction.[120] These trials either indicate the lack of early coronary patency as a determinant of benefit or may reflect the need to individualize adjunctive treatments to achieve previously documented increments in patency and survival. Alternative dosage regimens and combination regimens are undergoing current investigation to determine the benefits and risks of such strategies. Chapter 9 on acute myocardial infarction contains a discussion of thrombolytic agents that reflects results of the "megatrials" of thrombolytic therapy.

Thrombolytic agents available in the early 1990s are compared in Table 2. Note that this is an area of active research and rapid developments. Manufacturers' directions should be consulted for changes and dosing updates, and the clinical literature should be monitored for new data on the optimum use of adjunctive drugs.

Since clot formation is an ongoing process and is exacerbated by the administration of thrombolytic agents,[136,137] the adjunctive use of anticoagulant therapy should be helpful in achieving early coronary recanalization.[92,94,136] Studies show that continued activation of thrombin despite intense fibrinolysis may be a predisposing factor to both apparent initial failure of recanalization

Table 2. Comparison of Thrombolytic Agents

Agent	Half-life	Dose	Systemic Lytic State	Reperfusion Rate in Original Studies	Reocclusion Rate in Original Studies	Advantages	Disadvantages
Anistreplase	105 min	30 U bolus	++++	60-70%	10%	Long acting	Antigenicity, "lytic" effect, expensive
Streptokinase	90 min	1.5 million U over 1 hour	++++	50-60%	15%	Proven value, inexpensive	Antigenicity, "lytic" effect
Alteplase*	36 min	100 mg over 3 hours *Front-loaded regimen†:* • Give 15-mg bolus • Then 0.75 mg/kg over next 30 min (not to exceed 50 mg) • Then 0.50 mg/kg over next 60 min (not to exceed 35 mg) • Total dose ≤100 mg	+	65-75%	20%	Proven value, clot selective, nonantigenic	Expensive, inconvenient regimen, concurrent heparin

*Requires concurrent heparin administration.
†The front-loaded approach has shown success in controlled experimental trials but has not yet been approved by FDA for routine clinical use.
Adapted from Sherry.[135]

and overt early reocclusion.[136,137] Although alteplase may produce a sustained fibrinolysis despite its short half-life in the circulation,[138] the adjunctive use of anticoagulant therapy is useful in preventing reocclusion, especially with clot-specific activators (eg, alteplase).[92,94,139]

Indications

Thrombolytic therapy should be initiated as soon as possible after the onset of pain. Studies have not established a definite limit beyond which thrombolytics should not be given. It is indicated in young patients (eg, less than 70 years old) who have chest pain consistent with acute myocardial infarction with at least two 0.1 mV of ST-segment elevation in at least two contiguous ECG leads and have no contraindication to thrombolytics. In other patients, decisions on thrombolytic therapy are based on age, clarity of the diagnosis, presence of relative contraindications, and time from onset of chest pain (ie, between 6 and 12 hours).

Dosages

Anistreplase

To administer anistreplase, slowly add 5 mL of sterile water for injection to the vial containing anistreplase. Gently roll—do not shake—the vial to mix the powder with liquid. The reconstituted solution should be administered within 30 minutes. The 30-unit dose is administered over 5 minutes. The reconstituted solution should not be further diluted before administration or added mixed with other IV medications.

Streptokinase

Streptokinase powder for injection should be reconstituted with 5% dextrose injection or 0.9% sodium chloride injection. Gently roll—do not shake—the vial to mix the powder with liquid. For acute myocardial infarction, the IV dose of streptokinase is 750 000 to 1 500 000 IU, diluted to 45 mL. The dose is administered by infusion over 30 to 60 minutes. Do not mix with other IV medications.

Alteplase

Reconstitute the alteplase powder with diluent provided (sterile water for injection). Do not use bacteriostatic water for injection. Gently roll—do not shake—the vial to mix the powder with liquid. If further dilution to a concentration of 0.5 mg/mL is desired, use only 5% dextrose injection or 0.9% sodium chloride injection. Do not use other solution or preservative-containing solutions when further diluting the reconstituted solution, and do not mix with other IV medications. The alteplase solution should be used within 8 hours.

The standard regimen calls for a 10-mg bolus over 2 minutes, then 50 mg over 1 hour, then 20 mg over the second hour, and 20 mg over the third hour for a total dose of 100 mg. For patients weighing less than 65 kg, a dose of 1.25 mg/kg is given over 3 hours. An accelerated or front-loading regimen of alteplase delivers the total 100-mg dose over 90 minutes and achieves earlier patency of the infarct-related artery.[140]

Precautions

Bleeding is the major complication of thrombolytic therapy. Most commonly, bleeding occurs at puncture sites and can be treated locally. The risk of bleeding is not reduced by administration of clot-specific agents. Furthermore, lytic activity persists in plasma for many hours after thrombolytics are cleared from the circulation.[138] Chest pain or reperfusion arrhythmias (ie, accelerated idioventricular rhythms are most common, sinus bradycardia, second- and third-degree block) may occur during or following thrombolytic therapy in patients with acute myocardial infarction. Hypotension may occur with agents containing streptokinase. If hypotension is due to streptokinase, a reduction in the infusion rate will reduce the fall in blood pressure. Nausea and vomiting have also been reported during thrombolytic therapy. Allergic reactions (eg, difficulty in breathing, bronchospasm, periorbital swelling, angioneurotic edema, urticaria, itching, flushing, hypotension) may occur with agents containing streptokinase. These reactions can be treated with diphenhydramine, corticosteroids, or both.

References

1. Ahlquist RP. A study of adrenotropic receptors. *Am J Physiol.* 1948;153:586-600.
2. Lands AM, Arnold A, McAuliff JP, Luduena FP, Brown TG Jr. Differentiation of receptor systems activated by sympathomimetic amines. *Nature.* 1967;214:597-598.
3. Langer SZ. Sixth Gaddum memorial lecture, National Institute for Medical Research, Mill Hill, January 1977. Presynaptic receptors and their role in the regulation of transmitter release. *Br J Pharmacol.* 1977;60:481-497.
4. Lefkowitz RJ. Beta-adrenergic receptors: recognition and regulation. *N Engl J Med.* 1976;295:323-328.
5. Schumann HJ, Wagner J, Knorr A, Reidemeister JC, Sadony V, Schramm G. Demonstration in human atrial preparations of alpha-adrenoceptors mediating positive inotropic effects. *Naunyn Schmiedebergs Arch Pharmacol.* 1978;302:333-336.
6. Langer SZ, Hicks PE. Alpha-adrenoreceptor subtypes in blood vessels: physiology and pharmacology. *J Cardiovasc Pharmacol.* 1984;6(suppl 4):S547-S558.
7. Mehta J, Lopez LM. Calcium-blocker withdrawal phenomenon: increase in affinity of alpha 2 adrenoceptors for agonist as a potential mechanism. *Am J Cardiol.* 1986;58:242-246.
8. Haeusler G. Cardiovascular regulation by central adrenergic mechanisms and its alteration by hypotensive drugs. *Circ Res.* 1975;36(suppl 1):223-232.
9. Shaw J, Hunyor SN, Korner PI. The peripheral circulatory effects of clonidine and their role in the production of arterial hypotension. *Eur J Pharmacol.* 1971;14:101-111.
10. Brown MJ, Brown DC, Murphy MB. Hypokalemia from beta2-receptor stimulation by circulating epinephrine. *N Engl J Med.* 1983;309:1414-1419.
11. Leier CV, Heban PT, Huss P, Bush CA, Lewis RP. Comparative systemic and regional hemodynamic effects of dopamine and dobutamine in patients with cardiomyopathic heart failure. *Circulation.* 1978;58:466-475.
12. Haddy FJ. Physiology and pharmacology of the coronary circulation and myocardium, particularly in relation to coronary artery disease. *Am J Med.* 1969;47:274-286.
13. Dempsey PJ, Cooper T. Pharmacology of the coronary circulation. *Annu Rev Pharmacol.* 1972;12:99-110.
14. King MP, Angelakos ET, Uzgiris I. Innervation of the coronaries. *Fed Proc.* 1971;30:613. Abstract.
15. Berne RM. Regulation of coronary blood flow. *Physiol Rev.* 1964;44:1-29.
16. Feigl EO. Sympathetic control of coronary circulation. *Circ Res.* 1967;20:262-271.
17. Katori M, Berne RM. Release of adenosine from anoxic hearts: relationship to coronary flow. *Circ Res.* 1966;19:420-425.
18. Mudge GH Jr, Goldberg S, Gunther S, Mann T, Grossman W. Comparison of metabolic and vasoconstrictor stimuli on coronary vascular resistance in man. *Circulation.* 1979;59:544-550.
19. Levy MN, Martin PJ, Stuesse SL. Neural regulation of the heart beat. *Annu Rev Physiol.* 1981;43:443-453.
20. Vedernikov YP. Mechanisms of coronary spasm of isolated human epicardial coronary segments excised 3 to 5 hours after sudden death. *J Am Coll Cardiol.* 1986;8(suppl A):42A-49A.
21. Shepherd JT, Vanhoutte PM. Mechanisms responsible for coronary vasospasm. *J Am Coll Cardiol.* 1986;8(suppl A):50A-54A.
22. Weiner N. Norepinephrine, epinephrine, and the sympathomimetic amines. In: Gilman AG, Goodman LS, Rall TW, Murad F, eds. *Goodman and Gilman's The Pharmacological Basis of Therapeutics.* 7th ed. New York, NY: Macmillan Publishing Co Inc; 1985:145-180.
23. Sobel BE, Braunwald E. The management of acute myocardial infarction. In: Braunwald E, ed. *Heart Disease: A Textbook of Cardiovascular Medicine.* 2nd ed. Philadelphia, Pa: WB Saunders Co; 1984:1301-1333.
24. Ross J Jr, Frahm CJ, Braunwald E. The influence of intracardiac baroreceptors on venous return, systemic vascular volume and peripheral resistance. *J Clin Invest.* 1961;40:563-572.
25. Cohn JN. Blood pressure measurement in shock: mechanism of inaccuracy in auscultatory and palpatory methods. *JAMA.* 1967;199:118-122.
26. Mueller HS, Evans R, Ayres SM. Effect of dopamine on hemodynamics and myocardial metabolism in shock following acute myocardial infarction in man. *Circulation.* 1978;57:361-365.
27. Gonzalez ER, Ornato JP, Levine RL. Vasopressor effect of epinephrine with and without dopamine during cardiopulmonary resuscitation. *Drug Intell Clin Pharm.* 1988;22:868-872.
28. Lindner KH, Ahnefeld FW, Bowdler IM. Comparison of epinephrine and dopamine during cardiopulmonary resuscitation. *Intensive Care Med.* 1989;15:432-438.
29. Keung EC, Siskind SJ, Sonneblick EH, Ribner HS, Schwartz WJ, LeJemtel TH. Dobutamine therapy in acute myocardial infarction. *JAMA.* 1981;245:144-146.
30. Anderson JL. Bretylium tosylate: profile of the only available class III antiarrhythmic agent. *Clin Ther.* 1985;7:205-224.
31. Bivins BA, Rapp RP, Griffen WO Jr, Blouin R, Bustrack J. Dopamine-phenytoin interaction: a cause of hypotension in the critically ill. *Arch Surg.* 1978;113:245-249.
32. Newton DW, Fung EY, Williams DA. Stability of five catecholamines and terbutaline sulfate in 5% dextrose injection in the absence and presence of aminophylline. *Am J Hosp Pharm.* 1981;38:1314-1319.
33. Leier CV. Acute inotropic support. In: Leier CV, ed. *Cardiotonic Drugs: A Clinical Survey.* New York, NY: Marcel Dekker; 1986:49-84.
34. Stoner JD III, Bolen JL, Harrison DC. Comparison of dobutamine and dopamine in treatment of severe heart failure. *Br Heart J.* 1977;39:536-539.
35. Gillespie TA, Ambos HD, Sobel BE, Roberts R. Effects of dobutamine in patients with acute myocardial infarction. *Am J Cardiol.* 1977;39:588-594.
36. Francis GS, Sharma B, Hodges M. Comparative hemodynamic effects of dopamine and dobutamine in patients with acute cardiogenic circulatory collapse. *Am Heart J.* 1982;103:995-1000.
37. Richard C, Ricome JL, Rimailho A, Bottineau G, Auzepy P. Combined hemodynamic effects of dopamine and dobutamine in cardiogenic shock. *Circulation.* 1983;67:620-626.
38. Maekawa K, Liang CS, Hood WB Jr. Comparison of dobutamine and dopamine in acute myocardial infarction: effects of systemic hemodynamics, plasma catecholamines, blood flows and infarct size. *Circulation.* 1983;67:750-759.
39. Dell'Italia LJ, Starling MR, Blumhardt R, Lasher JC, O'Rourke RA. Comparative effects of volume loading, dobutamine, and nitroprusside in patients with predominant right ventricular infarction. *Circulation.* 1985;72:1327-1335.
40. Niemann JT, Haynes KS, Garner D, Rennie CJ III, Jagels G, Stormo O. Postcountershock pulseless rhythms: response to CPR, artificial cardiac pacing, and adrenergic agonists. *Ann Emerg Med.* 1986;15:112-120.
41. Mancini D, LeJemtel T, Sonnenblick E. Intravenous use of amrinone for the treatment of the failing heart. *Am J Cardiol.* 1985;56:8B-15B.

42. Taylor SH, Verma SP, Hussain M, Reynolds G, Jackson NC, Hafizullah M, Richmond A, Silke B. Intravenous amrinone in left ventricular failure complicated by acute myocardial infarction. *Am J Cardiol.* 1985;56:29B-32B.

43. Klein NA, Siskind SJ, Frishman WH, Sonnenblick EH, LeJemtel TH. Hemodynamic comparison of intravenous amrinone and dobutamine in patients with chronic congestive heart failure. *Am J Cardiol.* 1981;48:170-175.

44. Rude RE, Kloner RA, Maroko PR, Khuri S, Karaffa S, DeBoer LW, Braunwald E. Effects of amrinone on experimental acute myocardial ischemic injury. *Cardiovasc Res.* 1980;14:419-427.

45. Hoffman BF, Bigger JT Jr. Digitalis and allied cardiac glycosides. In: Gilman AG, Rall TW, Nies AS, Taylor P, eds. *Goodman and Gilman's The Pharmacological Basis of Therapeutics.* 8th ed. New York, NY: Macmillan Publishing Co Inc; 1993:814-839.

46. Fawaz G. Effect of reserpine and pronethalol on the therapeutic and toxic actions of digitalis in the dog heart-lung preparation. *Br J Pharmacol.* 1967;29:302-308.

47. Smith TW, Antman EM, Friedman PL, Blatt CM, Marsh JD. Digitalis glycosides: mechanisms and manifestations of toxicity: part 2. *Prog Cardiovasc Dis.* 1984;26:495-540.

48. Ordog GJ, Benaron S, Bhasin V, Wasserberger J, Balasubramanium S. Serum digoxin levels and mortality in 5,100 patients. *Ann Emerg Med.* 1987;16:32-39.

49. Goldstein RA, Passamani ER, Roberts R. A comparison of digoxin and dobutamine in patients with acute infarction and cardiac failure. *N Engl J Med.* 1980;303:846-850.

50. Packer M, Gheorghaide M, Young JB, et al. Randomized, double blind, placebo controlled, withdrawal study of digoxin in patients with chronic heart failure treated with converting-enzyme inhibitors. *J Am Coll Cardiol.* 1992;19:260A. Abstract.

51. Young JB, Urestsky BF, Shahidi FE, et al. Multicenter, double-blind, placebo controlled, randomized withdrawal trial of the efficacy and safety of digoxin in patients with mild to moderate chronic heart failure not treated with converting-enzyme inhibitors. *J Am Coll Cardiol.* 1992;19:259A. Abstract.

52. Smith TW, Antman EM, Friedman PL, Blatt CM, Marsh JD. Digitalis glycosides: mechanisms and manifestations of toxicity: part 1. *Prog Cardiovasc Dis.* 1984;26:413-458.

53. Sodeman WA. Diagnosis and treatment of digitalis toxicity. *N Engl J Med.* 1965;273:35-37,93-95.

54. Chung EK. *Digitalis Intoxication.* Baltimore, Md: Williams & Wilkins Co; 1969.

55. Lang TW, Bernstein H, Barbieri F, Gold H, Corday E. Digitalis toxicity: treatment with diphenylhydantoin. *Arch Intern Med.* 1965;116:573-580.

56. Hilmi KI, Regan TJ. Relative effectiveness of antiarrhythmic drugs in treatment of digitalis-induced ventricular tachycardia. *Am Heart J.* 1968;76:365-369.

57. Kleiger R, Lown B. Cardioversion and digitalis, II: clinical studies. *Circulation.* 1966;33:878-887.

58. Smith TW, Butler VP Jr, Haber E, Fozzard H, Marcus FI, Bremner WF, Schulman IC, Phillips A. Treatment of life-threatening digitalis intoxication with digoxin-specific Fab antibody fragments: experience in 26 cases. *N Engl J Med.* 1982;307:1357-1362.

59. Bismuth C, Gaultier M, Conso F, Efthymiou ML. Hyperkalemia in acute digitalis poisoning: prognostic significance and therapeutic implications. *Clin Toxicol.* 1973;6:153-162.

60. Cohn JN, Burke LP. Nitroprusside. *Ann Intern Med.* 1979;91:752-757.

61. Franciosa JA, Dunkman WB, Wilen M, Silverstein SR. 'Optimal' left ventricular filling pressure during nitroprusside infusion for congestive heart failure. *Am J Med.* 1983;74:457-464.

62. Guiha NH, Cohn JN, Mikulic E, Franciosa JA, Limas CJ. Treatment of refractory heart failure with infusion of nitroprusside. *N Engl J Med.* 1974;291:587-592.

63. Miller RR, Vismara LA, Williams DO, Amsterdam EA, Mason DT. Pharmacological mechanisms for left ventricular unloading in clinical congestive heart failure: differential effects of nitroprusside, phentolamine, and nitroglycerin on cardiac function and peripheral circulation. *Circ Res.* 1976;39:127-133.

64. Flaherty JT. Comparison of intravenous nitroglycerin and sodium nitroprusside in acute myocardial infarction. *Am J Med.* 1983;74:53-60.

65. Franciosa JA, Limas CJ, Guiha NH, Rodriguera E, Cohn JN. Improved left ventricular function during nitroprusside infusion in acute myocardial infarction. *Lancet.* 1972;1:650-654.

66. Chatterjee K, Parmley WW, Ganz W, Forrester J, Walinsky P, Crexells C, Swan HJ. Hemodynamic and metabolic responses to vasodilator therapy in acute myocardial infarction. *Circulation.* 1973;48:1183-1193.

67. Fuch RM, Rutler DL, Powell WJ. Effects of dobutamine on venous capacity. *Clin Res.* 1976;24:218a. Abstract.

68. Grossman W, Brodie B, Mann T, McLaurin L. Effects of sodium nitroprusside on left ventricular diastolic pressure-volume relations. *Circulation.* 1975;52(suppl 2):II-35. Abstract.

69. Mookherjee S, Waner R, Keighley J, et al. Worsening of ventilation perfusion relationship in the lungs in the face of hemodynamic improvement during nitroprusside infusion. *Am J Cardiol.* 1977;39:282. Abstract.

70. Brodie TS, Gray R, Swan HJC, et al. Effect of nitroprusside on arterial oxygenation, intrapulmonic shunts, and oxygen delivery. *Am J Cardiol.* 1976;37:123. Abstract.

71. Yacobi A, Amann AH, Baaske DM. Pharmaceutical considerations of nitroglycerin. *Drug Intell Clin Pharm.* 1983;17:255-263.

72. Jaffe AS, Roberts R. The use of intravenous nitroglycerin in cardiovascular disease. *Pharmacotherapy.* 1982;2:273-280.

73. Murad F. Drugs used for the treatment of angina: organic nitrates, calcium-channel blockers, and β-adrenergic antagonists. In: Gilman AG, Rall TW, Nies AS, Taylor P, eds. *Goodman and Gilman's The Pharmacological Basis of Therapeutics.* 8th ed. New York, NY: Macmillan Publishing Co Inc; 1993:764-783.

74. Hill NS, Antman EM, Green LH, Alpert JS. Intravenous nitroglycerin: a review of pharmacology, indications, therapeutic effects and complications. *Chest.* 1981;79:69-76.

75. Horwitz LD, Herman MV, Gorlin R. Clinical response to nitroglycerin as a diagnostic test for coronary artery disease. *Am J Cardiol.* 1972;29:149-153.

76. Cohen MV, Downey JM, Sonnenblick EH, Kirk ES. The effects of nitroglycerin on coronary collaterals and myocardial contractility. *J Clin Invest.* 1973;52:2836-2847.

77. Malindzak GS Jr, Green HD, Stagg PL. Effects of nitroglycerin on flow after partial constriction of the coronary artery. *J Appl Physiol.* 1970;29:17-22.

78. Hillis LD, Braunwald E. Coronary-artery spasm. *N Engl J Med.* 1978;299:695-702.

79. Kotter V, von Leitner ER, Wunderlich J, Schroder R. Comparison of haemodynamic effects of phentolamine, sodium nitroprusside, and glyceryl trinitrate in acute myocardial infarction. *Br Heart J.* 1977;39:1196-1204.

80. Miller RR, Vismara LA, Williams DO, Amsterdam EA, Mason DT. Pharmacological mechanisms for left ventricular unloading in clinical congestive heart failure: differential effects of nitroprusside, phentolamine, and nitroglycerin on cardiac function and peripheral circulation. *Circ Res.* 1976;39:127-133.

81. Gold HK, Leinbach RC, Sanders CA. Use sublingual nitroglycerin in congestive failure following acute myocardial infarction. *Circulation.* 1972;46:839-845.

82. Kovick RB, Tillisch JH, Berens SC, Bramowitz AD, Shine KI. Vasodilator therapy for chronic left ventricular failure. *Circulation.* 1976;53:322-328.

83. Gray R, Chatterjee K, Vyden JK, Ganz W, Forrester JS, Swan HJ. Hemodynamic and metabolic effects of isosorbide dinitrate in chronic congestive heart failure. *Am Heart J.* 1975;90:346-352.

84. Greenberg H, Dwyer EM Jr, Jameson AG, Pinkernell BH. Effects of nitroglycerin on the major determinants of myocardial oxygen consumption: an angiographic and hemodynamic assessment. *Am J Cardiol.* 1975;36:426-432.

85. Leier CV, Bambach D, Thompson MJ, Cattaneo SM, Goldberg RJ, Unverferth DV. Central and regional hemodynamic effects of intravenous isosorbide dinitrate, nitroglycerin and nitroprusside in patients with congestive heart failure. *Am J Cardiol.* 1981;48:1115-1123.

86. Bussmann WD, Schofer H, Kaltenbach M. Effects of intravenous nitroglycerin on hemodynamics and ischemic injury in patients with acute myocardial infarction. *Eur J Cardiol.* 1978;8:61-74.

87. Curfman GD, Heinsimer JA, Lozner EC, Fung HL. Intravenous nitroglycerin in the treatment of spontaneous angina pectoris: a prospective, randomized trial. *Circulation.* 1983;67:276-282.

88. Bussman WD, Passek D, Seidel W, Kaltenbach M. Reduction of CK and CK-MB indexes of infarct size by intravenous nitroglycerin. *Circulation*. 1981;63:615-622.

89. Jaffe AS, Geltman EM, Tiefenbrunn AJ, Ambos HD, Strauss HD, Sobel BE, Roberts R. Reduction of infarct size in patients with inferior infarction with intravenous glyceryl trinitrate: a randomized study. *Br Heart J.* 1983;49:452-460.

90. Flaherty JT, Becker LC, Bulkley BH, Weiss JL, Gerstenblith G, Kallman CH, Silverman KJ, Wei JY, Pitt B, Weisfeldt ML. A randomized prospective trial of intravenous nitroglycerin in patients with acute myocardial infarction. *Circulation*. 1983;68:576-588.

91. Standards and guidelines for Cardiopulmonary Resuscitation (CPR) and Emergency Cardiac Care (ECC). *JAMA*. 1986;255:2905-2989.

92. Gunnar RM, Passamani ER, Bourdillon PD, Pitt B, Dixon DW, Rapaport E, Fuster V, Reeves TJ, Karp RB, Russell RO Jr, Kennedy JW, Sobel BE, Klocke FJ, Winters WL Jr, Fisch C, Beller GA, DeSanctis RW, Dodge HT, Weinberg SL. Guidelines for the early management of patients with acute myocardial infarction: a report of the American College of Cardiology/American Heart Association Task Force on Assessment of Diagnostic and Therapeutic Cardiovascular Procedures (Subcommittee to Develop Guidelines for the Early Management of Patients With Acute Myocardial Infarction). *J Am Coll Cardiol*. 1990;16:249-292.

93. Yusuf S, Wittes J, Friedman L. Overview of results of randomized clinical trials in heart disease, I: treatments following myocardial infarction. *JAMA*. 1988;260:2088-2093.

94. Gonzalez ER, Jones LA, Ornato JP, Bleecker GC, Strauss MJ. Adjunctive medications in patients receiving thrombolytic therapy: a multicenter prospective assessment. The Virginia Multicenter Thrombolytic Study Group. *Ann Pharmacother*. 1992;26:1383-1384.

95. Lichtenthal PR, Rossi EC, Louis G, Rehnberg KA, Wade LD, Michaelis LL, Fung HL, Patrignani P. Dose-related prolongation of the bleeding time by intravenous nitroglycerin. *Anesth Analg*. 1985;64:30-33.

96. Gonzalez ER, Jones HD, Graham S, Elswick RK. Assessment of the drug interaction between intravenous nitroglycerin and heparin. *Ann Pharmacother*. 1992;26:1512-1514.

97. Habbab MA, Haft JI. Heparin resistance induced by intravenous nitroglycerin: a word of caution when both drugs are used concomitantly. *Arch Intern Med*. 1987;147:857-860.

98. Mehta JL, Nicolini FA, Nichols WW, Saldeen TG. Concurrent nitroglycerin administration decreases thrombolytic potential of tissue-type plasminogen activator. *J Am Coll Cardiol*. 1991;17:805-811.

99. Mikolich JR, Nicoloff NB, Robinson PH, Logue RB. Relief of refractory angina with continuous intravenous infusion of nitroglycerin. *Chest*. 1980;77:375-379.

100. Leinbach RC, Gold HK. Intermittent and continuous nitroglycerin infusions for control of myocardial ischemia. *Circulation*. 1977;56 (suppl 3):III-194. Abstract.

101. Abrams J. Tolerance to organic nitrates. *Circulation*. 1986;74:1181-1185.

102. Flaherty JT. Nitrate tolerance: a review of the evidence. *Drugs*. 1989;37:523-550.

103. Come PC, Pitt B. Nitroglycerin-induced severe hypotension and bradycardia in patients with acute myocardial infarction. *Circulation*. 1976;54:624-628.

104. Weygandt GR, Kopman EA, Bauer S, et al. The cause of hypoxemia induced by nitroglycerin. *Am J Cardiol*. 1979;43:427. Abstract.

105. Shand DG. Drug therapy: propranolol. *N Engl J Med*. 1975;293:280-285.

106. Koch-Weser J. Drug therapy: metoprolol. *N Engl J Med*. 1979;301:698-703.

107. Prichard BN. The second Lilly Prize Lecture, University of Newcastle, July 1977: beta-adrenergic receptor blockade in hypertension, past, present and future. *Br J Clin Pharmacol*. 1978;5:379-399.

108. Nordrehaug JE. Malignant arrhythmia in relation to serum potassium in acute myocardial infarction. *Am J Cardiol*. 1985;56:20D-23D.

109. Davis LD, Temte JV. Effects of propranolol on the transmembrane potentials of ventricular muscle and Purkinje fibers of the dog. *Circ Res*. 1968;22:661-677.

110. Woosley RL, Kornhauser D, Smith R, Reele S, Higgins SB, Nies AS, Shand DG, Oates JA. Suppression of chronic ventricular arrhythmias with propranolol. *Circulation*. 1979;60:819-827.

111. Gonzalez ER, Sypniewski E. Acute myocardial infarction: diagnosis and treatment. In: DiPiro JT, Talbert R, Hays M, Yee W, Posey M, eds. *Pharmacotherapy: A Pathophysiologic Approach*. 2nd ed. New York, NY: Elsevier Inc; 1992:231-255.

112. Koch-Weser J, Frishman WH. Beta-adrenoceptor antagonists: new drugs and new indications. *N Engl J Med*. 1981;305:500-506.

113. Peter T, Norris RM, Clarke ED, Heng MK, Singh BN, Williams B, Howell DR, Ambler PK. Reduction of enzyme levels by propranolol after acute myocardial infarction. *Circulation*. 1978;57:1091-1095.

114. Hjalmarson A, Herlitz J, for the Göteborg Metoprolol Trial Group. The Göteborg Metoprolol Trial in acute myocardial infarction. *Am J Cardiol*. 1984;53:(suppl 1):1D-50D.

115. Metoprolol in acute myocardial infarction (MIAMI): a randomized placebo-controlled intervention trial. The MIAMI Trial Research Group. *Eur Heart J*. 1985;6:199-226.

116. Acute myocardial infarct size reduction by timolol administration: the International Collaborative Study Group. *Am J Cardiol*. 1986;57:28F-33F.

117. Randomized trial of intravenous atenolol among 16,027 cases of suspected acute myocardial infarction: ISIS-1. First International Study of Infarct Survival Collaborative Group. *Lancet*. 1986;2:57-66.

118. Frishman WH, Furberg CD, Friedewald WT. Beta-adrenergic blockade for survivors of acute myocardial infarction. *N Engl J Med*. 1984;310:830-837.

119. Rydén L, Ariniego R, Arnman K, Herlitz J, Hjalmarson A, Holmberg S, Reyes C, Smedgard P, Svedberg K, Vedin A, Waagstein F, Waldenstrom A, Wilhelmsson C, Wedel H, Yamamoto M. A double-blind trial of metoprolol in acute myocardial infarction: effects on ventricular tachyarrhythmias. *N Engl J Med*. 1983;308:614-618.

120. Norris RM, Barnaby PF, Brown MA, Geary GG, Clarke ED, Logan RL, Sharpe DN. Prevention of ventricular fibrillation during acute myocardial infarction by intravenous propranolol. *Lancet*. 1984;2:883-886.

121. GISSI-2: a factorial randomized trial of alteplase versus streptokinase and heparin versus no heparin among 12,490 patients with acute myocardial infarction. Gruppo Italiano per lo Studio della Sopravvivenza nell'Infarto Miocardico. *Lancet*. 1990;336:65-71.

122. Yusuf S, Wittes J, Friedman L. Overview of results of randomized clinical trials in heart disease, I: treatments following myocardial infarction. *JAMA*. 1988;260:2088-2093.

123. Comparison of invasive and conservative strategies after treatment with intravenous tissue plasminogen activator in acute myocardial infarction: results of the thrombolysis in myocardial infarction (TIMI) phase II Trial. The TIMI Study Group. *N Engl J Med*. 1989;320:618-627.

124. Randomized trial of intravenous streptokinase, oral aspirin, both, or neither among 17,187 cases of suspected acute myocardial infarction: ISIS-2. ISIS-2 (Second International Study of Infarct Survival) Collaborative Group. *Lancet*. 1988;2:349-360.

125. Weiner IM. Diuretics and other agents employed in the mobilization of edema fluid. In: Gilman AG, Rall TW, Nies AS, Taylor P, eds. *Goodman and Gilman's The Pharmacological Basis of Therapeutics*. 8th ed. New York, NY: Macmillan Publishing Co Inc; 1993:713-731.

126. Dikshit K, Vyden JK, Forrester JS, Chatterjee K, Prakash R, Swan HJ. Renal and extrarenal hemodynamic effects of furosemide in congestive heart failure after acute myocardial infarction. *N Engl J Med*. 1973;288:1087-1090.

127. Biddle TL, Yu PN. Effect of frusemide on hemodynamics and lung water in acute pulmonary edema secondary to myocardial infarction. *Am J Cardiol*. 1979;43:86-90.

128. Schuster CJ, Weil MH, Besso J, Carpio M, Henning RJ. Blood volume following diuresis induced by furosemide. *Am J Med*. 1984;76:585-592.

129. Francis GS, Siegel RM, Goldsmith SR, Olivari MT, Levine TB, Cohn JN. Acute vasoconstrictor response to intravenous furosemide in patients with chronic congestive heart failure: activation of the neurohumoral axis. *Ann Intern Med*. 1985;103:1-6.

130. Lawson DH, Gray JM, Henry DA, Tillstone WJ. Continuous infusion of frusemide in refractory oedema. *Br Med J*. 1978;2:476.

131. Copeland JG, Campbell DW, Plachetka JR, Salomon NW, Larson DF. Diuresis with continuous infusion of furosemide after cardiac surgery. *Am J Surg.* 1983;146:796-799.

132. Amiel SA, Blackburn AM, Rubens RD. Intravenous infusion of furosemide as treatment for ascites in malignant disease. *Br Med J.* 1984;288:1041.

133. Krasna MJ, Scott GE, Scholz PM, Spotnitz AJ, Mackenzie JW, Penn F. Postoperative enhancement of urinary output in patients with acute renal failure using continuous furosemide therapy. *Chest.* 1986;89:294-295.

134. Lahav M, Regev A, Ra'anani P, Theodor E. Intermittent administration of furosemide vs continuous infusion preceded by a loading dose for congestive heart failure. *Chest.* 1992;102:725-731.

135. Sherry S. Appraisal of various thrombolytic agents in the treatment of acute myocardial infarction. *Am J Med.* 1987;83:31-37.

136. Eisenberg PR, Sherman L, Rich M, Schwartz D, Schechtman K, Geltman EM, Sobel BE, Jaffe AS. Importance of continued activation of thrombin reflected by fibrinopeptide A to the continued efficacy of thrombolysis. *J Am Coll Cardiol.* 1986;7:1255-1262.

137. Eisenberg PR, Sherman LA, Jaffe AS. Paradoxic elevation of fibrinopeptide A after streptokinase: evidence for continued thrombosis despite intense fibrinolysis. *J Am Coll Cardiol.* 1987;10: 527-529.

138. Eisenberg PR, Sherman LA, Tiefenbrunn AJ, Ludbrook PA, Sobel BE, Jaffe AS. Sustained fibrinolysis after administration of t-PA despite its short half-life in the circulation. *Thromb Haemost.* 1987;57:35-40.

139. Hsia J, Hamilton WP, Kleiman N, Roberts R, Chaitman BR, Ross AM. A comparison between heparin and low-dose aspirin as adjunctive therapy with tissue plasminogen activator for acute myocardial infarction. Heparin-Aspirin Reperfusion Trial (HART) Investigators. *N Engl J Med.* 1990;323:1433-1437.

140. Vaughan DE, Braunwald E. Front-loaded accelerated infusions of tissue plasminogen activator: putting a better foot forward. *J Am Coll Cardiol.* 1992;19:1076-1078.

Myocardial Infarction

Chapter 9

This chapter presents clinical guidelines for the early management of the patient with acute myocardial infarction (MI). The chapter reviews the clinical principles of the early management of such patients, focusing on the first 30 to 60 minutes, and presents the principles of thrombolytic therapy for acute MI. A more detailed discussion of these issues can be found in the appropriate references and the ACC/AHA task force report on management of acute MI.[1]

Myocardial infarction refers to necrosis of heart muscle caused by an inadequate blood supply. In the majority of patients, it is the result of severe atherosclerotic narrowing of one or more of the coronary arteries. Factors that have been implicated in the pathogenesis of MI include atherosclerotic plaque rupture (fissuring or hemorrhage)[2-4] and spasm.[5,6] During the early hours of an acute transmural MI, one or more of these factors are usually associated with thrombosis of the involved coronary artery. Understanding of this pathophysiology has led to the development of thrombolytic therapy as a therapeutic strategy in patients with acute transmural infarction. Nontransmural infarction may be less frequently associated with thrombosis.[7] Coronary spasm and coronary embolism are uncommon causes of MI. Rarely MI can occur in the absence of coronary artery narrowing if there is a marked disparity between myocardial oxygen supply and demand. Cocaine abuse has been implicated as a possible cause of such a disparity.[8] The prompt recognition that an infarction is occurring is critical since most deaths associated with acute infarction are due to electrical instability and occur suddenly, often before arrival at the hospital.[9] As such, they are potentially preventable.[10]

Clinical Presentation

Precipitating Events

Most patients suffer the onset of infarction at rest or with moderate activity. In one study 59% were either at rest or asleep. Forty-one percent were involved in some activity, most engaged in mild to moderate or usual exertion.[11] Research studies conflict on a cause-and-effect relationship between vigorous exertion and MI.[12-17] A daily pattern (circadian rhythm)[18,19] in the onset of acute infarction, which peaks from 6 AM to noon, and a seasonal pattern with 15% to 20% more cases during the winter[20] suggest that factors other than activity may be critical. Nonetheless, the combination of severe exertion and excessive fatigue or unusual emotional stress has been associated with precipitation of MI.[13] Emotional stress and life events with a powerful impact on the individual, eg, death of a significant other person, divorce, or loss of job,

are common before MI and in the long run may prove to have some relationship to causing MI.[21,22]

Symptom Recognition and Response

Acute MI can cause many symptoms. In association with acute MI these symptoms carry a risk of sudden death and must be recognized and treated promptly:

- New onset of chest pain suspicious for myocardial ischemia (see below) either at rest or with ordinary or usual activity
- A change in a previously stable pattern of anginal pain, such as an increase in frequency or severity or occurrence at rest for the first time
- Chest pain suspicious for myocardial ischemia, in a patient with known coronary heart disease, that is unrelieved by rest and/or nitroglycerin

Chest pain or discomfort due to myocardial ischemia may be central (substernal) or more diffuse.[23] The pain is commonly described as crushing, pressing ("like a vise"), constricting, oppressive, or heavy ("like an elephant on my chest"), but in some patients it may be mild. It tends to increase in intensity over a period of minutes. The pain may radiate to one (more often the left) or both shoulders and arms or to the neck, lower jaw, or back. Less commonly, high epigastric discomfort may be a manifestation of myocardial ischemia and may be dismissed as "indigestion." Any unusual or prolonged "indigestion" should raise suspicion, particularly in a person at high risk. Rarely will the chest discomfort be described as sharp or achy. Discomfort in the arms, shoulders, neck, jaw, epigastrium, or back may also be due to myocardial ischemia or infarction, even in the absence of substernal chest discomfort.

New discomfort in the chest or in the areas described above that persists more than a few minutes should be evaluated, especially in a patient known to be at risk. The AHA recommends that a patient with known angina pectoris seek emergency medical care if chest pain is not relieved by three nitroglycerin tablets over 10 minutes. In a person with previously unrecognized coronary disease, the persistence of suspicious chest pain for longer than a few minutes is an indication for emergency medical assistance.[24] In some patients, especially those with diabetes, acute MIs may not cause chest discomfort, and symptoms may range from vague uneasiness to severe shortness of breath. Recent data indicate that women and elderly patients are also more likely to have atypical presentations.[25] A high level of suspicion is necessary when evaluating patients with coronary risk factors and typical or atypical chest discomfort or shortness of breath.

It is important to respond vigorously to patients who have symptoms of myocardial ischemia. Ventricular fibrillation (VF) is 15 times more frequent during the first hour after symptoms than during the subsequent 12 hours.[10] In one study 36% of MI patients who experienced VF had the arrhythmia within the first hour.[26] Despite these facts the average delay between onset of symptoms of acute MI and the decision to call for medical assistance is 2 to 4 hours.[27-29] People who are aware of their illness and who are taking cardiac medications are even less prompt in calling for medical assistance.[30] This unnecessary delay not only places the patient at higher risk of death from VF but also diminishes the effectiveness of interventions that limit the size of the infarction. Patients, families, and communities must be educated about the need for prompt response. Training the patient's family and the community in general in cardiopulmonary resuscitation continues to be critical in reducing prehospital death from coronary artery disease.

General Management Approaches

Suspicion of acute MI is based on the patient's symptoms. If the history is consistent with the diagnosis, the patient must be treated rapidly and appropriately. Although the electrocardiogram (ECG) often confirms the diagnosis, it also may be entirely normal. Therefore, a single normal ECG cannot be relied on to exclude the diagnosis. A succinct history and physical examination, which can be done in 7 to 10 minutes or less, can provide the key to correct management of the acute MI victim. Some prehospital EMS systems have successfully used a questionnaire to rapidly screen patients and evaluate them for thrombolytic therapy.[31] Onset and duration of symptoms, use of concurrent medicines, and recent (less than 6 months) history of trauma, surgery, and bleeding should be rapidly determined. Examination should focus on the patient's general condition, vital signs, lung examination, heart sounds, carotid bruits, and evidence of trauma or bleeding. This simple initial evaluation will guide care, including potential thrombolytic therapy.

Electrocardiographic Monitoring

Because of the high incidence of VF and other serious arrhythmias during the first hour of acute infarction,[9,26] begin ECG monitoring immediately on suspicion of the diagnosis. If an AED with a monitor is available, apply AED electrodes and thus monitor the patient, but never place the AED in analysis mode unless the patient becomes unconscious in arrest.

Establishing Intravenous Access

Since pharmacologic therapy may be needed rapidly, secure intravenous (IV) access must be placed, preferably a large-bore IV line in an arm vein. The percutaneous puncture of veins that are noncompressible (eg,

subclavian vein) should be discouraged since this is a contraindication to the use of thrombolytic agents for several days.[32]

Oxygen in Myocardial Infarction

Hypoxemia in patients with uncomplicated acute MI is usually caused by ventilation-perfusion abnormalities[33,34] and is exacerbated by left ventricular failure. Significant hypoxemia may occur even in patients with uncomplicated infarction. Begin therapy with supplemental oxygen even when the patient possesses a normal arterial oxygen tension (Pao_2). There is some evidence that an elevation of Pao_2 may limit the ultimate size of the infarction.[35,36] However, superphysiological levels of oxygen may increase systemic vascular resistance and arterial pressure, lowering cardiac output and possibly compromising peripheral oxygen delivery.[37-39] Even at high concentrations, this concern is hypothetical and should not discourage the administration of oxygen to all patients with MI. When oxygen is used, it should be administered by mask or nasal cannula at a flow rate of 4 to 6 L/min, or as described in chapter 7. In patients with chronic obstructive pulmonary disease (COPD), lower flow rates of oxygen are appropriate to avoid carbon dioxide retention. In such patients with suspected infarction and documented hypoxia, however, oxygen should be administered at rates sufficient to reverse the hypoxia, and rescuers should be prepared to support ventilation if hypoventilation occurs. Further increase in the concentration of delivered oxygen is necessary only if serious left ventricular failure or pulmonary complications develop. Arterial blood gas determinations should be discouraged during the early stages of an acute MI if thrombolytic agents may be administered.[40] This minimizes bleeding complications. Pulse oximetry can be used to monitor oxygen saturation.

Relief of Pain: Role of Nitroglycerin and Morphine

Place a high priority on relief of pain. Try sublingual nitroglycerin first unless the patient is hypotensive (systolic blood pressure less than 90 mm Hg). If chest pain and ECG changes resolve promptly and completely, infarction is less likely. In the presence of ongoing ischemia and blood pressure less than 90 mm Hg, a single tablet of sublingual nitroglycerin may be tried with caution if IV access is available. However, when infarction is present, nitroglycerin alone may not be adequate.[41] Prolonged attempts to relieve pain with multiple doses of nitroglycerin are to be discouraged if they delay the time to initiation of thrombolysis or other methods of coronary reperfusion.

Morphine sulfate is the drug of choice for the pain associated with acute MI. Morphine is administered 1 to 3 mg IV over 1 to 5 minutes (see chapter 7). It may be repeated at short intervals until pain is relieved. In addition to its analgesic properties, morphine exerts favorable though mild hemodynamic effects by increasing venous capacitance (thereby reducing venous return and preload) and by reducing systemic vascular resistance (thereby reducing impedance to left ventricular emptying or afterload). The result of both effects is a reduction in myocardial oxygen demand. In addition, relief of pain alleviates anxiety and thus lowers secretion of catecholamines.[42] Hypotension may occur after administration of morphine, occasionally with an inappropriate heart rate response.[43] This is even more likely if the patient has also been given nitroglycerin or a diuretic, and it usually resolves with fluid (with or without positioning the patient with head down and legs elevated). It is rarely necessary to use a pressor agent. If bradycardia and hypotension occur, atropine should be given after volume administration.[43] In patients with ongoing chest pain and hypotension, morphine analogs that have excellent analgesic properties but few vasodilatory or central sedative effects (eg, nalbuphine) may be useful.

Inappropriate or large doses of nitroglycerin may reduce the mean arterial blood pressure (with a resultant fall in coronary perfusion pressure) and cause a reflex tachycardia (with a possible increase in myocardial oxygen demand).[37] Sublingual or IV nitroglycerin must be used with particular caution in patients with right ventricular infarction because of the associated risks of hypotension. Hence, blood pressure must be monitored closely. Even if blood pressure is normal when the patient is supine, there is a danger of orthostatic hypotension. If hypotension occurs, patients should be placed in the supine position and/or have their legs raised. Intravenous fluids may also be required. Pressor agents should be avoided if possible. If hypotension occurs with IV nitroglycerin, decreasing the dose or stopping the infusion usually results in a prompt increase in blood pressure. If significant bradycardia (less than 50 to 60) also occurs with the hypotension, atropine 0.5 to 1.0 mg IV should be considered.[44]

Other benefits of nitroglycerin may be a reduction in myocardial oxygen demand, an increase in collateral flow to the ischemic myocardium,[45] and a reduction of coronary artery spasm.[46] This may reduce the extent of infarction if carefully titrated.[41,47,48] Recent data suggest that the early institution of IV nitroglycerin titrated to a 10% reduction in mean systolic arterial pressure can significantly reduce infarct size and the incidence of congestive heart failure.[49] It has also been suggested that nitroglycerin decreases the susceptibility of the ischemic myocardium to VF.[50] Meta-analysis results show that early nitroglycerin therapy also reduces mortality in acute MI.[51] However, indiscriminate use may reduce coronary blood flow and produce significant arrhythmias if hypotension ensues. Hence, it cannot be recommended for use in all patients with MI. It appears to be most useful in patients with ongoing ischemia, heart failure, or hypertension.

Management of Arrhythmias and Heart Rate

Premature Ventricular Complexes and Ventricular Rhythms

The routine use of prophylactic antiarrhythmic agents in all patients with suspected acute MI is no longer recommended.[52,53] Treatment with antiarrhythmic agents has previously been recommended in patients with definite acute MI whenever "warning arrhythmias" occur (Class IIb). These arrhythmias include

- Six or more premature ventricular complexes (PVCs) per minute
- PVCs that are closely coupled (QR/QT less than 0.85)
- PVCs that fall on the T wave of the preceding beat (R-on-T phenomenon)
- PVCs that occur in pairs (couplets) or in runs of three or more (ie, ventricular tachycardia)
- PVCs that are multiform[54,55]

Before widespread use of thrombolytic and β-blocker therapy, early lidocaine (within 6 hours of onset of chest pain) was noted to reduce the incidence of primary VF (VF without pump failure or hypotension), even in the absence of warning arrhythmias.[56,57] However, the understanding that VF is infrequently preceded by such warning arrhythmias[58] and that VF may occur in their absence, together with the lack of mortality benefit of such therapy, has called routine prophylactic antiarrhythmic therapy into question.[52,53,59,60] In addition, recent data indicate an increased incidence of asystole with lidocaine.[61] Therefore, lidocaine should be reserved for patients with symptomatic ventricular ectopy that produces symptoms such as angina or hypotension. Many patients who are to receive thrombolytic agents are treated with prophylactic antiarrhythmic agents[62] before administration of thrombolytic therapy (Class IIb). However, no randomized study has specifically evaluated the benefit of routine prophylactic antiarrhythmics in such patients.

There is a lower incidence of PVCs and ventricular tachycardia during the first several hours of acute MI[63] but a higher incidence of VF.[64] Thus, factors other than warning arrhythmias must play an important role in the genesis of VF during the initial hours of acute MI. There are several possibilities. The autonomic nervous system is abnormal during these early hours.[65] The pharmacologic inhibition of adrenergic influences on the acutely ischemic myocardium may explain the apparent efficacy of β-adrenergic blockade in improving survival after MI.[65-67] Furthermore, tachycardia when it occurs will lower the threshold for VF in the ischemic left ventricle. Thus, it is important to immediately correct significant tachycardia and avoid stimuli that might increase the heart rate in patients with acute MI.[68]

Hypokalemia and hypomagnesemia are also associated with ventricular arrhythmias during the early stage of MI.[69] Prior diuretic therapy or elevated levels of circulating catecholamines may contribute to hypokalemia. When known or strongly suspected, hypokalemia and hypomagnesemia should be corrected. Hypokalemia is present in 9% to 25% of patients with acute MI and may predispose these patients to VF.[70] Ornato and colleagues[71] found a 49% incidence of hypokalemia in their out-of-hospital cardiac arrest victims. Potassium should be measured and hypokalemia corrected in patients with acute MI by giving 10 mEq potassium chloride diluted in 100 mL of D_5W over 60 minutes. This dosage can be repeated as necessary, rechecking the serum potassium every hour until it measures 4.0 to 4.6 mEq/L.

The role of magnesium in cardiac disease is well described.[72] Magnesium deficiency is associated with a high frequency of cardiac arrhythmias, symptoms of cardiac insufficiency, and sudden cardiac death.[73] Hypomagnesemia, often accompanied by hypokalemia, is usually caused by diuretics.[74] Transient hypomagnesemia not induced by diuresis has been observed in patients with acute MI.[75] Because hypomagnesemia can precipitate refractory VF and hinder the replacement of intracellular potassium, it must be corrected if present. It must be understood that serum magnesium is only a small percentage of total body magnesium and that patients can have a normal serum magnesium and yet have total body depletion. One or two grams of magnesium sulfate (2 to 3 mL of a 50% solution) is diluted in 100 mL of D_5W and administered over 60 minutes. Magnesium supplementation is relatively safe and reduces the incidence of post-infarction ventricular arrhythmias.[76] In many centers 2 g of magnesium is given empirically to all acute MI patients upon admission, though definitive data to support this approach is lacking. In late 1993 a large "mega-trial" observed that routine empiric treatment with magnesium does not improve long-term mortality.

Bradycardias

Controversy exists about the management of bradycardia (heart rates less than 60 beats per minute) during acute MI.[55,68,77,78] In early studies in nonischemic hearts, bradycardia favored the development of VF.[79] Investigations of ischemic myocardium, however, indicated that slow heart rates exert a protective effect.[77] These concepts are not mutually exclusive, and both must be considered when treating patients with MI.

Bradycardia is particularly prevalent during the first hour after onset of symptoms. This bradycardia is likely due to autonomic dysfunction.[22,26,64] Commonly encountered mechanisms for bradycardia are sinus bradycardia, sinus bradycardia with junctional escape rhythm, and sinus rhythm with second- or third-degree atrioventricular (AV) block.[55] These rhythms are most often the result of increased parasympathetic tone and are particularly likely to be associated with inferior and posterior MI. If the ventricular rate falls below 60 beats per minute and is associated with symptoms, hypotension, or ventricular ectopy, treatment with atropine (0.5 to 1.0 mg IV) is indicated.[68] In theory, some patients with Mobitz II second-degree heart block and third-degree heart block may respond adversely to atropine with a paradoxical ventricular slowing. In the absence of symptoms, hypotension, or ventricular ectopy, bradycardia does not require therapy. Increased vagal tone may contribute to improved electrical stability as long as blood pressure and coronary perfusion are maintained.[80-83] As the rate falls below 50 beats per minute, more intense observation is necessary since such low rates may not maintain an adequate cardiac output in patients with compromised cardiac function.[84,85]

Ventricular escape rhythms (*idioventricular rhythms*) with low rates can be treated either with atropine, which promotes escape of supraventricular pacemakers, or by pacemakers, which increase the rate of the ventricular pacemaker.[86,87] Accelerated idioventricular rhythm (AIVR) is often seen with rates well above 40 beats per minute but less than 100. Ventricular escape rhythms do not require treatment unless they are associated with symptoms. Occasionally AIVR suddenly increases its rate with the same QRS morphology. Such a rhythm is presumed to represent ventricular tachycardia with varying exit block and should be treated as ventricular tachycardia.[88] In many cases, however, AIVR represents an escape ventricular rhythm that develops when the sinus rhythm is too slow. This may also be a rhythm of reperfusion. Atropine or atrial pacing may be needed if hemodynamic consequences occur. Rhythmic precordial percussion or repetitive coughing may be effective as an interim measure in patients with symptomatic bradycardia, pending administration of atropine.

During the prehospital phase, bradycardia requiring therapy that is refractory to atropine may be managed with an external pacemaker.[89]

After atropine the preferred agents for symptomatic bradycardia are dopamine and epinephrine infusions, which are discussed in the section on bradycardia in chapter 1. Some clinicians still use low doses of IV isoproterenol, although isoproterenol may worsen myocardial ischemia and provoke ventricular ectopy. Isoproterenol should be used, if at all, with extreme caution. At low doses (2 to 10 µg/min) it is Class IIb (possibly helpful). At higher doses it is Class III (harmful). The lowest dose that is effective must be used. A constant infusion of 2 to 10 µg/min can be titrated to achieve an adequate heart rate until a transvenous pacemaker can be inserted.

Sinus Tachycardia

Sinus tachycardia (heart rate greater than 100 beats per minute) is a physiological response to stress. In the patient with acute MI, tachycardia alerts the clinician to the likelihood of heart failure or hypovolemia, but other causes (eg, fever, pericarditis, anemia, infection) must be excluded. Appropriate therapeutic decisions may require hemodynamic monitoring to guide proper therapy. In a small but significant number of cases, pain or anxiety or both may be responsible for sinus tachycardia. If so, analgesia and sedation may be the only therapy required. Young patients with anterior MI may have sinus tachycardia plus a hyperdynamic state, including hypertension. This is caused by an increase in circulating catecholamines as well as local increases in catecholamines in injured areas of the heart.[90] Once this hyperdynamic state is diagnosed, the early use of β-adrenergic receptor blocking agents may be useful because excessive catecholamines have negative effects on myocardial ischemia, automaticity, cardiac work, and the threshold for VF. ACE inhibitors have had variable effects on mortality.[91] Hence their early use is discouraged. In many instances tachycardia is due to massive myocardial damage, heart failure, or hypovolemia. In these circumstances β-adrenergic receptor blockade is contraindicated. When hypovolemia is suspected to cause tachycardia, a fluid challenge may be used.

Supraventricular Arrhythmias

Premature atrial complexes per se do not require therapy, but they may be manifestations of occult heart failure or excessive adrenergic tone, for which treatment with diuretics, analgesia, sedation, or β blockade may be appropriate. Atrial tachycardia, flutter, or fibrillation may be due to atrial ischemia,[92] but most often they are associated with left ventricular failure due to increases in left atrial pressure (and pulmonary artery occlusive pressure).[93] These rhythms are seen more often after anterior wall infarction and are associated with increased mortality.[94] The success of therapy frequently depends on correction of the underlying abnormality.

When hemodynamic compromise occurs as a result of supraventricular arrhythmias, the prompt restoration of normal sinus rhythm and rate must be the immediate goal.

Synchronized cardioversion is the treatment of choice for symptomatic supraventricular tachycardias in the setting of acute MI. Adenosine, IV verapamil, or IV diltiazem may be effective in terminating paroxysmal supraventricular tachycardias and in slowing the ventricular response in atrial flutter or fibrillation. Adenosine has the advantage of a very short half-life (as compared with verapamil or diltiazem). If two or three repeat doses of adenosine are unsuccessful, consider verapamil or diltiazem. If verapamil or diltiazem is not immediately successful, cardioversion should be perfomed. If cardioversion is successful but supraventricular tachycardia recurs, do not repeat cardioversion until after underlying abnormalities are corrected and pharmacologic therapy has been instituted to prevent recurrence (eg, procainamide). Diltiazem and verapamil should not be used if hypotension or left ventricular failure is present or if a wide-complex tachycardia is noted.

Atrioventricular Junctional Rhythms

Atrioventricular junctional rhythms may compromise ventricular function. These rhythms reduce ventricular filling caused by the loss of atrial contraction. AV dyssynchrony causes atrial stretch, atrial natriuretic peptide secretion, and reflex systemic hypotension. This is particularly likely when left ventricular failure or right ventricular infarction is present. Sequential AV pacing may help restore the contribution of atrial contraction in this setting. Unless the rate is slow and symptoms or signs of hemodynamic compromise are present, a junctional rhythm with a narrow QRS complex does not require pacemaker placement.

Ventricular Tachycardia

Ventricular tachycardia must be treated promptly. If the patient is hemodynamically stable and asymptomatic, lidocaine may be tried first. Rarely ventricular tachycardia may "break" with vigorous coughing.[95] The precordial thump may cause the rhythm to degenerate to VF, so it is recommended only when collapse occurs and a monitor/defibrillator is not immediately available. Cardioversion (chapter 4) with sedation of the patient, if possible, should be employed without delay if these approaches are unsuccessful or if the patient is unstable in any way.

Atrioventricular Block

First-degree AV block alone does not require treatment. The possibility of progression to higher degrees of block is always present and should be a primary concern. Careful monitoring is essential.[96,97]

Similarly, second-degree AV block of the Mobitz type I (Wenckebach) variety does not require therapy in the absence of hemodynamically significant slowing of the ventricular rate. If treatment is required, atropine (0.5 mg IV) should be tried first. A temporary pacemaker may occasionally be necessary if atropine is not effective or if hemodynamically significant slowing occurs.

When second-degree AV block of the Mobitz type II variety is associated with probable acute MI, it carries a significant risk of progression to complete heart block. Therefore, Mobitz type II heart block is an indication for placement of a transvenous pacemaker.[97,98] The prognosis for patients who develop complete heart block (infranodal) is poor because of its usual association with extensive myocardial injury. The reestablishment of sequential AV contraction may be of value in these patients.

Intraventricular Block

Clinically significant forms of intraventricular block (such as right bundle-branch block plus left anterior or posterior fascicular block, or any of the various forms of trifascicular block[99]) are more likely to occur with anterior MI and are an adverse prognostic sign. The prognostic significance of new isolated right bundle- or left bundle-branch block is less adverse.[100,101] Prognosis associated with intraventricular conduction disturbances is determined predominantly by the extent of myocardial damage rather than by the conduction disturbance.[98] Pacing and aggressive management of hemodynamic abnormalities remain the only therapeutic alternatives. Pacing should be used in all patients with right bundle-branch block unless it is clear that the right bundle-branch block is old. The need for pacing is less clear with left bundle-branch block.[102]

Ventricular Fibrillation

Although the risk of VF is highest during the first few hours of infarction, the risk continues for the first 48 hours and even after discharge from the coronary care unit. High-dose lidocaine administered prophylactically does not reduce mortality and is no longer recommended.[53,56,103-105] When primary VF in the setting of acute infarction is treated promptly with defibrillation, prognosis may not be affected adversely. The likelihood of successful restoration of an effective cardiac rhythm declines rapidly with time. Thus, electrical countershock should be performed at the earliest possible moment.

Secondary VF (VF preceded and apparently provoked by severe ischemia, pump failure, or hypotension) is associated with high mortality: only 20% to 25% of patients survive hospitalization.[106,107] Such patients must be aggressively treated with appropriate anti-ischemic agents and early intra-aortic balloon support and considered for cardiac catheterization and revascularization.

Management of Abnormal Blood Pressure Responses in Myocardial Infarction

Hypotension

During acute infarction hypotension may occur for several reasons. Cardiac output may be decreased (because of low stroke volume or because the heart rate is too slow or too fast), or intravascular volume depletion (hypovolemia) may be present. On occasion systemic vascular resistance may be transiently low because of enhanced vagal tone in association with bradycardia. When hypotension is associated with pulmonary congestion (cardiogenic shock), usually at least 35% of the left ventricular myocardium has been destroyed. Right ventricular damage may also cause hypotension acutely and merit

volume infusion (see below). Treatment is determined by identifying the cause of the hypotension and planning therapy accordingly (see below). Dopamine is the most common pressor used in cardiogenic shock, and clinicians should remember that hypotension in the setting of acute MI is an indication for percutaneous transluminal coronary angioplasty.

Hypertension

Patients who have been previously normotensive or mildly hypertensive may be significantly hypertensive during the evolution of acute MI. This response may be transient and self-limited, but persistent elevation of systolic blood pressure above 140 mm Hg harms recovery because it results in increased myocardial oxygen demand and is associated with mechanical complications such as myocardial rupture and infarct expansion.[108]

Initial therapy consists of relief of pain and anxiety and administration of oxygen. These measures may be sufficient to control mild hypertension. For more severe hypertension, IV nitroglycerin is recommended, especially if concomitant heart failure is present.[109] β-Receptor blockade is indicated in hypertensive patients without evidence of heart failure or heart block. During the first few hours of infarction, blood pressure can be reduced with a short-acting IV agent such as metoprolol or esmolol. The effects of short-activity β blockers can be reversed if hypotension develops. After initial management, you may usually substitute an oral antihypertensive drug.

Management of Heart Failure in Acute Myocardial Infarction

Myocardial infarction may affect the pumping function of the heart in either a generalized or localized manner. When the left ventricle is affected diffusely, there is a decrease in wall motion with a proportionate fall in the amount of blood pumped with each heart beat (stroke volume). As stroke volume falls, left ventricular volume and pressure increase. This increases the myocardial oxygen requirements, and the wall stress reduces subendocardial perfusion. This occurs at a time when blood pressure and coronary perfusion have fallen. These changes adversely affect the relation of myocardial oxygen supply to demand, aggravate myocardial ischemia, and extend infarction. This process begins a pernicious cycle that may end with myocardial necrosis so extensive that the pumping mechanism of the heart is compromised (pump failure). When a critical amount of left ventricular myocardium is destroyed, pump failure may be recognized clinically as pulmonary congestion or by systemic hypotension, or both. In extreme pump failure, pulmonary edema may occur. These syndromes, from mild to severe, are the major determinants of survival in hospitalized patients.[110,111] Thus, aggressive management is recommended.[112] The combination of hypotension with pump failure and pulmonary edema is known as *cardiogenic shock.* The impact of thrombolytic therapy on heart failure in acute MI has not yet been determined.

Clinical Classification

A useful classification to guide the clinical management of patients with acute MI was developed by Killip and Kimball[113]:

Class I. Patients with uncomplicated infarction without evidence of heart failure as judged by the absence of rales and a ventricular filling sound (third heart sound)

Class II. Patients with mild to moderate heart failure as evidenced by pulmonary rales in the lower half of the lung field and a ventricular filling sound

Class III. Patients with severe left ventricular failure or pulmonary edema

Class IV. Patients with cardiogenic shock, defined as systolic blood pressure less than 90 mm Hg (in previously normotensive patients) with oliguria and other evidence of poor peripheral perfusion, such as mental obtundation[113]

Although this classification is a relatively poor predictor of exact hemodynamic status, it continues to be useful in determining which patients are likely to need therapeutic decisions that require hemodynamic monitoring and more aggressive interventions.

Mortality in acute MI is obviously greater for the more severe clinical and hemodynamic classes, exceeding 75% for patients in Class IV. For Class II patients, prompt treatment with diuretics and/or IV nitroglycerin usually results in clinical improvement. Class III heart failure (pulmonary edema) and Class IV (cardiogenic shock) will be discussed in greater detail.

Acute Pulmonary Edema
(See chapter 1, Fig 8)

Pulmonary edema indicates severe left ventricular dysfunction. It is characterized by extreme respiratory distress. Signs of adrenergic stimulation are usually present (eg, tachycardia, diaphoresis). Hypertension or hypotension may be present. In the most severely ill patients, a pink frothy material is exuded from the mouth or nose. Generally either pulmonary edema improves rapidly or the patient dies.

First-line Actions

Initial measures in the management of patients with pulmonary edema include placing the patient in a sitting or semisitting position and providing supplementary oxygen. If IV access is not immediately available, sublingual nitroglycerin can be effective in increasing venous capacitance and decreasing blood pressure and thus significantly decreasing ischemia and myocardial work. Intravenous furosemide is effective in patients with pulmonary edema. Since its primary effect is to increase venous capacitance, pulmonary edema usually resolves before the induction of diuresis.[114] Morphine in a dose of 1 to 5 mg has also been used to increase venous capacitance and to relieve anxiety.

Second-line Actions

If the patient is normotensive or hypertensive, IV nitroglycerin can be used to reduce blood pressure and thereby improve heart failure due to impedance (afterload) reduction.[115] Proper titration is important to avoid hypotension and impaired coronary perfusion, especially if interventions that reduce preload (furosemide and morphine) have been undertaken as well (see above, "Role of Nitroglycerin and Morphine").[112] If the patient is hypotensive, dopamine may be helpful.

In the absence of hypotension, parenteral vasodilators and/or inotropes are the drugs of choice. Since nitroglycerin benefits ischemia and may reduce infarct size[41,47,48] and there is controversy concerning beneficial versus detrimental effects with nitroprusside,[108,116] IV nitroglycerin is preferred for patients with acute infarction. If arterial pressure is inadequate to permit therapy with vasodilators, dobutamine may be used. In general, dobutamine improves contractility, resulting in increases in stroke volume and reflex decreases in systemic vascular resistance. At doses that do not increase heart rate by more than 10%, dobutamine appears unlikely to exacerbate myocardial ischemia.[117,118]

Cardiogenic Shock

The diagnosis of cardiogenic shock is based on depression of blood pressure (usually systolic pressure below 80 to 90 mm Hg or a reduction of 70 mm Hg or more), clinical signs of hypoperfusion (eg, oliguria, mental obtundation, pallor, sweating, and tachycardia) and pulmonary congestion. In the setting of acute MI, it is usually a consequence of extensive infarction, ventricular septal rupture, papillary muscle rupture or dysfunction with acute mitral insufficiency, or free wall rupture. Rarely hypovolemia or right ventricular infarction can present in a similar fashion.[119]

Cardiogenic shock is associated with a mortality rate of 50% to 80%. The lower rates are associated with aggressive treatment, such as cardiac catheterization, PTCA, intra-aortic balloon pump, and coronary artery bypass grafting. When cardiogenic shock is due to loss of a large area (more than 35%) of the left ventricle (myocardiogenic shock), survival is not expected. With prompt treatment patients with surgically correctable complications (eg, ventricular septal rupture and papillary muscle dysfunction) or severe coronary artery disease with preserved left ventricular function may have a slightly better prognosis.[120] Other causes of shock, such as aortic dissection, massive pulmonary embolism, and septic shock, also should be considered in the differential diagnosis.

The cornerstone of therapy is rapid diagnosis and hemodynamic stabilization of the patient. If hypovolemia is found, volume expansion with dextran, blood, or saline may be beneficial. Hypotension unresponsive to a fluid challenge should be treated with pressor support. Usually dopamine is titrated to maintain systolic blood pressure at 80 to 100 mm Hg. If a mechanical abnormality such as acute mitral insufficiency or a left-to-right shunt with a ventricular septal defect is identified or if global ischemia with consequent "stunning" (myocardial hypofunction) is suspected, intra-aortic balloon counterpulsation, cardiac catheterization, and revascularization should be considered. These interventions have been shown to improve outcome.[120]

Cardiogenic shock may also require cardiac catheterization, angioplasty, intra-aortic balloon counterpulsation, and revascularization. If severe hypotension is not present, dobutamine can be tried to improve cardiac output. For severe hypotension, dopamine is recommended. The lowest dose consistent with the desired result should be used. Careful monitoring of cardiac rhythm is essential because of the risk of serious ventricular arrhythmias with greater doses of dopamine. If all else fails, norepinephrine may be added. Early endotracheal intubation is recommended for patients in cardiogenic shock to optimize ventilation, especially if hypoxemia exists.

Right Ventricular Infarction

Shock may occur in the course of MI when the right ventricle is so damaged that it cannot pump blood through the pulmonary circulation into the left ventricle. This syndrome occurs predominantly in patients with inferior infarction. Noninvasive studies have suggested that as many as 30% of patients with acute inferior infarction have associated right ventricular infarction.[121] Hemodynamically significant right ventricular infarction occurs in only about half of these patients. Right ventricular infarction should be suspected in patients with inferior infarction, hypotension, distended neck veins, and relatively clear lungs on auscultation. Right-sided precordial leads often will demonstrate ST-segment elevation.[122,123]

Treatment requires judicious though often vigorous fluid therapy to raise left ventricular filling pressure (PAOP); dobutamine may also be required.[124] Vasodilator drugs should be strictly avoided.

Other Causes of Hemodynamic Collapse to Be Distinguished From Acute Infarction

Massive Pulmonary Embolism

Massive pulmonary embolism may result in shock and cardiovascular collapse. The precipitating event is critical obstruction of the pulmonary arterial system, resulting in

hypoxemia, pulmonary hypertension, and acute right ventricular failure, ie, acute cor pulmonale.[125,126] Patients with pulmonary embolism may have ischemic-type chest pain and ECG abnormalities consistent with myocardial ischemia and, more rarely, pseudoinfarction. The clinical hallmarks of acute cor pulmonale — depression of cardiac output, systemic hypotension, tachycardia, hypoxemia — may be secondary to cardiogenic shock or right ventricular infarction. The initial management of the patient is the same as outlined above, ie, correction of hypoxemia and consideration for intubation, hemodynamic stabilization with IV fluids if there is no pulmonary congestion, and pressors to support blood pressure. The diagnosis can be clarified by specific diagnostic tests. Abnormal nuclear perfusion lung scans and evidence of deep venous thrombosis in the legs favors the diagnosis of pulmonary embolism, which can be a complication of MI, although the routine use of IV and low-dose subcutaneous heparin in the early stages of MI has decreased the likelihood of the complication.[127]

Hypovolemic and Septic Shock

Hypovolemic shock may be associated with the clinical indices of hypoperfusion and hypotension. In contrast to cardiogenic shock, volume loss can be diagnosed through history and clinical evaluation. The explanation for low cardiac output is inadequate left ventricular filling. Emergency personnel must recognize this syndrome because it is readily treatable. Hypotension may lead to changes on the ECG and hence diagnostic confusion. If there is no significant pulmonary congestion on clinical evaluation or chest x-ray, shock should first be treated with volume replacement. When the hematocrit is normal, crystalloid or colloid solution should be used to correct hypovolemia. If the hematocrit is low, whole blood or packed red blood cells are preferable.

In septic shock, hypotension is caused by a marked reduction in systemic vascular resistance, and cardiac output is characteristically increased. Findings are similar in anaphylactic and neurogenic shock. In circumstances where decreased systemic vascular resistance causes shock, treatment with volume replacement dopamine or norepinephrine can help. Definitive therapy is to correct the underlying cause.

Cardiac Tamponade

Acute pericarditis can mimic acute MI. When present, acute pericarditis must be detected, especially if treatment with thrombolytic agents is considered.

Hemodynamic compromise associated with pericarditis occurs only when tamponade is present. Suspect cardiac tamponade when any of these signs exist: persistent tachycardia, pulsus paradoxus (an inspiratory drop in systolic blood pressure greater than 10 to 12 mm Hg), pulsatile neck veins (often with inspiratory distention), an enlarging heart shadow on x-ray, or falling blood pressure. An echocardiogram will help make this diagnosis if time permits.[128,129] If the patient is in shock, immediate augmentation of circulatory blood volume with volume infusion will improve cardiac output. Emergency pericardiocentesis is warranted if the patient's condition is deteriorating and a definitive surgical procedure cannot be performed immediately.[130]

Cardiac rupture after acute MI can also cause tamponade. Patients who sustain cardiac rupture are characteristically aged 60 years and older, with hypertension during the acute phase of their infarction. Cardiac rupture after acute MI can occur as early as day 1 or after the first week.[131] It is more common in women and in patients with no prior history of cardiac disease who are experiencing an uncomplicated recovery after their first infarction.[131] Pericardiocentesis may allow them to survive long enough to undergo emergency surgical repair.

Aortic Dissection

Acute aortic dissection may cause pain similar to that of acute MI. It can cause infarction, acute cardiac tamponade, shock due to acute aortic rupture, or left ventricular failure due to sudden aortic valve regurgitation.

Aortic dissection occurs when a tear of the aortic intima allows blood to enter the aortic wall and strip the intima away from the outer wall of the aorta, driven by the force of the aortic blood pressure. When dissection occurs in the ascending aorta, it may occlude a coronary artery and cause MI. Occlusion of other vessels can cause neurological abnormalities and pulse deficits. Dissection may involve the aortic valve itself and provoke severe regurgitation of the aortic valve. It may dissect into the pericardial space and cause cardiac tamponade. Rupture of the dissection into the pleural space, mediastinum, or retroperitoneal space will cause hypovolemia and shock.[132]

Without recognition and proper therapy, aortic dissection almost always proves fatal. Inappropriate treatment with thrombolytic therapy, in the mistaken belief that one is treating an acute MI, can cause prompt exsanguination. Therefore, the physician must consider aortic dissection early in patients suspected of having an acute MI. History, physical examination, and chest x-ray alert the clinician to the possibility of aortic dissection.

The pain of dissection usually is intense and located in the same area and with the same radiation patterns as that of MI. Dissection of the descending aorta is more likely to cause intrascapular pain or pain radiating to the abdomen. Often the pain of dissection is as severe at its onset as it ever becomes. In contrast, the pain at the beginning of an MI usually increases progressively (crescendo pattern). The clinician should be alert to the possibility of dissection by a history of hypertension or by congenital lesions, such as Marfan's syndrome, that weaken the aortic wall. The physical examination in dissection may reveal pulse deficits, neurological deficits, aortic regurgitation, pericardial rubs, or tamponade. The

chest x-ray usually demonstrates a widened mediastinum.[133] Echocardiography, especially transesophageal echo, may confirm the diagnosis of ascending aortic dissection.[134] Aortography, computed tomography (CT scan) with contrast, or magnetic resonance imaging (MRI) is needed to confirm or exclude the diagnosis when the clinical presentation suggests dissection.[135]

If the patient is hypertensive or normotensive, the initial therapy for dissection should be to lower the blood pressure and the contractile force of the left ventricle. This will stop progressive dissection by the column of aortic blood. Use IV antihypertensive agents — specifically β blockers. Ascending aortic dissections are best treated with early surgical repair. Descending aortic dissections need not be operated on unless (1) pain continues despite medical therapy, (2) there is a threat of infarction of bowel, kidney, or extremities, or (3) rupture occurs.[136,137]

Special Therapeutic Considerations

β-Receptor Blockers

β-Adrenergic blocking agents have been used in the setting of acute MI to decrease myocardial oxygen demand and thus attempt to limit myocardial damage.[138-140] β-Receptor blockers improve long-term survival when used after acute MI,[66,67,141,142] and recent results with metoprolol[143,144] and atenolol[145] have shown that early institution of IV β-receptor blockade in a subgroup of patients with high sympathetic tone has a beneficial effect on mortality.[143,144] In the first day of acute MI, β-receptor blockers also decrease the incidence of and mortality from VF.[145-147] In patients receiving thrombolytic therapy, the institution of early IV β blockers within 2 hours of onset of chest pain significantly decreases mortality and reinfarction.[143,144] In patients treated after 4 to 6 hours of chest pain, the benefits are less striking, although reinfarction rates are lower. Recent data also suggest that metoprolol may help reduce the incidence of intracranial bleeding and myocardial rupture in patients receiving thrombolytic therapy.[148] β Blockers must be used with caution in patients with first-degree heart block and are contraindicated in the presence of more advanced heart block, heart failure, pre-existing bradycardia (less than 60 beats per minute), systolic blood pressure less than 100 mm Hg, severe chronic obstructive lung disease, or peripheral hypoperfusion. In patients with hypertension, ongoing ischemia, or atrial tachyarrhythmias, β blockers are often useful. β Blockers with intrinsic sympathomimetic activity, such as pindolol, should not be used in acute MI.

Nitroglycerin

Nitroglycerin is a potent vasodilator discussed earlier in this chapter (see "Relief of Pain," "Role of Nitroglycerin"). When used early in MI, it can reduce infarct size,[49] incidence of heart failure, and ischemia. It is extremely effective in the early treatment of MI patients with pulmonary congestion, hypertension, or discrete ischemia.

Calcium Channel Blockers

Although there is laboratory evidence that calcium channel blockers reduce infarct size in transmural infarction, these results have not been observed under clinical conditions. Currently there is no reason to recommend general treatment with calcium channel blockers to reduce infarct size.[149] Intravenous diltiazem or verapamil may be used to control rapid ventricular rate in patients with atrial fibrillation if other agents are thought to be contraindicated or unsuitable. They should be used with caution in patients with heart failure or heart block.

Aspirin, Heparin

The ISIS-2 study demonstrated the dramatic mortality benefit of aspirin therapy in acute MI.[150] In this study 160 mg of chewable aspirin achieved a mortality reduction comparable to that of streptokinase. Side effects were few. Given this potential benefit and the minimal side effects, treat virtually all patients with suspected MI with a chewable 160-mg aspirin tablet. Although the optimal dose is in dispute, most authorities recommend a dosage of 150 to 325 mg per day for treating patients during acute MI. Pediatric aspirin preparations may be more palatable than conventional aspirin and are thus preferable when chewable aspirin is used. A daily long-term aspirin dose (80 mg/d) should be continued.[150] It is particularly beneficial in preventing reinfarction.

The role and optimal route of heparin administration remains controversial. Although anticoagulation with heparin has not unequivocally decreased mortality after acute infarction, it appears to prevent embolic complications, infarct extension, deep venous thrombosis, pulmonary emboli, and arterial emboli from cardiac mural thrombi.[151] Low-dose heparin (5000 U subcutaneously or IV every 12 hours) safely and effectively reduces the risk of pulmonary embolization and cerebrovascular accident after infarction.[151] Among patients with transmural anterior MI, 30% to 40% develop left ventricular thrombi. Early anticoagulation with full-dose heparin may prevent mural thrombus formation and subsequent embolization in these patients.[151] Inferior wall MI is much less frequently complicated by thrombus formation or cerebrovascular accident. The ACC/AHA task force report on the management of acute MI recommends the routine use of IV heparin in all patients with transmural MI, except those receiving anistreplase. It is essential with alteplase (see below).[1]

Thrombolytic Therapy

Since the previous edition of this textbook, thrombolytic agents have been confirmed as a revolutionary therapeutic intervention. Numerous studies over the last 10 years have established the clinical benefit of prompt thrombolytic therapy for acute transmural MI. Consider all patients with symptoms and ECG findings suggestive of acute transmural MI for treatment with thrombolytic agents.[152] This section focuses on specific issues that the ACLS provider needs to know to better screen and evaluate patients for thrombolytic therapy.

Thrombolytic Agents: Clinical Features

Several thrombolytic agents have been studied extensively in acute MI: streptokinase, anistreplase, urokinase, prourokinase, and single- and double-stranded recombinant tissue plasminogen activator (rt-PA). The major thrombolytic agents currently available (streptokinase, anistreplase, alteplase) significantly reduce mortality and improve left ventricular function in patients with acute transmural MI.[153] Chapter 8, Table 2 compares the relative features of the various thrombolytic agents.

No thrombolytic agent can be singled out as the overall agent of choice.[153-155] So-called "mega-trials" of the currently available thrombolytic agents have enlisted tens of thousands of patients and have established subtle differences in outcomes.[156] One recent study of more than 41 000 patients in 15 countries observed a significant benefit when alteplase was administered in an "accelerated" fashion.[157] Although this "front-loaded" regimen appears to offer some benefit over previous standard regimens, newer agents and alternative combinations of agents are being developed constantly.[154,155] In addition, researchers are studying new adjunctive antiplatelet and antithrombin agents that should improve the efficacy and safety of thrombolysis even more.[154,155] The major contemporary challenge is not selection of the "best" thrombolytic agent but rather how to reduce excessive patient delay in seeking care.[1,153,154]

The major complication of thrombolytic therapy is bleeding. The incidence of intracranial bleeding is 0.9% to 1.0% in patients aged less than 75 years.[155] This may serve as a deterrent for treatment; however, this risk must be compared with the 3% incidence of in-hospital strokes from all causes in patients with acute MI before the advent of thrombolytic therapy.[155] In addition, randomized placebo-controlled trials of thrombolytic agents have confirmed a comparable incidence of stroke in treatment and placebo groups, with more intracranial hemorrhage reported with thrombolytic agents and more thromboembolic events reported in the placebo group.[155] The incidence of major bleeding (greater than 10-point hematocrit drop or hemorrhage requiring transfusion) is less than 5%. Allergic responses are also common with streptokinase and anistreplase and may require prompt treatment with IV diphenhydramine. Intravenous steroids should be avoided if possible in such patients because of the risk of aneurysm formation.[158] Most patients who have received streptokinase or anistreplase will be sensitized to the drug and should not be re-treated if there is recurrent infarction for fear of drug neutralization or, to a lesser extent, anaphylaxis.[159] Allergic reactions have not been reported with alteplase and are rare with urokinase.

Though early (90-minute) infarct artery patency differs for the available thrombolytic agents (84% for rt-PA, 62% for urokinase, and 48% for streptokinase), 24-hour patency is comparable for all agents (approximately 84% to 85%). Intravenous heparin is essential to maintain the early patency of rt-PA because of its short half-life.[155] Intravenous heparin is recommended but less critical with the other thrombolytic agents. Recent data suggest that heparin should not be used following administration of anistreplase because of the increased risk of bleeding.[155] Despite intense research in this area, questions remain about the clinical value of early artery patency, the desirable "treatment window" for optimal results, the relative safety of the various thrombolytic agents, and optimal adjunctive therapy.

Rapid Diagnosis, Therapy Initiation, Patient Selection

The therapeutic benefit of thrombolytic agents is markedly time-dependent. Strategies must be developed and implemented to achieve rapid initiation of therapy. Healthcare professionals involved in the care of patients with acute MI must prospectively develop written plans and protocols appropriate for their resources. Protocols require input from emergency department physicians, cardiologists, internists, pharmacists, nurses, and the prehospital EMS program.

The protocol should address the following: identification of patients with chest pain in the prehospital setting (if EMS systems are involved), triage of patients in the emergency department, a mechanism to rapidly obtain a 12-lead ECG, determination of contraindications to thrombolytic therapy, location of thrombolytic drugs and how mixed, designation of who decides to order thrombolytic therapy, and consultation for atypical cases. Finally, healthcare professionals must develop a standard time interval from emergency department arrival to treatment administration and prospective monitoring of procedures and times to assess performance. An interval of 30 to 60 minutes is a widely recommended goal.

The National Heart, Lung, and Blood Institute publication *Emergency Department: Rapid Identification and Treatment of Patients With Acute Myocardial Infarction* (NIH publication 93-3278; September 1993) provides an excellent series of protocols and recommendations consistent with the AHA guidelines and should be reviewed by all providers who treat patients with chest pain.

EMS systems can be assigned responsibility for prehospital evaluation and screening of patients. The following information should be obtained for patients complaining of chest pain:

- Pain of probable cardiac origin
- Age greater than 30 years
- Systolic blood pressure less than 180 mm Hg; diastolic blood pressure less than 110 mm Hg
- Persistent pain for 15 minutes or longer
- Lack of cerebrovascular accident or other serious central nervous system problems in preceding 6 months
- No surgery or major trauma in preceding 2 weeks
- No bleeding problems
- No pregnancy

If the answer to all questions is *yes*, a 12-lead ECG should be obtained and either verbally or directly transmitted to the emergency department. If an ECG cannot be obtained, then the patient should be transported immediately to the emergency department.

A number of studies have addressed prehospital administration of thrombolytic therapy.[160-165] European researchers have established the feasibility and safety of starting thrombolytic therapy in the prehospital setting, using physicians as emergency personnel.[166] Similar results have been observed in US studies where paramedics rather than physicians assessed the patients and initiated thrombolytic therapy.[164] If circumstances routinely delay in-hospital administration of thrombolytic therapy, then prehospital initiation of thrombolytic agents is acceptable and definitely helpful.[153,164]

Several trials have demonstrated that the maximal reduction of mortality occurs in patients who see a physician within 3 hours of chest pain.[153,155] The emergency department must make every effort to rapidly identify patients with suspected acute MI when they enter the department. Patients with chest pain, chest tightness, acute epigastric distress, and other symptoms suggestive of MI must be evaluated quickly and, when appropriate, placed on a protocol. These patients should have ECG monitoring from time of entry, an immediate full ECG, and frequent measurement of vital signs, and they must be seen by a physician within the first few minutes of arrival in the emergency department. Delays in evaluation and treatment related to hospital administrative procedures, such as establishing insurance coverage, must not occur.

The diagnosis of acute transmural MI is based on the patient's history and ECG findings. In patients in whom the clinical presentation and ECG are characteristic of acute MI, the initial therapy should be started by appropriately trained emergency physicians and staff. This includes appropriate use of thrombolytic therapy. When the diagnosis of acute MI is less certain, consult with an immediately available cardiologist or internist. Prolonged efforts to consult with the patient's private physician are inappropriate if likely to result in a delay in therapy.

The maximum clinical benefit is realized in patients with acute anterior or inferior transmural MI (ST-segment elevation greater than 1 to 2 mm in two or more leads) treated within 90 minutes from onset of acute MI symptoms. Most clinical benefit occurs in patients treated 6 hours or less after the onset of acute MI symptoms.[153] Two recent studies, however, have established that thrombolytic therapy produces significant benefit to patients when administered up to 12 hours[167] and even 24 hours from symptom onset.[168]

The mechanism of benefit for patients treated after the first 2 hours is unclear. The major benefit may follow the restoration of an open artery sooner than might occur from spontaneous reperfusion. Other proposed mechanisms include superior ventricular healing and remodeling, improved collateral vessels, and improved electrophysiological stability.

Most studies initially restricted the use of thrombolytic therapy to patients less than 75 years old because of concern about excessive hemorrhagic complications. Older MI patients, however, experience a high mortality from their acute MI that outweighs their increased risks of complications. Two studies published in 1993 eliminated age restrictions on patients receiving thrombolytic therapy and demonstrated significant clinical benefits for persons aged more than 75 years.[167,168] The risk of hemorrhagic complications is highest in elderly patients who are female, diabetic, and/or hypertensive.[148,169] Similarly, treatment benefits patients with new left bundle-branch block or right bundle-branch block.[170] The value of thrombolytic therapy in patients with non–Q-wave MI has not been established and is the focus of a large multicenter National Institutes of Health trial (TIMI III). Patients with sustained systolic blood pressure greater than 180 mm Hg systolic or greater than 110 mm Hg diastolic, recent surgery or major trauma (less than 2 weeks), known history of recent gastrointestinal or genitourinary bleeding, known bleeding diathesis, pregnancy, chest pain of more than 12 hours' duration, or prolonged or traumatic CPR should not receive thrombolytic therapy, although each case is unique and clinicians must always make a risk-benefit assessment based on the therapeutic options and perceived consequences of alternate strategies.

In patients deemed to be candidates for thrombolytic therapy, two large-bore peripheral IV lines should be started and baseline blood samples drawn for analysis before administration of the thrombolytic agent.

Adjunctive Therapy

The major adjunctive agents to consider for patients with acute MI are β blockers, morphine, aspirin, heparin, ACE inhibitors, nitroglycerin, magnesium sulfate, and calcium channel blockers. Virtually every patient who you suspect is having an acute MI should be given an aspirin to chew as soon as possible. Aggressive pain control should be achieved with nitroglycerin and morphine.

Control elevated blood pressure and heart rates with β blockers. The other adjunctive agents have particular indications and counterindications and are discussed in chapter 1 and the pharmacology chapters.

Treatment of Complications With Thrombolytic Therapy

Allergic reactions may occur in 5% to 10% of patients following treatment with streptokinase or anistreplase. Early allergic reactions may manifest in several ways, ranging from itching to hypotension. If the patient develops hives, IV diphenhydramine is useful and steroids may also be used, although data from studies of laboratory animals suggest that early use of steroids predisposes patients to infarct expansion.[171] Hypotension, if observed, usually responds to fluids or placing the patient in a Trendelenburg position (head down, feet up) if there is no pulmonary congestion. Pressors are seldom needed.

Major gastrointestinal, genitourinary, or intracranial bleeding can occur in approximately 1% of patients, and bleeding may occur early in patients with undetected underlying pathology. If major bleeding occurs, the thrombolytic infusion and heparin should be discontinued and blood samples drawn to measure hematocrit and fibrinogen. Blood loss should be replaced with whole blood/packed red cells if needed. Coagulation abnormalities that are a consequence of thrombolytic therapy (ie, fibrinogen depletion, decrease in factors V and VIII) can be corrected to a large extent by giving fresh frozen plasma and cryoprecipitate. For patients receiving streptokinase, aminocaproic acid (Amicar) can also be used. Arrhythmias are treated in the usual fashion.

References

1. ACC/AHA guidelines for the early management of patients with acute myocardial infarction: a report of the American College of Cardiology/American Heart Association Task Force on Assessment of Diagnostic and Therapeutic Cardiovascular Procedures (Subcommittee to Develop Guidelines for the Early Management of Patients with Acute Myocardial Infarction). Gunnar RM, Bourdillon PDV, Dixon DW, et al. Special report. *Circulation.* 1990;82:664-707.
2. Chapman I. Morphogenesis of occluding coronary artery thrombosis. *Arch Path.* 1965;80:256-261.
3. Ambrose JA, Winters SL, Stern A, et al. Angiographic morphology and the pathogenesis of unstable angina pectoris. *J Am Coll Cardiol.* 1985;5:609-616.
4. Wilson RF, Holida MD, White CW. Quantitative angiographic morphology of coronary stenoses leading to myocardial infarction or unstable angina. *Circulation.* 1986;73:286-293.
5. Maseri A, L'Abbate A, Baroldi G, et al. Coronary vasospasm as a possible cause of myocardial infarction: a conclusion derived from the study of 'preinfarction' angina. *N Engl J Med.* 1978;299:1271-1277.
6. Oliva PB, Breckinridge JC. Arteriographic evidence of coronary arterial spasm in acute myocardial infarction. *Circulation.* 1977;56:366-374.
7. DeWood MA, Stifter WF, Simpson CS, et al. Coronary arteriographic findings soon after non–Q-wave myocardial infarction. *N Engl J Med.* 1986;315:417-423.
8. Howard RE, Hueter DC, Davis GJ. Acute myocardial infarction following cocaine abuse in a young woman with normal coronary arteries. *JAMA.* 1985;254:95-96.

9. Kuller LH. Sudden death — definition and epidemiologic considerations. *Prog Cardiovasc Dis.* 1980;23:1-12.

10. Pantridge JF, Geddes JS. A mobile intensive-care unit in the management of myocardial infarction. *Lancet.* 1967;2:271-273.

11. Phipps C. Contributory causes of coronary thrombosis. *JAMA.* 1936;106:761-762.

12. Master AM, Dack S, Jaffe HL. Factors and events associated with onset of coronary artery thrombosis. *JAMA.* 1937;109:546-549.

13. Fitzhugh G, Hamilton BE. Coronary occlusion and fatal angina pectoris: study of the immediate causes and their prevention. *JAMA.* 1933;100:475-480.

14. Smith C, Sauls HC, Ballew J. Coronary occlusion: clinical study of 100 patients. *Ann Intern Med.* 1942;17:681-692.

15. French AJ, Dock W. Fatal coronary arteriosclerosis in young soldiers. *JAMA.* 1944;124:1233-1237.

16. Boas EP. Some immediate causes of cardiac infarction. *Am Heart J.* 1942;23:1-15.

17. Levine HD. Acute myocardial infarction following wasp sting: report of two cases and critical survey of the literature. *Am Heart J.* 1976;91:365-374.

18. Muller JE, Stone PH, Turi ZG, et al. Circadian variation in the frequency of onset of acute myocardial infarction. *N Engl J Med.* 1985;313:1315-1322.

19. Levine RL, Pepe PE, Fromm RE Jr, Curka PA, Clark PA. Prospective evidence of a circadian rhythm for out-of-hospital cardiac arrest. *JAMA.* 1992;267:2935-2937.

20. Marchant B, Ranjadayalan K, Stevenson R, Wilkinson P, Timmis AD. Circadian and seasonal factors in the pathogenesis of acute myocardial infarction: the influence of environmental temperature. *Br Heart J.* 1993;69:385-387.

21. Jenkins CD. Recent evidence supporting psychologic and social risk factors for coronary disease. *N Engl J Med.* 1976;294:1033-1038.

22. Rahe RH, Romo M, Bennett L, Siltanen P. Recent life changes, myocardial infarction, and abrupt coronary death: studies in Helsinki. *Arch Intern Med.* 1974;133:221-228.

23. Paraskos JA. Approach to the patient with chest pain. In: Rippe JM, Irwin RS, Alpert JS, Fink MP, eds. *Intensive Care Medicine.* 2nd ed. Boston, Mass: Little Brown and Co; 1991:359-364.

24. *Heart Attack: Signals and Actions for Survival.* Dallas, Tex: American Heart Association; 1976.

25. Peberdy M, Ornato JP. Coronary artery disease in women. *Heart Dis Stroke.* 1992;1:315-319.

26. Rose RM, Lewis AJ, Fewkes J, Clifton JF, Criley JM. Occurrence of arrhythmias during the first hour in acute myocardial infarction. *Circulation.* 1974;50(suppl 3):III-121. Abstract.

27. Moss AJ, Goldstein S. The pre-hospital phase of acute myocardial infarction. *Circulation.* 1970;41:737-742.

28. Goldberg RJ, Gurwitz J, Yarzebski J, et al. Patient delay and receipt of thrombolytic therapy among patients with acute myocardial infarction from a community-wide perspective. *Am J Cardiol.* 1992;70:421-425.

29. Gonzalez ER, Jones LA, Ornato JP, Bleecker GC, Strauss MJ. Hospital delays and problems with thrombolytic administration in patients receiving thrombolytic therapy: a multicenter prospective assessment. Virginia Thrombolytic Study Group. *Ann Emerg Med.* 1992;21:1215-1221.

30. Turi ZG, Stone PH, Muller JE, et al. Implications for acute intervention related to time of hospital arrival in acute myocardial infarction. *Am J Cardiol.* 1986;58:203-209.

31. Weaver WD, Eisenberg MS, Martin JS, et al. Myocardial infarction triage and intervention project — phase I: patient characteristics and feasibility of prehospital initiation of thrombolytic therapy. *J Am Coll Cardiol.* 1990;15:925-931.

32. Standards and guidelines for cardiopulmonary resuscitation (CPR) and emergency cardiac care (ECC). *JAMA.* 1986;255:2905-2984.

33. Valentine PA, Fluck DC, Mounsey JP, Reid D, Shillingford JP, Steiner RE. Blood-gas changes after acute myocardial infarction. *Lancet.* 1966;2:837-841.

34. Fillmore SJ, Shapiro M, Killip T. Arterial oxygen tension in acute myocardial infarction: serial analysis of clinical state and blood gas changes. *Am Heart J.* 1970;79:620-629.

35. Maroko PR, Radvany P, Braunwald E, Hale SL. Reduction of infarct size by oxygen inhalation following acute coronary occlusion. *Circulation.* 1975;52:360-368.

36. Madias JE, Hood WB Jr. Reduction of precordial ST-segment elevation in patients with anterior myocardial infarction by oxygen breathing. *Circulation.* 1976;53(suppl 1):I-198-I-200.

37. Thomas M, Malmcrona R, Shillingford J. Haemodynamic effects of oxygen in patients with acute myocardial infarction. *Br Heart J.* 1965;27:401-407.

38. Sukumalchantra Y, Levy S, Danzig R, Rubins S, Alpern H, Swan HJ. Correcting arterial hypoxemia by oxygen therapy in patients with acute myocardial infarction: effect on ventilation and hemodynamics. *Am J Cardiol.* 1969;24:838-852.

39. Ganz W, Donoso R, Marcus H, Swan HJ. Coronary hemodynamics and myocardial oxygen metabolism during oxygen breathing in patients with and without coronary artery disease. *Circulation.* 1972;45:763-768.

40. Eisenberg PR, Jaffe AS. Coronary thrombolysis: practical considerations. *Cardiol Clin.* 1987;5:129-141.

41. Jaffe AS, Geltman EM, Tiefenbrunn AJ, et al. Reduction of infarct size in patients with inferior infarction with intravenous glyceryl trinitrate. *Br Heart J.* 1983;49:452-460.

42. Zelis R, Mansour EJ, Capone RJ, Mason DT. The cardiovascular effects of morphine: the peripheral capacitance and resistance vessels in human subjects. *J Clin Invest.* 1974;54:1247-1258.

43. Semenkovich CF, Jaffe AS. Adverse effects due to morphine sulfate: challenge to previous clinical doctrine. *Am J Med.* 1985;79:325-330.

44. Come PC, Pitt B. Nitroglycerin-induced severe hypotension and bradycardia in patients with acute myocardial infarction. *Circulation.* 1976;54:624-628.

45. Epstein SE, Borer JS, Kent KM, Redwood DR, Goldstein RE, Levitt B. Protection of ischemic myocardium by nitroglycerin: experimental and clinical results. *Circulation.* 1976;53:(suppl 1):I-191-I-198.

46. Dalen JE, Ockene IS, Alpert JS. Coronary spasm, coronary thrombosis, and myocardial infarction: a hypothesis concerning the pathophysiology of acute myocardial infarction. *Am Heart J.* 1982;104:1119-1124.

47. Bussmann WD, Passek D, Seidel W, Kaltenbach M. Reduction of CK and CK-MB indexes of infarct size by intravenous nitroglycerin. *Circulation.* 1981;63:615-622.

48. Flaherty JT, Becker LC, Bulkley BH, et al. A randomized prospective trial of intravenous nitroglycerin in patients with acute myocardial infarction. *Circulation.* 1983;68:576-588.

49. Jugdutt BI. Role of nitrates after acute myocardial infarction. *Am J Cardiol.* 1992;70:828-878.

50. Stockman MB, Verrier RL, Lown B. Effect of nitroglycerin on vulnerability to ventricular fibrillation during myocardial ischemia and reperfusion. *Am J Cardiol.* 1979;43:233-238.

51. Antman EM, Lau J, Kupelnick B, Mostellar F, Chalmers TC. A comparison of results of meta-analyses of randomized control trials and recommendations of clinical experts: treatments for myocardial infarction. *JAMA.* 1992;268:240-248.

52. Jaffe AS. Prophylactic lidocaine for suspected acute myocardial infarction? *Heart Disease Stroke.* 1992;1:179-183.

53. Jaffe AS. The use of antiarrhythmics in advanced cardiac life support. *Ann Emerg Med.* 1993;22:307-316.

54. DeSanctis RW, Block P, Hutter AM Jr. Tachyarrhythmias in myocardial infarction. *Circulation.* 1972;45:681-702.

55. Kimball JT, Killip T. Aggressive treatment of arrhythmias in acute myocardial infarction: procedures and results. *Prog Cardiovasc Dis.* 1968;10:483-504.

56. Lie KI, Wellens HJ, van Capelle FJ, Durrer D. Lidocaine in the prevention of primary ventricular fibrillation: a double-blind, randomized study of 212 consecutive patients. *N Engl J Med.* 1974;291:1324-1326.

57. Wyman MG, Hammersmith L. Comprehensive treatment plan for the prevention of primary ventricular fibrillation in acute myocardial infarction. *Am J Cardiol.* 1974;33:661-667.

58. Lawrie DM. Ventricular fibrillation in acute myocardial infarction. *Am Heart J.* 1969;78:424-426.

59. Lie KI, Wellens HJ, Downar E, Durrer D. Observations on patients with primary ventricular fibrillation complicating acute myocardial infarction. *Circulation.* 1975;52:755-759.

60. Dhurandhar RW, MacMillan RL, Brown KW. Primary ventricular fibrillation complicating acute myocardial infarction. *Am J Cardiol.* 1971;27:347-351.

61. Gonzalez ER. Pharmacologic controversies in CPR. *Ann Emerg Med.* 1993;22:317-323.
62. Jaffe A. Putting it all together: resuscitation of the patient. In: Jaffe A, ed. *Textbook of Advanced Cardiac Life Support.* 2nd ed. Dallas, Tex: American Heart Association, 1990:235-248.
63. Oliver MF. Significance of ventricular arrhythmias during myocardial ischemia. *Circulation.* 1976;53(suppl 1):I-155-I-157.
64. Adgey AA, Allen JD, Geddes JS, et al. Acute phase of myocardial infarction. *Lancet.* 1971;2:501-504.
65. Lucchesi BR, Kniffen FJ. Pharmacological modification of arrhythmias after experimentally induced acute myocardial infarction: drugs acting on the nervous system. *Circulation.* 1975;52 (suppl 3):III-241-III-247.
66. β-Blocker Heart Attack Trial Group. A randomized trial of propranolol in patients with acute myocardial infarction, I: mortality results. *JAMA.* 1982;247:1707-1714.
67. Pedersen TR. Six-year follow-up of the Norwegian Multicenter Study on Timolol after acute myocardial infarction. *N Engl J Med.* 1985;313:1055-1058.
68. Rotman M, Wagner GS, Wallace AG. Bradyarrhythmias in acute myocardial infarction. *Circulation.* 1972;45:703-722.
69. Nordrehaug JE, Johannessen A, von der Lippe G. Serum potassium concentration as a risk factor of ventricular arrhythmias early in acute myocardial infarction. *Circulation.* 1985;71:645-649.
70. Kafka H, Langevin L, Armstrong PW. Serum magnesium and potassium in acute myocardial infarction: influence on ventricular arrhythmias. *Arch Intern Med.* 1987;147:465-469.
71. Ornato JP, Gonzalez ER, Starke H, Morkunas A, Coyne MR, Beck CL. Incidence and causes of hypokalemia associated with cardiac resuscitation. *Am J Emerg Med.* 1985;3:503-506.
72. Dyckner T, Wester PO. Potassium/magnesium depletion in patients with cardiovascular disease. *Am J Med.* 1987;82:11-17.
73. Hollifield JW. Electrolyte disarray and cardiovascular disease. *Am J Cardiol.* 1989;63:21B-26B.
74. Whang R, Whang DD, Ryan MP. Refractory potassium repletion: a consequence of magnesium deficiency. *Arch Intern Med.* 1992;152:40-45.
75. Rasmussen HS, Grønbaek M, Cintin C, Balsløv S, Nørregård P, McNair P. One-year death rate in 270 patients with suspected acute myocardial infarction, initially treated with intravenous magnesium or placebo. *Clin Cardiol.* 1988;11:377-381.
76. Rasmussen HS, Cintin C, Aurup P, Breum L, McNair P. The effect of intravenous magnesium therapy on serum and urine levels of potassium, calcium and sodium in patients with ischemic heart disease, with and without acute myocardial infarction. *Arch Intern Med.* 1988;148:1801-1805.
77. Epstein SE, Goldstein RE, Redwood DR, et al. The early phase of acute myocardial infarction: pharmacologic aspects of therapy. *Ann Intern Med.* 1973;78:918-936.
78. Grauer LE, Gershen BJ, Orlando MM, Epstein SE. Bradycardia and its complications in the prehospital phase of acute myocardial infarction. *Am J Cardiol.* 1973;32:607-611.
79. Han J, Millet D, Chizzonitti B, Moe GK. Temporal dispersion of recovery of excitability in atrium and ventricle as a function of heart rate. *Am Heart J.* 1966;71:481-487.
80. Corr PB, Gillis RA. Effect of autonomic neural influences on the cardiovascular changes induced by coronary occlusion. *Am Heart J.* 1975;89:767-774.
81. Goldstein RE, Karsh RB, Smith ER, et al. Influence of atropine and of vagally mediated bradycardia on the occurrence of ventricular arrhythmias following acute coronary occlusion in closed-chest dogs. *Circulation.* 1973;47:1180-1190.
82. Scherlag BJ, Helfant RH, Haft JI, Damato AN. Electrophysiology underlying ventricular arrhythmias due to coronary ligation. *Am J Physiol.* 1970;219:1665-1671.
83. Kent KM, Smith ER, Redwood DR, Epstein SE. Electrical stability of acutely ischemic myocardium: influences of heart rate and vagal stimulation. *Circulation.* 1973;47:291-298.
84. James TN. The coronary circulation and conduction system in acute myocardial infarction. *Prog Cardiovasc Dis.* 1968;10:410-449.
85. Gregory JJ, Grance WJ. The management of sinus bradycardia, nodal rhythm and heart block for the prevention of cardiac arrest in acute myocardial infarction. *Prog Cardiovasc Dis.* 1968;10:505-517.
86. Massumi RA, Mason DT, Amsterdam EA, et al. Ventricular fibrillation and tachycardia after intravenous atropine for treatment of bradycardias. *N Engl J Med.* 1972;287:336-338.
87. Higgins CB, Vatner SF, Braunwald E. Parasympathetic control of the heart. *Pharmacol Rev.* 1973;25:119-155.
88. de Soyza N, Bissett JK, Kane JJ, Murphy ML, Doherty JE. Association of accelerated idioventricular rhythm and paroxysmal ventricular tachycardia in acute myocardial infarction. *Am J Cardiol.* 1974;34:667-670.
89. Zoll PM, Zoll RH, Falk RH, Clinton JE, Eitel DR, Antman EM. External noninvasive temporary cardiac pacing: clinical trials. *Circulation.* 1985;71:937-944.
90. Corr PB, Gillis RA. Autonomic neural influences on the dysrhythmias resulting from myocardial infarction. *Circ Res.* 1978;43:1-9.
91. Yusuf S. Clinical experience in protecting the failing heart. *Clin Cardiol.* 1993;16 (suppl 2):II-25-II-29.
92. Hod H, Lew AS, Keltai M, et al. Early atrial fibrillation during evolving myocardial infarction: a consequence of impaired left atrial perfusion. *Circulation.* 1987;75:146-150.
93. Sugiura T, Iwasaka T, Ogawa A, et al. Atrial fibrillation in acute myocardial infarction. *Am J Cardiol.* 1985;56:27-29.
94. Cristal N, Szwarcberg J, Gueron M. Supraventricular arrhythmias in acute myocardial infarction: prognostic importance of clinical setting; mechanism of production. *Ann Intern Med.* 1975;82:35-39.
95. Wei JY, Greene HL, Weisfeldt ML. Cough-facilitated conversion of ventricular tachycardia. *Am J Cardiol.* 1980;45:174-176.
96. Kitchen MG III, Kastor JA. Pacing in acute myocardial infarction: indications, methods, hazards and results. In: Brest AN, Wiener L, Chung EK, et al, eds. *Innovations in the Diagnosis and Management of Acute Myocardial Infarction.* Philadelphia, Pa: FA Davis Co; 1975;7(No. 1):219. Cardiovascular Clinics Series.
97. Norris RM, Mercer CJ. Significance of idioventricular rhythms in acute myocardial infarction. *Prog Cardiovasc Dis.* 1974;16:455-468.
98. Haft J. I: Clinical implications of atrioventricular and intraventricular conduction abnormalities. II: Acute myocardial infarction. In: Rios JC, ed. *Clinical-Electrocardiographic Correlations.* Philadelphia, Pa: FA Davis Co; 1977;8(No. 3):65. Cardiovascular Clinics Series.
99. Hindman MC, Wagner GS, JaRo M, et al. The clinical significance of bundle branch block complicating acute myocardial infarction, II: indications for temporary and permanent pacemaker insertion. *Circulation.* 1978;58:689-699.
100. Hollander G, Nadiminti V, Lichstein E, Greengart A, Sanders M. Bundle branch block in acute myocardial infarction. *Am Heart J.* 1983;105:738-743.
101. Klein RC, Vera Z, Mason DT. Intraventricular conduction defects in acute myocardial infarction: incidence, prognosis, and therapy. *Am Heart J.* 1984;108:1007-1013.
102. Jaffe AS. Complications of acute myocardial infarction. *Cardiol Clin.* 1984;2:79-94.
103. Antman EM, Berlin JA. Declining incidence of ventricular fibrillation in myocardial infarction: implications for the prophylactic use of lidocaine. *Circulation.* 1992;86:764-773.
104. Gao R. Reperfusion arrhythmias in acute myocardial infarction [in Chinese]. *Chung Hua Hsin Hsueh Kuan Ping Tsa Chih.* 1992;20:84-86, 133.
105. Berntsen RF, Rasmussen K. Lidocaine to prevent ventricular fibrillation in the prehospital phase of suspected acute myocardial infarction: the North-Norwegian Lidocaine Intervention Trial. *Am Heart J.* 1992;124:1478-1483.
106. Bigger JT Jr, Dresdale FJ, Heissenbuttel RH, Weld FM, Wit AL. Ventricular arrhythmias in ischemic heart disease: mechanism, prevalence, significance, and management. *Prog Cardiovasc Dis.* 1977;19:255-300.
107. Goldberg RJ, Gore JM, Haffajee CI, Alpert JS, Dalen JE. Outcome after cardiac arrest during acute myocardial infarction. *Am J Cardiol.* 1987;59:251-255.
108. Durrer JD, Lie KI, van Capelle FJ, Durrer D. Effect of sodium nitroprusside on mortality in acute myocardial infarction. *N Engl J Med.* 1982;306:1121-1128.
109. Flaherty JT. Role of nitrates in acute myocardial infarction. *Am J Cardiol.* 1992;70:73B-81B.
110. Resnekov L. Management of acute myocardial infarction. *Cardiovasc Med.* 1977;2:949.

111. Hamosh P, Cohn JN. Left ventricular function in acute myocardial infarction. *J Clin Invest.* 1971;50:523-533.

112. Genton R, Jaffe AS. Management of congestive heart failure in patients with acute myocardial infarction. *JAMA.* 1986;256: 2556-2560.

113. Killip T III, Kimball JT. Treatment of myocardial infarction in a coronary care unit: a two-year experience with 250 patients. *Am J Cardiol.* 1967;20:457-464.

114. Dikshit K, Vyden JK, Forrester JS, Chatterjee K, Prakash R, Swan HJ. Renal and extrarenal hemodynamic effects of furosemide in congestive heart failure after acute myocardial infarction. *N Engl J Med.* 1973;288:1087-1090.

115. Cohn JN, Franciosa JA. Vasodilator therapy of cardiac failure. *N Engl J Med.* 1977;297:254-258.

116. Cohn JN, Franciosa JA, Francis GS, et al. Effect of short-term infusion of sodium nitroprusside on mortality rates in acute myocardial infarction complicated by left ventricular failure: results of a Veterans Administration cooperative study. *N Engl J Med.* 1982;306:1129-1135.

117. Gillespie TA, Ambos HD, Sobel BE, Roberts R. Effects of dobutamine in patients with acute myocardial infarction. *Am J Cardiol.* 1977;39:588-594.

118. Rude RE, Izquierdo C, Buja LM, Willerson JT. Effects of inotropic and chronotropic stimuli on acute myocardial ischemic injury, I: studies with dobutamine in the anesthetized dog. *Circulation.* 1982;65:1321-1328.

119. Rackley CE, Russell RO Jr, Mantle JA, Moraski RE. Cardiogenic shock: recognition and management. *Cardiovasc Clin.* 1975;7:251-258.

120. Jaffe AS. Who is likely to survive cardiogenic shock? *Clin Management.* 1982;7:699-713.

121. Dell'Italia LJ, Starling MR, Crawford MH, Boros BL, Chaudhuri TK, O'Rourke RA. Right ventricular infarction: identification by hemodynamic measurements before and after volume loading and correlation with noninvasive techniques. *J Am Coll Cardiol.* 1984; 4:931-939.

122. Lopez-Sendon J, Coma-Canella I, Alcasena S, Seoane J, Gamallo C. Electrocardiographic findings in acute right ventricular infarction: sensitivity and specificity of electrocardiographic alterations in right precordial leads V_4R, V_3R, V_1, V_2, and V_3. *J Am Coll Cardiol.* 1985;6:1273-1279.

123. Reddy GV, Schamroth L. The electrocardiology of right ventricular myocardial infarction. *Chest.* 1986;90:756-760.

124. Dell'Italia LJ, Starling MR, Blumhardt R, Lasher JC, O'Rourke RA. Comparative effects of volume loading, dobutamine, and nitroprusside in patients with predominant right ventricular infarction. *Circulation.* 1985;72:1327-1335.

125. McIntyre KM, Sasahara AA. The hemodynamic response to pulmonary embolism in patients without prior cardiopulmonary disease. *Am J Cardiol.* 1971;28:288-294.

126. Paraskos JA. Pulmonary heart disease including pulmonary embolism. In: Parmley WW, Chatterjee K, eds. *Cardiology.* Philadelphia, Pa: JB Lippincott Co; 1987.

127. Warlow C, Terry G, Kenmure AC, Beattie AG, Ogston D, Douglas AS. A double-blind trial of low doses of subcutaneous heparin in the prevention of deep-vein thrombosis after myocardial infarction. *Lancet.* 1973;2:934-936.

128. Feigenbaum H. Echocardiographic diagnosis of pericardial effusion. *Am J Cardiol.* 1970;26:475-479.

129. D'Cruz IA, Cohen HC, Prabhu R, Glick G. Diagnosis of cardiac tamponade by echocardiography: changes in mitral valve motion and ventricular dimensions, with special reference to paradoxical pulse. *Circulation.* 1975;52:460-465.

130. Spodick DH. Acute cardiac tamponade: pathologic physiology, diagnosis and management. *Prog Cardiovasc Dis.* 1967;10:64-96.

131. Bates RJ, Beutler S, Resnekov L, Anagnostopoulos CE. Cardiac rupture — challenge in diagnosis and management. *Am J Cardiol.* 1977;40:429-437.

132. Roberts WC. Aortic dissection: anatomy, consequences, and causes. *Am Heart J.* 1981;101:195-214.

133. Slater EE, DeSanctis RW. The clinical recognition of dissecting aortic aneurysm. *Am J Med.* 1976;60:625-633.

134. Victor MF, Mintz GS, Kotler MN, Wilson AR, Segal BL. Two-dimensional echocardiographic diagnosis of aortic dissection. *Am J Cardiol.* 1981;48:1155-1159.

135. Lardé D, Belloir C, Vasile N, Frija J, Ferrané J. Computed tomography of aortic dissection. *Radiology.* 1980;136:147-151.

136. Dalen JE, Alpert JS, Cohn LH, Black H, Collins JJ. Dissection of the thoracic aorta: medical or surgical therapy? *Am J Cardiol.* 1974;34:803-808.

137. Doroghazi RM, Slater EE, DeSanctis RW, Buckley MJ, Austen WG, Rosenthal S. Long-term survival of patients with treated aortic dissection. *J Am Coll Cardiol.* 1984;3:1026-1034.

138. Maroko PR, Kjekshus JK, Sobel BE, et al. Factors influencing infarct size following experimental coronary artery occlusions. *Circulation.* 1971;43:67-82.

139. International Collaborative Study Group. Reduction of infarct size with the early use of timilol in acute myocardial infarction. *N Engl J Med.* 1984;310:9-15.

140. Rude RE, Muller JE, Braunwald E. Efforts to limit the size of myocardial infarcts. *Ann Intern Med.* 1981;95:736-761.

141. The Norwegian Multicenter Study Group. Timolol-induced reduction in mortality and reinfarction in patients surviving acute myocardial infarction. *N Engl J Med.* 1981;304:801-807.

142. Herlitz J, Elmfeldt D, Holmberg S, et al. Göteborg Metoprolol Trial: mortality and causes of death. *Am J Cardiol.* 1984;53:9D-14D.

143. The MIAMI Trial Research Group. Metoprolol in acute myocardial infarction: development of myocardial infarction. *Am J Cardiol.* 1985;56:23G-26G.

144. The MIAMI Trial Research Group. Metoprolol in acute myocardial infarction: enzymatic estimation of infarct size. *Am J Cardiol.* 1985;56:27G-29G.

145. Smith LF, Heagerty AM, Bing RF, Barnett DB. Intravenous infusion of magnesium sulphate after acute myocardial infarction: effects on arrhythmias and mortality. *Int J Cardiol.* 1986;12:175-183.

146. Norris RM, Barnaby PF, Brown MA, et al. Prevention of ventricular fibrillation during acute myocardial infarction by intravenous propranolol. *Lancet.* 1984;2:883-886.

147. Hjalmarson A, Elmfeldt D, Herlitz J, et al. Effect on mortality of metoprolol in acute myocardial infarction: a double-blind randomised trial. *Lancet.* 1981;2:823-827.

148. Bovill EG, Terrin ML, Stump DC, et al. Hemorrhagic events during therapy with recombinant tissue-type plaminogen activator, heparin, and aspirin for acute myocardial infarction: results of the Thrombolysis in Myocardial Infarction (TIMI), Phase II Trial. *Ann Intern Med.* 1991;115:256-265.

149. Held PH, Yusuf S, Furberg CD. Calcium channel blockers in acute myocardial infarction and unstable angina: an overview. *BMJ.* 1989;299:1187-1192.

150. ISIS-2 Collaborative Group. Randomised trial of intravenous streptokinase, oral aspirin, both, or neither among 17 187 cases of suspected acute myocardial infarction: ISIS-2. *Lancet.* 1988;2:349-360.

151. Turpie AG, Robinson JG, Doyle DJ, et al. Comparison of high-dose with low-dose subcutaneous heparin to prevent left ventricular mural thrombosis in patients with acute transmural anterior myocardial infarction. *N Engl J Med.* 1989;320:352-357.

152. Franzosi MG, Maggioni AP, Tognoni G. GISSI update: which patients with myocardial infarction should receive thrombolysis: *Chest.* 1992;101(suppl 4):116S-123S.

153. Eisenberg MS, Aghababian RV, Bossaert L, Jaffe AS, Ornato JP, Weaver WD. Thrombolytic therapy. *Ann Emerg Med.* 1993;22:417-427.

154. Fuster V. Coronary thrombolysis — a perspective for the practicing physician. *N Engl J Med.* 1993;329:723-725.

155. Anderson HV, Willerson JT. Thrombolysis in acute myocardial infarction. *N Engl J Med.* 1993;329:703-709.

156. Ridker PM, O'Donnell C, Marder VJ, Hennekens CH. Large-scale trials of thrombolytic therapy for acute myocardial infarction: GISSI-2, ISIS-3 and GUSTO-1. *Ann Intern Med.* 1993;119:530-532. Editorial.

157. Topol EJ and the GUSTO Investigators. An International randomized trial comparing four thrombolytic strategies for acute myocardial infarction. *N Engl J Med.* 1993;329:673-682.

158. Metz CA, Stubbs DF, Hearron MS. Significance of infarct site and methylprednisolone on survival following acute myocardial infarction. *J Int Med Res.* 1986;14(suppl 1):11-14.

159. Brugemann J, van der Meer J, Bom VJ, van der Schaaf W, de Graeff PA, Lie KI. Anti-streptokinase antibodies inhibit fibrinolytic effects of anistreplase in acute myocardial infarction. *Am J Cardiol.* 1993;72:462-464.

160. Cummins RO, Eisenberg MS. From pain to reperfusion: what role for the prehospital 12-lead ECG? *Ann Emerg Med.* 1990;19: 1343-1346.

161. Aufderheide TP, Hendley GE, Thakur RK, et al. The diagnostic impact of prehospital 12-lead electrocardiography. *Ann Emerg Med.* 1990;19:1280-1287.

162. Kudenchuk PJ, Ho MT, Weaver WD, et al. Accuracy of computer-interpreted electrocardiography in selecting patients for thrombolytic therapy. *J Am Coll Cardiol.* 1991;17:1486-1491.

163. Weaver WD, Kudenchuk P, Ho M. Computerized electrocardiography for selection of patients for prehospital initiated thrombolysis. *J Electrocardiol.* 1992;24(suppl):1.

164. Weaver WD, Cerqueira M, Hallstrom AP, et al. Prehospital-initiated vs hospital-initiated thrombolytic therapy: the Myocardial Infarction Triage and Intervention Trial. *JAMA.* 1993;270: 1211-1216.

165. Weaver WD, Eisenberg MS, Martin JS, et al. Myocardial Infarction Triage and Intervention Project — phase I: patient characteristics and feasibility of prehospital initiation of thrombolytic therapy. *J Am Coll Cardiol.* 1990;15:925-931.

166. The European Myocardial Infarction Project Group. Prehospital thrombolytic therapy in patients with suspected acute myocardial infarction. *N Engl J Med.* 1993;329:383-389.

167. Late Assessment of Thrombolytic Efficacy (LATE) study with alteplase 6-24 hours after onset of acute myocardial infarction. *Lancet.* 1993;342:759-766.

168. EMERAS (Estudio Multicentrico Estreptoquinasa Republicas de America del Sur) Collaborative Group. Randomised trial of late thrombolysis in patients with suspected acute myocardial infarction. *Lancet.* 1993;342:767-772.

169. Califf RM, Topol EJ, George BS, et al. Hemorrhagic complications associated with the use of intravenous tissue plasminogen activator in treatment of acute myocardial infarction. *Am J Med.* 1988;85:353-359.

170. Roth A, Miller HI, Glick A, Barbash GI, Laniado S. Rapid resolution of new right bundle branch block in acute anterior myocardial infarction patients after thrombolytic therapy. *PACE Pacing Clin Electrophysiol.* 1993;16(1, pt 1):13-18.

171. Mannisi JA, Weisman HF, Bush DE, Dudeck P, Healy B. Steroid administration after myocardial infarction promotes early infarct expansion: a study in the rat. *J Clin Invest.* 1987;79:1431-1439.

Special Resuscitation Situations

Chapter 10

Stroke, acute myocardial infarction, heart failure, and cardiac arrest are each part of the wide spectrum of cardiovascular disease. The informed ACLS provider should know the initial management of each of these conditions.

Several special situations associated with cardiopulmonary arrest require rescuers to change their approach to resuscitation. Emergency personnel should note carefully the differences in triage, emphasis, and techniques. These special situations are

- Stroke
- Hypothermia
- Near-drowning
- Cardiac arrest associated with trauma
- Electric shock and lightning strike
- Cardiac arrest associated with pregnancy
- Toxicologic cardiac emergencies, including emergencies caused by
  - Cocaine toxicity
  - Tricylic antidepressant overdose
  - Digitalis overdose
  - Calcium channel blocker overdose
  - β Blocker overdose
  - Narcotics overdose

Stroke

Stroke results from occlusion or rupture of a blood vessel supplying the brain. It is the most common serious central nervous system pathology of sudden onset. Approximately 500 000 Americans suffer a new or recurrent stroke each year, and in 1989 (the latest statistics) more than 145 000 people died of stroke.[1] Emergency healthcare providers should be adept in evaluating and treating patients with suspected stroke because stroke can produce signs and symptoms similar to those of other cardiovascular emergencies — airway compromise, hypotension or hypertension, and unconsciousness.

Approximately 75% of strokes are ischemic, resulting from complete occlusion of an artery that deprives the brain of essential nutrients. Cerebrovascular occlusions result from a blood clot that develops within the brain artery itself (cerebral thrombosis) or from a clot that arises elsewhere in the body and then migrates to the brain (cerebral embolism). Other strokes are due to rupture of an artery with secondary bleeding into the brain (intracerebral hemorrhage) or adjacent to the brain (subarachnoid hemorrhage). This classification of stroke must be understood because the management of hemorrhagic stroke and ischemic stroke is markedly different. Fortunately much of the supportive treatment in an emergency is similar for the major groups of stroke.

Although stroke can rapidly lead to death, it rarely leads to death within the first hour, in contrast to cardiac arrest. On the other hand, worsening brain damage, which may result in permanent disability, can evolve quickly. Stroke is an emergency condition that can be helped: several medical and surgical therapies will lessen the consequences of stroke. Successful treatment of the person with acute stroke is linked to rapid transport to the hospital, because specific treatments cannot be given in the field.

Warning Signs of Stroke

Major stroke can be prevented in many cases, but only if warning signs are heeded. These signs may be subtle or transient, but they foretell a potentially life-threatening neurological illness. Emergency healthcare providers should recognize the importance of these symptoms and respond quickly with medical or surgical measures of proven efficacy in stroke prevention. *The two most important forecasters of stroke are a transient ischemic attack (TIA) for brain infarction and a "warning leak" for subarachnoid hemorrhage.*

Transient Ischemic Attack

A TIA is a brief, reversible episode of focal dysfunction of the brain or eye that is secondary to transient occlusion of an artery.[2,3] *It is the most important forecaster of brain infarction.* Approximately 10% of patients with brain infarction have a preceding TIA, and approximately 30% of patients with TIA will have a major stroke.[4] The risk of stroke is greatest in the first few days and weeks after the TIA.[5,6] Evaluation to determine the likely cause of TIA and institution of an appropriate treatment can significantly reduce the risk of stroke. Carotid endarterectomy is of proven benefit among patients with recent TIA who have a severe (greater than 70%) narrowing of the origin of the internal carotid artery.[7,8] Aspirin and ticlopidine are effective in preventing stroke among some patients with TIA.[9-12] Oral anticoagulants are usually prescribed to prevent embolism to the brain among patients with cardiac causes of stroke, particularly those with atrial fibrillation.[13-15]

Patients with minor strokes are at risk for major stroke, and they should be treated like those with TIA. *The key to the treatment of a patient with a TIA or minor stroke is prompt recognition.* Transient loss of consciousness, syncope, seizures, global wooziness, giddiness, confusion, and generalized collapse are often due to TIA or minor stroke. The symptoms of TIA result from poor blood flow in either the carotid or vertebrobasilar circulation (Table 1). This distinction is important because, as noted, carotid endarterectomy is of proven value among patients with severe carotid stenosis and recent TIA in the carotid distribution.[7,8]

Patients with TIA or minor stroke should be treated as an emergency because of the significant risk of a major, disabling stroke. Remember, 30% will go on to experience brain infarction. Evaluation should be prompt, and patients with a recent TIA (within 7 days) should be admitted. Computed tomography (CT) or magnetic resonance imaging (MRI) should be performed to help eliminate nonvascular causes of the neurological symptoms.[16] Other diagnostic studies, such as arteriography or cardiac imaging, are performed to determine the likely cause of

Table 1. Symptoms of Transient Ischemic Attack

Carotid Circulation

Monocular blindness. — Painless visual loss in one eye; may involve loss of all or part of the eye's vision, often described as a scum, fog, grayout or blackout of vision. The involved eye is on the same side as the diseased artery.

Visual disturbance. — Blurred or indistinct vision to one side of the field of vision in both eyes. The involved visual field is opposite the side of the diseased artery.

Paralysis. — Weakness, clumsiness, or heaviness. Involves hand, arm, face, or leg, alone or in combination, most commonly the hand and face. Sagging of one side of the face may occur. The involved body parts are opposite the side of the diseased artery.

Numbness. — Sensory loss, tingling, or abnormal sensation. Involves hand, arm, face, or leg, alone or in combination, most commonly the hand and face. Usually occurs simultaneously with weakness. The involved body parts are opposite the side of the diseased artery.

Speech disturbance. — Slurred or indistinct speech, abnormal pronunciation of words and articulation. Trouble selecting correct words, incomprehensible or nonsense speech, trouble understanding others' speech, trouble writing or reading.

Vertebrobasilar Distribution

Vertigo. — Sense of spinning or whirling, persisting at rest. Should be differentiated from dizziness, lightheadedness, or giddiness, which are not symptoms of TIA. Vertigo is also a common symptom of a number of nonvascular diseases, and therefore one of the other symptoms listed should also be present to make the diagnosis of TIA.

Visual disturbance. — Blurred or indistinct vision in the left or right visual field or both, involving both eyes simultaneously.

Diplopia. — Seeing two images instead of one; may have a sense of bouncing and moving visual images.

Paralysis. — Weakness, clumsiness, heaviness, or dysfunction of the arm, leg, face, and hand. Can involve one half of the body or all four limbs. The face can be involved on one side and the limbs on the other. A "drop attack" is the sudden onset of paralysis of all four limbs without loss of consciousness. This results in collapse and is rarely due to a TIA.

Numbness. — Sensory loss, tingling or loss of feeling of the arm, leg, face, and hand. Can involve one half of the body or all four limbs. It usually occurs simultaneously with the motor symptoms.

Dysarthria. — Slurred or indistinct speech, poor articulation, mumbling.

Ataxia. — Poor balance, stumbling gait, staggering, incoordination of a side of the body.

TIA and to guide treatment.[3] Because of the high risk of stroke after recent TIA, heparin is frequently prescribed as an interim therapy, although its value in this situation has not been established.[5,17] Heparin should not be prescribed until imaging studies have eliminated brain hemorrhage or nonvascular diseases as the cause of the neurological symptoms. Aspirin, warfarin, and ticlopidine are medical options for long-term prevention and may be started within the first few days after TIA.[9-15]

Subarachnoid Hemorrhage: The "Warning Leak"

Approximately one fourth of patients with subarachnoid hemorrhage secondary to rupture of an intracranial aneurysm will have had warning symptoms secondary to a minor bleed — the "warning leak."[18,19] Patients with minor hemorrhages have the best prognosis and are most effectively treated by medical measures and early operation. Without treatment a second serious hemorrhage is likely in the next 2 to 3 weeks. Unfortunately the nature of these symptoms is often not recognized, particularly by emergency medical personnel, and delays in treatment occur in 25% of cases.[20-22] The symptoms of a warning leak are the same as those of a subarachnoid hemorrhage but milder.[20] The most common symptom is a sudden headache of sufficient severity that it prompts a patient to seek medical attention. It is often described as the worst headache or pain in the patient's life. The headache usually occurs suddenly, often during exertion, and immediately reaches maximal severity. It is usually holocranial and often radiates to the neck or face. A headache associated with transient loss of consciousness should be particularly alarming. Associated symptoms of a warning leak include nausea, vomiting, and intolerance of noise or light.

Clinical Presentation of Stroke

Stroke should be considered in any patient who has *sudden* onset of focal neurological deficits or an alteration in consciousness. The symptoms of stroke (Table 2) can occur alone or in any combination. The findings can worsen, wax and wane, or be of maximal severity at onset.

The histories and physical findings of hemorrhagic and ischemic stroke overlap, and emergency personnel should not depend solely on the clinical presentation for diagnosis. In general, patients with hemorrhagic stroke appear more seriously ill and have a more rapid course of deterioration than those with ischemic stroke. Headaches, disturbances in consciousness, nausea, and vomiting are also more prominent with hemorrhagic stroke. The loss of consciousness may be transient and may have resolved by the time the patient receives medical attention. Patients with subarachnoid hemorrhage may have only an intense headache without focal neurological signs such as paralysis. Examination of patients with recent stroke may change considerably over time, with neurological signs worsening or improving spontaneously.

Table 2. Symptoms of Acute Stroke and Subarachnoid Hemorrhage

Impaired consciousness. — Coma, unresponsiveness, confusion, delirium, stupor, drowsiness.

Seizures. — New onset, single or recurrent, focal or generalized. Focal seizures usually involve motor activity.

Headache. — Sudden or rapid onset, intense or unusually severe, "the worst headache of my life." May be associated with loss of consciousness, unusual and severe facial or neck pain, or neck stiffness (nuchal rigidity).

Cognitive impairment/aphasia. — Impaired memory, difficulty thinking clearly, trouble producing or comprehending language, mutism, monotonous speech, difficulty writing, reading, or performing calculations. May be unable to name objects or parts of objects or cannot repeat sentences. May be unable to perform skilled motor acts in the absence of paralysis. May not recognize nature of problem and even deny the illness or body parts.

Paralysis. — Weakness — partial or complete inability to move body parts. Often involves one half of the body. May be asymmetrical, with the arm much weaker than the leg. Reflexes are usually hyperactive in the involved limbs, and a Babinski response usually is present. Facial weakness may be on the same or opposite side of the limb paralysis. The facial weakness is usually noted when the patient speaks or smiles and may be accompanied by problems with drooling on that side. Paralysis can occur without associated sensory loss.

Ataxia. — Incoordination of one side of the body. Poor balance, difficulty walking, and clumsiness. Incoordination and poor control of limbs should not be attributable to paralysis or sensory loss.

Visual loss. — Partial or complete loss of vision in both eyes. A part of the visual field is often involved. A homonymous hemianopia or even total blindness.

Diplopia. — Double visual images. Two images can be vertical, horizontal, or oblique. Sensation of movement, spinning, or jumping vision. Intense vertigo may occur. Abnormal ocular rotations are seen, including nystagmus. Abnormal position of the eyes at rest or dysconjugate eye movements. Abnormalities in the pupillary responses in light may be present. Of particular concern is inequality in size or reactivity of the pupils.

Sensory loss. — Numbness, tingling, loss of sensation to touch, pin, temperature, position in one or more body parts. Usually on one half of the body. Facial sensory loss can be on the same side as sensory loss in the limbs or on the opposite side. Sensory loss without any paralysis can occur.

Dysarthria. — Slurred or indistinct speech. Speech that is hard to understand because of poor articulation. May be associated with trouble swallowing or facial asymmetry.

Dysphagia. — Inability to swallow that is most pronounced with attempts to swallow clear liquids. May be associated with nasal regurgitation of liquids. Absent gag reflex.

Other stroke symptoms. — Nausea, vomiting, malaise, feeling unwell. Light and noise intolerance, neck or face pain, low back pain.

Initial Examination of the Patient With Stroke

The evaluation (examination and baseline diagnostic studies) should be done as quickly as possible — a goal should be 1 hour.[23] Some assessments and studies can be obtained while the patient is being transported to an emergency department. The ABCs of critical care are applicable to the patient with stroke. Cardiac decompensation is unusual, but airway and respiratory problems are always important concerns, particularly in a comatose patient.

Airway

Paralysis of the muscles of the throat, tongue, or mouth can lead to partial or complete upper airway obstruction. Saliva pools in the throat and may be aspirated. Vomiting occurs, particularly with hemorrhagic stroke, and aspiration of vomitus is a concern. Tracheal obstruction or bronchial obstruction can result. Comatose patients are at particular risk for problems with the airway.

The airway can be supported by repositioning the head or placing an oropharyngeal or nasopharyngeal airway. Endotracheal intubation is usually needed for comatose patients. Frequent suctioning of the oropharynx or nasopharynx is also indicated. Turning the patient into a lateral decubitus position or preferably the "recovery position" may ease removal of vomitus.

Patients with recurrent epileptic seizures and stroke also have airway obstruction, which is worsened by abundant saliva, vomiting, and buccal or tongue lacerations. Periods of apnea are common during the clonic phase of the seizure, and cyanosis is frequent. Repositioning the head or placing the patient in the "rescue" position (on one side with the arm used to sustain neck extension) will help. Do not place foreign objects, including fingers, into the patient's mouth during a seizure. Injuries to the patient or healthcare provider can occur. Suction of secretions should be performed to clear the airway.

Caution in moving the neck should be exercised if there is a possibility of cervical trauma. Most patients with stroke will be able to relate a history of recent injuries, but this information may be lacking in a comatose patient. Rarely a patient will have a stroke in conjunction with a head or neck injury, or the patient will fall with the onset of stroke and have a secondary cervical injury. In such cases the neck should not be hyperextended or the patient turned until a firm cervical collar is placed.

Vital Signs

Vital signs (pulse, respirations, blood pressure) should be checked frequently to detect changes or abnormalities. Disturbances in these signs are frequent.

Breathing

Breathing abnormalities are uncommon except in patients with severe stroke, and rescue breathing is seldom needed. However, abnormal respirations are prominent in comatose patients and portend serious brain injury.[24] Irregular respiratory rates include prolonged pauses, Cheyne-Stokes respirations, or neurogenic hyperventilation. Shallow respirations or inadequate air exchange as the result of paralysis can also occur. Rescue breathing, assisted ventilation, and supplemental oxygen may be helpful. Severe, coma-producing brain injuries can lead to respiratory arrest, but this is usually preceded by other abnormalities in respiratory pattern. Rescue breathing or assisted ventilation is required with respiratory arrest, although the probability of a favorable outcome is low.

Circulation

Cardiac arrest is an uncommon complication of stroke and usually follows respiratory arrest. Therefore, very few stroke patients will require chest compressions. However, cardiovascular disturbances are frequent, and monitoring of both blood pressure and cardiac rhythm should be part of the early assessment and treatment of a patient with stroke. Hypotension or shock is rarely due to stroke, and other causes should be sought. Hypertension is often found after stroke and may represent prestroke hypertension, a stress reaction to the brain injury, or a physiological response to improve brain perfusion. Cardiac arrhythmias may point to an underlying cardiac cause of stroke or may be the consequence of the stroke. Bradycardia may indicate hypoxia or elevation of intracranial pressure. The electrocardiographic changes secondary to stroke, in particular with hemorrhage, include prolongation of the QT interval and alterations of the P, T, and U waves. ST segment depression or elevation can mimic myocardial infarction.[25,26] Other abnormalities include paroxysmal supraventricular tachycardia, atrial fibrillation, sinus bradycardia, ventricular tachycardia (VT), premature atrial or ventricular contractions, and atrioventricular conduction[27] defects or blocks.[28] More serious arrhythmias such as torsades de pointes and ventricular fibrillation are rare.[29]

General Medical Assessment

In patients with signs and symptoms of stroke, check for hypoglycemia, narcotic or other drug overdoses, and electrolyte and osmolality problems. Empiric treatment with glucose and naloxone hydrochloride is appropriate with any suspicion of these conditions.

In an emergency, patients with altered consciousness should be examined for evidence of cranial or cervical trauma. A hemotympanum, Battle's sign (ecchymosis over the mastoid), or orbital ecchymosis point to a skull or orbital fracture. Skull tenderness, spine tenderness, or pericervical muscle spasm also suggest a fracture.

Cardiac examination may demonstrate an irregular rhythm, friction rub, murmur, click, or gallop that might suggest a cardiac cause of emboli. Abdominal or flank tenderness or peripheral skin lesions may also be seen with cardiogenic embolism. Fever, Roth's spots, Janeway lesions, splinter hemorrhages, or Osler nodes can be seen in a patient with cerebral embolism secondary to infective endocarditis.

An absent pulse or cool limb can also suggest multisystem embolism. A weak carotid pulse can be found with carotid occlusion, and this may be accompanied by bounding facial or superficial temporal artery pulses. A carotid bruit favors an atherosclerotic lesion as the cause of ischemic stroke. Bruits over the head or neck can occasionally be heard in patients with hemorrhage secondary to a large cerebral vascular malformation.

Petechiae or ecchymoses point to a hemorrhagic stroke secondary to a blood dyscrasia or coagulopathy. Preretinal (subhyaloid) hemorrhages allow early identification of an intracranial hemorrhage in a comatose patient. Papilledema is rarely seen during the first hours after stroke. If it is present, a nonvascular intracranial mass should be considered.

Neurological Assessment

Clinical examinations should be performed frequently so that any worsening or improvement can be detected. They do not need to be exhaustive. *The most important finding is the patient's level of consciousness,* because a depressed consciousness usually represents a major brain event, often a large intracerebral or subarachnoid hemorrhage or a basilar artery occlusion. These stroke patients are at greatest risk of dying in the first few hours. The Glasgow Coma Scale (Table 3) is useful in appraising the severity of neurological injury in patients with altered alertness. It can be performed by every healthcare provider. The range of scores is 3 through 15 and is based on the best responses for eye opening, movement, and verbal responses.[30] In general, a patient with a Glasgow Coma Scale score of 8 or less has a very poor prognosis.

Coma is secondary to dysfunction of the brain stem; therefore, the emergency physician should focus on the examination of this vital structure.[31] The examiner should evaluate the size, equality, and reactivity of the pupils; corneal reflexes; gag; and the position of the eyes at rest and in response to the doll's eyes maneuver. The doll's eyes test should not be performed if a cervical spine fracture is suspected. A unilateral dilated and unreactive pupil

Table 3. Glasgow Coma Scale

Eye opening	
Spontaneous	4
To speech	3
To pain	2
None	1
Best motor response	
Obeys	6
Localizes	5
Withdraws	4
Abnormal flexion	3
Abnormal extension	2
None	1
Best verbal response	
Oriented conversation	5
Confused conversation	4
Inappropriate words	3
Incomprehensible sounds	2
None	1

in a comatose stroke patient is usually due to uncal herniation ("coning"). The same pupillary changes in an alert patient complaining of an intense headache can be seen with a ruptured aneurysm. Retinal hemorrhages are an important clue for intracranial bleeding as a cause of coma.[32]

Nuchal rigidity is an important finding in patients with hemorrhagic stroke. However, it may take several hours to develop and may be missed in a comatose patient. Passive flexion of the neck should be performed but only if there is no suggestion of a coincidental cervical spine injury. If there is any doubt about the possibility of neck trauma, the best course is not to check for nuchal rigidity.

Examination of an alert patient with a suspected stroke should include assessments of language, motor responses, and sensation. The type and severity of neurological deficits should be recorded as a baseline for future changes. Language can be tested by asking the patient to name objects, by asking him or her to repeat a sentence of at least seven words, by listening to spontaneous speech, and by observing the patient's responses to commands. Assessment of limb movements and testing the strength of wrist extensors, deltoids, hip flexors, and ankle dorsiflexors can be done quickly. Sensation to pinprick should also be checked. Reflexes and limb coordination can also be evaluated.

Differential Diagnosis of Acute Stroke

Very few nonvascular neurological diseases will cause the sudden onset of focal brain dysfunction that is the hallmark of stroke. The most important alternative diagnosis for brain infarction is brain hemorrhage, and vice versa. The separation is crucial because prognosis and treatment of these two major categories of stroke are radically different. Unfortunately the clinical presentations overlap, and the diagnosis of one type of stroke or the other cannot, with certainty, be made based on the clinical findings. MRI or CT, however, does help differentiate brain infarction from brain hemorrhage.

The list of potential alternative diagnoses is larger if the patient is comatose and no history of the course of the current illness is available (Table 4). If the course is one of a gradual worsening over several days, a nonvascular neurological disease may be present.

Hypoglycemia can cause focal neurological signs, such as aphasia or hemiparesis, with or without an altered mental status. Hypoglycemia is an important consideration in any diabetic patient who has a "stroke."[33] Seizures may be unwitnessed and the patient found with only postictal neurological signs. Signs such as paresis or aphasia can persist for several hours after a seizure, but many patients will also have some clouding of consciousness. Lacerations along the lateral aspect of the tongue or inside the cheek, signs of urinary or fecal incontinence, or evidence of trauma all point to a seizure. However, seizures can also accompany stroke. Approximately 1%

Table 4. Differential Diagnosis — Stroke

Hemorrhagic stroke
Ischemic stroke
Craniocerebral/cervical trauma
Meningitis/encephalitis
Intracranial mass
    Tumor
    Subdural hematoma
Seizure with persistent neurological signs
Migraine with persistent neurological signs
Metabolic
    Hyperglycemia (nonketotic hyperosmolar coma)
    Hypoglycemia
    Post–cardiac arrest ischemia
    Drug/narcotic overdose

of patients with cerebral thrombosis, 5% to 10% of patients with cerebral embolism, and 15% of patients with subarachnoid hemorrhage will have convulsions at the time of stroke.[34,35]

Emergent Diagnostic Studies

Diagnostic studies ordered in the emergency department are aimed at establishing stroke as the cause of the patient's symptoms, differentiating brain infarction from brain hemorrhage, and determining the most likely cause of the stroke. See Table 5 and Fig 1.

CT is the single most important test and should be obtained as soon as possible. It should be done initially without contrast enhancement to avoid confusing blood and contrast. Some experts, however, recommend contrast studies to look for enhancing lesions. Almost all patients with a recent intracranial hemorrhage will have an abnormal study.[36-39] An area of increased density (white on CT) will be seen in the location of the bleeding. Blood density may also be seen in the ventricles and the subarachnoid space. The cause of hemorrhage is often suggested by specific CT features. Blood in the basal cisterns is particularly common with ruptured aneurysms, but the CT findings may be subtle. Only a thin white layer

Table 5. Initial Evaluation of a Patient With Stroke

CT of the brain without contrast (with contrast or MRI may be
    necessary)
Lumbar puncture (selected cases of suspected subarachnoid
    hemorrhage)
Lateral cervical spine and skull x-rays (in comatose patients without
    a clearcut history to suspect hemorrhage)
Chest x-ray
Electrocardiogram
Hematologic studies
    Complete blood count
    Platelet count
    Prothrombin time
    Partial thromboplastin time
Serum electrolytes (Na, K, Cl, bicarbonate)
Blood glucose
Other chemistries (osmolality, calcium, liver, and renal tests)
Arterial blood gas levels (comatose patient)

adjacent to the brain may be present.[36,40] CT is usually normal during the first hours after brain infarction.[39] However, larger infarctions may rapidly obscure the gray-white matter junction or lead to a hypodensity (gray to black) on CT. Often CT misses small infarctions or ischemic lesions in the cerebellum or brain stem. Acute intracranial complications of stroke such as hydrocephalus, edema, mass effect, or shift of normal brain structures can be seen with CT. If CT is not available at a community hospital, the patient with suspected stroke should be stabilized and transferred to an institution where this technology is available. A patient with suspected stroke should not be given anticoagulants or thrombolytic drugs until CT has eliminated a brain hemorrhage.

Patients with a small subarachnoid hemorrhage may have a normal CT.[36] Such patients are usually alert and have no focal neurological deficits. Lumbar puncture to search for blood in the cerebrospinal fluid (CSF) is indicated in these cases. The risk of major complications of lumbar puncture in such patients is very low. Lumbar puncture should be avoided if a patient has altered consciousness, focal findings, or major neurological deficits. If CT demonstrates blood in a patient with stroke, there is no need to perform a lumbar puncture.

If bloody CSF is found, the appearance of the fluid in successive tubes should be compared. Bloody CSF secondary to subarachnoid hemorrhage should not change. The CSF should also be immediately centrifuged. If the supernatant fluid is xanthochromic, a traumatic tap is unlikely. However, it may take 12 hours after subarachnoid hemorrhage for the fluid to become yellow; therefore, delaying lumbar puncture may be warranted.[41]

Electrocardiography can demonstrate cardiac arrhythmias that reflect the cause of stroke. Clinically silent myocardial infarction can also be detected. Chest x-ray is done to look for cardiomegaly, pulmonary edema, or aspiration. In comatose patients, skull and lateral cervical spine x-rays are performed to search for a fracture or dislocation.

A complete blood count, platelet count, prothrombin time, and partial thromboplastin time are good general screens for a hematologic cause of stroke or a blood dyscrasia. These tests are also important in the screening of patients who may need a neurosurgical procedure. In comatose patients with a suspected "surgical" lesion, a blood sample for typing, screening, and possibly cross-matching for blood transfusion should also be obtained. Measurement of fibrinogin, bleeding time, and hemoglobin SS or SC and specialized studies of coagulation can be performed after admission to the hospital. The emergency physician should order pulse oximetry or arterial blood gas analyses in comatose patients and other stroke patients as clinically indicated. A chemistry screen, including electrolytes and glucose, is also important.

Magnetic resonance imaging (MRI) is not part of the initial evaluation of stroke. MRI is very sensitive and will detect some lesions (small or brain stem) missed by CT; it is not superior to CT in detecting hemorrhage, the most important emergency indication for CT. MRI is time-consuming, and the acutely ill patient may be sequestered from emergency medical personnel. It can be ordered after initial stabilization. Likewise, after admission to the hospital other studies can be done, including arteriography, electroencephalography, echocardiography, non-invasive studies of the carotid artery, and transcranial Doppler.

Stroke may be a complication of drug or alcohol abuse. Urinary or blood specimens for cocaine, amphetamines, opiates, or alcohol should be obtained if clinically indicated.

Emergency Treatment of Stroke

General Care

Patients should have an intravenous line placed to receive either normal saline or lactated Ringer's solution at a rate of 30 mL/h. Unless the patient is hypotensive, *rapid infusions of fluids are avoided* because of the risk of potentiating brain edema. Because 5% dextrose and water is hypo-osmolar, it can aggravate cerebral edema and should be avoided. Electrolyte disturbances should be corrected. A bolus of 50% dextrose and water with 50 mg of thiamine should be administered if hypoglycemia is demonstrated on rapid blood glucose determinations. Thiamine (100 mg) should be administered empirically to all cachectic, malnourished, or chronic alcoholic patients with suspected stroke.

There is experimental evidence that elevated blood sugar levels can potentiate the severity of brain ischemia.[42] In patients the relation between hyperglycemia and severe stroke is less clear, and an elevated blood glucose may be a stress response to a major brain insult.[43] In an emergency a moderately elevated blood sugar in a patient with stroke need not be corrected, although markedly elevated levels warrant treatment. There is little reason to risk hypoglycemia through attempts to lower the blood sugar to normal values.

Volume of infused fluids and urinary output should be recorded. Most patients with stroke do not need an indwelling bladder catheter, and its placement should be avoided if possible. During the first few hours after stroke, patients should not be given food or drink. Paralysis of bulbar muscles, decreased alertness, and vomiting can all lead to aspiration or airway obstruction.

Management of Elevated Blood Pressure

Most patients have hypertension after either ischemic or hemorrhagic stroke. A moderately elevated blood pressure after stroke does not constitute a hypertensive emergency unless the patient has acute myocardial ischemia or an aortic dissection. In most patients the blood pres-

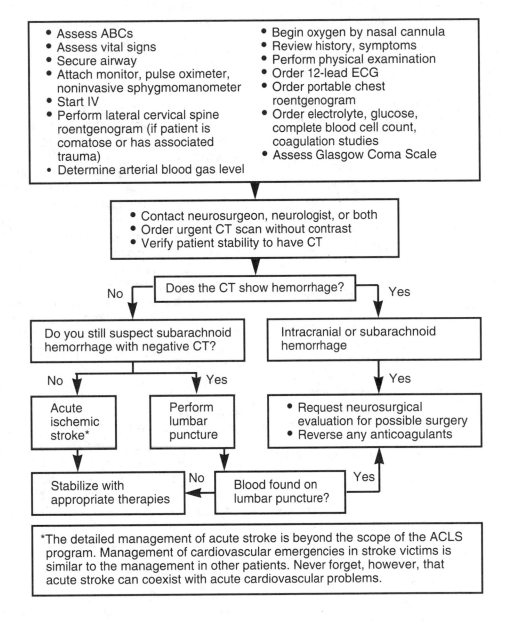

Fig. 1. Algorithm for initial evaluation of suspected stroke.

sure will spontaneously fall as pain, agitation, vomiting, or increased intracranial pressure are controlled.

Vigorous antihypertensive therapy can lower cerebral perfusion and lead to worsening of the stroke. In addition, the response of stroke patients to antihypertensive therapy can be exaggerated. Elevated arterial pressures are often treated more aggressively after brain hemorrhage because of concerns about rebleeding or extension of bleeding. For patients with an arterial occlusion, maintenance of adequate collateral flow is of paramount concern. Generally, aggressive antihypertensive treatment is reserved for patients with a markedly elevated blood pressure.

Markedly elevated blood pressure (above 200 mm Hg systolic or above 130 calculated mean) after stroke should be treated, but cautiously, because response to therapy may be exaggerated (Table 6). Results of the emergency CT scan provide the guiding distinction for antihypertensive therapy — whether the stroke is ischemic or hemorrhagic. For *ischemic stroke*, elevated systolic or diastolic pressures do not require treatment unless specific medical indications are present, such as acute myocardial infarction or left ventricular failure. There is no evidence that pressures even as high as 230 mm Hg systolic or 120 mm Hg diastolic are harmful, and up to 80% of patients will have a spontaneous and substantial decline in blood pressure within the first 2 hours after symptom onset.[44]

For *hemorrhagic stroke*, acute elevations in blood pressure may be associated with early rebleeding after subarachnoid hemorrhage or with continued bleeding after intracerebral hemorrhage. Pressures above 160 mm Hg systolic or above 105 mm Hg diastolic require venous sodium nitroprusside (0.5 to 10 μg/kg per minute) may be necessary. Labetalol is an alternative parenteral treatment. For patients with severe blood pressure elevations and a large volume of intracranial blood, intravenous

Table 6. Emergency Antihypertensive Therapy for Hemorrhagic Stroke

---

1. If systolic blood pressure (BP) is >230 mm Hg or if diastolic BP is >120 mm Hg on two readings 5 min apart, start an infusion pump of sodium nitroprusside, 0.5 to 10 μg/kg per min, or nitroglycerin, 10 to 20 μg/min.

2. If systolic BP is >160 mm Hg or diastolic BP is >105 mm Hg, or both, on two readings 10 min apart, consider labetalol, 10 mg IV over 1 to 2 min. The labetalol dose may be repeated or doubled every 20 min until a satisfactory BP reduction is achieved or until a cumulative dose of 300 mg has been administered via this minibolus technique. Labetalol is avoided in patients with asthma, cardiac failure, or severe cardiac conduction abnormalities. Alternative therapy may be considered with sodium nitroprusside or esmolol for refractory hypertension.

3. If systolic BP is <160 mm Hg and diastolic BP is <105 mm Hg but prehemorrhage blood pressure is estimated to have been considerably lower (eg, 120/80), then antihypertensive therapy may be appropriate to approximate premorbid pressures, particularly in the first hours after subarachnoid hemorrhage.

---

sodium nitroprusside (0.5 to 10 μg/kg per minute) may be necessary. Labetalol is an alternative parenteral therapy for less severe elevations. It has rapid onset without causing cerebral vasodilation or decreases in cerebral blood flow.

There is no unanimity about which parenteral antihypertensive drugs should be given after stroke. Continuous blood pressure monitoring should be performed to judge responses to treatment. Sodium nitroprusside has the attributes of an immediate effect and short duration of action, but it causes cerebral vasodilation, which could worsen intracranial pressure. Intravenous nitrates, β-blocking agents, or a calcium channel blocker are alternative intravenous drugs.

Management of Seizures

Recurrent seizures are a potentially life-threatening complication of stroke. The seizures can worsen the stroke and should be controlled. Protection of the airway, supplemental oxygen, and maintenance of normothermia are part of supportive care. Patients should also be protected against skeletal or soft tissue injuries.

Intravenous diazepam (5 mg over 2 minutes or up to 10 mg for most adults) or lorezapam (1 to 4 mg over 2 to 10 minutes) will usually stop seizures, but the patient should be observed for respiratory depression.[45] Lorezapam, with a short half-life, may be the superior agent. These benzodiazepines can be repeated, but they should be followed by a longer-acting anticonvulsant. Intravenous phenytoin (loading dose 1000 mg or 16 mg/kg, followed by 100 mg every 8 hours) is usually prescribed, but the infusion should not exceed 50 mg/min to avoid cardiac-depressant side effects.[45] In less urgent situations use a slower rate (25 mg/min). Subsequent doses of phenytoin can be adjusted to the results of serum concentration testing. Phenobarbital (usual loading dose in adults 1000 mg or 20 mg/kg) is followed by 30 to 60 mg every 6 to 8 hours. Phenobarbital may potentiate the respiratory-depressant effects of diazepam, and intubation may be needed. For intractable seizures not responding to phenytoin and phenobarbital, pentobarbital is an alternative. These patients should have intensive care, artificial ventilation, and electroencephalographic monitoring to help judge therapeutic response.

Treatment of Increased Intracranial Pressure

Increased intracranial pressure is an important neurological complication of stroke that results from the mass effect of the stroke (especially a hematoma), hydrocephalus, or secondary cerebral edema. Intracranial hypertension can lead to impaired cerebral perfusion and worsen ischemia. Variable levels of pressure in different parts of the cranial vault may lead to herniation of brain tissue with secondary brain stem compromise. Increased intracranial pressure during the first hours after stroke is more likely to occur with hemorrhages. In general, the level of consciousness is the best clinical measure of intracranial pressure. Progressive stupor suggests critically high levels of intracranial pressure. Increased intracranial pressure is not a major concern in an alert patient who has minimal neurological deficits.

Measures to lower intracranial pressure include moderate fluid restriction, elevation of the head of the bed, avoidance of hypoventilation and hypercarbia, and control of agitation and pain. Corticosteroids are not effective in controlling ischemic stroke-related cerebral edema.[46] More vigorous methods are needed.

Hyperventilation. Hyperventilation is a temporarily effective measure to lower pressure in a patient who is developing signs of herniation. The Pco_2 can be safely lowered to a value of approximately 25 mm Hg, but greater reductions can cause ischemia. The effects of hyperventilation, by reducing the intracranial intravascular volume, are immediate but short-lived.

Mannitol. Hyperventilation should be supplemented with mannitol (0.5 mg/kg in a 20% solution given over 20 minutes).[47] Mannitol is an osmotic agent that will extract water from normal brain tissue; its effects begin within 20 minutes and persist for 4 to 6 hours. Additional doses of mannitol (0.25 mg/kg) can be administered every 4 to 6 hours as needed. If several doses of mannitol are given, careful monitoring of the fluid status and osmolarity is required: serum osmolarity should not exceed 310 mOsm.

Other Approaches. Monitoring of intracranial pressure with a subdural transducer or intraventricular catheter eases management of intracranial pressure. Furosemide, acetazolamide, and barbiturate-induced coma are also possible treatments. Placement of a ventricular drainage system will allow removal of CSF in patients with acute hydrocephalus and increased intracranial pressure after stroke.

Medical management of intracranial pressure is of limited value in long-term control of increased intracranial pressure. Patients with large hematomas or infarction may need neurosurgical intervention. Superficial hematomas and hemorrhages in the cerebellum can be successfully evacuated. Deep hemispheric hematomas and major infarctions can have surgical resection as a life-saving measure, although major neurological sequelae are found among survivors.

Anticoagulant Therapy

Heparin is frequently prescribed for patients with acute ischemic stroke, but its value is unproven.[48,49] There are no data that establish the usefulness or lack of usefulness of anticoagulants in acute stroke. Heparin may be helpful in preventing recurrent embolism or propagation of a thrombus, but it may lead to bleeding complications, including brain hemorrhage. Heparin should not be given to a patient with suspected endocarditis, and therapy should not be initiated until a CT has ruled out any intracranial bleeding. There is no unanimity about when

to start heparin, the desired level of anticoagulation, or if a loading bolus dose should be given. *In light of all the uncertainty about heparin after stroke, the most prudent course for an emergency physician is **not** to start heparin therapy,* unless the patient's neurologist or the responsible attending physician concurs with the decision.

Low-molecular-weight anticoagulants have more selective antithrombotic actions than heparin, which might be an advantage in stroke management.[50] This therapy is being tested in a clinical trial but is not yet available for general use. While aspirin, ticlopidine, and oral anticoagulants are of proven value in stroke prevention, their utility in acute stroke is unknown.

Thrombolytic Therapy

In theory, thrombolysis for acute thrombotic stroke should prove to be a potentially effective therapy. Thrombolytic drugs are being tested in clinical trials of stroke, but they should not be used outside such research studies.[51-53] The best thrombolytic agent for stroke, the optimal route of administration, the required dose, and the maximal interval from stroke onset to treatment have not been determined. The potential risk of bleeding complications also is unknown.

Other Treatment

A neurologist or neurosurgeon should be consulted about the management of most patients with stroke. If necessary, the emergency physician should refer patients to an institution that has the facilities and personnel to manage these critically ill patients. These centers may also be testing new and promising therapies that will be beneficial to the patient. If necessary, air transportation can be used to quickly transfer the patient — the interval since stroke onset becomes critical in many new treatments for stroke.

Patients with subarachnoid or intracerebral hemorrhage often need emergent arteriography, and if a saccular aneurysm is detected, early intracranial operation with clipping of the aneurysm is usually advised.[54-57] Large intracerebral or cerebellar hematomas also often need operative therapy.[58] The calcium channel blocking drug nimodipine (60 mg orally every 4 hours) is of proven benefit in improving outcome after subarachnoid hemorrhage.[59,60] Correction of hyponatremia and water loss after subarachnoid hemorrhage is also important, although strict fluid restriction (as for inappropriate secretion of antidiuretic hormone) should be avoided.[61,62] Other causes of intracerebral hemorrhage (vascular malformations, hypertension, neoplasia, vasculitis) will need specific surgical or medical interventions.

No demonstrable benefit in easing ischemic stroke has been shown for calcium channel blocking drugs, volume expansion, hypertension-hypervolemia hemodilution, and low-molecular-weight dextran.

Hypothermia

Severe accidental hypothermia (body temperature below 30°C, 86°F) is associated with marked depression of cerebral blood flow and oxygen requirement, reduced cardiac output, and decreased arterial pressure. Victims can appear to be clinically dead because of marked depression of brain and cardiovascular function, and the potential for full resuscitation with intact neurological recovery is possible, although unusual.[63] The victim's peripheral pulses and respiratory efforts may be difficult to detect, but lifesaving procedures should not be withheld based on clinical presentation.

Fig 2 presents a recommended hypothermia treatment algorithm, with recommended actions that providers should take for all possible victims of hypothermia. Note that these recommendations should be applied to all drowning and near-drowning victims as well.

Basic Life Support

If the victim is not breathing, rescue breathing should be initiated. Basic life support (CPR) in the pulseless patient should be begun immediately, although pulse and respirations may need to be checked for longer periods to detect minimal cardiopulmonary efforts. The previous recommendation that pulse and respirations be checked for 1 to 2 minutes before beginning CPR[64,65] is excessive. Take 30 to 45 seconds to confirm pulselessness or profound bradycardia. CPR will be required if no pulse is felt in 30 to 45 seconds. It is important to prevent further heat loss from the core by removing any wet garments, insulating the victim, shielding from wind, and ventilating with warm, humidified oxygen.[63,66] For victims not in cardiac arrest with core temperatures of 30°C to 34°C (86°F to 93°F), apply external warming devices to truncal areas only (warm packs to neck, armpits, and groin). After stabilization, cautiously ready the patient for transportation to a hospital.

Treatment of severe hypothermia (temperature less than 30°C, 86°F) in the field remains controversial. Many providers do not have the equipment or time to adequately assess core body temperature or to institute rewarming with warm, humidified oxygen or warm fluids, although these methods should be initiated if possible to help prevent afterdrop.[63,66-68] Cardiac monitoring and intravenous access should be rapidly established if possible, and core temperature should be determined in the field with either tympanic membrane sensors or rectal probes, but none of these should delay transfer. Airway management and transportation should be performed as gently as possible to avoid precipitating ventricular fibrillation (VF). The patient should be moved in the horizontal position to avoid aggravating hypotension through orthostatic mechanisms.

If the hypothermic victim is in cardiac arrest, follow the hypothermia treatment algorithm (Fig 2). If VF is detected, emergency personnel should deliver three shocks to determine fibrillation responsiveness. If VF persists after three shocks, further shocks should be avoided until after rewarming to above 30°C (86°F). CPR, rewarming, and rapid transport should immediately follow the initial three defibrillation attempts. If core temperature is below 30°C (86°F), successful defibrillation may not be possible until rewarming is accomplished.[68]

Advanced Cardiac Life Support

In the hypothermic victim who has not yet developed cardiac arrest, many physical manipulations (including endotracheal or nasogastric intubation, temporary pacemaker, or pulmonary artery catheter insertion) have been reported to precipitate VF.[63,68] However, when specifically and urgently indicated, such procedures should not be withheld. In a prospective multicenter study of hypothermia victims, careful endotracheal intubation did not result in a single incident of VF.[69] Endotracheal intubation to provide effective ventilation with warm, humidified oxygen and to prevent aspiration should be performed in the unconscious hypothermic patient with inadequate ventilation. In such cases, prior ventilation with 100% oxygen via adjunct devices is recommended. Conscious victims who are cold with only mild symptoms of hypothermia may be rewarmed with external active and passive rewarming techniques (eg, warm packs, warmed sleeping bags, and warm baths).

Management of cardiac arrest due to hypothermia differs from management of normothermic arrest. The hypothermic heart may be unresponsive to cardioactive drugs, pacemaker stimulation, and defibrillation,[68] and drug metabolism is reduced. Administered medications, including epinephrine, lidocaine, and procainamide, can accumulate to toxic levels if used repeatedly in the severely hypothermic victim. Active core rewarming techniques are the primary therapeutic modality in hypothermic victims in cardiac arrest or unconscious with a slow heart rate.

If the patient fails to respond to initial defibrillation attempts or initial drug therapy, subsequent defibrillations or additional boluses of medication should be avoided until the core temperature rises above 30°C (86°F). Bradycardia may be physiological in severe hypothermia, and cardiac pacing is usually not indicated unless bradycardia persists after rewarming. The temperature at which defibrillation should first be attempted and how often it should be tried in the severely hypothermic patient has not been firmly established. There are also conflicting reports about the efficacy of bretylium tosylate in this setting,[70,71] although it may prove helpful in VF by raising the fibrillation threshold.

Treatment of severely hypothermic victims in cardiac arrest in the hospital setting should be directed at rapid core rewarming. Techniques that can be used include the administration of heated, humidified oxygen (42°C to

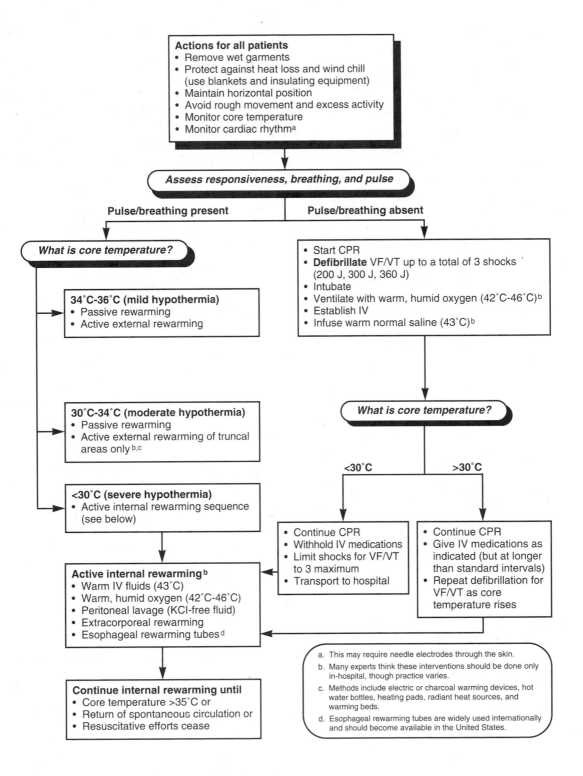

Actions for all patients
- Remove wet garments
- Protect against heat loss and wind chill (use blankets and insulating equipment)
- Maintain horizontal position
- Avoid rough movement and excess activity
- Monitor core temperature
- Monitor cardiac rhythm[a]

Assess responsiveness, breathing, and pulse

Pulse/breathing present

What is core temperature?

34°C-36°C (mild hypothermia)
- Passive rewarming
- Active external rewarming

30°C-34°C (moderate hypothermia)
- Passive rewarming
- Active external rewarming of truncal areas only [b,c]

<30°C (severe hypothermia)
- Active internal rewarming sequence (see below)

Active internal rewarming[b]
- Warm IV fluids (43°C)
- Warm, humid oxygen (42°C-46°C)
- Peritoneal lavage (KCl-free fluid)
- Extracorporeal rewarming
- Esophageal rewarming tubes[d]

Continue internal rewarming until
- Core temperature >35°C or
- Return of spontaneous circulation or
- Resuscitative efforts cease

Pulse/breathing absent

- Start CPR
- **Defibrillate** VF/VT up to a total of 3 shocks (200 J, 300 J, 360 J)
- Intubate
- Ventilate with warm, humid oxygen (42°C-46°C)[b]
- Establish IV
- Infuse warm normal saline (43°C)[b]

What is core temperature?

<30°C

- Continue CPR
- Withhold IV medications
- Limit shocks for VF/VT to 3 maximum
- Transport to hospital

>30°C

- Continue CPR
- Give IV medications as indicated (but at longer than standard intervals)
- Repeat defibrillation for VF/VT as core temperature rises

a. This may require needle electrodes through the skin.

b. Many experts think these interventions should be done only in-hospital, though practice varies.

c. Methods include electric or charcoal warming devices, hot water bottles, heating pads, radiant heat sources, and warming beds.

d. Esophageal rewarming tubes are widely used internationally and should become available in the United States.

Fig 2. Algorithm for treatment of hypothermia.

46°C, 108°F to 115°F), warmed intravenous fluids (normal saline) at 43°C (109°F) infused centrally at rates of approximately 150 to 200 mL/h (*note*: avoid overhydration), peritoneal lavage with warmed (43°C, 109°F) potassium-free fluid administered 2 L at a time, or extracorporeal blood warming with partial bypass.[63,65,66,68,72] Esophageal rewarming tubes have been used extensively and with great success in Europe[73] and are now available in the United States. Pleural lavage with warm saline instilled through a chest tube has also been used successfully.[69] The routine administration of steroids, barbiturates, or antibiotics has not been documented to help increase survival or decrease postresuscitative damage.[74]

Some clinicians believe that patients who appear dead after prolonged exposure to cold temperatures should not be considered dead until they are near normal core temperatures and are still unresponsive to CPR.[75] If drowning preceded the victim's becoming hypothermic, successful resuscitation may be quite limited. Physicians in the hospital setting should use their clinical judgment to decide when resuscitative efforts should cease in a hypothermic arrest victim. Complete rewarming is not indicated for all victims.

Severe accidental hypothermia is a serious and preventable health problem. Clinicians should look for "urban" hypothermia in inner city areas, where it has a high association with poverty and drug and alcohol use.[76,77] In some rural areas more than 90% of hypothermic deaths are associated with elevated blood alcohol levels.[78] Successful treatment of hypothermia requires optimal training of emergency personnel and appropriate resuscitation methods at each institution. Since severe hypothermia is frequently preceded by other disorders (eg, drug overdose, alcohol use, or trauma), the clinician must look for and treat these underlying conditions while simultaneously treating the hypothermia. All cachectic, malnourished, or alcoholic patients should receive thiamine (100 mg IV) early during rewarming procedures.

Near-Drowning

The most important consequence of prolonged underwater submersion without ventilation is hypoxemia. The duration of hypoxia is the critical factor in determining the victim's outcome. Therefore, rescuers must restore ventilation and perfusion as rapidly as possible.

Basic Life Support

Rescue From the Water

When attempting to rescue a near-drowning victim, the rescuer should get to the victim as quickly as possible, preferably with some conveyance (boat, raft, surfboard, or flotation device). Always be aware of personal safety in attempting a rescue, and exercise caution to minimize the danger.

Rescue Breathing

Initial treatment of the near-drowning victim consists of rescue breathing with the mouth-to-mouth technique. Rescue breathing should be started as soon as the victim's airway can be opened and protected and the rescuer's safety can be ensured. This is usually achieved when the victim is in shallow water or out of the water.

Appliances (such as a snorkel for the mouth-to-snorkel technique or buoyant aids) may permit specially trained rescuers to perform rescue breathing in deep water. However, rescue breathing should not be delayed for lack of such equipment if it can be provided safely. Untrained rescuers should not attempt to use such adjuncts.

In diving trauma neck injury should be suspected. The victim's neck should be supported in a neutral position (without flexion or extension), and the victim should be floated supine on a back support before being removed from the water. If the victim must be turned, the head, neck, chest, and body should be aligned, supported, and turned as a unit to the horizontal, supine position. If artificial respiration is required, rescue breathing should be provided with the head maintained in a neutral position; ie, jaw thrust without head tilt or chin lift without head tilt should be used.

Immediate ventilation and rescue breathing should be initiated if the submersion victim is not breathing. Management of the airway and ventilation of the submersion victim is similar to that of any victim in cardiopulmonary arrest. There is no need to clear the airway of aspirated water. Usual airway management with adjuncts, such as bag-mask ventilation and intubation, can be accomplished in the near-drowning victim.[79,80] At most only a modest amount of water is aspirated by the majority of both freshwater and seawater drowning victims, and it is rapidly absorbed from the lungs into the circulation.[81] Furthermore, 10% to 12% of victims do not aspirate at all because of laryngospasm or breath-holding.[81,82] An attempt to remove water from the breathing passages by any means other than suction is usually unnecessary and apt to be dangerous because it may eject gastric contents and cause aspiration.[82]

A subdiaphragmatic abdominal thrust (Heimlich maneuver) delays initiation of ventilation and breathing. The Heimlich maneuver's value for the drowning victim has not been proven scientifically. Support comes only from personal testimony and anecdotal evidence, and its risk-benefit ratio is untested. Therefore, a subdiaphragmatic abdominal thrust should be used only if the rescuer suspects that foreign matter is obstructing the airway or if the victim does not respond appropriately to mouth-to-mouth ventilation. Then, if necessary, CPR should be reinstituted after the Heimlich maneuver has been performed.[79,83,84] The Heimlich maneuver is performed on the near-drowning victim as described in the treatment of foreign-body airway obstruction (unconscious supine) except that in near-drowning the victim's head should be turned sideways unless cervical trauma is suspected.

Chest Compressions

Chest compressions should not be attempted in the water unless special equipment is available to support the back and the rescuer has had special training in techniques of in-water CPR. The brain is not perfused effectively unless the victim is maintained in the horizontal position and the back is supported. It is usually not possible to keep the victim's body horizontal and the head above water in position for rescue breathing.

Removal From the Water

Maintain the victim in a horizontal position at all times. Extrication methods that place the victim in a vertical position (harnesses, lifts) can reduce the blood supply to the brain and heart because victims will have peripheral pooling of their intravascular volume. After removal from the water, the victim must be immediately assessed for adequacy of circulation. The pulse may be difficult to appreciate in a near-drowning victim because of peripheral vasoconstriction and a low cardiac output. If a pulse cannot be felt, chest compressions should be started at once.

Associated Hypothermia

Almost all drowning and near-drowning victims will have some degree of hypothermia. Always treat these patients as combined drowning-hypothermia victims. The algorithm recommendations for hypothermia should be followed for drowning and near-drowning victims. See Fig 2 and below.

Advanced Cardiac Life Support

The near-drowning victim in cardiac arrest should be given ACLS including intubation without delay. Every submersion victim, even one who requires only minimal resuscitation and regains consciousness at the scene, should be transferred to a medical facility for follow-up care. It is imperative that monitoring of life support measures be continued en route and that oxygen be administered if it is available in the transport vehicle since pulmonary injury may develop up to several hours after submersion.

Although survival is unlikely in victims who have undergone prolonged submersion and require prolonged resuscitation,[80] successful resuscitation with full neurological recovery has occurred in near-drowning victims with prolonged submersion in extremely cold water.[75,85-87] Since it is often difficult for rescuers to obtain an accurate time of submersion, attempts at resuscitation should be initiated by rescuers at the scene unless there is obvious physical evidence of death (such as putrefaction, dependent lividity, or rigor mortis). The victim should be transported with continued CPR to an emergency facility where a physician can decide whether to continue resuscitation. End-tidal CO_2 determinations may be helpful in making the decision to continue resuscitative efforts. Aggressive attempts at resuscitation in the hospital should be continued for the victim of icy water submersion.[88]

Cardiac Arrest Associated With Trauma

General Considerations

Patients who develop cardiac arrest in association with trauma are treated differently from patients with a primary cardiac or respiratory arrest. Cardiopulmonary arrest associated with trauma has several possible causes, and prognosis and treatment vary. These causes include

1. Severe central neurological injury with secondary cardiovascular collapse
2. Hypoxia resulting from neurological injury, airway obstruction, large open pneumothorax, or severe tracheobronchial laceration or crush
3. Direct and severe injury to vital structures, such as the heart or aorta
4. Underlying medical problems that led to the injury, such as sudden VF
5. Severely diminished cardiac output from tension pneumothorax or pericardial tamponade
6. Exsanguination leading to hypovolemia and severely diminished oxygen delivery
7. Injuries in a cold environment (eg, fractured leg) complicated by secondary severe hypothermia

With the exception of injuries with massive physical damage, the reversibility of cardiac arrest in the injured patient cannot be estimated on initial assessment. Long-term survival may occur in certain patients with respiratory arrest through aggressive early airway management and ventilatory support. Underlying VF may be treatable with early defibrillation. If identified and treated early, severely diminished cardiac output from a tension pneumothorax or pericardial tamponade can be reversed. However, when an injured patient becomes pulseless as a result of exsanguination, long-term survival is unlikely except when single organ hemorrhage is rapidly identified and controlled, along with appropriate volume resuscitation, blood transfusions, and circulatory support.

In cases of cardiac arrest associated with uncontrolled internal hemorrhage or cardiac tamponade, a favorable outcome requires that the victim be rapidly transported to an emergency facility with immediate operative capabilities.[89] Despite a rapid and otherwise effective out-of-hospital and trauma center response, patients with prehospital cardiopulmonary arrest due to multiple-organ hemorrhage (as commonly seen with the blunt trauma of motor vehicle accidents) will rarely survive neurologically intact.[89-92] Patients who survive a prehospital cardiopulmonary arrest associated with trauma generally are young, have penetrating injuries, have received endotracheal intubation, and undergo prompt transport by highly skilled paramedics to a definitive care facility.[90,91]

The recognition that the mechanism that led to pulselessness in a particular patient cannot always be immediately identified suggests the following approach to the injured patient in cardiac arrest:

- Treat the patient in VF as if the rhythm abnormality were the primary cause of cardiac arrest and the injury was secondary to the cardiac arrest. This means, at a minimum, three shocks to persistent VF. Further treatment for VF can be provided en route.
- Identify and treat potentially reversible injuries that adversely affect ventilation, oxygenation, or cardiac output.
- Provide rapid transport for definitive in-hospital therapy for life-threatening injuries.
- Provide rewarming therapy for patients whose arrest may have been due to or complicated by hypothermia.

Out-of-Hospital Approaches to Cardiac Arrest Associated With Injuries

The injured patient without a pulse requires immediate assessment. Despite the bleak outlook, resuscitative efforts should be initiated when the patient appears to have some potential for survival. Resuscitation should not be attempted in cardiac arrest patients with hemicorporectomy, decapitation, or total body burns, nor in patients with obvious, severe blunt trauma who are without vital signs, pupillary response, or an organized or shockable cardiac rhythm at the scene. Patients in cardiac arrest with deep penetrating cranial injuries and patients with penetrating cranial or truncal wounds associated with asystole and a transport time of more than 15 minutes to a definitive care facility are unlikely to benefit from resuscitative efforts. Most EMS systems have developed guidelines that permit the withholding of cardiac resuscitative efforts in such futile situations. EMS personnel should work within such guidelines when available.

In patients for whom resuscitative efforts are attempted, rapid extrication should be paramount with preparation for rapid evacuation to and notification of a facility that provides definitive trauma care. Simultaneously the ECG rhythm of an injured and pulseless patient should be checked immediately using a quick-look paddle, lead paddle, or adhesive monitor leads. Alternatively, when an automatic defibrillator is the only device available, it should be used to look for VF. Patients in VF should be immediately defibrillated. During the evacuation, airway assessment and ventilation should follow, with intubation of the trachea a priority.[89-91] While chances of survival are inversely proportional to the period of pulselessness and time required for basic CPR, toleration of pulselessness may be extended in patients who receive endotracheal intubation.[91] During airway procedures when the potential for cervical injury exists, in-line stabilization of the neck by an assistant should be used.[89] For such patients, use of lateral neck supports, strapping, and backboards is recommended to minimize exacerbation of an occult neck injury during transport.[93]

Chest compressions are of unknown value in the victims of trauma-associated cardiac arrest. Compressions were used in studies that demonstrated favorable outcomes following out-of-hospital cardiac arrest in injured patients.[89-91] Chest compressions should be initiated for pulseless trauma patients but only after defibrillation or airway control is provided. The value of cardiac medications and crystalloid volume resuscitation in the injured cardiac arrest patient is uncertain. Unless other circumstances prohibit immediate evacuation (eg, prolonged extrication), intravenous line placement should not be attempted until the patient is being transported to the receiving trauma center.[89,94]

In injuries to the chest, the thorax should be vented if asymmetry of breath sounds or increased airway resistance is noted. One should seek and seal any significant open pneumothorax, and monitoring for (and relief of) tension pneumothorax should be performed. Although pericardiocentesis is theoretically useful, efforts to relieve cardiac tamponade generally should be undertaken only by properly trained and qualified personnel.

Emergency Facility Approach to Cardiac Arrest Associated With Injuries

At the emergency facility, the care of the injured patient who has sustained a cardiac arrest is based on the principles mentioned above. Further resuscitative efforts for normothermic patients who deteriorate to asystole during transportation generally are futile. If the patient meets criteria for a potentially meaningful survival, definitive care should be initiated immediately. The patient with VF should be defibrillated. The airway should be secured (if not already done) with an endotracheal tube or surgical airway if needed.

Clinical suspicion of a tension pneumothorax should be treated immediately by thoracic decompression followed by tube thoracostomy. In the absence of an immediate hemodynamic response to thoracic decompression or, alternatively, in the presence of a penetrating thoracic wound, more aggressive interventions may be warranted. During concurrent volume resuscitation, prompt emergency thoracotomy will permit direct massage of the heart and indicated surgical procedures. Such procedures may include relief of cardiac tamponade, direct cardiac volume loading, control of thoracic and extrathoracic hemorrhage, and aortic cross-clamping.

In any event, performing prolonged closed-chest resuscitation for the normothermic, traumatized cardiac arrest patient, either at the emergency facility or in the out-of-hospital setting, is of no benefit, even with out-of-hospital intubation. Thus, delays in the out-of-hospital setting must be minimized and the receiving resuscitation team prepared to immediately initiate full invasive resuscitative efforts when justified by the patient's condition.[94]

Triage and Treatment of Multiple Critically Injured Patients

When multiple patients receive serious injuries, emergency personnel must establish priorities for care. When the number of patients with critical injuries exceeds the capability of the EMS system, traumatized patients without a pulse should be considered the lowest priority for care and triage.

The only exception to this rule is when confronted with multiple victims of lightning strike or electric injuries. In these events use "reverse trauma triage" and treat the nonbreathing pulseless victims first.

Most EMS systems have developed mass casualty guidelines that permit the out-of-hospital pronouncement of death or withholding of cardiac resuscitative efforts for multiple patients with critical injuries incompatible with life. EMS personnel should work within such guidelines when available.

Electric Shock and Lightning Strike

Electric Shock

Electric shock is associated with a fatality rate of 0.5 per 100 000 population per year in the United States.[95] It accounts for approximately 1000 deaths annually and causes an additional 5000 patients to require emergency treatment.[96,97] Victims of electric shock encompass a wide spectrum of injury, ranging from a transient unpleasant sensation from brief exposure to low-intensity current to instantaneous cardiac arrest from accidental electrocution.

Electric injuries result from the direct effects of current and the conversion of electric energy into heat energy as current passes through body tissues. Factors that determine the nature and severity of electric trauma include the magnitude of energy delivered, resistance to current flow, type of current, duration of contact with the current source, and current pathway. High-tension current (more than 1000 V) causes the most serious injuries, although fatal electrocutions may occur with low-voltage household current (110 V).[98] Bone and skin are most resistant to the passage of electric current; muscle, blood vessels, and nerves conduct with least resistance.[96,97] Skin resistance, the most important factor impeding current flow, can be reduced substantially by moisture, thereby converting what ordinarily might be a minor low-voltage injury into a life-threatening shock.[99]

Alternating current at 60 cycles per second (the frequency used in most US household and commercial sources of electricity) is much more dangerous than direct current of the same magnitude. Contact with alternating current may cause tetanic skeletal muscle contractions and prevent victims from releasing the source of the electricity. This leads to prolonged exposure and increased current delivery. The repetitive frequency of alternating current also increases the likelihood of current delivered to the myocardium during the vulnerable recovery period of the cardiac cycle and can precipitate VF, analogous to the R-on-T phenomenon.[100]

Transthoracic current flow, such as a hand-to-hand pathway, is more likely to be fatal than a vertical (hand-to-foot) or straddle (foot-to-foot) current path.[101] However, the vertical pathway has been associated with an increased incidence of cardiac muscle damage, possibly due to longer tissue transit of electricity and wider path of current spread.[102] Myocardial injury has been documented following both high-voltage and low-voltage electric shock and has been attributed to the direct effects of current and coronary artery spasm.[103,104]

Cardiac and Respiratory Arrest

Cardiopulmonary arrest is the primary cause of immediate death due to electric injury.[105] Ventricular fibrillation or ventricular asystole may occur as a direct result of electric shock. Ventricular fibrillation occurs more commonly following contact with alternating current, whereas asystole is more common with direct current.[106] Other serious cardiac arrhythmias, including VT that may progress to VF, may result from exposure to low- or high-voltage current.[107]

Respiratory arrest may occur secondary to (1) electric current passing through the brain and causing inhibition of medullary respiratory center function; (2) tetanic contraction of the diaphragm and chest wall musculature during current exposure; or (3) prolonged paralysis of respiratory muscles, which may continue for minutes after the shock current has terminated. If respiratory arrest persists, hypoxic cardiac arrest may occur.

Basic Life Support

Immediately after accidental electrocution, failure of either respiration or circulation, or both, may result. The patient may be apneic, mottled, unconscious, and in circulatory collapse from VF or asystole. The prognosis for recovery from electric shock is not readily predictable because the amplitude and duration of the charge usually are not known. However, because many victims are young and without preexisting cardiopulmonary disease, they have a reasonable chance for survival, and vigorous resuscitative measures are indicated, even for those who appear dead on initial evaluation.

It is critically important that the rescuer be certain that rescue efforts will not put him or her in danger of electric shock. After authorized personnel have shut off the power or the victim is clear of the electric source, the rescuer should determine the victim's cardiopulmonary status. If spontaneous respiration or circulation is absent, BLS techniques should be initiated immediately.

As soon as possible, secure airway patency and provide ventilation and supplemental oxygen. If electric shock occurs at a site that is not readily accessible, such as on a utility pole, rescue breathing should be started at once, and the victim must be lowered to the ground as quickly as possible. Ventilations and chest compressions should be instituted immediately for victims of cardiac arrest. Spinal protection and immobilization should be maintained during extrication, airway control, and initial resuscitation if there is any likelihood of head or neck trauma. Smoldering clothing, shoes, and belts should be removed to prevent further thermal damage.

Advanced Life Support

Resuscitation of electric shock victims requires aggressive and sustained resuscitative measures and necessitates application of advanced cardiac and advanced trauma life support techniques to achieve initial stabilization and to overcome associated complications.[108] Ventricular fibrillation, ventricular asystole, and other serious arrhythmias should be treated with standard advanced life support techniques and cardiac drug therapy. If defibrillation or cardioversion is necessary, currently recommended defibrillation energy levels and dosage schedules should be used. Establishing an artificial airway may be difficult in patients with electrical burns of the face, mouth, or anterior neck. Extensive soft tissue swelling may develop rapidly and complicate airway control measures, such as endotracheal intubation.

Victims with electric trauma, especially those with significant underlying tissue destruction or hypovolemic shock, require rapid intravenous fluid administration to correct ongoing fluid losses, counteract shock, and maintain a diuresis to avoid renal shutdown due to myoglobinuria. Normal saline or lactated Ringer's solution should be administered to maintain a urinary output of at least 50 to 100 mL/h. When myoglobinuria is suspected, urinary alkalinization and osmotic agents enhance the clearance of myoglobin and help prevent renal failure. Normal saline with one ampule (50 mEq) sodium bicarbonate added to each liter is the recommended fluid and should be administered to maintain urinary output at 1.0 to 1.5 mL/kg per hour and maintain blood pH at 7.45 or greater.[108] Mannitol should also be given if myoglobinuria is present, with an initial dose of 25 g followed by 12.5 g/h.

Continuous monitoring of respiratory and hemodynamic status, cardiac rhythm, and urinary output, along with a thorough evaluation for associated complications and injuries, is indicated for all victims of electric injuries. Acute complications of electric shock that may interfere with resuscitative efforts include neurological disturbances, such as coma, severe agitation, and seizures; hypovolemia and metabolic acidosis resulting from electric burns and widespread underlying tissue destruction; injuries to the head, spinal cord, chest, or abdomen secondary to falling or being thrown from the electric source; and vascular complications, including arterial spasm and thrombosis, making pulses difficult to palpate, and thrombosis of peripheral veins, precluding their use for intra-

venous access. Finally, because electrothermal burns and underlying tissue injury may require surgical attention, early consultation with a physician skilled in treatment of electric injury is encouraged.

Lightning Strike

Lightning strike, which accounts for more deaths than any other natural phenomenon, causes approximately 50 to 300 fatalities per year in the United States, with about twice that number of persons sustaining serious injury.[109,110] Lightning injuries have a 30% mortality rate, and up to 70% of survivors have significant residual damage.[111]

Lightning has a much higher magnitude of energy than electric shock, a substantially shorter duration of exposure, and a different current pathway. The lightning current may range as high as 100 million to 2 billion V and 200 A.[112,113] The instantaneous duration of current flow frequently results in the lightning current "flashing over" the outside of the victim, a phenomenon that may account for the relatively high survival rate considering the magnitude of current involved. However, a small amount of current may enter the victim, disrupt cardiac and respiratory center function, and induce immediate cardiopulmonary arrest.[114]

Cardiac and Respiratory Arrest

The primary cause of death in lightning victims is cardiac arrest, which may be due to primary ventricular asystole or VF.[115] Lightning acts as a massive direct current countershock, depolarizing the entire myocardium at once and producing asystole. In many cases, cardiac automaticity may restore organized cardiac activity, and sinus rhythm may return spontaneously. However, concomitant respiratory arrest due to thoracic muscle spasm and suppression of the medullary respiratory center persist even after spontaneous heartbeats return. Unless ventilatory assistance is provided, a secondary hypoxic cardiac arrest from inadequate respirations may occur.

Patients most likely to die of lightning injury are those who suffer immediate cardiac arrest. Patients who do not experience immediate arrest have an excellent chance of recovery.[111] Therefore, when multiple victims are struck simultaneously by lightning, "reverse triage" should be performed. The usual triage priorities are reversed and rescuers should give highest priority to patients in cardiac or respiratory arrest. Victims who appear clinically dead after the strike should be treated before other victims showing signs of life.

Basic Life Support

For victims in cardiopulmonary arrest, basic and advanced life support measures should be instituted immediately. The goal is to oxygenate the heart and brain adequately until cardiac activity is restored. Victims with respiratory arrest may require only ventilation and oxygenation to avoid secondary hypoxic cardiac arrest.

Resuscitative attempts may have higher success rates in lightning victims than in patients with other causes of cardiac arrest, and efforts may be effective even when the interval before resuscitation or the resuscitative attempt is prolonged.

Advanced Life Support

Advanced resuscitative measures, including indications and energy levels for defibrillation as well as dosages and administration schedules for cardiac medications, are the same as for victims of cardiac arrest from other causes. As with electric shock, victims of lightning strike require careful hemodynamic and cardiac monitoring along with thorough evaluation for associated injuries to the head, spine, chest, or abdomen and fractures or dislocations. However, unlike victims of electric shock, patients with lightning strike seldom have significant cutaneous damage, underlying tissue destruction, or associated myoglobinuria, and fluid loading is rarely necessary. As soon as spontaneous circulation and adequate blood pressure are established, fluid administration should be restricted to prevent exacerbation of cerebral edema, elevated intracranial pressure, and intracranial injuries that may accompany lightning strike.[116-118]

Cardiac Arrest Associated With Pregnancy

CPR of expectant mothers is unique because of dramatic alterations in maternal cardiovascular and respiratory physiology. During normal pregnancy, maternal cardiac output and blood volume increase up to 50%. Maternal heart rate, minute ventilation, and oxygen consumption also increase.[119] Pulmonary functional residual capacity, systemic and pulmonary vascular resistance, colloid oncotic pressure, and the ratio of colloid oncotic pressure to pulmonary capillary wedge pressure all decrease.[119,120] Together these changes render the pregnant woman more susceptible to and less tolerant of major cardiovascular and respiratory insults. Also, when the mother is supine, the gravid uterus may compress the iliac vessels, the inferior vena cava, and the abdominal aorta, resulting in hypotension and as much as a 25% reduction in cardiac output.[121] Precipitating events for cardiac arrest during pregnancy include pulmonary embolism, trauma, peripartum hemorrhage with hypovolemia, amniotic fluid embolism, congenital and acquired cardiac disease, and complications of tocolytic therapy, including arrhythmia, congestive heart failure, and myocardial infarction.[122]

When cardiac arrest occurs in a pregnant woman, standard resuscitative measures and procedures should be taken without modification. If VF is present, it should be treated with defibrillation according to the VF algorithm. Closed-chest compressions and support of ventilation should be done in accord with usual protocols. To minimize the effects of the gravid uterus on venous return and cardiac output, a wedge, such as a pillow, should be placed under the right abdominal flank and hip to displace the uterus to the left side of the abdomen.[123] One practical proposal is for a second rescuer to form a "human wedge" to help relieve aortocaval compression.[124] In this maneuver the back of the victim is rolled onto the thighs of a kneeling second rescuer, who can then stabilize the shoulders and pelvis of the victim. Alternatively, continuous manual displacement to the left may be used. Standard pharmacologic therapy should also be used without modification. Specifically, vasopressors such as epinephrine, norepinephrine, and dopamine should not be withheld when clinically indicated.

If there is potential fetal viability, prompt performance of a perimortem cesarean section should be considered if initial attempts at CPR, leftward displacement of the gravid uterus, fluid volume restoration, and standard application of the ACLS algorithms have failed to restore effective circulation. Several authors now recommend that the decision to perform a perimortem cesarean section should be made rapidly, with delivery effected within 4 to 5 minutes of the arrest. This approach will maximize the chances of both maternal and infant survival.[125,126] Delivery of the fetus is thought to obviate the effects of aortocaval compression and allow recovery of venous return to the heart.

The decision to perform a perimortem cesarean section is complex. The circumstances precipitating the arrest, the gestational age and potential for survival of the fetus, the availability of trained personnel, and the amount of time since the onset of the arrest should be considered. Obstetric and neonatal personnel should be in attendance if available. While the optimum interval from arrest to delivery is within 5 minutes, there are case reports of intact infant survival after more than 20 minutes of complete maternal arrest.[125,127]

Summary

- Perform CPR with the patient rolled toward her left side. Use one of the following:
  — A pillow, rolled sheets, or towels
  — Manual displacement
  — Cardiff wedge (specially constructed solid device)
  — Human wedge (thighs of second rescuer)
- Provide defibrillation, intubation, and pharmacologic agents in the usual manner
- Consider emergency cesarean section if pulse has not been restored in 4 to 5 minutes. The factors to consider in this decision are
  — Potential fetal viability
  — Personnel trained in the procedure
  — Appropriate support for mother and fetus after the procedure

Toxicologic Cardiac Emergencies

Cocaine

Millions of people in the United States use cocaine. The crystalline form of the drug may be inhaled nasally or injected intravenously.[128] The free base form of the drug, commonly known as "crack," is usually smoked.[129] Although arrhythmias and cardiac arrest from cocaine are relatively rare, cocaine use of any type by any route may cause disastrous complications.[128-136]

The toxicity of cocaine relates to its pharmacologic properties. Cocaine stimulates the release and blocks the reuptake of norepinephrine, epinephrine, dopamine, and serotonin.[128,132] This results in an elevation in blood pressure, tachycardia, and feelings of euphoria coupled with decreased fatigue. Cocaine toxicity is dose-dependent. However, numerous seizures, myocardial infarctions, and deaths have been reported in both new and experienced users who used only small quantities of the drug.[128,131,137]

Serious cardiac toxicity from cocaine is due to cocaine's direct effect on the heart coupled with central nervous system stimulatory effects on the cardiovascular system.[138-142] Cocaine's β effects increase heart rate and myocardial contractility.[138,139] Cocaine's α effects decrease coronary blood flow and may induce coronary artery spasm.[139,141,143,144] Thus, there is decreased coronary artery perfusion at a time of increased myocardial oxygen demand. Hypoxia from pulmonary edema and acidosis from cocaine-induced seizures may also exacerbate cocaine's cardiotoxicity.[130,136,140]

Arrhythmias Due to Cocaine

Supraventricular arrhythmias due to cocaine include paroxysmal supraventricular tachycardia, rapid atrial fibrillation, and atrial flutter.[135] These arrhythmias are short-lived and usually do not require immediate therapy.[145-147] Hemodynamically stable patients with persistent supraventricular arrhythmias should be treated with a benzodiazepine, such as diazepam, in a dose of 5 to 20 mg IV over 5 to 20 minutes. Benzodiazepines work by modulating the stimulatory effects of cocaine on the central nervous system and therefore blunt the patient's hypersympathetic state.[148-150]

Ventricular arrhythmias due to cocaine include ventricular ectopy, runs of VT, and in rare instances cardiac arrest due to VF.[139,140,151] As in the case of supraventricular arrhythmias, ventricular ectopy is usually very transient and should be treated with careful observation supplemented by a titrated dose of a benzodiazepine.

Ventricular Tachycardia Due to Cocaine

Malignant ventricular ectopy and VT due to cocaine should initially be treated by standard ACLS guidelines. Patients should be well oxygenated and receive lidocaine at a dose of 1 to 1.5 mg/kg. A defibrillator should be brought to the bedside. The decision to use lidocaine must be carefully weighed against the increased risk of seizure due to the synergistic toxic effects of lidocaine in the presence of cocaine.[149,152] Although controversial, judicious use of a β blocker[128,149,153,154] (propranolol 0.5 to 1 mg IV every 5 minutes) or a combined α- and β-blocking agent such as labetalol may be used to treat ventricular ectopy.[155]

Ventricular Fibrillation Due to Cocaine

Ventricular fibrillation due to cocaine should initially be treated by the ACLS algorithm.

Although cocaine and epinephrine have similar cardiovascular effects and there are theoretical arguments against administering epinephrine to cocaine-induced VF, there is no good evidence to suggest eliminating the initial epinephrine dose in treating cocaine-induced VF. Clinicians should, however, increase the interval between subsequent doses of epinephrine to every 5 to 10 minutes and avoid high-dose epinephrine (greater than 1 mg per dose) in refractory patients.

If VF continues, treat with a bolus of lidocaine at a dose of 1.5 mg/kg and reshock the patient in standard fashion. The treatment of choice for refractory patients is not well defined.

Propranolol at a dose of 1 mg every minute, to a total of 3 to 5 mg, appears to be the next most appropriate therapy for refractory VF. This recommendation is based on animal data and empiric reports but is not supported by any controlled human studies.[128,140,149,154] The risk of β blockade in cocaine toxicity is that of unopposed α stimulation.[153] This is not a primary concern when compared with the potential benefit of successfully reverting refractory VF. Patients should be reshocked immediately before each propranolol administration. Other antiarrhythmic options include magnesium sulfate, procainamide, and bretylium tosylate.

Summary: Treatment of Cocaine-Induced Arrhythmias

Supraventricular arrhythmias requiring therapy should be treated with

- Oxygen
- An escalating dose of 5 to 20 mg of diazepam

Malignant ventricular arrhythmias and VT with hemodynamic stability should be treated with

- Oxygen
- Lidocaine 1 to 1.5 mg/kg
- An escalating dose of 5 to 20 mg of diazepam
- If needed, a titrated dose of a β blocker (propranolol 0.5 to 1 mg IV every 5 minutes) or labetalol

Ventricular fibrillation should initially be treated in standard fashion:

- Give three successive shocks (200 J, 300 J, and 360 J).
- Oxygenate and hyperventilate nonresponders and administer a single dose of epinephrine 1 mg.

- Treat patients with continued VF with lidocaine 1.5 mg/kg and reshock.

The following modifications to the standard ACLS VF algorithm should be made:

- Give propranolol at a dose of 1 mg each minute for refractory VF.
- Limit epinephrine to 1 mg every 5 to 10 minutes.
- Avoid repeat doses of lidocaine.

Hypertension and Pulmonary Edema

Cocaine toxicity may result in hypertensive emergency because of the drug's effects on the central nervous system and its peripheral α-agonist effects.[128,132,140] Hypertensive patients should initially be treated with a benzodiazepine in an attempt to minimize the stimulatory effects of cocaine on the central nervous system.[142,149,150] Patients who require additional therapy are best treated with a vasodilator, such as a titrated dose of nitroglycerin or nitroprusside. Nitroglycerin is preferred in those patients with superimposed chest pain. β-Blocking agents such as propranolol or esmolol should be avoided.[153,156] Both have the potential to raise, rather than lower, blood pressure by allowing unopposed cocaine-induced α stimulation. Labetalol, a combined α and β blocker, has been used with mixed results and appears to be inferior to nitroglycerin or nitroprusside.[155,157] A pure α blocker, such as phentolamine (1 to 10 mg) may also be used, although it too is not yet well studied for treatment of cocaine toxicity.

Cocaine effects on pulmonary dynamics may result in pulmonary edema. Pulmonary edema may also occur secondary to a subarachnoid hemorrhage, from a cocaine-induced myocardial infarction, or as a consequence of additional drugs of abuse such as heroin.[130,136,158,159] Most patients respond to standard medical management. Positive-pressure ventilation with a continuous positive airway pressure (CPAP) mask or intubation supplemented by positive end-expiratory pressure (PEEP) will usually rapidly correct medically resistant hypoxemia.

Cocaine Chest Pain and Myocardial Infarction

Chest pain is one of the most common complaints of cocaine users.[145-147] The vast majority of patients have only transient chest pain and no evidence of acute ischemia on their ECG. Unfortunately, abnormal, nondiagnostic ECGs are common in the young adults who use cocaine.[160] Although rare, acute myocardial infarctions do occur in cocaine users.[134,137,161,162] Most cocaine-related infarctions occur in patients who also smoke cigarettes or who have other cardiac risk factors,[134,137,161] though some infarctions occur in active healthy patients with no risk factors for ischemic heart disease.[134,161-163]

Cocaine-related myocardial ischemia should be treated with oxygen, aspirin, nitrates, and a titrated dose of a benzodiazepine.[150,164] β Blockers should not be used. β-Blocking agents may increase the probability of α-mediated vasospasm.[144] Because of its antispasm effects and its beneficial role in myocardial infarction, magnesium should also be used for cocaine-related ischemia and infarction.[165-167] Morphine should be administered for continued pain.

Thrombolytic therapy in conjunction with heparin has the potential to restore relatively normal coronary arterial flow to these predominantly young, previously healthy patients.[161] Its use, however, must be weighed against its increased risk in patients who have likely had multiple episodes of uncontrolled hypertension due to the repeated smoking of cocaine.[130,137] An additional concern is that up to one half of all cocaine-related myocardial infarctions appear to be due to spasm and not thrombus.[134,161-163] Thrombolytic use must also be tempered by the common ECG variants that mimic infarction in cocaine users, such as early repolarization and QRS complexes with elevated J points.[160] Before thrombolysis some clinicians may choose to perform an echocardiogram, have isoenzyme evidence of infarction via a rapid assay technique, or take the patient to a cardiac catheterization laboratory where a decision to use lytic therapy or angioplasty can be made with certainty.

Tricyclic Antidepressants

When taken in excess, the tricyclic antidepressants are among the most cardiotoxic medications.[168,169] Although tricyclic antidepressants rarely cause cardiovascular side effects when taken in therapeutic amounts, they are the number one cause of death from overdose in patients who arrive at the hospital alive.[167,170]

The toxic side effects of tricyclic antidepressants are due to the interplay of their four major pharmacologic properties.[171,172] Tricyclics (1) stimulate catecholamine release and then block reuptake, (2) have central and peripheral anticholinergic actions, (3) have quinidine-like membrane stabilizing effects, and (4) have direct α-blocking actions.

Warning signs of tricyclic toxicity include alterations in mental status, tachycardia (especially in association with a rightward QRS axis),[173] prolongation of the QT interval, and evidence of anticholinergic effects, such as delirium, mydriasis, and gastric atony.[168,169,174] Coma, seizures, QRS widening, or ventricular arrhythmias are ominous findings and require immediate therapy.[168,174-176] Hypotension, though not usually a life-threatening complication, also requires immediate therapy.[176,177] Usually serum levels are not readily available and are of little prognostic or therapeutic value in acute overdoses.[168] Most patients will manifest some sign of toxicity within 2 hours of ingestion, and patients who are asymptomatic after 6 hours of continuous monitoring are at essentially no risk for toxicity.[168,174]

Bicarbonate for Tricyclic Antidepressant Overdose

Alkalinization with sodium bicarbonate is the mainstay of therapy for treating seriously ill tricyclic antidepressant overdoses.[168,174,176,178-180] Alkalinization decreases the free, nonprotein-bound form of the tricyclic molecule and overrides the tricyclic-induced sodium channel blockade of phase 1 of the action potential.[168,178] Alkalinization is not required in patients who have only a mild resting tachycardia or prolongation of the QT interval. However, patients with prolongation of the QRS to greater than 100 ms, ventricular arrhythmias, or hypotension unresponsive to a saline bolus of 500 to 1000 mL should have their serum pH elevated to 7.5 to 7.55.

Alkalinization for Unstable Patients

- Raise pH to 7.45 to 7.55 with 1 mEq/kg of sodium bicarbonate given over 1 to 2 minutes.
- Analyze arterial blood gas levels to confirm pH elevation.
- Place patients on an infusion of two ampules (50 to 100 mEq) of sodium bicarbonate in normal saline solution (0.9 NS).
- Run the infusion at 150 to 200 mL/h until the patient stabilizes, evidenced by QRS less than 100 ms, arrhythmia cessation, and blood pressure normalization.
- Maintain the patient's pH at 7.45 to 7.55 by routine venous or arterial pH measurements.

Seizing patients and those with respiratory arrest should initially be hyperventilated to a pH of 7.5 to 7.55.[181]

Magnesium for Tricyclic Antidepressant Overdose

Some patients may develop arrhythmias due to tricyclic actions on phase 2 of the action potential.[171,172,182] The phase 2 effects are initially manifest by a prolongation of the QT interval, but it may result in the torsades de pointes variant of VT.[182,183] Magnesium sulfate is the drug of choice for this select group of patients.[183-185] The dose of magnesium is 2 g as an IV bolus in unstable patients (up to 5 to 10 grams IV may be used), or over 1 to 5 minutes in patients with hemodynamic stability.[185,186]

Cardiac Arrest in Tricyclic Antidepressant Overdose

Cardiac arrest from tricyclic overdose is usually due to myocardial depression resulting in pulseless electrical activity (PEA) or due to VF.[168,176,178,187]

PEA should initially be treated with hyperventilation and sodium bicarbonate infusion to a pH of at least 7.50 to 7.55. A saline infusion with normal saline running at a rate greater than 1 L/h should also be begun. Epinephrine should be used if alkalinization and the saline infusion do not immediately reverse the patient's status. Other causes of PEA should also be considered.

Ventricular ectopy that does not respond to sodium bicarbonate therapy should be treated with 1 to 1.5 mg/kg of lidocaine. Responders should be maintained on a continuous infusion. Nonresponders should be treated with either 2 g of magnesium sulfate over 1 to 5 minutes[186] or phenytoin[188,189] at 25 to 50 mg/min. Ventricular tachycardia that does not respond to sodium bicarbonate should be

treated similarly if the patient remains conscious and maintains hemodynamic stability. Procainamide should not be used in tricyclic-induced arrhythmias because of its tricyclic-like pharmacologic properties.[171,172]

The protocol for treating VF due to tricyclic antidepressant overdose requires some modification of the standard ACLS algorithm:

- Defibrillate with escalating energy levels in the standard fashion.
- Then intubate, oxygenate, give epinephrine 1 mg, and immediately defibrillate at 360 J.
- Rapidly alkalinize patient by administering sodium bicarbonate 1 mEq/kg IV push. If bicarbonate is not readily available, hyperventilate the patient.

Lidocaine is the initial antiarrhythmic of choice for tricyclic-induced VF and VT in pulseless or unconscious patients, although there are no studies proving its effectiveness. Refractory VF and VT may be treated with bretylium tosylate (500 mg IV push), magnesium sulfate (2 g IV push), and/or repeat doses of lidocaine (0.5 mg/kg IV push).

Seizures and Hypotension

Seizures due to tricyclic antidepressant overdose should be terminated immediately. Uncontrolled seizure activity usually results in hypoxia, acidosis, tachycardia, hypotension, and electrolyte fluxes, all of which increase morbidity and mortality from tricyclic antidepressant overdose.[168,176,190]

Hypotension is usually responsive to infusions of 500 to 1000 mL of normal saline. Alkalinization with sodium bicarbonate is recommended for nonresponders. Patients with refractory hypotension may be treated with dopamine or norepinephrine.[191]

General Management

Gastric decontamination with activated charcoal should be considered in all patients with an acute tricyclic antidepressant overdose.[192] Orogastric lavage should be used in all unconscious patients and considered in those with 1 to 2 hours of overdose with a life-threatening amount of a tricyclic.[193] Syrup of ipecac is unnecessary in the hospital care of tricyclic antidepressant overdose patients because superior gastric emptying techniques are readily available.[194]

Digitalis Overdose and Cardiac Toxicity

Digitalis-induced cardiac toxicity occurs usually in chronic users of this widely prescribed medication. It may also be due to an acute accidental or intentional overdose in a previously healthy patient.

Many of the early symptoms of digitalis intoxication are nonspecific manifestations of central nervous system and gastrointestinal toxicity. Fatigue, visual symptoms, weakness, nausea, vomiting, and abdominal pain are quite common.[195,196] Cardiac arrhythmias occur in the vast majority of toxic patients. Arrhythmias most commonly seen include ventricular ectopy and bradycardia, often in association with varying degrees of heart block.[195,196] Some rhythm disturbances should immediately suggest digitalis intoxication. These include paroxysmal atrial tachycardia with block, nonparoxysmal accelerated junctional tachycardia, bidirectional VT, new onset bigeminy, and regularized atrial fibrillation.[197]

The cardiac toxicity of digitalis is due to the combination of its inhibitory effects on nodal conduction and its excitatory effects on individual atrial and ventricular fibers.[195,196] Life-threatening digitalis toxicity is usually due to bradyarrhythmias, with resultant congestive heart failure, malignant ventricular arrhythmias, and hyperkalemia, the last a manifestation of digitalis poisoning of the sodium-potassium adenosine triphosphatase pump.[198-200]

The treatment of arrhythmias due to digitalis toxicity is based on whether the overdose is acute or chronic and whether the patient is maintaining hemodynamic stability.

Digitalis intoxication in chronic users generally develops in association with hypokalemia, hypomagnesemia, dehydration, declining renal function, or loss of muscle mass.[196,201] Patients on non–potassium-sparing diuretics are especially prone to developing toxicity. Cardiotoxicity in these patients is best treated by replenishing total body potassium and magnesium stores.[195] Hypokalemic patients should be presumed to be hypomagnesemic until proven otherwise.[202] Potassium and magnesium therapy in association with volume replacement will usually correct most arrhythmias over a period of hours.

Digitalis-Induced Bradycardias

Patients with symptomatic bradycardia and heart block should initially receive atropine in doses starting at 0.5 mg IV. Because of the vagally mediated effects of digitalis, atropine may temporarily reverse digitalis intoxication.[195,203] Digitalis-toxic patients are more prone to pacemaker-induced ventricular rhythm disturbances, so that the use of pacemakers should be highly selective.[195]

Digoxin-Specific Fab Fragment Therapy

The availability of digoxin-specific antibodies (Fab fragments) to treat severe chronic and acute toxicity has dramatically reduced morbidity and mortality from digitalis intoxication.[198,199,204,205] Fab fragments bind to free digoxin, resulting in an inactive compound that is excreted in the urine. Their use results in lowered free serum digoxin levels, and this concentration gradient pulls free digoxin out of myocardial tissue. Effects begin in minutes, and complete reversal of digitalis-mediated effects usually occurs within 30 minutes of administration.[205] The high cost per vial for Fab fragment therapy must be weighed against the decreased need for prolonged and expensive intensive care therapy.

The specific dose of Fab fragment is determined by the patient's weight and serum digoxin level if known, or in the case of acute toxicity, by the estimated milligrams ingested. Each 40-mg vial of Fab fragments binds 0.6 mg of digoxin. Dosing charts are available from the pharmacy, the drug insert, or a regional poison control center (Tables 7, 8, and 9). Serum digoxin levels after Fab fragment therapy rise dramatically and should not be obtained to guide a patient's therapy.[198,199]

The specific indications for Fab fragment therapy are presumed digoxin toxicity in association with (1) life-threatening arrhythmias refractory to conventional therapy, (2) shock or fulminant congestive heart failure, (3) hyperkalemia (K >5.0), (4) steady state serum levels above 10 to 15 ng/mL in adults or 5 ng/mL in children and infants, and (5) cardiac arrest.[198,199,205] Additional indications for cases of acute ingestion are ingestions

Table 7. Approximate Digibind Dose for Reversal of a Single Large Digoxin Overdose

Number of Digoxin Tablets or Capsules Ingested*	Digibind Dose (No. of Vials)
25	9
50	17
75	25
100	34
150	50
200	67

*0.25 mg tablets with 80% bioavailability or 0.2 mg Lanoxicaps capsules with 100% bioavailability

Table 8. Adult Dose Estimate of Digibind (in No. of Vials) From Steady-State Serum Digoxin Concentration

Patient Weight (kg)	Serum Digoxin Concentration (ng/mL) (Vials)						
	1	2	4	8	12	16	20
40	0.5	1	2	3	5	7	8
60	0.5	1	3	5	7	10	12
70	1	2	3	5	9	11	14
80	1	2	3	7	10	13	16
100	1	2	3	8	12	15	20

Table 9. Infants and Small Children Dose Estimates of Digibind (in mg) From Steady-State Serum Digoxin Concentration

Patient Weight (kg)	Serum Digoxin Concentration (ng/mL) (mg)						
	1	2	4	8	12	16	20
1	0.4*	1*	1.5*	3	5	7	8
3	1*	3*	5	10	15	19	24
5	2*	4	8	16	24	32	40
10	4	8	16	32	48	64	80
20	8	15	32	64	96	128	160

*Dilution of reconstituted vial to 1 mg/mL may be desirable.
Tables 7, 8, and 9 were reproduced by permission of Burroughs Wellcome Company.

greater than 10 mg in adults or 0.3 mg/kg in infants and children.[204]

In general, 3 to 5 vials are effective in patients with chronic intoxication. Hemodynamically significant brady-arrhythmias and life-threatening heart block in acute over-dose require much greater quantities of Fab fragments. The dosing nomogram is used for the correct dosage of antibody. Massive overdoses may require as many as 20 vials.

Digitalis-Induced Ventricular Arrhythmias

Ventricular ectopy unresponsive to conservative ther-apy with replacement amounts of potassium, magnesium, and crystalloid may be treated with lidocaine, magne-sium, or phenytoin. Lidocaine may be rapid acting and has little acute toxicity when used in the recommended dose of 1 to 1.5 mg/kg.[195,196,203] Care must be taken in elderly patients with congestive heart failure and coexis-tent renal impairment who are placed on a lidocaine maintenance infusion.

In the past phenytoin was the preferred antiarrhythmic for digitalis-induced ventricular arrhythmias.[203] It has the advantage of causing fewer central nervous system side effects than lidocaine and has little effect on AV conduc-tion. Recent case reports suggest that magnesium may be the initial drug of choice for digitalis-induced ventricu-lar arrhythmias.[206,207] A dose of 2 g of magnesium sulfate over 1 to 5 minutes may be used as first-line therapy for ventricular arrhythmia due to digitalis toxicity. Others may choose to use it only in patients with malignant ventricular rhythms unresponsive to lidocaine or phenytoin. A con-tinuous magnesium infusion of 1 to 2 g (8 to 16 mEq) per hour may be required for continued arrhythmia suppression. Patients with arrhythmias refractory to pharmacologic ther-apy should be treated with Fab fragment antibodies.[198,204]

Digitalis-Induced Ventricular Tachycardia

Ventricular tachycardia not accompanied by shock or cardiac arrest should be treated by Fab fragment anti-bodies combined with a rapidly active antiarrhythmic.[195] A lidocaine bolus of 1.5 mg/kg is the best initial antiarrhyth-mic therapy.[195] Responders should be placed on a lido-caine infusion of 3 mg/min until the Fab fragment therapy becomes effective. Nonresponders to lidocaine are best treated by a rapid infusion of 2 g of magnesium sulfate over 1 to 2 minutes. Responders should be placed on a constant infusion of 1 to 2 g (8 to 16 mEq) per hour for the next 30 to 60 minutes to allow for Fab fragment administration and effects.

Hemodynamically unstable VT requires immediate cardioversion, administration of 10 to 20 vials of Fab frag-ments, and antiarrhythmic therapy. Cardioversion is prob-ably best begun at 25 to 50 J because of the increased likelihood of postcountershock rhythm deterioration in digitalis-toxic patients.[195,203] Patients who do not respond to 25 to 50 J should be immediately reshocked at 200 J

and then at 300 J if a third conversion is required. Stan-dard ACLS guidelines should be followed concerning the "sync" mode setting. Lidocaine and magnesium are both appropriate choices in unstable patients and should be used as previously described for stable patients. Mag-nesium may be given as a dose of 2 g IV push for un-stable patients and those in cardiac arrest. Up to 5 g over 2 to 5 minutes seems appropriate for unstable patients with digitalis-induced VT.

Digitalis-Induced Ventricular Fibrillation

Ventricular fibrillation due to digitalis overdose requires some modification of standard ACLS guidelines. The ini-tial steps of electrical reversion, intubation and oxygena-tion, and epinephrine administration should be performed in standard fashion. Two additional therapies should be administered as *rapidly as possible* after the lidocaine bolus of 1.5 mg/kg:

- Magnesium sulfate 2 g IV push
- 20 vials (or as many as available up to 20) of Fab fragment antibodies

While awaiting the Fab fragment therapy to become effective, clinicians may give additional magnesium at a dose of 1 g every 1 minute for a total dose up to 5 to 10 g and repeat boluses of lidocaine 0.5 mg/kg every 8 to 10 minutes for a total loading dose not to exceed 3 mg/kg. Attempts at defibrillation should occur approximately every minute until conversion is achieved or the arrest terminated.

General Management: Digitalis Overdose

Gastric decontamination with activated charcoal should be considered in all patients with an acute digitalis overdose.[192,193] Orogastric lavage should be used in all unconscious patients and considered in those with 1 to 2 hours of overdose with a life-threatening amount of digoxin.[193] Syrup of ipecac is not useful in the hospital care of digitalis-overdose patients where other gastric emptying techniques are available.[194]

Calcium Blocker and β-Blocker Cardiotoxicity

Calcium channel blocker and β-blocker cardiotoxicity should be considered together. Calcium channel blockers have negative inotropic and chronotropic effects and pos-sess varying degrees of direct vasodilatory properties.[208] Their actions are mediated by blocking slow calcium channels. β-Blocking agents also have negative inotropic and chronotropic effects but are not direct vasodilators.[209]

Toxicity from either group of agents presents as depression of myocardial contractility, a declining heart rate, or alterations in mental status.[208,209] Patients usually have varying degrees of hypotension and sinus bradycar-dia, which may be complicated by heart block and decline in mental status ranging from lethargy to coma. Seizures may occur and are usually due to central nervous system hypoperfusion.[210,211] On occasion seizures may be the initial sign of serious toxicity.[211,212] Many patients suffer acute decompensation and go from relative stability to profound shock within minutes.[208-211] Cardiac arrests are due to refractory heart block or PEA. Hypoglycemia and hyperkalemia may be seen in β-blocker overdose, while hyperglycemia has been associated with calcium blocker overdose.[210,211]

Signs and symptoms of overdose from either group of agents are usually seen within 2 hours.[208,209] Failure to observe symptomatology within 4 to 6 hours is an indication of a minor ingestion. Unfortunately, controlled release and long-acting preparation may not exert significant toxic effects for up to 6 to 12 hours after ingestion.[208]

The optimal therapy for calcium channel and β-blocker overdoses has not been clearly defined. Variable responses have been reported with all of the available therapies.

Patients should initially be treated with oxygen, have a bedside finger stick glucose determination, and have two large-bore IV lines started. Hypotension should initially be treated by a fluid challenge of 500 to 1000 mL of normal saline.[210,211] Gastric decontamination with activated charcoal should be performed in acute overdoses.[192,193] Ipecac is contraindicated because of its delayed onset and the ability of calcium blockers and β blockers to cause rapid declines in hemodynamic stability, altered mental status, and seizures.[194] Whole bowel irrigation should be considered when large quantities of time-released medications have been consumed.[193]

Specific Calcium Blocker Overdose Therapy

Calcium appears to be the next best therapy for calcium blocker overdose patients who are unresponsive to saline.[208,210,212,213] The dose of calcium chloride is 1 to 4 g in adults, which should be titrated to hemodynamic effect.[212] Maximal effects are not achieved until the serum calcium level is elevated by 1 to 2 mg/dL.[212] Adult patients should initially receive 5 to 10 mL of calcium chloride. Initial doses are to be titrated to effect, but no more than 2 to 4 g of calcium chloride should be used during the acute phase of the patient's resuscitation.[210,212] Epinephrine and other α_1 agonists may sensitize the vasculature to calcium's effects.[212] Patients who were initially refractory to calcium should receive an additional 10 mL of calcium chloride after epinephrine has been administered.

Atropine may be tried in bradycardias due to calcium channel blocker overdose but is unlikely to be successful.[208,210,212] Patients with calcium-unresponsive bradycardia are best treated with pacing; patients with hypotension are best treated with a carefully titrated epinephrine infusion beginning with a dose of 2 µg/min. Hypotensive patients who do not respond to epinephrine should also begin receiving a titrated infusion of dopamine. Transcutaneous or transvenous pacemakers should be considered. If necessary, other agents should be used to supplement the effects of epinephrine and

dopamine. Dobutamine, norepinephrine, and/or isoproterenol should also be tried in refractory patients.[210,212] Glucagon has also been reported to be effective in some cases of calcium blocker overdose.[212,214] 4-Aminopyridine is used in Europe to treat calcium blocker overdose and is presently being evaluated for use in the United States.[212]

In summary, symptomatic calcium blocker overdoses should be treated with

- Oxygen
- Normal saline boluses 500 to 1000 mL
- Calcium chloride 5 to 10 mL IV
- Epinephrine infusion 2 to 100 µg/min or a combination of epinephrine and dopamine
- Repeat calcium administration
- Glucagon 1 to 5 mg IV
- Additional pressor agents: dobutamine, norepinephrine, and/or isoproterenol
- Consider pacing (either transvenous or transcutaneous)

Specific Therapies in β-Blocker Overdose

Patients with β-blocker cardiotoxicity who do not respond to saline infusions should probably next be treated with glucagon.[211] Glucagon directly stimulates cyclic AMP in cardiac tissue via non-α, non-β receptors.[211,215] The dose of glucagon is 1 to 5 mg in adults (0.015 to 0.1 mg/kg in children). Glucagon's major side effects are vomiting and, occasionally, hyperglycemia.[215]

Epinephrine has been used successfully in β-blocker overdoses.[211] Clinicians may choose to use it before, after, or in conjunction with glucagon. Infusions should be begun at approximately 2 µg/min and titrated to effect. Patients who do not respond to epinephrine should also begin receiving a titrated infusion of dopamine. Significant improvement with the potent β agonist isoproterenol is uncommon, and it should not be used as a first-line agent.[211] Isoproterenol may be carefully used in conjunction with an epinephrine infusion or used in combination with other agents.[215,216] Calcium chloride should also be tried in refractory patients.[217] Isoproterenol, dobutamine, and/or norepinephrine should be administered to patients who do not regain hemodynamic stability with epinephrine. Atropine is rarely effective in β-blocker–induced bradycardia or in reversing symptomatic heart block.[211]

In summary, symptomatic β-blocker overdoses should be treated with

- Oxygen
- Normal saline boluses 500 to 1000 mL
- Pacing (either transcutaneous or transvenous)
- Glucagon 1 to 5 mg IV
- Epinephrine infusion 2 to 100 µg/min or a combination of epinephrine and dopamine
- Calcium chloride 5 to 20 mL IV
- Additional pressor agents: isoproterenol, dobutamine, and/or norepinephrine

Pacemaker Therapy and Cardiopulmonary Bypass for Calcium and β-Blocker Overdoses

Patients with large overdoses may not respond to pharmacologic therapy. Transvenous or transcutaneous pacing may be attempted for refractory bradycardia or heart block.[211,212] Cardiopulmonary bypass for cases of refractory shock has also met with variable success.[218]

Narcotic Overdose

Overdoses with narcotics may result in a number of cardiopulmonary emergencies. Advanced life support may be required because of hypotension, pulmonary edema, or ventricular arrhythmias due to narcotic-induced respiratory depression.[219-221] Concomitant abuse of alcohol, cocaine, or other drugs of abuse increases the likelihood of cardiac complications.[219]

High doses of narcotics result in depression of the central nervous system with resultant hypoventilation, myocardial depression, vasodilation, and bradycardia.[219,220] Coma in association with hypotension, pinpoint pupils, or needle tracks on the skin is highly suggestive of narcotic abuse.[222] Pulmonary edema is a very common complication of intravenous narcotic abuse. It may be caused by adulterants, hypersensitivity, or neurogenic mechanisms or be the result of anoxia.[219] Hypothermia or seizures may also be seen.

The initial treatment for narcotic overdoses with cardiopulmonary compromise is as follows:

- Secure the airway and provide high-flow oxygen.
- Administer IV naloxone, a narcotic antagonist, beginning with a dose of 2 mg. Pediatric patients should initially receive 0.01 to 0.03 mg/kg.[219,223]
- Give adult nonresponders up to 10 mg IV over a short period of time. Increase the next pediatric dose to approximately 0.1 mg/kg.[219,223]
- Treat refractory patients in accordance with standard ACLS protocols.

Naloxone may precipitate narcotic withdrawal.[223,224] Suction should be available if the patient begins to vomit. For known narcotic abusers not in cardiac arrest, a lower starting dose of naloxone may be chosen to decrease the risk of agitation on arousal and to decrease the risk of patient violence.[219] The effective half-life of naloxone is patient-dependent and ranges from 15 to 45 minutes.[224] A continuous naloxone infusion may be required for patients who have overdosed on long-acting narcotic preparations such as methadone.[224,225] A mixture of 8 mg of naloxone in 1000 mL of D_5W should be started at 100 mL/h (0.8 mg/h) and titrated to effect.[224]

Intravenous drug abusers are at very high risk for being HIV positive.[219] It is imperative that blood and body fluid precautions be strictly followed.

Malnourished patients are at increased risk for protein, calorie, vitamin, and mineral deficiencies. All unconscious patients should have an immediate bedside finger stick glucose analysis. Hypoglycemia should be treated with hypertonic glucose (50 mL of $D_{50}W$ for adults, 2 mL/kg of $D_{25}W$ for children). Thiamine 100 mg IV should be administered to all cachectic and malnourished patients to avoid precipitating Wernicke's syndrome.[226]

Summary

Potentially cardiotoxic overdoses and their treatments are summarized in Table 10.

Table 10. Potentially Cardiotoxic Overdoses and Their Treatments

Toxin	Specific Antidote	Adjunctive Therapy
Benzodiazepine	Flumazenil	Airway support
β Blocker	...	Saline, epinephrine, glucagon
Calcium channel blocker	Calcium	Saline, epinephrine, glucagon
Carbon monoxide	Oxygen	Hyperbaric oxygen
Cocaine	...	Benzodiazepine, labetalol
Cyclic antidepressant	...	Bicarbonate, saline
Digitalis	Fab fragment antibodies	...
Ethanol	...	Supportive care
Isoniazid (INH)	Pyridoxine	Diazepam
Organophosphate	Atropine	Protopam sulfate
Narcotic	Naloxone	...

References

1. *1993 Heart and Stroke Facts Statistics.* Dallas, Tex: American Heart Association; 1992.
2. Fisher CM. Intermittent cerebral ischemia. In: Wright JS, Millikan CH, eds. *Vascular Diseases, Transactions of the Second Princeton Conference.* New York, NY: Grune & Stratton Inc; 1958:81-97.
3. Barnett HJ. The pathophysiology of transient cerebral ischemic attacks. *Med Clin North Am.* 1979;63:649-679.
4. Whisnant JP. A population study of stroke and TIA in Rochester, Minnesota. In: Gillingham FJ, Mawdsley C, Williams AE, eds. *Stroke.* Edinburgh, Scotland: Churchill Livingstone Inc; 1976:21-39.
5. Putman SF, Adams HP Jr. Usefulness of heparin in initial management of patients with recent transient ischemic attacks. *Arch Neurol.* 1985;42:960-962.
6. Sandok BA, Furlan AJ, Whisnant JP, Sundt TM Jr. Guidelines for the management of transient ischemic attacks. *Mayo Clin Proc.* 1978;53:665-674.
7. European Carotid Surgery Trialists' Collaborative Group. MRC European Carotid Surgery Trial: interim results for symptomatic patients with severe (70-99%) or with mild (0-29%) carotid stenosis. *Lancet.* 1991;337:1235-1243.
8. North American Symptomatic Carotid Endarterectomy Trial Collaborators. Beneficial effect of carotid endarterectomy in symptomatic patients with high-grade carotid stenosis. *N Engl J Med.* 1991;325:445-453.
9. Antiplatelet Trialists' Collaboration. Secondary prevention of vascular disease by prolonged antiplatelet treatment. *BMJ.* 1988;296:320-331.
10. The Dutch TIA Trial Study Group. A comparison of two doses of aspirin (30 mg vs 283 mg a day) in patients after a transient ischemic attack or minor ischemic stroke. *N Engl J Med.* 1991;325:1261-1266.
11. Barnett HJ. Aspirin in stroke prevention: an overview. *Stroke.* 1990;21(suppl 12):IV-40-IV-43.
12. Hass WK, Easton JD, Adams HP Jr, Pryse-Phillips W, Molony BA, Anderson S, Kamm B. Ticlopidine Aspirin Stroke Study Group. A randomized trial comparing ticlopidine hydrochloride with aspirin for the prevention of stroke in high-risk patients. *N Engl J Med.* 1989;321:501-507.

13. Stroke Prevention in Atrial Fibrillation Study Group Investigators. Preliminary report of the Stroke Prevention in Atrial Fibrillation Study. *N Engl J Med*. 1990;322:863-868.

14. The Boston Area Anticoagulation Trial for Atrial Fibrillation Investigators. The effect of low-dose warfarin on the risk of stroke in patients with nonrheumatic atrial fibrillation. *N Engl J Med*. 1990; 323:1505-1511.

15. Petersen P, Boysen G, Godtfredsen J, Andersen ED, Andersen B. Placebo-controlled, randomised trial of warfarin and aspirin for prevention of thromboembolic complications in chronic atrial fibrillation: the Copenhagen AFASAK study. *Lancet*. 1989;1:175-179.

16. Baker HL Jr, Campbell JK, Houser OW, Reese DF, Sheedy PF, Holman CB. Computer assisted tomography of the head: an early evaluation. *Mayo Clin Proc*. 1974;49:17-27.

17. Biller J, Bruno A, Adams HP Jr, Godersky JC, Loftus CM, Mitchell VL, Banwart KJ, Jones MP. A randomized trial of aspirin or heparin in hospitalized patients with recent transient ischemic attacks: a pilot study. *Stroke*. 1989;20:441-447.

18. Waga S, Otsubo K, Handa H. Warning signs in intracranial aneurysms. *Surg Neurol*. 1975;3:15-20.

19. Hauerberg J, Andersen BB, Eskesen V, Rosenörn J, Schmidt K. Importance of the recognition of a warning leak as a sign of a ruptured intracranial aneurysm. *Acta Neurol Scand*. 1991;83:61-64.

20. Kassell NF, Kongable GL, Torner JC, Adams HP Jr, Mazuz H. Delay in referral of patients with ruptured aneurysms to neurosurgical attention. *Stroke*. 1985;16:587-590.

21. Ferro JM, Lopes J, Melo TP, et al. Investigation into the causes of delayed diagnosis of subarachnoid hemorrhage. *Cerebrovasc Dis*. 1991;1:160-164.

22. Adams HP Jr, Jergenson DD, Kassell NF, Sahs AL. Pitfalls in the recognition of subarachnoid hemorrhage. *JAMA*. 1980;244:794-796.

23. Barsan WG, Brott TG, Olinger CP, Marler JR. Early treatment for acute ischemic stroke. *Ann Intern Med*. 1989;111:449-451.

24. Hijdra A, Vermeulen M, van Gijn J, van Crevel H. Respiratory arrest in subarachnoid hemorrhage. *Neurology*. 1984;34:1501-1503.

25. Stober T, Kunze K. Electrocardiographic alterations in subarachnoid hemorrhage: correlation between spasm of the arteries of the left side on the brain and T inversion and QT prolongation. *J Neurol*. 1982;227:99-113.

26. Harries AD. Subarachnoid haemorrhage and the electrocardiogram: a review. *Postgrad Med J*. 1981;57:294-296.

27. Oppenheimer SM, Cechetto DF, Hachinski VC. Cerebrogenic cardiac arrhythmias: cerebral electrocardiographic influences and their role in sudden death. *Arch Neurol*. 1990;47:513-519.

28. Estañol Vidal B, Badui Dergal E, Cesarman E, Marin San Martin O, Loyo M, Vargas Lugo B, Pérez Ortega R. Cardiac arrhythmias associated with subarachnoid hemorrhage: prospective study. *Neurosurgery*. 1979;5:675-680.

29. Di Pasquale G, Pinelli G, Andreoli A, Manini G, Grazi P, Tognetti F. Holter detection of cardiac arrhythmias in intracranial subarachnoid hemorrhage. *Am J Cardiol*. 1987;59:596-600.

30. Teasdale G, Jennett B. Assessment of coma and impaired consciousness: a practical scale. *Lancet*. 1974;2:81-84.

31. Plum F, Posner JB. *The Diagnosis of Stupor and Coma*. 3rd ed. Philadelphia, Pa: FA Davis Co; 1980:313-328.

32. Keane JR. Retinal hemorrhages: its significance in 100 patients with acute encephalopathy of unknown cause. *Arch Neurol*. 1979;36:691-694.

33. Wallis WE, Donaldson I, Scott RS, Wilson J. Hypoglycemia masquerading as cerebrovascular disease (hypoglycemic hemiplegia). *Ann Neurol*. 1985;18:510-512.

34. Hart RG, Byer JA, Slaughter JR, Hewett JE, Easton JD. Occurrence and implications of seizures in subarachnoid hemorrhage due to ruptured intracranial aneurysms. *Neurosurgery*. 1981;8:417-421.

35. Mohr JP, Caplan LR, Melski JW, Goldstein RJ, Duncan GW, Kistler JP, Pessin MS, Bleich HL. The Harvard Cooperative Stroke Registry: a prospective registry. *Neurology*. 1978;28:754-762.

36. Adams HP Jr, Kassell NF, Torner JC, Sahs AL. CT and clinical correlations in recent aneurysmal subarachnoid hemorrhage: a preliminary report of the Cooperative Aneurysm Study. *Neurology*. 1983;33:981-988.

37. Scott WR, New PF, Davis KR, Schnur JA. Computerized axial tomography of intracerebral and intraventricular hemorrhage. *Radiology*. 1974;112:73-80.

38. Lukin RR, Chambers AA, Tomsick TA. Cerebral vascular lesions: infarction, hemorrhage, aneurysm, and arteriovenous malformation. *Semin Roentgenol*. 1977;12:77-89.

39. Davis KR, Ackerman RH, Kistler JP, Mohr JP. Computed tomography of cerebral infarction: hemorrhagic, contrast enhancement, and time of appearance. *Comput Tomogr*. 1977;1:71-86.

40. Davis KR, New PF, Ojemann RG, Crowell RM, Morawetz RB, Roberson GH. Computed tomographic evaluation of hemorrhage secondary to intracranial aneurysm. *Am J Roentgenol*. 1976;127:143-153.

41. Vermeulen M, van Gijn J. The diagnosis of subarachnoid haemorrhage. *J Neurol Neurosurg Psychiatry*. 1990;53:365-372.

42. Pulsinelli WA, Waldman S, Rawlinson D, Plum F. Moderate hyperglycemia augments ischemic brain damage: a neuropathologic study in the rat. *Neurology*. 1982;32:1239-1246.

43. Candelise L, Landi G, Orazio EN, Boccardi E. Prognostic significance of hyperglycemia in acute stroke. *Arch Neurol*. 1985;42:661-663.

44. Broderick J, Brott T, Barsan W, et al. Blood pressure during the first hours of acute focal cerebral ischemia. *Neurology*. 1990;40 (suppl 1):145.

45. Delgado-Escueta AV, Wasterlain C, Treiman DM, Porter RJ. Current concepts in neurology: management of status epilepticus. *N Engl J Med*. 1982;306:1337-1340.

46. Norris JW, Hachinski VC. Megadose steroid therapy in ischemic stroke. *Stroke*. 1985;16:150. Abstract.

47. Marshall LF, Smith RW, Rauscher LA, Shapiro HM. Mannitol dose requirements in brain-injured patients. *J Neurosurg*. 1978;48:169-172.

48. Marsh EE III, Adams HP Jr, Biller J, Wasek P, Banwart K, Mitchell V, Woolson R. Use of antithrombotic drugs in the treatment of acute ischemic stroke: a survey of neurologists in practice in the United States. *Neurology*. 1989;39:1631-1634.

49. Gilles Geraud AB. Is anticoagulant therapy too frequently used in ischemic stroke? *Cerebrovasc Dis*. 1991;1(suppl 1):120-123.

50. Gordon DL, Linhardt R, Adams HP Jr. Low-molecular-weight heparins and heparinoids and their use in acute or progressing ischemic stroke. *Clin Neuropharmacol*. 1990;13:522-543.

51. del Zoppo GJ, Ferbert A, Otis S, Brückmann H, Hacke W, Zyroff J, Harker LA, Zeumer H. Local intra-arterial fibrinolytic therapy in acute carotid territory stroke: a pilot study. *Stroke*. 1988;19:307-313.

52. Brott T, Haley C, Levy D, Barsan W, Sheppard G, Broderick J, Reed R, Marler J. Safety and potential efficacy of tissue plasminogen activator (tPA) for stroke. *Stroke*. 1990;21:181. Abstract.

53. Okada Y, Sadoshima S, Nakane H, Utsunomiya H, Fujishima M. Early computed tomographic findings for thrombolytic therapy in patients with acute brain embolism. *Stroke*. 1992;23:20-23.

54. Kassell NF, Torner JC, Haley EC Jr, Jane JA, Adams HP, Kongable GL. The International Cooperative Study on the Timing of Aneurysm Surgery, I: overall management results. *J Neurosurg*. 1990;73:18-36.

55. Kassell NF, Torner JC, Jane JA, Haley EC Jr, Adams HP. The International Cooperative Study on the Timing of Aneurysm Surgery, II: surgical results. *J Neurosurg*. 1990;73:37-47.

56. Auer LM. Acute operation and preventive nimodipine improve outcome in patients with ruptured cerebral aneurysms. *Neurosurgery*. 1984;15:57-66.

57. Sundt TM Jr, Kobayashi S, Fode NC, Whisnant JP. Results and complications of surgical management of 809 intracranial aneurysms in 722 cases: related and unrelated to grade of patient, type of aneurysm, and timing of surgery. *J Neurosurg*. 1982;56:753-765.

58. Ojemann RG, Mohr JP. Hypertensive brain hemorrhage. *Clin Neurosurg*. 1976;23:220-244.

59. Petruk KC, West M, Mohr G, Weir BK, Benoit BG, Gentili F, Disney LB, Khan MI, Grace M, Holness RO, et al. Nimodipine treatment in poor-grade aneurysm patients: results of a multicenter double-blind placebo-controlled trial. *J Neurosurg*. 1988;68:505-517.

60. Pickard JD, Murray GD, Illingworth R, Shaw MD, Teasdale GM, Foy PM, Humphrey PR, Lang DA, Nelson R, Richards P, et al. Effect of oral nimodipine on cerebral infarction and outcome after subarachnoid haemorrhage: British aneurysm nimodipine trial. *BMJ*. 1989;298:636-642.

61. Wijdicks EF, Vermeulen M, van Gijn J. Hyponatraemia and volume status in aneurysmal subarachnoid haemorrhage. *Acta Neurochir Suppl (Wien)*. 1990;47:111-113.

62. Wijdicks EF, Vermeulen M, ten Haaf JA, Hijdra A, Bakker WH, van Gijn J. Volume depletion and natriuresis in patients with a ruptured intracranial aneurysm. *Ann Neurol*. 1985;18:211-216.

63. Schneider SM. Hypothermia: from recognition to rewarming. *Emerg Med Rep*. 1992;13:1-20.

64. Steinman AM. Cardiopulmonary resuscitation and hypothermia. *Circulation*. 1986;74(suppl 4):IV-29-IV-32.

65. Zell SC, Kurtz KJ. Severe exposure hypothermia: a resuscitation protocol. *Ann Emerg Med*. 1985;14:339-345.

66. Weinberg AD, Hamlet MP, Paturas JL, White RD, McAninch GW. *Cold Weather Emergencies: Principles of Patient Management*. Branford, Conn: American Medical Publishing Co; 1990:10-30.

67. Romet TT. Mechanism of afterdrop after cold water immersion. *J Appl Physiol*. 1988;65:1535-1538.

68. Reuler JB. Hypothermia: pathophysiology, clinical settings, and management. *Ann Intern Med*. 1978;89:519-527.

69. Hall KN, Syverud SA. Closed thoracic cavity lavage in the treatment of severe hypothermia in human beings. *Ann Emerg Med*. 1990;19:204-206.

70. Elenbaas RM, Mattson K, Cole H, Steele M, Ryan J, Robinson W. Bretylium in hypothermia-induced ventricular fibrillation in dogs. *Ann Emerg Med*. 1984;13:994-999.

71. Buckley JJ, Bosch OK, Bacaner MB. Prevention of ventricular fibrillation during hypothermia with bretylium tosylate. *Anesth Analg*. 1971;50:587-593.

72. Althaus U, Aeberhard P, Schüpbach P, Nachbur BH, Mühlemann W. Management of profound accidental hypothermia with cardiorespiratory arrest. *Ann Surg*. 1982;195:492-495.

73. Kristensen G, Drenck NE, Jordening H. A simple system for central rewarming of hypothermic patients. *Lancet*. 1986;2:1467-1468. Letter.

74. Moss J. Accidental severe hypothermia. *Surg Gynecol Obstet*. 1986;162:501-513.

75. Southwick FS, Dalglish PH Jr. Recovery after prolonged asystolic cardiac arrest in profound hypothermia: a case report and literature review. *JAMA*. 1980;243:1250-1253.

76. Woodhouse P, Keatinge WR, Coleshaw SR. Factors associated with hypothermia in patients admitted to a group of inner city hospitals. *Lancet*. 1989;2:1201-1205.

77. Danzl DF, Pozos RS, Auerbach PS, Glazer S, Goetz W, Johnson E, Jui J, Lilja P, Marx JA, Miller J, et al. Multicenter hypothermia survey. *Ann Emerg Med*. 1987;16:1042-1055.

78. Gallaher MM, Fleming DW, Berger LR, Sewell CM. Pedestrian and hypothermia deaths among Native Americans in New Mexico: between bar and home. *JAMA*. 1992;267:1345-1348.

79. Heimlich HJ. Subdiaphragmatic pressure to expel water from the lungs of drowning persons. *Ann Emerg Med*. 1981;10:476-480.

80. Quan L, Wentz KR, Gore EJ, Copass MK. Outcome and predictors of outcome in pediatric submersion victims receiving prehospital care in King County, Washington. *Pediatrics*. 1990;86:586-593.

81. Modell JH, Davis JH. Electrolyte changes in human drowning victims. *Anesthesiology*. 1969;30:414-420.

82. Modell JH, Davis JH. Is the Heimlich maneuver appropriate as first treatment for drowning? *Emerg Med Serv*. 1981;10:63-66.

83. Patrick EA. A case report: the Heimlich maneuver. *Emergency*. 1981;13:45-47.

84. Heimlich HJ. The Heimlich maneuver: first treatment for drowning victims. *Emerg Med Serv*. 1981;10:58-61.

85. Siebke H, Rod T, Breivik H, Link B. Survival after 40 minutes: submersion without cerebral sequelae. *Lancet*. 1975;1:1275-1277.

86. Bolte RG, Black PG, Bowers RS, Thorne JK, Corneli HM. The use of extracorporeal rewarming in a child submerged for 66 minutes. *JAMA*. 1988;260:377-379.

87. Bierens JJ, van der Velde EA, van Berkel M, van Zanten JJ. Submersion cases in The Netherlands. *Ann Emerg Med*. 1989;18:366-373.

88. Bierens JJ, van der Velde EA, van Berkel M, van Zanten JJ. Submersion in The Netherlands: prognostic indicators and results of resuscitation. *Ann Emerg Med*. 1990;19:1390-1395.

89. Pepe PE, Copass MK. Prehospital care. In: Moore EE, Ducker TB. American College of Surgeons, Committee on Trauma, eds. *Early Care of the Injured Patient*. 4th ed. Philadelphia, Pa: BC Decker Inc; 1990:34-55.

90. Copass MK, Oreskovich MR, Bladergroen MR, Carrico CJ. Prehospital cardiopulmonary resuscitation of the critically injured patient. *Am J Surg*. 1984;148:20-26.

91. Durham LA III, Richardson RJ, Wall MJ Jr, Pepe PE, Mattox KL. Emergency center thoracotomy: impact of prehospital resuscitation. *J Trauma*. 1992;32:775-779.

92. Lorenz HP, Steinmetz B, Lieberman J, Schecoter WP, Macho JR. Emergency thoracotomy: survival correlates with physiologic status. *J Trauma*. 1992;32:780-788.

93. Daya MR, Mariani RJ, Dick T. Prehospital splinting. In: Roberts JR, Hedges JR, eds. *Clinical Procedures in Emergency Medicine*. Philadelphia, Pa: WB Saunders Co; 1991:716-743.

94. O'Gorman M, Trabulsy P, Pilcher DB. Zero-time prehospital IV. *J Trauma*. 1989;29:84-86.

95. Wright RK, Davis JH. The investigation of electrical deaths: a report of 220 fatalities. *J Forensic Sci*. 1980;25:514-521.

96. Cooper MA. Electrical and lightning injuries. *Emerg Med Clin North Am*. 1984;2:489-501.

97. Kobernick M. Electrical injuries: pathophysiology and emergency management. *Ann Emerg Med*. 1982;11:633-638.

98. Budnick LD. Bathtub-related electrocutions in the United States, 1979 to 1982. *JAMA*. 1984;252:918-920.

99. Wallace JF. Electrical injuries. In: Wilson JD, Braunwald E, Isselbacher KJ, Petersdorf RG, et al, eds. *Harrison's Principles of Internal Medicine*. 12th ed. New York, NY: McGraw-Hill Book Co, Health Professions Division; 1991:2202-2204.

100. Geddes LA, Bourland JD, Ford G. The mechanism underlying sudden death from electric shock. *Med Instrum*. 1986;20:303-315.

101. Thompson JC, Ashwal S. Electrical injuries in children. *Am J Dis Child*. 1983;137:231-235.

102. Chandra NC, Siu CO, Munster AM. Clinical predictors of myocardial damage after high voltage electrical injury. *Crit Care Med*. 1990;18:293-297.

103. Ku CS, Lin SL, Hsu TL, Wang SP, Chang MS. Myocardial damage associated with electrical injury. *Am Heart J*. 1989;118:621-624.

104. Xenopoulos N, Movahed A, Hudson P, Reeves WC. Myocardial injury in electrocution. *Am Heart J*. 1991;122:1481-1484.

105. Homma S, Gillam LD, Weyman AE. Echocardiographic observations in survivors of acute electrical injury. *Chest*. 1990;97:103-105.

106. Browne BJ, Gaasch WR. Electrical injuries and lightning. *Emerg Med Clin North Am*. 1992;10:211-229.

107. Jensen PJ, Thomsen PE, Bagger JP, Nørgaard A, Baandrup U. Electrical injury causing ventricular arrhythmias. *Br Heart J*. 1987;57:279-283.

108. Cooper MA, Johnson K. Electrical injuries. In: Rosen P, Barkin RM, Braen CR, et al, eds. *Emergency Medicine — Concepts and Clinical Practice*. 3rd ed. St Louis, Mo: Mosby Year Book; 1992:969-978.

109. Epperly TD, Stewart JR. The physical effects of lightning injury. *J Fam Pract*. 1989;29:267-272.

110. Duclos PJ, Sanderson LM. An epidemiological description of lightning-related deaths in the United States. *Int J Epidemiol*. 1990;19:673-679.

111. Cooper MA. Lightning injuries: prognostic signs for death. *Ann Emerg Med*. 1980;9:134-138.

112. Moran KT, Thupari JN, Munster AM. Lightning injury: physics, pathophysiology and clinical features. *Ir Med J*. 1986;79:120-122.

113. Cwinn AA, Cantrill SV. Lightning injuries. *J Emerg Med*. 1984;2:379-388.

114. Cooper MA. Lightning injuries. In: Rosen P, Barkin RM, Braen CR, et al, eds. *Emergency Medicine — Concepts and Clinical Practice*. 3rd ed. St Louis, Mo: Mosby Year Book; 1992:979-985.

115. Kleiner JP, Wilkin JH. Cardiac effects of lightning stroke. *JAMA*. 1978;240:2757-2759.

116. Lehman LB. Successful management of an adult lightning victim using intracranial pressure monitoring. *Neurosurgery*. 1991;28:907-910.

117. Frayne JH, Gilligan BS. Neurological sequelae of lightning stroke. *Clin Exp Neurol*. 1987;24:195-200.

118. Cherington M, Yarnell P, Lammereste D. Lightning strikes: nature of neurological damage in patients evaluated in hospital emergency departments. *Ann Emerg Med*. 1992;21:575-578.

119. Lee W, Cotton DB. Cardiorespiratory changes during pregnancy. In: Clark SL, Cotton DB, Hankins GDV, Phelan JP, eds. *Critical Care Obstetrics*. 2nd ed. Boston, Mass: Blackwell Scientific Publications Inc: 1991:2-34.

120. Clark SL, Cotton DB, Lee W, Bishop C, Hill T, Southwick J, Pivarnik J, Spillman T, DeVore GR, Phelan J, et al. Central hemodynamic assessment of normal term pregnancy. *Am J Obstet Gynecol*. 1989;161:1439-1442.

121. Kerr MG. The mechanical effects of the gravid uterus in late pregnancy. *J Obstet Gynaec Brit Comm*. 1965;72:513-529.

122. Satin AJ, Hankins GDV. Cardiopulmonary resuscitation in pregnancy. In: Clark SL, Cotton DB, Hankins GDV, Phelan JP, eds. *Critical Care Obstetrics*. 2nd ed. Boston, Mass: Blackwell Scientific Publications Inc; 1991:579.

123. Rees GA, Willis BA. Resuscitation in late pregnancy. *Anaesthesia*. 1988;43:347-349.

124. Goodwin AP, Pearce AJ. The human wedge: a manoeuvre to relieve aortocaval compression during resuscitation in late pregnancy. *Anaesthesia*. 1992;47:433-434.

125. Katz VL, Dotters DJ, Droegemueller W. Perimortem cesarean delivery. *Obstet Gynecol*. 1986;68:571-576.

126. Strong TH Jr, Lowe RA. Perimortem cesarean section. *Am J Emerg Med*. 1989;7:489-494.

127. Lopez-Zeno JA, Carlo WA, O'Grady JP, Fanaroff AA. Infant survival following delayed postmortem cesarean delivery. *Obstet Gynecol*. 1990;76:991-992.

128. Cregler LL, Mark H. Medical complications of cocaine abuse. *N Engl J Med*. 1986;315:1495-1500.

129. Jekel JF, Allen DF, Podlewski H, Clark N, Dean-Patterson S, Cartwright P. Epidemic free-base cocaine abuse: case study from the Bahamas. *Lancet*. 1986;1:459-462.

130. Mody CK, Miller BL, McIntyre HB, Cobb SK, Goldberg MA. Neurologic complications of cocaine abuse. *Neurology*. 1988;38:1189-1193.

131. Lowenstein DH, Massa SM, Rowbotham MC, Collins SD, McKinney HE, Simon RP. Acute neurologic and psychiatric complications associated with cocaine abuse. *Am J Med*. 1987;83:841-846.

132. Farrar HC, Kearns GL. Cocaine: clinical pharmacology and toxicology. *J Pediatr*. 1989;115:665-675.

133. Roth D, Alarcón FJ, Fernandez JA, Preston RA, Bourgoignie JJ. Acute rhabdomyolysis associated with cocaine intoxication. *N Engl J Med*. 1988;319:673-677.

134. Amin M, Gabelman G, Karpel J, Buttrick P. Acute myocardial infarction and chest pain syndromes after cocaine use. *Am J Cardiol*. 1990;66:1434-1437.

135. Barth CW III, Bray M, Roberts WC. Rupture of the ascending aorta during cocaine intoxication. *Am J Cardiol*. 1986;57:496.

136. Allred RJ, Ewer S. Fatal pulmonary edema following intravenous "freebase" cocaine use. *Ann Emerg Med*. 1981;10:441-442.

137. Gradman AH. Cardiac effects of cocaine: a review. *Yale J Biol Med*. 1988;61:137-147.

138. Goldfrank LR, Hoffman RS. The cardiovascular effects of cocaine. *Ann Emerg Med*. 1991;20:165-175.

139. Kloner RA, Hale S, Alker K, Rezkalla S. The effects of acute and chronic cocaine use on the heart. *Circulation*. 1992;85;407-419.

140. Catravas JD, Waters IW. Acute cocaine intoxication in the conscious dog: studies on the mechanism of lethality. *J Pharmacol Exp Ther*. 1981;217:350-356.

141. Billman GE. Mechanisms responsible for the cardiotoxic effects of cocaine. *FASEB J*. 1990;4:2469-2475.

142. Wilkerson RD. Cardiovascular effects of cocaine in conscious dogs: importance of fully functional autonomic and central nervous systems. *J Pharmacol Exp Ther*. 1988;246:466-471.

143. Lange RA, Cigarroa RG, Yancy CW Jr, Willard JE, Popma JJ, Sills MN, McBride W, Kim AS, Hillis LD. Cocaine-induced coronary-artery vasoconstriction. *N Engl J Med*. 1989;321:1557-1562.

144. Lange RA, Cigarroa RG, Flores ED, McBride W, Kim AS, Wells PJ, Bedotto JB, Danziger RS, Hillis LD. Potentiation of cocaine-induced coronary vasoconstriction by beta-adrenergic blockade. *Ann Intern Med*. 1990;112:897-903.

145. Brody SL, Slovis CM, Wrenn KD. Cocaine-related medical problems: consecutive series of 233 patients. *Am J Med*. 1990;88:325-331.

146. Derlet RW, Albertson TE. Emergency department presentation of cocaine intoxication. *Ann Emerg Med*. 1989;18:182-186.

147. Rich JA, Singer DE. Cocaine-related symptoms in patients presenting to an urban emergency department. *Ann Emerg Med*. 1991;20:616-621.

148. Jonsson S, O'Meara M, Young JB. Acute cocaine poisoning: importance of treating seizures and acidosis. *Am J Med*. 1983;75:1061-1064.

149. Gay GR. Clinical management of acute and chronic cocaine poisoning. *Ann Emerg Med*. 1982;11:562-572.

150. Silverstein W, Lewin NA, Goldfrank L. Management of the cocaine-intoxicated patient. *Ann Emerg Med*. 1987;16:234-235. Letter.

151. Isner JM, Estes NA III, Thompson PD, Costanzo-Nordin MR, Subramanian R, Miller G, Katsas G, Sweeney K, Sturner WQ. Acute cardiac events temporally related to cocaine abuse. *N Engl J Med*. 1986;315:1438-1443.

152. Derlet RW, Albertson TE, Tharratt RS. Lidocaine potentiation of cocaine toxicity. *Ann Emerg Med*. 1991;20:135-138.

153. Ramoska E, Sacchetti AD. Propranolol-induced hypertension in treatment of cocaine intoxication. *Ann Emerg Med*. 1985;14:1112-1113.

154. Robin ED, Wong RJ, Ptashne KA. Increased lung water and ascites after massive cocaine overdosage in mice and improved survival related to beta-adrenergic blockage. *Ann Intern Med*. 1989;110:202-207.

155. Gay GR, Loper KA. The use of labetalol in the management of cocaine crisis. *Ann Emerg Med*. 1988;17:282-283.

156. Sand IC, Brody SL, Wrenn KD, Slovis CM. Experience with esmolol for the treatment of cocaine-associated cardiovascular complications. *Am J Emerg Med*. 1991;9:161-163.

157. Briggs RS, Birtwell AJ, Pohl JE. Hypertensive response to labetalol in phaeochromocytoma. *Lancet*. 1978;1:1045-1046. Letter.

158. Hoffman CK, Goodman PC. Pulmonary edema in cocaine smokers. *Radiology*. 1989;172:463-465.

159. Cucco RA, Yoo OH, Cregler L, Chang JC. Nonfatal pulmonary edema after "freebase" cocaine smoking. *Am Rev Respir Dis*. 1987;136:179-181.

160. Gitter MJ, Goldsmith SR, Dunbar DN, Sharkey SW. Cocaine and chest pain: clinical features and outcome of patients hospitalized to rule out myocardial infarction. *Ann Intern Med*. 1991;115:277-282.

161. Hollander JE, Hoffman RS. Cocaine-induced myocardial infarction: an analysis and review of the literature. *J Emerg Med*. 1992;10:169-177.

162. Smith HW III, Liberman HA, Brody SL, Battey LL, Donohue BC, Morris DC. Acute myocardial infarction temporally related to cocaine use: clinical, angiographic, and pathophysiologic observations. *Ann Intern Med*. 1987;107:13-18.

163. Minor RL Jr, Scott BD, Brown DD, Winniford MD. Cocaine-induced myocardial infarction in patients with normal coronary arteries. *Ann Intern Med*. 1991;115:797-806.

164. Brogan WC III, Lange RA, Kim AS, Moliterno DJ, Hillis LD. Alleviation of cocaine-induced coronary vasoconstriction by nitroglycerin. *J Am Coll Cardiol*. 1991;18:581-586.

165. Kimura T, Yasue H, Sakaino N, Rokutanda M, Jougasaki M, Araki H. Effects of magnesium on the tone of isolated human coronary arteries: comparison with diltiazem and nitroglycerin. *Circulation*. 1989;79:1118-1124.

166. Woods KL, Fletcher S, Roffe C, Haider Y. Intravenous magnesium sulphate in suspected acute myocardial infarction: results of the second Leicester Intravenous Magnesium Intervention Trial (LIMIT-2). *Lancet*. 1992;339:1553-1558.

167. Mayer DB, Miletich DJ, Feld JM, Albrecht RF. The effects of magnesium salts on the duration of epinephrine-induced ventricular tachyarrhythmias in anesthetized rats. *Anesthesiology*. 1989;71:923-928.

168. Callaham M, Kassel D. Epidemiology of fatal tricyclic antidepressant ingestion: implications for management. *Ann Emerg Med*. 1985;14:1-9.

169. Wedin GP, Oderda GM, Klein-Schwartz W, Gorman RL. Relative toxicity of cyclic antidepressants. *Ann Emerg Med*. 1986;15:797-804.

170. Litovitz TL, Holm KC, Bailey KM, Schmitz BF. 1991 annual report of the American Association of Poison Control Centers National Data Collection System. *Am J Emerg Med*. 1992;10:452-505.

171. Glassman AH. Cardiovascular effects of tricyclic antidepressants. *Annu Rev Med*. 1984;35:503-511.

172. Marshall JB, Forker AD. Cardiovascular effects of tricyclic antidepressant drugs: therapeutic usage, overdose, and management of complications. *Am Heart J.* 1982;103:401-414.

173. Wolfe TR, Caravati EM, Rollins DE. Terminal 40-ms frontal plane QRS axis as a marker for tricyclic antidepressant overdose. *Ann Emerg Med.* 1989;18:348-351.

174. Frommer DA, Kulig KW, Marx JA, Rumack B. Tricyclic antidepressant overdose: a review. *JAMA.* 1987;257:521-526.

175. Foulke GE, Albertson TE, Walby WF. Tricyclic antidepressant overdose: emergency department findings as predictors of clinical course. *Am J Emerg Med.* 1986;4:496-500.

176. Braden NJ, Jackson JE, Walson PD. Tricyclic antidepressant overdose. *Pediatr Clin North Am.* 1986;33:287-297.

177. Shannon M, Merola J, Lovejoy FH Jr. Hypotension in severe tricyclic antidepressant overdose. *Am J Emerg Med.* 1988;6: 439-442.

178. Sasyniuk BI, Jhamandas V, Valois M. Experimental amitriptyline intoxication: treatment of cardiac toxicity with sodium bicarbonate. *Ann Emerg Med.* 1986;15:1052-1059.

179. Hoffman JR, McElroy CR. Bicarbonate therapy for dysrhythmia and hypotension in tricyclic antidepressant overdose. *West J Med.* 1981;134:60-64.

180. Nattel S, Mittleman M. Treatment of ventricular tachyarrythmias resulting from amitriptyline toxicity in dogs. *J Pharmacol Exp Ther.* 1984;231:430-435.

181. Bessen HA, Niemann JT. Improvement of cardiac conduction after hyperventilation in tricyclic antidepressant overdose. *J Toxicol Clin Toxicol.* 1985-1986;23:537-546.

182. Liberatore MA, Robinson DS. Torsade de pointes: a mechanism for sudden death associated with neuroleptic drug therapy? *J Clin Psychopharmacol.* 1984;4:143-146.

183. Keren A, Tzivoni D, Gavish D, Levi J, Gottlieb S, Benhorin J, Stern S. Etiology, warning signs and therapy of torsade de pointes: a study of 10 patients. *Circulation.* 1981;64:1167-1174.

184. Perticone F, Adinolfi L, Bonaduce D. Efficacy of magnesium sulfate in the treatment of torsade de pointes. *Am Heart J.* 1986;112: 847-849.

185. Tzivoni D, Banai S, Schuger C, Benhorin J, Keren A, Gottlieb S, Stern S. Treatment of torsade de pointes with magnesium sulfate. *Circulation.* 1988;77:392-397.

186. Iseri LT, Chung P, Tobis J. Magnesium therapy for intractable ventricular tachyarrhythmias in normomagnesemic patients. *West J Med.* 1983;138:823-828.

187. Goldberg RJ, Capone RJ, Hunt JD. Cardiac complications following tricyclic antidepressant overdose: issues for monitoring policy. *JAMA.* 1985;254:1772-1775.

188. Hagerman GA, Hanashiro PK. Reversal of tricyclic-antidepressant-induced cardiac conduction abnormalities by phenytoin. *Ann Emerg Med.* 1981;10:82-86.

189. Mayron R, Ruiz E. Phenytoin: does it reverse tricyclic-antidepressant-induced cardiac conduction abnormalities? *Ann Emerg Med.* 1986;15:876-880.

190. Ellison DW, Pentel PR. Clinical features and consequences of seizures due to cyclic antidepressant overdose. *Am J Emerg Med.* 1989;7:5-10.

191. Vernon DD, Banner W Jr, Dean M. Dopamine and norepinephrine are equally effective for treatment of shock in amitriptyline intoxication. *Crit Care Med.* 1990;18:S239.

192. Park GD, Spector R, Goldberg MJ, Johnson GF. Expanded role of charcoal therapy in the poisoned and overdosed patient. *Arch Intern Med.* 1986;146:969-973.

193. Kulig K. Initial management of ingestions of toxic substances. *N Engl J Med.* 1992;326:1677-1681.

194. Wrenn K, Rodewald L, Dockstader L. Potential misuse of ipecac. *Ann Emerg Med.* 1993;22:1408-1412.

195. Dick M, Curwin J, Tepper D. Digitalis intoxication recognition and management. *J Clin Pharmacol.* 1991;31:444-447.

196. Antman EM, Smith TW. Digitalis toxicity. *Annu Rev Med.* 1985;36: 357-367.

197. Moorman JR, Pritchett EL. The arrhythmias of digitalis intoxication. *Arch Intern Med.* 1985;145:1289-1292.

198. Antman EM, Wenger TL, Butler VP Jr, Haber E, Smith TW. Treatment of 150 cases of life-threatening digitalis intoxication with digoxin-specific Fab antibody fragments: final report of a multicenter study. *Circulation.* 1990;81:1744-1752.

199. Martiny SS, Phelps SJ, Massey KL. Treatment of severe digitalis intoxication with digoxin-specific antibody fragments: a clinical review. *Crit Care Med.* 1988;16:629-635.

200. Ordog GJ, Benaron S, Bhasin V, Wasserberger J, Balasubramanium S. Serum digoxin levels and mortality in 5100 patients. *Ann Emerg Med.* 1987;16:32-39.

201. Sonnenblick M, Abraham AS, Meshulam Z, Eylath U. Correlation between manifestations of digoxin toxicity and serum digoxin, calcium, potassium, and magnesium concentrations and arterial pH. *BMJ.* 1983;286:1089-1091.

202. Whang R, Oei TO, Watanabe A. Frequency of hypomagnesemia in hospitalized patients receiving digitalis. *Arch Intern Med.* 1985;145:655-656.

203. Sharff JA, Bayer MJ. Acute and chronic digitalis toxicity: presentation and treatment. *Ann Emerg Med.* 1982;11:327-331.

204. Woolf AD, Wenger T, Smith TW, Lovejoy FH Jr. The use of digoxin-specific Fab fragments for severe digitalis intoxication in children. *N Engl J Med.* 1992;326:1739-1744.

205. Smith TW, Butler VP Jr, Haber E, Fozzard H, Marcus FI, Bremner WF, Schulman IC, Phillips A. Treatment of life-threatening digitalis intoxication with digoxin-specific Fab antibody fragments: experience in 26 cases. *N Engl J Med.* 1982;307:1357-1362.

206. Cohen L, Kitzes R. Magnesium sulfate and digitalis-toxic arrhythmias. *JAMA.* 1983;249:2808-2810.

207. Reisdorff EJ, Clark MR, Walters BL. Acute digitalis poisoning: the role of intravenous magnesium sulfate. *J Emerg Med.* 1986;4: 463-469.

208. Pearigen PD, Benowitz NL. Poisoning due to calcium antagonists: experience with verapamil, diltiazem and nifedipine. *Drug Saf.* 1991;6:408-430.

209. Jackson CD, Fishbein L. A toxicological review of beta-adrenergic blockers. *Fundam Appl Toxicol.* 1986;6:395-422.

210. Erickson FC, Ling LJ, Grande GA, Anderson DL. Diltiazem overdose: case report and review. *J Emerg Med.* 1991;9:357-366.

211. Weinstein RS. Recognition and management of poisoning with beta-adrenergic blocking agents. *Ann Emerg Med.* 1984;13:1123-1131.

212. Horowitz BZ, Rhee KJ. Massive verapamil ingestion: a report of two cases and a review of the literature. *Am J Emerg Med.* 1989; 7:624-631.

213. Herrington DM, Insley BM, Weinmann GG. Nifedipine overdose. *Am J Med.* 1986;81:344-346.

214. Zaritsky AL, Horowitz M, Chernow B. Glucagon antagonism of calcium channel blocker-induced myocardial dysfunction. *Crit Care Med.* 1988;16:246-251.

215. Hall-Boyer K, Zaloga GP, Chernow B. Glucagon: hormone or therapeutic agent? *Crit Care Med.* 1984;12:584-589.

216. Agusa ED, Wexler LL, Witzburg RA. Massive propranolol overdose: successful treatment with high dose isopropanenol and glucagon. *Am J Med.* 1986;180:755-757.

217. Langemeijer J, de Wildt D, de Groot G, Sangster B. Calcium interferes with the cardiodepressive effects of beta-blocker overdose in isolated rat hearts. *J Toxicol Clin Toxicol.* 1986;24:111-133.

218. Hendren WG, Schieber RS, Garrettson LK. Extracorporeal bypass for the treatment of verapamil poisoning. *Ann Emerg Med.* 1989; 18:984-987.

219. Ford M, Hoffman RS, Goldfrank LR. Opioids and designer drugs. *Emerg Med Clin North Am.* 1990;8:495-511.

220. Sternbach G, Moran J, Eliastam M. Heroin addiction: acute presentation of medical complications. *Ann Emerg Med.* 1980;9: 161-169.

221. Lusk JA, Maloley PA. Morphine-induced pulmonary edema. *Am J Med.* 1988;84:367-368. Letter.

222. Hoffman JR, Schriger DL, Luo JS. The empiric use of naloxone in patients with altered mental status: a reappraisal. *Ann Emerg Med.* 1991;20:246-252.

223. Handal KA, Schauben JL, Salamone FR. Naloxone. *Ann Emerg Med.* 1983;12:438-445.

224. Opiates antagonists. In: Ellenhorn MJ, Barceloux DG, eds. *Medical Toxicology: Diagnosis and Treatment of Human Poisoning.* New York, NY: Elsevier Science Publishing Co Inc; 1988:752-759.

225. Goldfrank L, Weisman RS, Errick JK, Lo MW. A dosing nomogram for continuous infusion intravenous naloxone. *Ann Emerg Med.* 1986;15:566-570.

226. Wrenn KD, Murphy F, Slovis CM. A toxicity study of parenteral thiamine hydrochloride. *Ann Emerg Med.* 1989;18:867-870.

Adjuncts for Artificial Circulation

Chapter 11

Cardiopulmonary resuscitation (CPR) provides blood flow to vital organs until more definitive care such as defibrillation can be provided. Cardiac output and perfusion pressures vary considerably with individual patients. Many patients, however, have very poor perfusion during CPR.[1,2] Circulatory adjuncts or changes in the technique of CPR that improve blood flow or perfusion pressures may improve resuscitation success for patients in cardiac arrest. This chapter reviews adjuncts that have been proposed to improve CPR techniques, mechanical CPR devices, invasive CPR, and aids for assessing the efficacy of CPR.

Alternative CPR Techniques

Several alterations in the technique of CPR have been proposed to improve hemodynamics. While each of these techniques has shown promise in individual studies, none has demonstrated enough consistent improvement in survival to replace the standard CPR technique.

Interposed Abdominal Compression CPR

The technique of interposed abdominal compression or counterpulsation CPR (IAC-CPR) (Fig 1) has been proposed as an alternative to standard CPR.[3-15] During IAC-CPR, a second person compresses the abdomen during the relaxation phase of chest compression. Pressure on the abdomen can be standardized to 100 mm Hg by the use of a blood pressure cuff. Pressure on the abdomen during the relaxation phase of CPR may augment the aortic diastolic pressure and improve myocardial blood flow. Experimental studies have demonstrated that IAC-CPR can improve systolic and diastolic pressures, cardiac output, and myocardial perfusion pressures compared with standard CPR.[3-7] Other laboratory studies have not shown improvement in 24-hour survival when IAC-CPR was compared with standard CPR.[15]

Human studies of IAC-CPR have shown mixed results. Two studies of in-hospital cardiac arrests demonstrated improved survival to hospital discharge for IAC-CPR compared with standard CPR.[10,11] Another clinical study found no improvement in resuscitation when IAC-CPR was compared with standard CPR for patients in cardiac arrest outside of the hospital.[8] Questions regarding the practicality and safety of IAC-CPR also must be considered. The technique requires three people, and most clinical studies have used the technique after the patient has been endotracheally intubated. The risk of abdominal injuries, hypoventilation, and aspiration if used in patients with unprotected airways must be further studied.

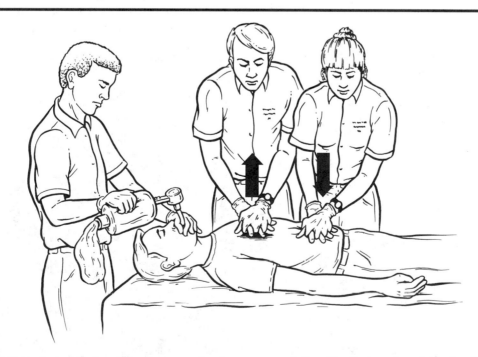

Fig 1. Interposed abdominal counterpulsation during human cardiopulmonary resuscitation. All patients undergo intubation. The abdominal compression rate is equal to the chest compression rate of 80/min to 100/min. The abdominal compression force is standardized at 100±20 mm Hg. Adapted from Sack.[10]

The technique of IAC-CPR shows promise in the treatment of patients in cardiac arrest. Further outcome studies must be done to determine its efficacy and safety. At present, IAC-CPR should be considered an experimental technique and should not be routinely used in the management of patients in cardiac arrest.

Simultaneous Ventilation-Compression CPR

The technique of simultaneous ventilation and chest compression CPR (SVC-CPR) takes advantage of the entire thorax as a pump to produce forward blood flow.[16-25] Pressure gradients are developed between intrathoracic and extrathoracic structures. Studies in experimental models demonstrated that SVC-CPR resulted in improved systolic pressures and carotid blood flows.[16-18] Based on these promising studies, a mechanical CPR device that provides simultaneous ventilation and chest compression was developed and tested in clinical studies. Survival studies demonstrated improvement when SVC-CPR was compared with standard CPR in some laboratories but not in others.[15,20,21,24,25] Clinical studies have shown standard CPR to be superior to SVC-CPR in hemodynamics and survival.[22,23,25] Therefore, SVC-CPR is not recommended for use in the resuscitation of patients in cardiac arrest.

High-Frequency ("Rapid Compression Rate") CPR

High-frequency or rapid manual CPR has been advocated as a technique for improving resuscitation from cardiac arrest.[26-30] Studies in some, but not all, laboratories have demonstrated that rapid compression rates improve cardiac output, aortic and myocardial perfusion pressures, and 24-hour survival compared with standard CPR.[26,27] Clinical studies on the use of high-frequency CPR are limited. There is evidence for improved hemodynamics using manual but not mechanical rapid chest compression rates in patients.[23,28-30] Thus, high-frequency CPR shows some promise for improving CPR technique. Outcome studies in humans are needed to determine the efficacy of this technique in the management of patients in cardiac arrest.

Mechanical Aids for CPR

Mechanical devices are available that can be used as substitutes for manual chest compression. Some also can provide ventilation that is synchronized with chest compressions. The advantages of such devices are that they can (1) standardize CPR technique, (2) eliminate rescuer fatigue, (3) free trained persons to participate in the delivery of ACLS when there is a limited number of rescuers, and (4) ensure adequacy of compression when a patient requires continued resuscitation during transportation. Mechanical CPR that is carefully and properly administered can be as effective as carefully administered manual CPR in adults.[31-34] In certain circumstances (such as during transportation or when CPR must be provided for prolonged periods), it may even be advantageous. Mechanically performed CPR should be used only for adults; its efficacy and safety have not been demonstrated in infants and children.

Cardiac Press

The simplest and least expensive adjunct is the cardiac press. This hinged, manually operated device gives the rescuer a mechanical advantage in performing chest compressions. The downstroke of the cardiac press can be adjusted to provide a stroke of 1½ to 2 inches (3.9 to 5.0 cm). It can be applied with only a brief interruption in manual CPR. Advantages include its relatively modest cost, its ease of storage, transportation, and assembly, its lightweight construction, and its simplicity, which reduces the possibility of mechanical breakdown. Problems related to its use include tendencies for the compressor head to shift position and for the tightening device to become loosened so that the plunger does not compress the chest adequately. Therefore, constant monitoring of the position of the press and the adequacy of compression is necessary.

Automatic Resuscitators

A mechanical resuscitator can provide chest compressions or ventilations during CPR. Devices currently available consist of a compressed-gas–powered plunger mounted on a backboard and a time-pressure–cycled ventilator (Fig 2). The devices are programmed to deliver standard AHA-recommended CPR in a 5:1 compression-ventilation ratio using a compression duration that is 50% of the cycle length.

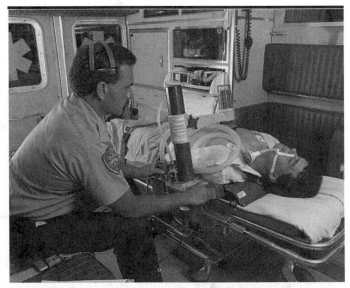

Fig 2. Compressed-gas–powered plunger and time-pressure–cycled ventilator.

This type of device does not require electrical power since it is powered by high-pressure 100% oxygen gas. The depth of plunger compression can be adjusted by the rescuer to compress the sternum 1½ to 2 inches with each cycle or 20% to 25% of the patient's anterior-posterior diameter (for patients with a large anterior-posterior diameter). When used properly, this device causes less injury to the chest wall and internal organs during patient transport (as in the back of a moving ambulance) than manually performed CPR because the patient can be "harnessed" to the device's backboard, fixing the position of the plunger on the sternum. An acceptable ECG can often be recorded with the compressor in operation, and the patient can be defibrillated or transported without interrupting CPR. Defibrillation is timed to occur during the downstroke of a chest compression when the lungs are relatively empty and chest impedance is low. This will result in more energy being delivered to the heart and, perhaps, more successful defibrillations.[35]

The principal disadvantage of the automatic resuscitator is its cost. Its disadvantage in size and weight is offset because it permits rescuers to perform other tasks and provides better access to the patient for procedures by reducing the number of rescuers at the patient's side.

One advantage often claimed for automatic resuscitators is their usefulness for prolonged periods of CPR, especially during transport of patients over long distance. However, current practice is changing in the direction of ending unsuccessful resuscitation attempts in the pre-hospital setting without continuing CPR during transport.

Pneumatic Antishock Garment

The pneumatic antishock garment (PASG) is a one-piece, double-layered fabric made into pants with inflatable bladders for each leg and the abdomen. These garments can maintain high internal pressures.[36-43] Physiologically, the PASG increases peripheral vascular resistance and mean arterial pressure while shunting blood to the upper half of the body.[37-39] Although its efficacy in improving outcome has not been demonstrated, the PASG is used primarily for patients in hypovolemic shock from traumatic injury in the lower half of the body.[42,43] Its effect in improving mean arterial pressure was thought to be useful for patients in cardiac arrest. However, studies have not demonstrated an improvement in survival or coronary perfusion pressures when PASG-CPR was compared with standard CPR.[40] In addition, injuries such as liver lacerations have been noted in animals when CPR was performed with the abdominal binder inflated.[41] In summary, the PASG is not indicated for use as an adjunct to CPR for patients in cardiac arrest.

Vest CPR

Vest CPR uses the same principles of moving blood by manipulation of intrathoracic pressure that SVC-CPR uses, but ventilation is asynchronous, and changes in intrathoracic pressure are produced by rhythmic inflation-deflation of a perithoracic pneumatic vest. Preliminary hemodynamic studies have shown that (depending on vest design) significant increases in arterial pressure occur, compared with conventional CPR. Preliminary studies of human use of vest CPR have been published.[44-46]

Active Compression-Decompression CPR (ACD-CPR)

A device for active compression and decompression of the chest during CPR has shown promise as an adjunct (Fig 3). The device applies suction to the chest during the relaxation phase of CPR. Studies in experimental models and humans have demonstrated improvement in some hemodynamic parameters when the device was compared with standard CPR.[47-49] Further outcome studies using the compression-decompression device are warranted.

Invasive CPR

Direct Cardiac Massage

Before the introduction in 1960 of closed-chest massage (ie, external compressions), direct cardiac massage

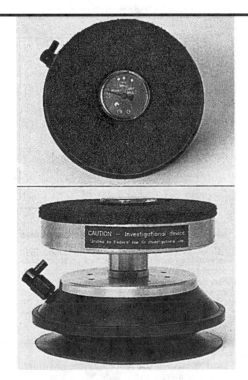

Fig 3. The active compression-decompression device consists of a corrugated suction header, bellows, and handle, with a resilient plastic compression area within the bellows. This device is placed midsternum at the level of the nipples and provides active manual compression of the chest as well as active chest expansion (decompression). Views are from above (top) and from the side (bottom). The compression phase is performed in accordance with the cardiopulmonary resuscitation guidelines of the American Heart Association.

was used frequently to treat patients with in-hospital cardiac arrest. Studies from the 1950s show survival rates ranging from 16% to 37%.[50,51] A large percentage of these arrests, however, occurred in the operating room. Following the introduction of closed-chest CPR, no studies were done comparing survival with both techniques. Closed-chest CPR seemed to be effective, was considerably less invasive, and quickly became the standard method for resuscitation.

It is now clear that properly performed direct cardiac massage provides better hemodynamics than closed-chest compression.[52-65] Cardiac index and coronary perfusion pressure often are improved by switching from closed- to open-chest CPR.[57,58] There are several case reports of patients who have been resuscitated after direct cardiac massage when attempts using closed-chest CPR had been unsuccessful.[58,66,67] Studies in animals also support the concept that survival is improved when open-chest CPR is used soon after the onset of cardiac arrest (15 minutes or less) (Fig 4).[59] When open-chest CPR is initiated after cardiac arrest has been treated with closed-chest CPR for 20 to 25 minutes or more, there is no improvement in outcome despite a significant improvement in hemodynamics.[55] In one of the few outcome studies on humans, open-chest CPR did not improve survival for patients with out-of-hospital arrest when performed 30 minutes after onset of arrest time.[68]

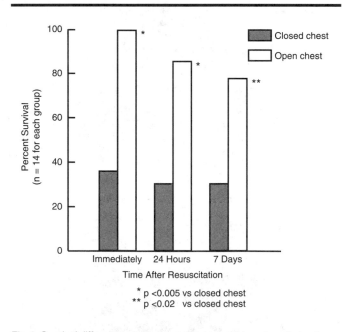

Fig 4. Survival differences between animals receiving closed-chest CPR and animals that received open-chest CPR after 12 minutes of closed-chest compressions. Immediate survival was determined at 30 minutes after resuscitation. From Kern.[59]

Few physicians today are skilled in the technique of direct cardiac massage. Since most cardiac arrests occur outside of the hospital and since most patients cannot be brought to a facility where a thoracotomy and direct cardiac massage can be performed in less than 15 minutes of total arrest time, the applicability of direct cardiac massage is limited. The risks and benefits of open-chest cardiac massage used early (within the first 15 minutes of cardiac arrest) in humans have not yet been adequately studied. Thoracotomy and direct cardiac massage cannot be recommended for the routine patient with cardiac arrest.

An exception is the victim with cardiac trauma due to penetrating chest trauma. Most studies indicate clear benefit from thoracotomy for victims of penetrating chest trauma who develop cardiac arrest.[69-72] A thoracotomy potentially allows rescuers to relieve pericardial tamponade and identify and control severe intrathoracic hemorrhage or treat concomitant abdominal hemorrhage by aortic cross-clamping.

Emergency thoracotomy is practical as a resuscitation technique in well-equipped trauma centers. A multidisciplinary team should be present to provide definitive surgical treatment in the operating room as soon as possible. If direct cardiac massage is used at all, it should be applied early. Opening the chest as a "last-ditch effort" to resuscitate a patient in cardiac arrest is of little or no value.

Although penetrating chest trauma is the only absolute indication for a thoracotomy and open-chest CPR, there are other specific instances in which open-chest CPR may be considered:

1. Cardiac arrest due to hypothermia, pulmonary embolism, pericardial tamponade, or abdominal hemorrhage
2. Chest deformity where closed-chest CPR is ineffective
3. Penetrating abdominal trauma with deterioration and cardiac arrest
4. Blunt trauma with cardiac arrest

In summary, even in properly equipped and staffed settings, open-chest direct cardiac massage is an underused technique in the treatment of patients in cardiac arrest. Prospective outcome studies are needed to determine the role of direct cardiac massage when used early in the treatment of cardiac arrest victims.

Emergency Cardiopulmonary Bypass

Cardiopulmonary bypass is an important adjunct for patients undergoing cardiac surgery. Cardiopulmonary bypass has been applied experimentally for the treatment of cardiac arrest without thoracotomy, using the femoral artery and vein for access to the circulation.[73-83] Animal models of cardiac arrest show improved hemodynamics and survival when cardiopulmonary bypass is used soon after the onset of cardiac arrest.[73-81]

Clinical studies have also demonstrated the feasibility of cardiopulmonary bypass in the treatment of selected patients in cardiac arrest.[82,83] Its implementation requires a coordinated resuscitation team. The role of cardiopulmonary bypass in the treatment of patients in cardiac arrest needs to be clearly defined by further clinical studies.

Mechanical Assist Devices

Direct mechanical assist devices and the intra-aortic balloon pump have been evaluated in experimental models of cardiac arrest and resuscitation.[84-90] Application of the mechanical assist device requires a thoracotomy and the attachment of suction directly to the myocardium. The device is designed to enhance ventricular diastole and coronary blood flow. Studies in experimental models have shown improvement in systolic and diastolic pressures, cardiac output, and cerebral blood flow when the direct mechanical assist device was compared with standard CPR or open-chest direct cardiac massage.[84-88] Similarly, use of the intra-aortic balloon pump during CPR demonstrated improved hemodynamics in experimental models.[89,90] Further outcome studies of these devices in experimental models are warranted.

Assessment of CPR

There are presently no good prognostic criteria clinicians can use to assess the efficacy of CPR. Outcome — either resuscitation or death — is often the only way to judge the adequacy of CPR efforts. Assessment of ongoing CPR efforts would allow clinicians to modify resuscitative efforts and individualize treatment protocols for patients in cardiac arrest. Ideally, clinicians could judge the value of specific adjuncts in individual patients. Several adjuncts may be useful in the assessment of ongoing CPR efforts.

Hemodynamics

Studies in experimental models have repeatedly demonstrated the importance of the aortic diastolic and myocardial perfusion (aortic-to–right atrial diastolic gradient) pressures during CPR for successful resuscitation from cardiac arrest.[1,91-99] The aortic diastolic and myocardial perfusion pressures have been correlated with coronary blood flow during CPR.[97] Much CPR research has focused on drugs or adjuncts that improve these pressures. While the placement of arterial and central venous lines during resuscitation efforts has been accomplished in some settings by a resuscitation research team, the placement of these lines in most clinical settings is not practical.[1,2,100] When arterial lines are available, the clinician should attempt to optimize the aortic diastolic and myocardial perfusion pressures during the resuscitative effort.

Pulses

As noted elsewhere, this textbook recommends Doppler ultrasound assessment of patients with pulseless electrical activity. Doppler ultrasound may detect spontaneous blood flow that cannot be detected by manual palpation. The presence or absence of pulses is frequently used by clinicians to assess the adequacy of artificial perfusion during CPR. While the presence of pulses does indicate some blood flow during chest compression, no studies have shown the clinical utility of checking pulses during ongoing CPR. A pulse represents the systolic-to-diastolic pressure gradient. It gives the clinician no information about important hemodynamic parameters, ie, the aortic diastolic and myocardial perfusion pressures. Finally, it is important to remember that since there are no valves in the inferior vena cava, retrograde blood flow may occur in the femoral vein. Thus, palpation of a pulse in the femoral area may be misleading and indicate venous rather than arterial blood flow. In summary, the presence of carotid pulses with CPR indicates the presence of some forward blood flow, but it cannot be used to gauge the efficacy of ongoing CPR efforts.

Respiratory Gas Measurements

Arterial blood gases are used by some clinicians to gauge the efficacy of ongoing CPR efforts. Physiologically, however, arterial blood gases do not reflect tissue pH and P_{CO_2}. Mixed venous gases often show severe hypercarbia despite normal arterial gases.[101] No correlation between arterial blood gases and resuscitation success has been demonstrated in experimental models of cardiac arrest.[102] Thus, arterial blood gases can be useful for evaluating oxygenation but should not be used to assess adequacy of CPR efforts.

Studies on the use of oximetry for assessing tissue perfusion during CPR have demonstrated that transconjunctival oxygen tension falls rapidly when a patient goes into cardiac arrest and returns to baseline when spontaneous circulation is restored.[103] However, oximetry has not been shown to be a useful prognostic guide for predicting resuscitation from cardiac arrest. Although pulse oximetry is commonplace in emergency departments and critical care units, it depends on the presence of a peripheral pulse and thus is unreliable for monitoring patients in cardiac arrest.

Capnometry shows promise as a noninvasive measure of cardiac output generated during ongoing CPR.[104] Blood flow to the lungs depends on cardiac output. In most patients in cardiac arrest, the CO_2 that reaches the lungs diffuses out. Capnometry measures CO_2 excretion through the endotracheal tube. In experimental models, end-tidal CO_2 concentration during ongoing CPR correlated with cardiac output, perfusion pressures, and successful resuscitation from cardiac arrest.[104-107] Clinical studies have demonstrated that patients who were successfully resuscitated from cardiac arrest had significantly higher end-tidal CO_2 levels than patients who could not be resuscitated.[108-112] Capnometry can also be used as an early indicator of return of spontaneous circulation.[108-110]

Despite these promising studies, a number of factors must be considered. Large changes in the minute ventilations will affect the end-tidal CO_2 reading.[113] Thus, ventilations must be held relatively constant during the resuscitation effort. The administration of bicarbonate will increase CO_2 excretion for several minutes before it returns to baseline measurements.[110,111] High doses of pressor agents such as epinephrine will increase myocardial perfusion pressure but decrease cardiac output. CO_2 excretion will decrease with decreased blood flow to the lungs.[114-117] Finally, for capnometry to be a truly useful prognostic indicator of successful resuscitation, clinical studies must demonstrate that strategies that improve end-tidal CO_2 levels will result in improved outcome from cardiac arrest. In summary, end-tidal CO_2 monitoring during cardiac arrest can be useful as a noninvasive indicator of cardiac output generated during CPR. Further research needs to be done to determine its use as a prognostic indicator in clinical practice.

References

1. Paradis NA, Martin GB, Rivers EP, et al. Coronary perfusion pressure and the return of spontaneous circulation in human cardiopulmonary resuscitation. *JAMA*. 1990;263:1106-1113.
2. Sanders AB, Ogle M, Ewy GA. Coronary perfusion pressure during cardiopulmonary resuscitation. *Am J Emerg Med*. 1985;3:11-14.
3. Babbs CF, Ralston SH, Voorhees WD III. Improved cardiac output during CPR with interposed abdominal compressions. *Ann Emerg Med*. 1983;12:527.
4. Voorhees WD, Niebauer MJ, Babbs CF. Improved oxygen delivery during cardiopulmonary resuscitation with interposed abdominal compressions. *Ann Emerg Med*. 1983;12:128-135.
5. Ralston SH, Babbs CF, Niebauer MJ. Cardiopulmonary resuscitation with interposed abdominal compressions in dogs. *Anesth Analg*. 1982;61:645-651.
6. Howard M, Carrubba C, Foss F, Janiak B, Hogan B, Guinness M. Interposed abdominal compression-CPR: its effects on parameters of coronary perfusion in human subjects. *Ann Emerg Med*. 1987; 16:253-259.
7. Lindner KH, Ahnefeld FW, Bowdler IM. Cardiopulmonary resuscitation with interposed abdominal compression after asphyxial or fibrillatory cardiac arrest in pigs. *Anesthesiology*. 1990;72:675-681.
8. Mateer JR, Stueven HA, Thompson BM, Aprahamian C, Darin JC. Prehospital IAC-CPR versus standard CPR: paramedic resuscitation of cardiac arrests. *Am J Emerg Med*. 1985;8:143-146.
9. Bircher NG, Abramson NS. Interposed abdominal compression CPR (IAC-CPR): a glimmer of hope. *Am J Emerg Med*. 1984;2:177-178.
10. Sack JB, Kesselbrenner MB, Bregman D. Survival from in-hospital cardiac arrest with interposed abdominal counterpulsation during cardiopulmonary resuscitation. *JAMA*. 1992;267:379-385.
11. Sack JB, Kesselbrenner MB, Jarrad A. Interposed abdominal compression-cardiopulmonary resuscitation and resuscitation outcome during asystole and electromechanical dissociation. *Circulation*. 1992;86:1692-1700.
12. Barranco F, Lesmes A, Irles JA, et al. Cardiopulmonary resuscitation with simultaneous chest and abdominal compression: comparative study in humans. *Resuscitation*. 1990;20:67-77.
13. Berryman CR, Phillips GM. Interposed abdominal compression-CPR in human subjects. *Ann Emerg Med*. 1984;13:226-229.
14. Ward KR, Sullivan RJ, Zelenak RR, Summer WR. A comparison of interposed abdominal compression CPR and standard CPR by monitoring end-tidal P_{CO_2}. *Ann Emerg Med*. 1989;18:831-837.
15. Kern KB, Carter AB, Showen RL, et al. Twenty-four hour survival in a canine model of cardiac arrest comparing three methods of manual cardiopulmonary resuscitation. *J Am Coll Cardiol*. 1986;7: 859-867.
16. Rudikoff MT, Maughan WL, Effron M, Freund P, Weisfeldt ML. Mechanisms of blood flow during cardiopulmonary resuscitation. *Circulation*. 1980;61:345-352.
17. Chandra N, Snyder LD, Weisfeldt ML. Abdominal binding during cardiopulmonary resuscitation in man. *JAMA*. 1981;246:351-353.
18. Chandra N, Rudikoff M, Weisfeldt ML. Simultaneous chest compression and ventilation at high airway pressure during cardiopulmonary resuscitation. *Lancet*. 1980;1:175-178.
19. Niemann JT, Rosborough JP, Hausknecht M, Garner D, Criley JM. Pressure-synchronized cineangiography during experimental cardiopulmonary resuscitation. *Circulation*. 1981;64:985-991.
20. Sanders AB, Ewy GA, Alferness CA, Taft T, Zimmerman M. Failure of one method of simultaneous chest compression, ventilation, and abdominal binding during CPR. *Crit Care Med*. 1982;10:509-513.
21. Niemann JT, Rosborough JP, Niskanen RA, Alferness C, Criley JM. Mechanical "cough" cardiopulmonary resuscitation during cardiac arrest in dogs. *Am J Cardiol*. 1985;55:199-204.
22. Krisher JP, Fine EG, Weisfeldt ML, Guerci AD, Nagel E, Chandra N. Comparison of prehospital conventional and simultaneous compression-ventilation cardiopulmonary resuscitation. *Crit Care Med*. 1989;17:1263-1269.
23. Swenson RD, Weaver WD, Niskanen RA, Martin J, Dahlberg S. Hemodynamics in humans during conventional and experimental methods of cardiopulmonary resuscitation. *Circulation*. 1988;78:630-639.
24. Kern KB, Carter AB, Showen RL, et al. Comparison of mechanical techniques of cardiopulmonary resuscitation: survival and neurologic outcome in dogs. *Am J Emerg Med*. 1987;5:190-195.
25. Martin GB, Carden DL, Nowak RM, Lewinter JR, Johnston W, Tomlanovich MC. Aortic and right atrial pressures during standard and simultaneous compression and ventilation CPR in human beings. *Ann Emerg Med*. 1986;15:125-130.
26. Feneley MP, Maier GW, Kern KB, et al. Influence of compression rate on initial success of resuscitation and 24-hour survival after prolonged manual cardiopulmonary resuscitation in dogs. *Circulation*. 1988;77:240-250.
27. Halperin HR, Tsitlik JE, Guerci AD, et al. Determinants of blood flow to vital organs during cardiopulmonary resuscitation in dogs. *Circulation*. 1986;73:539-550.
28. Kern KB, Sanders AB, Raife J, Milander MM, Otto CW, Ewy GA. A study of chest compression rates during cardiopulmonary resuscitation in humans: the importance of rate-directed chest compressions. *Arch Intern Med*. 1992;152:145-149.
29. Ornato JP, Gonzales ER, Garnett AR, Levine RL, McClung BK. Effect of cardiopulmonary resuscitation compression rate on end-tidal carbon dioxide concentration and arterial pressure in man. *Crit Care Med*. 1988;16:241-245. Abstract.
30. Martin GB, Gokli A, Paradis NA, et al. Effect of high compression rates during mechanical CPR in human beings: preliminary results. *Ann Emerg Med*. 1990;19:1223-1224. Abstract.
31. Taylor GJ, Rubin R, Tucker M, Greene HL, Rudikoff MT, Weisfeldt ML. External cardiac compression: a randomized comparison of mechanical and manual techniques. *JAMA*. 1978;240:644-646.
32. McDonald JL. Systolic and mean arterial pressures during manual and mechanical CPR in humans. *Ann Emerg Med*. 1982;11: 292-295.
33. Barkalow CE. Mechanized cardiopulmonary resuscitation: past, present and future. *Am J Emerg Med*. 1984;2:262-269.
34. Ward KR, Menegazzi JJ, Zelenak RR. A comparison of mechanical CPR and manual CPR by monitoring end-tidal P_{CO_2} in human cardiac arrest. *Ann Emerg Med*. 1990;19:456. Abstract.
35. Ewy GA, Hellman DA, McClung S, Taren D. Influence of ventilation phase on transthoracic impedance and defibrillation effectiveness. *Crit Care Med*. 1980;8:164-166.
36. Kaback KR, Sanders AB, Meislin HW. MAST suit update. *JAMA*. 1984;252:2598-2603.
37. McSwain NE. Pneumatic trousers and the management of shock. *J Trauma*. 1977;17:719-724.
38. Gaffney FA, Thal ER, Taylor WF, et al. Hemodynamic effects of Medical Anti-Shock Trousers (MAST garment). *J Trauma*. 1981;21:931-937.
39. Niemann JT, Stapczynski JS, Rosborough JP, Rothstein RJ. Hemodynamic effects of pneumatic external counterpressure in canine hemorrhagic shock. *Ann Emerg Med*. 1983;12:661-667.

40. Mahoney BD, Mirick MJ. Efficacy of pneumatic trousers in refractory prehospital cardiopulmonary arrest. *Ann Emerg Med.* 1983; 12:8-12.

41. Harris LC Jr, Kirimli B, Safar P. Augmentation of artificial circulation during cardiopulmonary resuscitation. *Anesthesiology.* 1967;28: 730-734.

42. Mattox KL, Bickell W, Pepe PE, Burch J, Feliciano D. Prospective MAST study in 911 patients. *Trauma.* 1989;29:1104-1111.

43. Bickell WH, Pepe PE, Bailey ML, Wyatt CH, Mattox KL. Randomized trial of pneumatic antishock garments in the prehospital management of penetrating abdominal injuries. *Ann Emerg Med.* 1987;16:653-658.

44. Halperin HR, Tsitlik JE, Gelfand M, et al. A preliminary study of cardiopulmonary resuscitation by circumferential compression of the chest with use of a pneumatic vest. *N Engl J Med.* 1993;329: 762-768.

45. Beattie C, Guerci AD, Hall T, et al. Mechanisms of blood flow during pneumatic vest cardiopulmonary resuscitation. *J Appl Physiol.* 1991;70:454-465.

46. Halperin HR, Weisfeldt ML. New approaches to CPR: four hands, a plunger, or a vest. *JAMA.* 1992;267:2940-2941.

47. Cohen TJ, Tucker KJ, Redberg RF, et al. Active compression-decompression resuscitation: a new method of cardiopulmonary resuscitation. *Circulation.* 1990;84(suppl 2):II-8. Abstract.

48. Cohen TJ, Tucker KJ, Lurie KG, et al. Active compression-decompression: a new method of cardiopulmonary resuscitation. *JAMA.* 1992;267:2916-2923.

49. Cohen TJ, Tucker KJ, Redberg RF, et al. Active compression-decompression resuscitation: a novel method of cardiopulmonary resuscitation. *Am Heart J.* 1992;124:1145-1150.

50. Stephenson HE Jr, Reid LC, Hinton JW. Some common denominators in 1200 cases of cardiac arrest. *Ann Surg.* 1953;137:731-744.

51. Turk LN III, Glenn WWL. Cardiac arrest: results of attempted resuscitation in 42 cases. *N Engl J Med.* 1954;251:795-803.

52. Weiser FM, Adler LN, Kuhn LA. Hemodynamic effects of closed and open chest cardiac resuscitation in normal dogs and those with acute myocardial infarction. *Am J Cardiol.* 1962;10:555-561.

53. Bircher N, Safar P. Comparison of standard and "new" closed-chest CPR and open-chest CPR in dogs. *Crit Care Med.* 1981;9:384-385.

54. Sanders AB, Kern KB, Ewy GA, Atlas M, Bailey L. Improved resuscitation from cardiac arrest with open-chest massage. *Ann Emerg Med.* 1984;13:672-675.

55. Sanders AB, Kern KB, Atlas M, Bragg S, Ewy GA. Importance of the duration of inadequate coronary perfusion pressure on resuscitation from cardiac arrest. *J Am Coll Cardiol.* 1985;6:113-118.

56. Bircher N, Safar P. Cerebral preservation during cardiopulmonary resuscitation. *Crit Care Med.* 1985;13:185-190.

57. Howard MA, Labadie LL, Martin GB, et al. Improvement in coronary perfusion pressures after open-chest cardiac massage in humans: preliminary report. *Ann Emerg Med.* 1986;15:664-665. Abstract.

58. Del Guercio LR, Feins NR, Cohn JD, et al. Comparison of blood flow during external and internal cardiac massage in man. *Circulation.* 1965;31(suppl 1):I-171-I-180.

59. Kern KB, Sanders AB, Badylak SF, et al. Long-term survival with open-chest cardiac massage after ineffective closed-chest compression in a canine preparation. *Circulation.* 1987;75:498-503.

60. Kern KB, Sanders AB, Ewy GA. Open-chest cardiac massage after closed-chest compression in a canine model: when to intervene. *Resuscitation.* 1987;15:51-57.

61. Sanders AB, Kern KB, Ewy GA. Open-chest massage for resuscitation from cardiac arrest. *Resuscitation.* 1988;16:153-154.

62. Eldor J, Frankel DZ, Davidson JT. Open-chest cardiac massage: a review. *Resuscitation.* 1988;16:155-162.

63. Kern KB, Sanders AB, Janas W, et al. Limitations of open-chest cardiac massage after prolonged, untreated cardiac arrest in dogs. *Ann Emerg Med.* 1991;20:761-767.

64. Robertson C. The value of open-chest CPR for non-traumatic cardiac arrest. *Resuscitation.* 1991;22:203-208.

65. Babbs CF. Hemodynamic mechanisms in CPR: a theoretical rationale for resuscitative thoracotomy in non-traumatic cardiac arrest. *Resuscitation.* 1987;15:37-50.

66. Shockett E, Rosenblum R. Successful open cardiac massage after 75 minutes of closed massage. *JAMA.* 1967;200:333-335.

67. Sykes MK, Ahmed N. Emergency treatment of cardiac arrest. *Lancet.* 1963;2:347-349.

68. Geehr EC, Lewis FR, Auerbach PS. Failure of open-heart massage to improve survival after prehospital nontraumatic cardiac arrest. *N Engl J Med.* 1986;314:1189-1190. Letter.

69. Bodai BI, Smith JP, Ward RE, O'Neill MB, Auborg R. Emergency thoracotomy in the management of trauma. *JAMA.* 1983;249: 1891-1896.

70. Cogbill TH, Moore EE, Millikan JS, Cleveland HC. Rationale for selective application of emergency department thoracotomy in trauma. *J Trauma.* 1983;23:453-460.

71. Danne PD, Finelli F, Champion HR. Emergency bay thoracotomy. *J Trauma.* 1984;24:796-802.

72. Roberge RJ, Ivatury RR, Stahl W, Rohman M. Emergency department thoracotomy for penetrating injuries: predictive value of patient classification. *Am J Emerg Med.* 1986;4:129-135.

73. Martin GB, Nowak RM, Carden DL, Eisiminger RA, Tomlanovich MC. Cardiopulmonary bypass vs CPR as treatment for prolonged canine cardiopulmonary arrest. *Ann Emerg Med.* 1987;16:628-636.

74. Levine R, Gorayeb M, Safar P, Abramson N, Stezoski W, Kelsey S. Cardiopulmonary bypass after cardiac arrest and prolonged closed-chest CPR in dogs. *Ann Emerg Med.* 1987;16:620-627.

75. Angelos MG, Gaddis ML, Gaddis GM, Leasure JE. Improved survival and reduced myocardial necrosis with cardiopulmonary bypass reperfusion in a canine model of coronary occlusion and cardiac arrest. *Ann Emerg Med.* 1990;19:1122-1128.

76. Angelos M, Safar P, Reich H. A comparison of cardiopulmonary resuscitation with cardiopulmonary bypass after prolonged cardiac arrest in dogs: reperfusion pressures and neurologic recovery. *Resuscitation.* 1991;21:121-135.

77. Hartz R, LoCicero J III, Sanders JH Jr, Frederiksen JW, Joob AW, Michaelis LL. Clinical experience with portable cardiopulmonary bypass in cardiac arrest patients. *Ann Thorac Surg.* 1990;50: 437-441.

78. Angelos MG, Gaddis M, Gaddis G, Leasure JE. Cardiopulmonary bypass in a model of acute myocardial infarction and cardiac arrest. *Ann Emerg Med.* 1990;19:874-880.

79. Safar P, Abramson NS, Angelos M, et al. Emergency cardiopulmonary bypass for resuscitation from prolonged cardiac arrest. *Am J Emerg Med.* 1990;8:55-67.

80. Angelos M, Safar P, Reich H. External cardiopulmonary resuscitation preserves brain viability after prolonged cardiac arrest in dogs. *Am J Emerg Med.* 1991;9:436-443.

81. DeBehnke DJ, Angelos MG, Leasure JE. Comparison of standard external CPR, open-chest CPR, and cardiopulmonary bypass in a canine myocardial infarct model. *Ann Emerg Med.* 1991;20: 754-760.

82. Tisherman SA, Safar P, Abramson NS, et al. Feasibility of emergency cardiopulmonary bypass for resuscitation from CPR-resistant cardiac arrest — a preliminary report. *Ann Emerg Med.* 1991;20:491. Abstract.

83. Martin GB, Paradis NA, Rivers EP, et al. Cardiopulmonary bypass in the treatment of cardiac arrest in humans. *Crit Care Med.* 1990;18:5247. Abstract.

84. Anstadt MP, Anstadt GL, Lowe JE. Direct mechanical ventricular actuation: a review. *Resuscitation.* 1991;21:7-23.

85. Skinner DB. Experimental and clinical evaluations of mechanical ventricular assistance. *Am J Cardiol.* 1971;27:146-154.

86. McCabe JB, Ventriglia WJ, Anstadt GL, Nolan DJ. Direct mechanical ventricular assistance during ventricular fibrillation. *Ann Emerg Med.* 1983;739-744.

87. Bartlett RL, Stewart NJ Jr, Raymond J, Anstadt GL, Martin SD. Comparative study of three methods of resuscitation: closed-chest, open-chest manual, and direct mechanical ventricular assistance. *Ann Emerg Med.* 1984;13(pt 2):773-777.

88. Griffith RF, Anstadt M, Hoekstra J, et al. Regional cerebral blood flow with manual internal cardiac massage versus direct mechanical ventricular assistance. *Ann Emerg Med.* 1992;21:137-141.

89. Emerman CL, Pinchak AC, Hagen JF, Hancock D. Hemodynamic effects of the intra-aortic balloon pump during experimental cardiac arrest. *Am J Emerg Med.* 1989;7:378-383.

90. Wesley RC Jr, Morgan DB. Effect of continuous intra-aortic balloon inflation in canine open-chest cardiopulmonary resuscitation. *Crit Care Med.* 1990;18:630-633.

91. Redding JS. Abdominal compression in cardiopulmonary resuscitation. *Anesth Analg.* 1971;50:668-675.

92. Crile G, Dolley DH. Experimental resuscitation of dogs killed by anesthetics and asphyxia. *J Exp Med.* 1906;6:713-720.

93. Redding JS, Pearson JW. Resuscitation from ventricular fibrillation: drug therapy. *JAMA*. 1968;203:255-260.

94. Redding JS, Pearson JW. Evaluation of drugs for cardiac resuscitation. *Anesthesiology*. 1963;24:203-207.

95. Pearson JW, Redding JS. Influence of peripheral vascular tone on cardiac resuscitation. *Anesth Analg*. 1965;44:746-752.

96. Sanders AB, Ewy GA, Taft TV. Prognostic and therapeutic importance of the aortic diastolic pressure in resuscitation from cardiac arrest. *Crit Care Med*. 1984;12:871-873.

97. Ditchey RV, Winkler JV, Rhodes CA. Relative lack of coronary blood flow during closed-chest resuscitation in dogs. *Circulation*. 1982;66:297-302.

98. Michael JR, Guerci AD, Koehler RC, et al. Mechanisms by which epinephrine augments cerebral and myocardial perfusion during cardiopulmonary resuscitation in dogs. *Circulation*. 1984;69:822-835.

99. Ralston SH, Voorhees WD, Babbs CF. Intrapulmonary epinephrine during prolonged cardiopulmonary resuscitation: improved regional flow and resuscitation in dogs. *Ann Emerg Med*. 1984;13:79-86.

100. Pierpont GL, Kruse JA, Nelson DH. Intra-arterial monitoring during cardiopulmonary resuscitation. *Cathet Cardiovasc Diagn*. 1985;11:513-520.

101. Weil MH, Rackow EC, Trevino R, Grundler W, Falk JL, Griffel MI. Difference in acid-base state between venous and arterial blood during cardiopulmonary resuscitation. *N Engl J Med*. 1986;315:153-156.

102. Sanders AB, Ewy GA, Taft TV. Resuscitation and arterial blood gas abnormalities during prolonged cardiopulmonary resuscitation. *Ann Emerg Med*. 1984;13:676-679.

103. Abraham E, Fink S. Conjunctival oxygen tension monitoring in emergency department patients. *Am J Emerg Med*. 1988;6:549-554.

104. Weil MH, Bisera J, Trevino RR, Rackow EC. Cardiac output and end-tidal carbon dioxide. *Crit Care Med*. 1985;13:907-909.

105. Sanders AB, Atlas M, Ewy GA, Kern KB, Bragg S. Expired P_{CO_2} as an index of coronary perfusion pressure. *Am J Emerg Med*. 1985;3:147-149.

106. Sanders AB, Ewy GA, Bragg S, Atlas M, Kern KB. Expired P_{CO_2} as a prognostic indicator of successful resuscitation from cardiac arrest. *Ann Emerg Med*. 1985;14:948-952.

107. Gudipati CV, Weil MH, Bisera J, Deshmukh HG, Rackow EC. Expired carbon dioxide: a non-invasive monitor of cardiopulmonary resuscitation. *Circulation*. 1988;77:234-239.

108. Kalenda Z. The capnogram as a guide to the efficacy of cardiac massage. *Resuscitation*. 1978;6:259-263.

109. Garnett AR, Ornato JP, Gonzales ER, Johnson EB. End-tidal carbon dioxide monitoring during cardiopulmonary resuscitation. *JAMA*. 1987;257:512-515.

110. Falk JL, Rackow EC, Weil MH. End-tidal carbon dioxide concentration during cardiopulmonary resuscitation. *N Engl J Med*. 1988;318:607-611.

111. Sanders AB, Kern KB, Otto CW, Milander MM, Ewy GA. End-tidal carbon dioxide monitoring during cardiopulmonary resuscitation: a prognostic indicator for survival. *JAMA*. 1989;262:1347-1351.

112. Callaham M, Barton C. Prediction of outcome of cardiopulmonary resuscitation from end-tidal carbon dioxide concentration. *Crit Care Med*. 1990;8:358-362.

113. Barton CW, Callaham ML. Possible confounding effect of minute ventilation on ET_{CO_2} in cardiac arrest. *Ann Emerg Med*. 1991;20:445-446. Abstract.

114. Paradis NA, Goetting MG, Rivers EP, et al. Increases in coronary perfusion pressure after high-dose epinephrine result in decreases in end-tidal CO_2 during CPR in human beings. *Ann Emerg Med*. 1990;19:491. Abstract.

115. Callaham M, Barton C. Effect of epinephrine administration on ability of end-tidal carbon dioxide readings to predict outcome of cardiac arrest. *Ann Emerg Med*. 1990;19:490. Abstract.

116. Chase PB, Kern KB, Sanders AB, et al. The effect of high and low dose epinephrine on myocardial perfusion, cardiac output and end-tidal carbon dioxide during prolonged CPR. *Ann Emerg Med*. 1990;19:466. Abstract.

117. Martin GB, Gentile NT, Paradis NA, Moeggenberg J, Appleton TJ, Nowak RM. Effect of epinephrine on end-tidal carbon dioxide monitoring during CPR. *Ann Emerg Med*. 1990;19:396-398.

Invasive Monitoring Techniques

Chapter 12

In the ACLS Provider's Course all invasive monitoring techniques are considered supplemental material. More advanced providers should master these techniques, particularly when their professional work requires them.

Introduction to Arterial Cannulation

Indications

Placement of an intra-arterial catheter allows the clinician to (1) continuously monitor arterial pressure accurately, (2) avoid the discomfort and injury from frequent arterial punctures, (3) sample arterial blood without disturbing the steady state, and (4) determine cardiac output using indocyanine green dye (this is becoming less necessary given modern noninvasive technology, such as blood pressure and oximetry devices). To use intra-arterial monitoring safely and effectively, the operator must be skilled in the technique, and the staff must be familiar with the catheter and transducer system so as to eliminate air bubbles, prevent clots and contamination, calibrate the system correctly, and avoid artifacts.

Rationale for Intra-arterial Pressure Monitoring

For patients who are in shock and have an elevated systemic vascular resistance there is often a significant difference between the pressure obtained by auscultatory or palpatory methods and pressures obtained by intra-arterial measurement.[1] Central intra-arterial systolic pressure may be as much as 150 mm Hg higher than the pressure recorded with a sphygmomanometer. In hypotensive patients with normal or decreased systemic vascular resistance, there should be no discrepancy between pressure obtained with a cuff and intra-arterial pressure unless localized atherosclerosis is present.

The Korotkoff sounds heard over the brachial artery as the arm cuff is deflated are probably due to vibrations of the arterial wall set in motion by intermittent flow through the compressed segment. Absence of these sounds indicates that either flow is insufficient or the vessel wall itself has been altered so that sounds are not transmitted. Diastolic runoff is slowed with increased arterial constriction in hypotensive states. After release of pressure in the cuff at the onset of flow, there is a decreased pressure gradient. With a decreased gradient there is no intermittent turbulence-producing jet flow through the obstructed segment, and therefore no sounds are produced. The increased wall tension from vasoconstriction may also make the wall less likely to vibrate and produce sounds.[1]

In patients with increased vascular resistance, low cuff pressure does not necessarily indicate arterial hypotension. Failure to recognize this may lead to dangerous errors in therapy.

Any patient who requires titrated intravenous (IV) vasopressors or vasodilators for improved hemodynamics should have blood pressure recorded continuously. An intra-arterial line is vitally important if intense vasoconstriction is present.

Direct vs Indirect Arterial Pressure Measurements[2-6]

Variance of 5 to 20 mm Hg

A disparity of 5 to 20 mm Hg is probably within the expected range for direct and indirect pressure measurements. Directly recorded pressure may be slightly higher than indirectly recorded pressure for several reasons. As the arterial pressure pulse wave passes to the periphery, its form changes markedly. The pulse wave arrives later, the ascending limb becomes steeper, and the systolic pressure becomes higher, while the diastolic pressure is lower. The mean arterial pressure, however, is unchanged. The major factors responsible for changes in the arterial pulse contour are

- Distortion of the components of the pulse waves as they travel peripherally
- Different rates of transmission of various components of the pulse wave
- Amplification or distortion of different components of the pulse by standing or reflected waves
- Differences in elastic behavior and in the caliber of the arteries
- Conversions of some kinetic energy to hydrostatic energy
- Changes that occur in the arterial catheter and the extension line from the catheter to the transducer

There may also be a disparity in measurements if cuff size and placement are inappropriate. Finally, the transducer may be improperly calibrated or zeroed.

When indirect pressure is recorded as greater than direct pressure, either equipment malfunction or technical error is likely. Damping of the arterial waveform suggests a problem with the direct technique: air bubbles or blood in the line or the transducer dome, clotting at the catheter tip, mechanical occlusion of the catheter or the tubing, or loose or open connections. If the arterial waveform is normal, other causes must be excluded: improper cuff size and placement, failure to calibrate the sphygmomanometer and the transducer, or an error in electrically and mechanically zeroing the transducer.

Variance of 20 to 30 mm Hg

When there is a disparity of 20 to 30 mm Hg between cuff pressure and intra-arterial pressure, all factors listed above may be responsible. In addition, the auscultatory method may lead to lower readings in the patient with severe vasoconstriction, such as in shock or hypothermia. Another possible source of error is that the cuff reads pressure from beat to beat, whereas the digital recording on the electronic monitor reads the highest pressure every 3 to 7 seconds. In the presence of occlusive peripheral disease, the pressure recorded in a peripheral artery, such as the radial or the dorsalis pedis, may be significantly lower than the cuff pressure taken more proximally.

Variance of Greater Than 30 mm Hg

When the disparity is greater than 30 mm Hg, the most common problem is overshoot of the apparent systolic pressure (Fig 1) caused by the resonance of the catheter system. This more commonly occurs when the heart rate is rapid, when the rate of rise of pressure (dP/dt) is rapid, and when the natural frequency of the catheter system is low. The longer and more compliant the extension tubing and the lower the natural frequency, the greater the error in measurement. This can be minimized by using stiff extension tubing kept as short as possible.

Intra-arterial pressure may be significantly higher than cuff pressure when a single end-hole catheter is in a narrow artery with high flow. When the catheter faces the flow, kinetic energy is converted to potential energy, falsely elevating the measured blood pressure.

The disparity between the direct and indirect pressure measurements can be minimized by the following procedures[2,6]:

1. Allow the transducer and amplifier to warm up for at least 10 minutes before starting to zero and calibrate the system.
2. Mechanically zero the transducer.
3. Purge all air from the pressure system.
4. Check all fittings for tightness.
5. Electrically zero and calibrate the system with a mercury manometer or a water column.[7]
6. Use stiff, noncompliant extension tubing of shortest possible length, and avoid use of more than one stopcock between catheter and transducer.
7. Avoid draining blood samples the full length of the plumbing system.
8. Maintain the catheter by continuous low-flow flushing so that clotting does not occur.
9. Place the extension tubing near the patient with care to prevent a pulsating line.
10. Recheck the mechanical and electrical zero position, and recalibrate the system if necessary when the level of the patient is changed.
11. Avoid making adjustments to the amplifier except at time of calibration.
12. Check the zero setting (both electrically and mechanically) and calibration at least once per shift.

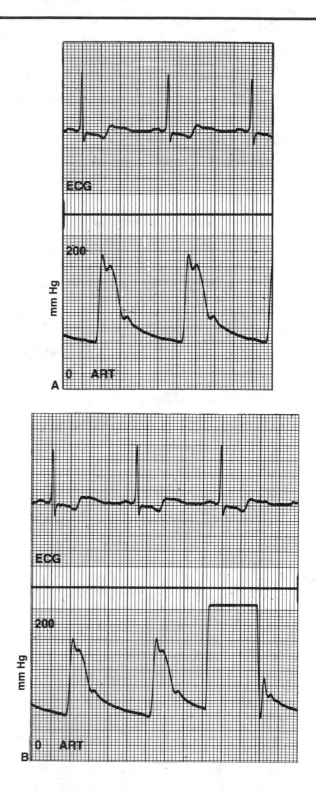

Fig 1. A, Overshoot of apparent systolic pressure (ART) due to resonance from 72-inch-long extension tubing. Recorded pressure is 195 mm Hg. B, Systolic pressure (ART) recorded with 6-inch extension tubing in same patient. The recorded systolic pressure is 175 mm Hg, which correlated with cuff systolic pressure of 170 mm Hg.

Use of Doppler Device for Blood Pressure Monitoring[8-10]

A Doppler device and an arm cuff may be used to measure blood pressure noninvasively. The Doppler transducer, which should be an instrument with high frequency output (10 MHz), is placed over the radial artery at the wrist, and a blood pressure cuff of appropriate size is placed around the upper arm. The cuff is inflated until the Doppler signal disappears and then is slowly deflated until blood flow is again audible; this is the systolic pressure. Diastolic readings are not possible with this technique.

The Doppler signal can be heard clearly and recorded, even at low levels of systolic pressure, when the Korotkoff sounds are not audible and the pulse is not palpable. Doppler measurement of blood pressure over the radial artery correlates well with intra-arterial pressure in the radial artery even in patients with hypotension. With intense vasoconstriction, neither the Doppler nor the intravascular radial arterial pressure will reflect aortic pressure, and a more centrally placed line, such as one in the femoral or the axillary artery, may be required.

Indirect Blood Pressure Monitoring by Automatic Oscillometry

These devices have become increasingly available in emergency departments, critical care units, and even prehospital care settings. They often incorporate several features, including pulse oximetry and electrocardiographic (ECG) monitoring. Automatic indirect blood pressure determinations can be performed via automatic oscillometry, a technique that uses a double air bladder enclosed in a cuff to determine the arterial blood pressure of the extremity within the cuff. The cuff is positioned over an artery, and the proximal bladder is inflated to occlude blood flow while residual air volume is maintained in the distal bladder. The proximal bladder is deflated stepwise, and restoration of blood flow causes arterial wall oscillations that are sensed by the distal bladder. A microprocessor then assesses the transmitted signals and determines systolic blood pressure, diastolic blood pressure, and mean blood pressure.[11] The accuracy of the data generated suffers from the same vagaries as do other nonautomatic blood pressure determinations. Cuff size and fit, extremes of blood pressure, and obesity may cause errors of measurement.[12-15]

Venus et al[16] compared indirect automatic blood pressure determination vs blood pressure determination via direct radial arterial cannulation. In 109 determinations there were no significant differences in mean arterial blood pressure between the two techniques. However, the indirect determination underestimated systolic blood pressure by 9.2±16.4 mm Hg and overestimated diastolic blood pressure by 8.7±10.6 mm Hg. The investigators concluded that automatic indirect blood pressure monitoring was adequate for routine monitoring of mean arterial pressure, but for hemodynamic titration of vasoactive drugs, direct intra-arterial measurements should be considered.

In a study by Johnson and Kerr[17] evaluating five automatic blood pressure monitors compared with measurements made from direct arterial line monitoring, the correlation coefficient ranged from .7 to more than .9. However, they concluded that in critically ill patients, especially those who were hypotensive and in whom peripheral recordings may themselves not correlate with central pressure, indirect monitorings were inadequate and direct monitoring necessary.

Site Selection for Indwelling Arterial Catheters

An artery suitable for placing an indwelling catheter for continuous monitoring of intra-arterial pressures should have the following characteristics:

- The vessel should be large enough to measure pressure accurately without the catheter occluding the artery or producing thrombosis.
- The artery should have adequate collateral circulation in case occlusion occurs.
- There should be easy access to the site for nursing care.
- It should not be in an area prone to contamination.

The axillary artery is large and has excellent collateral flow, so that thrombosis should not lead to any serious sequelae. It can be used to monitor central arterial pressure. However, embolism of air or thrombus that forms about the catheter tip may produce ischemic injury to the brain or the hand.

The femoral artery also can be used. The femoral pulse still may be palpable when the radial pulses are lost in patients with marked hypotension. It also reflects intra-aortic pressure better than peripheral arteries do.[1] Caution is advised in the presence of occlusive arterial disease.

The radial artery can be used for cannulation. It is usually safe for use if careful attention is directed toward demonstrating adequate ulnar collateral flow before cannulation. Even though thrombosis of the radial artery at the catheter site is common (as noted later), ischemic injury of the hand is rare if there is adequate ulnar collateral flow. (See "Modified Allen Test.")

The dorsal pedal arteries are without significant cannulation hazards if collateral flow is demonstrated to the remainder of the foot through the posterior tibial artery. *Cannulation of the brachial artery is not recommended because of the potential for thrombosis and ischemia of the lower arm and hand.[18] Alternative sites such as the radial, femoral, or axillary artery should be chosen.*

Complications of Arterial Catheterization

The major complications of arterial cannulation are ischemia and necrosis secondary to either thrombosis or embolism. Ischemia is manifested by pain (either at rest or when using the involved extremity), pallor, and paresthesias. Necrosis is manifested by obvious tissue death. Whether ischemia or necrosis distal to the area of obstruction occurs depends on the presence of collateral flow and the rate of recanalization. Other complications include hemorrhage, infection, vasovagal syncope, aneurysms, and arteriovenous fistula — the complications that may occur with cannulation of any artery. Complications following cannulation of specific arteries will be discussed as a separate topic in the sections pertaining to each artery.

Thrombosis

The longer the cannula is in place, the greater the incidence of thrombosis. Radial artery cannulas left in place longer than 48 hours markedly increase the incidence of thrombosis.[19-22] Yet cannulation of the femoral artery with a long, thin catheter for up to 16 days was not associated with any thrombotic complications in one published series of studies.[23,24] The larger the size of the cannula relative to the diameter of the arterial lumen, the greater the incidence of thrombosis. This may relate both to the fact that the larger cannula relative to vessel size may produce more intimal damage and that the larger cannula in a small vessel occupies most of the lumen and in itself obstructs the flow. A large 18-gauge catheter in a small vessel would occupy most of the lumen, whereas a smaller 20-gauge catheter in a large vessel might occupy only 15% to 20% of the lumen.[25] A 20-gauge catheter produces the lowest incidence of thrombosis in the radial artery.[25-27]

One study indicated that the incidence of dysfunction of the catheter as manifested by damping of the arterial waveform was the same with 18-gauge and 20-gauge catheters. However, the dysfunction was invariably due to thrombosis with the larger catheter; with the smaller catheter it was usually due to kinking.[25] The shape of the cannula and the material from which the cannula is made also influence the incidence of thrombosis. Nontapered catheters induce a lower incidence of thrombus formation compared with tapered catheters,[26,28] and catheters made of Teflon have been shown to invoke the lowest incidence of thrombosis.[25,27] Repeated attempts at puncturing the radial artery not only may lead to thrombosis in the absence of an indwelling catheter but also may increase the incidence of thrombosis with an indwelling catheter.[20,28] Hypotension and low cardiac output, the use of vasopressors, peripheral arteriosclerotic occlusive disease, diabetes mellitus, Raynaud's disease, hypothermia, autoimmune diseases with vasculitis, and excessive and prolonged pressure on the artery to control bleeding after catheter removal predispose to thrombosis and the ischemic sequelae of thrombosis.[20,29]

Intermittent flushing of the catheter increases the risk of thrombosis. A continuous flush system should be used to ensure catheter patency, prevent thrombosis, and mini-mize the incidence of embolism. Several systems are now available that provide continuous flow at 3.0 mL/h when the system is pressurized to 300 mm Hg. A valve can be opened that provides a flush at 1.5 mL/s.[30] With the flush valve closed, the resistance in the system is so high that the pressure measured within the system does not differ by more than 2% from the pressure at the tip of the catheter.[30,31] However, since air will pass easily through the flow system, it must be removed from the bag before pressurization. The solution for continuous irrigation should have heparin added; a concentration of 2 to 4 U/mL appears adequate. Opening the flush valve and then rapidly closing it generates a square wave on the arterial waveform that indicates that no clot or bubbles are present in the system (Fig 2A). If clots, bubbles, or loose connections are present, the square wave response will be damped significantly[32] (Fig 2B).

Embolism

Embolism from small clots that form around the tip of the catheter or from air and particulate matter introduced into the system may occur. Emboli are more common when intermittent flushing of the catheter is done by hand. If hand flushing is required, a few milliliters of blood should be withdrawn through the stopcock to clear the system of air or clot before flushing. A continuous flush system that eliminates the need for intermittent flushing minimizes the problem of embolism.[26,30]

Hemorrhage

If any connection in the arterial line between the patient and the transducer opens or becomes disconnected, rapid exsanguination of the patient may follow unless the situation is promptly recognized. A bleeding diathesis, due either to anticoagulation or a disease process, increases the incidence of hemorrhage from the puncture site. Bleeding may occur around the catheter if a needle larger than the catheter is used to introduce the catheter, or it may occur after catheter removal. Hypertension, especially with a rapid rise of the systolic upstroke (dP/dt) within the artery, may also increase the incidence of bleeding. Hematoma following removal of an arterial catheter is common, although it may not appear for 1 to 2 days after removal of the cannula, and may persist for 7 to 10 days. The incidence and size of the hematoma can be minimized with the application of pressure to the cannulation site for 10 minutes after withdrawal of the catheter.[29,30]

Infection

The most obvious risk factor for catheter-related infection appears to be the length of time the catheter resides in the vessel. Most infections are caused by arterial catheters left in place for more than 72 hours.[33] Arterial catheters inserted by cutdown involve an increased incidence of infection compared with catheters inserted percutaneously.[33] Infection also depends on bacterial exposure during placement of the catheter and the frequency of catheter-stopcock manipulation as well as a variety of host-related factors.

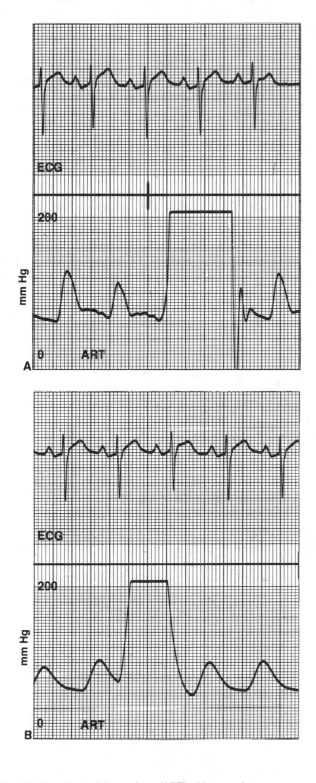

Fig 2. A, Normal arterial waveform (ART) with normal square wave response during rapid flushing with continuous flush system. B, Significantly damped square wave response in arterial waveform when clots, bubbles, or loose connections are present.

Vasovagal Reactions

Hypotension with bradycardia may occur during arterial puncture and can be reversed promptly with atropine.[34]

Arterial Cannulation Sites, Techniques, and Complications

Cannulation of the Femoral Artery

Anatomy

The femoral artery (Fig 3) is the continuation of the external iliac artery and traverses beneath the inguinal ligament in the leg. If a line is drawn from the antero-superior iliac spine to the symphysis pubis, the femoral artery generally passes through the midpoint of that line at the level of the inguinal ligament. Lateral to the femoral artery is the femoral nerve, and medial to the artery within the femoral sheath is the femoral vein.[35] See Figs 10 and 11, chapter 11.

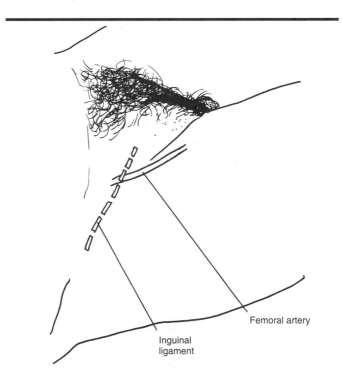

Fig 3. Anatomy of the femoral artery.

Equipment Needed

1. A 19- or 20-gauge Teflon catheter 16 cm long. The catheter should be long enough to extend through the skin well into the artery so that it does not become dislodged with movement of the patient.
2. A flexible guidewire small enough to pass through the catheter and needle
3. A 20-gauge needle 5 cm long
4. Other equipment as for any arterial cannulation

Technique (Fig 4)

1. Identify the femoral artery and choose a site approximately 2 cm below the inguinal ligament or near the inguinal fold.
2. Shave the groin and cleanse the skin with povidone-iodine.
3. Wear sterile gloves, mask, and hair cover.
4. Cover the area around the insertion site with sterile drapes. If the Seldinger technique is used, the sterile field should be large enough to allow manipulation of the guidewire and catheter without risk of contamination.
5. Place the index, middle, and ring fingers of one hand along the course of the femoral artery beyond the inguinal ligament. The use of three fingers not only indicates the location of the artery but also demonstrates its course. If the index finger is spread away from the middle and ring fingers, which are held together, the insertion site is between the index and the middle fingers.
6. Infiltrate the overlying skin with 1% lidocaine without epinephrine if the patient is awake.
7. If the Seldinger technique is used, enter the skin and artery at about a 45° angle. As soon as arterial blood is freely aspirated from the needle, remove the attached syringe, insert the wire through the needle well into the artery, and then remove the needle. If the artery is not entered with the initial attempt, insert the needle deeply until it can go no further through both the anterior and posterior walls of the artery and then slowly withdraw the needle until arterial blood is obtained. Some operators prefer to perform this technique without a syringe attached to the needle, watching for the free pulsation of arterial blood. The wire must pass without any resistance whatsoever to indicate that it is in the lumen of the artery. Inserting the wire

against resistance may lead to intramural insertion or dissection.

8. If the artery is not entered, withdraw the needle completely. Again determine the location of the femoral artery and make another attempt.
9. If the artery is entered with the needle but the wire cannot be passed, remove the needle and maintain pressure over the artery for at least 5 to 10 minutes before the next attempt is made.
10. If the wire passes easily into the artery, remove the needle and insert the catheter over the wire. Then remove the wire from the catheter and attach the connecting tubing to the end of the catheter. Be certain that the guidewire remains visible during these procedures at all times.
11. Suture the catheter in place with 3-0 silk or 4-0 nylon.
12. Cover the insertion site with povidone-iodine ointment and a sterile dressing.
13. If a catheter-over-needle device is used, insert both in the same manner as above. When free arterial flow is obtained through the end of the needle, advance the catheter into the artery while holding the needle in place. Finally, remove the needle. Subsequent care is the same as when the catheter is inserted via the Seldinger method.

Complications

Thrombosis. The larger the catheter used, the greater the incidence of thrombosis. When the femoral artery is used for cardiac catheterization via the Seldinger technique, thrombosis after catheterization may be as high as 1% to 4%.[36-40] Although rare with 19- or 20-gauge catheters,[23,24] thrombosis of the femoral artery may occur in the presence of peripheral vascular disease, after repeated attempts at insertion of catheters into the artery, or after prolonged, excessive pressure to control bleeding after catheter removal.

Embolism. A thrombus that forms about the catheter in the femoral artery may embolize to the lower leg and the foot, producing gangrene.[41] To detect emboli early, the pulses of the femoral, popliteal, posterior tibial, and dorsalis pedis arteries should be checked frequently, ideally with a Doppler flowmeter. If there is evidence of loss of pulses or diminution in peripheral pulses, the femoral artery catheter must be removed.

Hematoma and Hemorrhage. Hematoma is common after removal of the femoral arterial catheter but can be minimized by maintaining pressure over the femoral artery for approximately 10 minutes after removal of the catheter. However, the femoral pulse must not be completely obliterated by pressure since this will predispose the patient to thrombosis.[39,42] Above the inguinal ligament, the femoral artery joins the external iliac artery, which slopes abruptly backward as it ascends. If the artery is punctured above the inguinal ligament, it becomes difficult to tamponade the vessel to control bleeding. Since

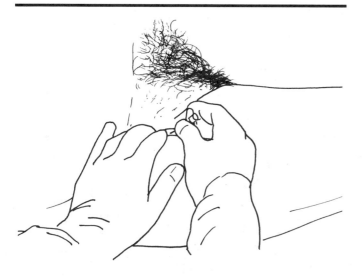

Fig 4. Cannulation of the femoral artery.

the posterior wall of the artery is commonly punctured during insertion, this occurrence may lead to unrecognized retroperitoneal hemorrhage.[40,43]

Arteriovenous Fistula: A fistula between the femoral artery and the femoral vein may be produced, especially with larger catheters such as are used for cardiac catheterization and angiography.[37,40] A false aneurysm ("pseudoaneurysm") may also follow femoral arterial catheterization.

Cannulation of the Axillary Artery

Anatomy

The axillary artery (Fig 5) is a continuation of the subclavian artery as it leaves the root of the neck at the lateral border of the first rib to enter the axilla. As the axillary artery leaves the axilla at the lower border of the teres major muscle, it enters the arm as the brachial artery. The axillary artery, vein, and the three cords of the brachial plexus form a neurovascular bundle within the axillary sheath. Because of the extensive collateral circulation that exists between the thyrocervical trunk of the subclavian artery and the subscapular artery, which is a branch of the distal axillary artery, ligation or thrombosis of the axillary artery usually will not lead to compromise of flow to the distal arm.[44,45] Since the axillary is a large artery (almost the size of the femoral artery) and is close to the aorta, pulsation and pressure are maintained even in the presence of peripheral vascular collapse with marked peripheral vasoconstriction.

Equipment Needed

1. Since the axillary artery may be cannulated with either the Seldinger technique or a catheter-over-needle device, the cannula required depends on the

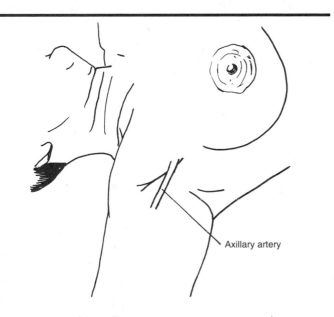

Fig 5. Anatomy of the axillary artery.

method used. For the Seldinger technique, a 19- or 20-gauge Teflon catheter 16 cm long, a flexible guidewire that fits both needle and catheter, and a 20-gauge needle 5 cm long will be necessary. The catheter-over-needle device should have a 20-gauge catheter at least 2½ inches (6.4 cm) long.
2. Other equipment is the same as for other arterial cannulation.

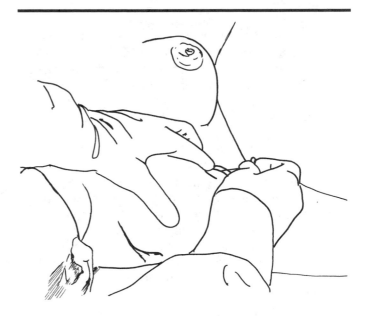

Fig 6. Cannulation of the axillary artery.

Technique[45,46] (Fig 6)

1. Immobilize the arm; it should be hyperabducted and externally rotated more than 90° from the patient's body.
2. Stand at the patient's side, either above or below the abducted arm.
3. Locate the artery within the axilla.
4. Shave and cleanse the skin with povidone-iodine solution.
5. Wear sterile gloves, mask, and hair cover and drape the area with sterile towels.
6. Infiltrate the skin with 1% lidocaine without epinephrine if the patient is awake.
7. Insert the needle into the artery as high as possible within the axilla.
8. If the Seldinger technique is used, once free arterial flow is obtained, pass the wire through the needle into the artery and remove the needle.
9. If the catheter-over-needle device is used, remove the needle and slowly withdraw the catheter once blood appears (indicating that the tip is in the lumen), then advance the catheter into the artery.
10. If after three attempts the artery is not entered, discontinue the procedure on that side and choose another site for arterial puncture.

11. If successful, secure the catheter in place with a 3-0 or 4-0 silk or 4-0 nylon suture.
12. Apply povidone-iodine ointment to the skin at the site of insertion and cover it with a sterile dressing.

Complications

Thrombosis. Because of extensive collateral circulation, thrombosis of the axillary artery should not lead to any ischemic or necrotic sequelae. Moreover, with 19- or 20-gauge catheters, thrombosis is rare.[24,45-47]

Embolism. Although thrombosis of the axillary artery may not lead directly to injury to the distal arm, it is still possible that a thrombus that forms about the catheter tip may embolize to the radial or ulnar circulation. In the absence of adequate collateral flow through the superficial palmar arch, this could produce ischemic injury to the hand.

Since the right axillary artery arises from the right brachiocephalic trunk in direct communication with the common carotid artery, it is quite possible that air, clot, or particulate matter may embolize to the brain during flushing. It may be safer to use the left axillary artery rather than the right, but in either instance, flushing should be performed gently, with minimum volume and with careful attention to prevent the introduction of air or clot into the system. Irrigation with a continuous flow system should be used.

Neurological Complications. During attempts at axillary arterial puncture, direct injury to the cords of the brachial plexus may occur, or an axillary sheath hematoma may lead to nerve compression and injury.[46] The axillary artery, therefore, should not be used for intra-arterial monitoring in patients with bleeding diatheses.

Cannulation of the Brachial Artery

Anatomy

The brachial artery (Fig 7) extends into the arm as a continuation of the axillary artery. It passes down the upper inner arm just under the medial edge of the biceps muscle. In the antecubital fossa, just above the elbow crease, it is easily palpable medial to the biceps tendon and lateral to the median nerve. In the lower part of the antecubital fossa, the brachial artery divides into the radial artery and the ulnar artery. There are anastomoses around the elbow from the inferior ulnar collateral artery above to branches of the ulnar artery below.[44] However, if collateral circulation is inadequate, obstruction of the brachial artery may be catastrophic, leading to loss of the forearm and hand. Therefore, this site should not be used unless other options have greater contraindications.

Equipment Needed

1. A 20-gauge Teflon catheter-over-needle, non-tapered shaft, 1½ to 2 inches (3.8 to 5.1 cm) in length (or a longer 20-gauge catheter may be inserted with the Seldinger technique)
2. Arm board to prevent the arm from flexing at the elbow
3. Other equipment the same as for radial artery cannulation

Technique (Fig 8)

1. Locate brachial artery medial to the biceps tendon above the elbow crease.
2. Cleanse the overlying skin with povidone-iodine solution.
3. Wear sterile gloves (plus mask and hair cover for optimal asepsis) and drape the area with sterile towels.
4. Infiltrate the overlying skin with 1% lidocaine without epinephrine if the patient is awake.
5. Immobilize the artery with two or three fingers.

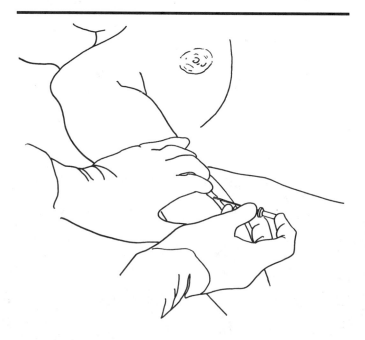

Fig 8. Cannulation of the brachial artery.

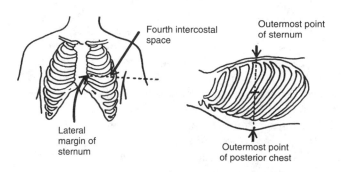

Fig 7. Anatomy of the brachial artery.

Fourth intercostal space

Outermost point of sternum

Lateral margin of sternum

Outermost point of posterior chest

6. Insert the catheter-over-needle device at about a 30° angle to the surface of the skin, and advance the catheter and needle stylet into the artery until blood appears in the hub of the needle.

7. While holding the needle in the fixed position, advance the catheter-over-needle into the artery.

8. Remove the needle and attach the hub of the catheter to connecting tubing.

9. Tie the catheter in place with 3-0 or 4-0 silk or 4-0 nylon sutures.

10. Apply povidone-iodine ointment to the skin at the site of insertion and cover it with a sterile dressing.

11. Make certain that the arm is immobilized to prevent flexion at the elbow.

Complications

Thrombosis and Embolism. Barnes et al[48] reported brachial artery catheterization in 1000 patients with no objective ischemia of the distal arm.[48] However, the duration of catheter placement was not described. The same group reported that of 54 patients who had brachial artery catheterization for 1 to 3 days with an 18-gauge Teflon catheter connected to a continuous flush system, 2 patients had evidence of ulnar artery obstruction and 1 had evidence of radial artery obstruction. Nevertheless, neither of the 2 patients had any symptoms or signs of ischemia of the hand. Another group reported a study of 25 patients in whom an 18-gauge polyethylene catheter was inserted in the brachial artery for an average of 11.5 hours.[18] Angiography, both before catheter removal and 6 months later, revealed a high incidence of early and late vascular abnormalities: 14 of the 25 subjects had absent peripheral pulses and vascular abnormalities after removal of the catheter. Of 11 patients who were studied 6 months later, 4 had evidence of vascular irregularities and narrowing of the brachial artery at the puncture site. They had, nonetheless, regained peripheral pulses.

Neurological Complications. Subfascial bleeding after percutaneous puncture of the artery has been reported[49] in patients on anticoagulant therapy and may lead to median nerve neuropathy and Volkman's contracture. Increasing pain, swelling, or minimal evidence of neuropathy in the area of distribution of the median nerve (such as paresthesias or weakness) are indications for both immediate reversal of anticoagulation treatment and fasciotomy. To prevent this complication, the brachial artery should not be used for cannulation in patients with bleeding diatheses.

Cannulation of the Radial Artery

Anatomy [35]

The radial artery (Fig 9), a branch of the brachial artery, extends down the anterior radial aspect of the forearm where, after sending a branch to the palm, it disappears deep to the abductor pollicis longus tendon just

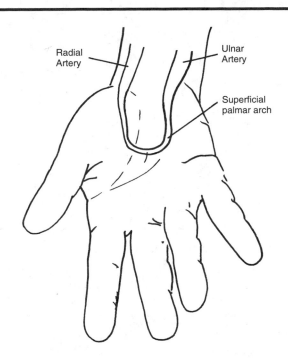

Fig 9. Anatomy of radial and ulnar arteries at wrist and superficial palmar arch.

beyond the distal end of the radius. From there it continues across the floor of the anatomical snuffbox into the dorsum of the hand. At the wrist the radial artery is palpable in a longitudinal groove formed by the tendon of the flexor carpi radialis medially and the distal radius laterally. The ulnar artery, the other major branch of the brachial artery, extends down the ulnar aspect of the forearm to the wrist, where it is sheltered by the tendon of the flexor carpi ulnaris. At the wrist the ulnar artery is palpable just lateral to this tendon. The superficial palmar arch is formed from a continuation of the ulnar artery into the hand; both the deep palmar arch and the dorsal arch are a continuation of the radial artery. Mozersky et al[50] studied 140 hands using a Doppler flow probe and found that the superficial palmar arch was predominantly supplied by the ulnar artery in only 88% of the cases; 12% of the hands had either poor collateral flow or an incomplete palmar arch with no collateral circulation whatsoever.

Assessment of Ulnar Collateral Circulation

Since radial artery cannulation is commonly associated with radial artery thrombosis, continued viability of the hand in such a situation depends on collateral flow via the superficial arch from the ulnar artery. If collateral flow is incomplete or absent, ischemic injury to the hand will follow radial artery thrombosis. It is therefore essential before cannulating a radial artery that the presence of collateral flow be demonstrated.[51] Four methods for determining the presence of collateral circulation are described.

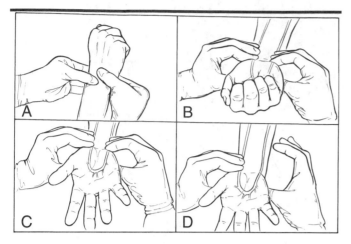

Fig 10. Modified Allen test. While patient's hand is held overhead with fist clenched to exsanguinate it, both radial and ulnar arteries are compressed (A). The hand is lowered (B) and opened (C). Pressure is then released over ulnar artery (D). Color should return to hand within 6 seconds, indicating patent ulnar artery and intact superficial palmar arch.

The Modified Allen Test.[52] The modified Allen test (Fig 10) differs from Allen's original description[53] in 1929 and is performed as follows:

1. If the patient's hands are not warm, they should be immersed in warm water to make pulsations more easily demonstrable.
2. Have the patient open and close his hand, held overhead or out in front, several times to exsanguinate it and then clench the fist tightly closed. If the patient is unconscious or under anesthesia, clench the fist passively for him.
3. Occlude both the radial and the ulnar artery; then have the patient lower and open his hand. When the hand is open, it should be relaxed; hyperextension of the wrist or hand should be avoided since it increases the tension of the palmar fascia, which compresses arterial microcirculation. Failure to relax the hand or hyperextending the hand at the wrist may cause a falsely abnormal Allen test.
4. Release the pressure over the ulnar artery and observe the open hand for return of color. Return within 6 seconds indicates patency of the ulnar artery and an intact arch. Delay of color from 7 to 15 seconds indicates that the ulnar artery filling is slow. Persistent blanching for up to 15 seconds or more indicates an incomplete ulnar arch. Those hands that have delayed or absent return of color with release of ulnar compression should not be used for radial artery cannulation.
5. To test for patency of the radial artery, repeat the test but release pressure over the radial artery instead of the ulnar artery.

Modified Allen Test With Doppler Plethysmography.[50,54] A Doppler instrument can be used to detect patency of the ulnar and radial artery by placing the probe over the artery to be examined. The normal arterial veloc-ity signal is multiphasic, with a prominent systolic component and one or more diastolic sounds. If the artery examined is obstructed, velocity distal to the obstruction is attenuated, with a resultant decrease in the systolic component and loss of the normal diastolic sounds.

The continuity of the palmar arch may be assessed by noting the response of the arterial velocity in either the radial or ulnar artery during a period of compression of the opposite artery. Normally the arterial velocity signal is increased in response to compression of the opposite artery at the wrist. If there is a lack of continuity between the radial and ulnar circulations in the hand, arterial compression will not result in an increase in velocity in the opposite artery. A similar response would result if the artery being compressed were congenitally absent or occluded by disease.

Doppler Assessment of the Superficial Palmar Arch (Fig 11).

1. Place the probe between the heads of the third and fourth metacarpals, acutely angulated in the transverse plane.
2. Advance the probe proximally until maximal signal is obtained. The superficial palmar arch is usually found proximal to a line drawn along the medial edge of the outstretched thumb; the superficial palmar arch is the more distal palmar arch.
3. Compress the radial artery once the arch is identified. If there is no change or an actual increase in the signal following compression, it confirms that the palmar arch is complete and that it could be supplied (to a greater or lesser degree) by the ulnar artery. If the signal disappears when the radial artery is compressed, the arch is incomplete with no antegrade collateral circulation.

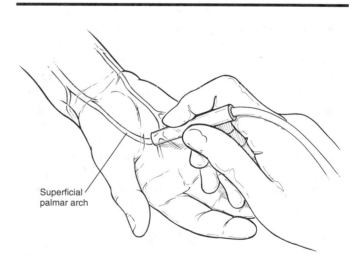

Superficial palmar arch

Fig 11. Assessment of the superficial palmar arch with Doppler instrument.

Method Using Plethysmography.[55]

1. Place a finger pulse transducer over the patient's thumb and observe the resulting pulse contour on an oscilloscope.
2. Compress both the radial and ulnar arteries, which should result in immediate loss of the pulse on the monitor.
3. Release the pressure over the ulnar artery. Normally there is an almost immediate return of the pulse contour on the monitor screen. The presence of pulsations in the thumb while the radial artery is still compressed is evidence of adequate ulnar artery circulation and an indication that the radial artery can be cannulated safely. Failure of the pulse to return after release of compression of the ulnar artery indicates that there is inadequate ulnar collateral circulation and that cannulation of that radial artery should be avoided.

Equipment Needed

1. A 20-gauge Teflon catheter-over-needle with non-tapered shaft 1¼ to 2 inches (3.2 to 5.1 cm) long. An alternative is a commercially prepared radial artery cannulation set that incorporates a guidewire, facilitating use of the Seldinger technique.
2. Short arm board and roll of gauze
3. Povidone-iodine solution
4. Lidocaine 1% without epinephrine and 3-mL syringe with 25-gauge needle
5. Sterile gloves and sterile drapes (face mask and hair cover for optimal asepsis)
6. Fluid-filled connecting tubing to transducer

Technique (Fig 12)

1. The patient's hand should be supported and dorsiflexed at the wrist approximately 60°, with both the hand and the lower forearm secured to a board. A roll of gauze behind the wrist will maintain dorsiflexion.

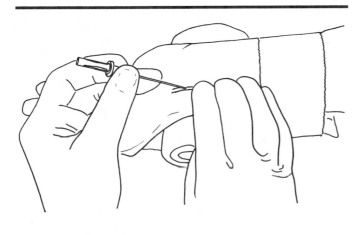

Fig 12. Cannulation of the radial artery.

2. Locate the radial artery just proximal to the head of the radius.
3. Cleanse the area with povidone-iodine solution.
4. Wear sterile gloves and drape the area with sterile towels.
5. Infiltrate the skin over and to the sides of the radial artery with 1% lidocaine without epinephrine if the patient is awake.
6. A small skin incision at the point of insertion may facilitate entry of the catheter-needle device, but with a 20-gauge needle this is usually unnecessary. Insert the catheter-over-needle device at about a 30° angle to the surface of the skin, and advance the catheter and needle stylet into the artery until blood appears in the hub of the needle.
7. While holding the needle in the fixed position, advance the catheter-over-needle into the artery.
8. Remove the needle and attach the hub of the catheter to connecting tubing.
9. Tie the catheter securely in place with 3-0 or 4-0 silk or 4-0 nylon sutures.
10. Remove packing from under the back of the wrist if used, and fix the wrist in a neutral position to the board. This is essential since one or two full flexions of the wrist joint can completely destroy an arterial line, and securing the hand in a dorsiflexed position for a prolonged period may lead to neuromuscular injury to the hand.
11. Apply povidone-iodine ointment to the skin at the site of insertion, and cover with a sterile dressing.

Complications

Thrombosis. Thrombosis is common, occurring in some series in more than 50% of radial artery cannulations.[17,21,25-28,34,56-58] Although the incidence of thrombosis is high, ischemic and necrotic complications are much less common, occurring in fewer than 1% of patients with radial artery cannulas. However, one study group reported persistent ischemic symptoms in the hands of 50% of patients with radial arterial thrombosis.[22] Patients with vasospastic (Raynaud's) disease and those with inadequate ulnar arches frequently exhibit ischemic and necrotic signs and symptoms following cannulation of radial arteries.[20,21,51] If there are frequent small emboli issuing from the site of catheter insertion to the distal vessels of the digits, they may lead to ischemic and necrotic symptoms even in the presence of an intact palmar collateral circulation. Thrombosis may occur several days following catheter removal. Although thrombosis of the radial artery is frequent, patients whose progress has been followed for several months generally show evidence of recanalization.[19,21,51]

To prevent complications that might follow thrombosis of the radial artery, it is important not only to demonstrate adequate ulnar collateral circulation before insertion of the radial catheter but also to monitor the radial artery daily at the site of insertion with a Doppler instrument.

Decreased or absent velocity signals may be due either to the catheter's obstructing flow in the radial artery or, more commonly, to the presence of a thrombus at the site of catheterization. If the Doppler signal is lost or ischemic changes appear, the cannula should be removed.

Spasm has been implicated as a cause of obstruction to flow in the hand and may occur both during cannulation and following removal of the cannula.[1,59] However, Crossland and Neviaser[51] reported that all instances of impaired circulation to the hand following radial artery cannulations were due to thrombosis rather than to spasm. Following catheter removal, if flow does not return to the hand after 1 hour, the artery should be explored for probable thrombectomy.[51,60] The radial pulse may still be palpable distal to a complete occlusion. In one series with a complete occlusion, the distal pulse was palpable in 64% of the research subjects, and 10% had a radial pulse equal to the opposite radial pulses.[27]

Embolism. Embolism, both distally and cephalad, occurs less commonly than thrombosis. Although distal emboli may be demonstrated with angiography in as many as 25% of patients after radial artery cannulation, objective and symptomatic digital ischemia is uncommon.[19,26,51,61] Whereas thrombosis with inadequate collateral flow to the hand is manifested by a pale or cold hand, emboli commonly produce cold and purple spots on the digits. These symptoms usually clear within approximately 1 week but may lead to digital gangrene, necessitating the amputation of fingers or, rarely, the entire hand.

Vigorous flushing with large volumes of flushing solution, especially when trying to correct a partially obstructed catheter with a damped arterial tracing, may allow the flushing solution to reach the central circulation and lead to either air or small-clot embolism in the brain. Lowenstein et al[61] showed that it took only 7 mL of fluid vigorously flushed as a bolus into a radial catheter to reach the central circulation of the aortic arch. The volume of flushed solution correlated with arm length and patient height. If intermittent flushing is performed, it is recommended that meticulous care be used to avoid introducing any air bubbles into the system and that no more than 2 mL of solution be flushed at any one time, and then at a relatively slow rate. Since a continuous flow system delivers approximately 1.5 mL/s when the flush valve is open, flushes should be restricted to 2 seconds or less.[30,61,62]

Necrosis of Overlying Skin. Necrosis of the skin proximal to the site of insertion may also occur. The blood supply to the skin of the distal forearm arises directly from small branches of the radial artery without any collateral circulation. If the tip of the catheter interferes with these small branches, ischemia to the overlying skin may follow.[63,64] If temporarily localized blanching of the skin appears with intermittent flushing, the tip of the catheter should be repositioned until blanching no longer occurs. The following steps should be used to decrease the incidence of skin necrosis:

1. The most distal site possible should be chosen for radial artery cannulation.
2. The smallest catheter size possible should be used to cause the least amount of obstruction of the lumen.
3. Prolonged cannulation should be avoided to prevent propagation of a thrombus from the catheter itself.

Aneurysm. Mathieu et al[65] reported an aneurysm of the radial artery in a patient cannulated with an 18-gauge catheter. The catheter, which was inserted after repeated attempts at puncture, remained in place for 10 days; 18 days after removal of the catheter, an aneurysm of the radial artery was noted. It was repaired without sequelae.

Cannulation of the Dorsalis Pedis Artery

Anatomy

The dorsalis pedis artery (Fig 13) extends subcutaneously as a continuation of the anterior tibial artery down the dorsum of the foot parallel and lateral to the extensor hallucis longus tendon. The lateral plantar artery, which is the terminal branch of the posterior tibial artery, is the other major artery supplying the foot. In most persons it supplies collateral flow via the main arterial arch of the foot, which is analogous to the palmar arch of the hand.

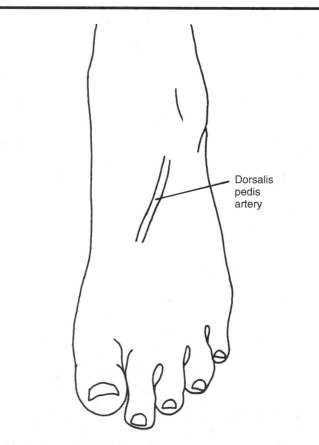

Dorsalis pedis artery

Fig 13. Anatomy of the dorsalis pedis artery.

However, in approximately 12% of the population, the dorsalis pedis artery is absent, usually bilaterally.[66-69]

Demonstration of Collateral Flow

Before cannulating the dorsalis pedis artery, it must be determined that adequate collateral flow to the distal foot is present. The foot should be warm, and immersion in water may be necessary. The simple procedure, which is analogous to the Allen test, follows:

1. Occlude the dorsalis pedis artery; then blanch the great toe by compressing the toenail for several seconds.
2. Release pressure on the nail and observe for flushing. A rapid return of color indicates adequate collateral flow.[67]

A Doppler flowmeter may also be used to assess flow in both the dorsalis pedis artery and the posterior tibial artery.[70]

Equipment Needed

1. A 20-gauge Teflon catheter-over-needle device with a nontapered shaft approximately 1½ inches (3.8 cm) long
2. Other equipment as for radial artery cannulation

Technique (Fig 14)

1. Check for presence of a dorsalis pedis artery pulse and for presence of adequate collateral flow as previously defined.
2. Cleanse the overlying skin with povidone-iodine solution.

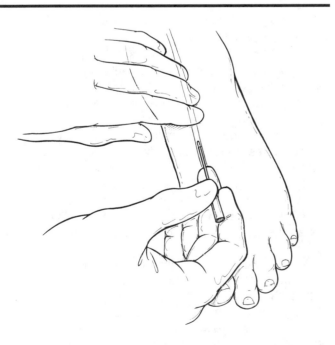

Fig 14. Cannulation of the dorsalis pedis artery.

3. Wear sterile gloves and drape the area with sterile towels.
4. Infiltrate the overlying skin with 1% lidocaine without epinephrine if the patient is awake.
5. Insert the catheter as for radial arterial cannulation.
6. Suture the catheter to the skin with 3-0 or 4-0 silk or 4-0 nylon.
7. Cover the insertion site with povidone-iodine ointment and a sterile dressing.
8. Tape the line to the catheter firmly to the foot.

Complication

Thrombosis.[70] Thrombosis may occur in approximately 7% of those arteries cannulated. It can be recognized during cannulation by noting blanching of the great and second toes lasting longer than 15 seconds with compression of the posterior tibial artery. Occlusion can be confirmed with the Doppler technique by demonstrating retrograde flow distal to the site of cannula insertion in the dorsalis pedis artery and with loss of the signal upon occlusion of the posterior tibial artery.

Bedside Pulmonary Artery Catheterization

Catheterization of the pulmonary artery can be performed easily and rapidly at the bedside using a balloon-tipped flow-directed thermodilution catheter. Continuous monitoring of the intravascular waveform allows the operator to follow the course of the catheter through the right heart and into the pulmonary artery to the wedge position. Although in a large number of patients this can be done without fluoroscopy, access to a fluoroscope is advised.

Indications[71-76]

There are several general indications for pulmonary artery catheterization in critically ill patients. These include the need to

1. Measure right atrial, pulmonary arterial, and pulmonary artery occlusive pressures (PAOP) or wedge pressures
2. Measure cardiac output by thermodilution (cardiac output also can be determined by the indocyanine green indicator dilution technique, with injection from either the right atrium or the pulmonary artery and sampling from a peripheral artery)
3. Sample pulmonary arterial (mixed venous) blood

With the data derived from the above measurements, one can evaluate both right and left ventricular function. This includes defining hemodynamic subsets,[77] separating cardiogenic from noncardiogenic pulmonary edema, diagnosing acute mitral regurgitation[77] and ruptured intraventricular septum,[78] and determining the response to therapeutic interventions with serial measurements.

Rationale

In the past, left heart filling or occlusive pressure was estimated from the level of central venous pressure, clinical examination, and chest x-ray; cardiac output from mixed venous oxygen saturation or content; and intrapulmonary shunt from the difference between calculated alveolar and the measured arterial oxygen tensions, ie, $P_{AO_2} - P_{aO_2}$ with A = alveolar and a = arterial. Direct measurement is more accurate. The following section will develop the rationale for pulmonary artery catheterization, which is based on the following principle: if one needs to know PAOP, cardiac output, or intrapulmonary shunt, each must be measured. Pulmonary artery catheterization allows this to be done.

Measurement of Occlusive Pressure

The level of the PAOP is a determinant of pulmonary congestion and the transfer of fluid from the pulmonary capillary bed to the interstitial space and alveoli. Measurement of PAOP allows one to differentiate between different causes of pulmonary edema and to monitor the physiological response to fluid.[79,80] In the absence of either mechanical ventilation with positive end-expiratory pressure (PEEP) or obstruction in the pulmonary veins, PAOP closely approximates left atrial mean pressure within ±2 mm Hg. In the absence of obstruction at the mitral valve, such as occurs with mitral stenosis or left atrial myxoma, PAOP also closely approximates mean left ventricular diastolic pressure.[81] However, in the presence of elevated left ventricular end-diastolic pressure (the height of ventricular filling pressure just before ventricular contraction) caused either by an increase in end-diastolic volume or a decrease in left ventricular compliance, PAOP does not as accurately reflect left ventricular end-diastolic pressure, which may significantly exceed mean PAOP. The height of the pulmonary artery A wave or the pulmonary capillary A wave, if recorded, is the most consistently accurate indirect index for sudden changes in actual left ventricular end-diastolic pressure.[82,83] Nevertheless, the PAOP reflects mean left ventricular diastolic pressure and is therefore a useful index to estimate not only the possible risk of the development of pulmonary edema[79,83] but also left ventricular preload. On the other hand, preload is defined as end-diastolic volume, not pressure. In critically ill patients, ventricular compliance is altered, and there may be no correlation between pressure and volume, making it impossible to estimate left ventricular preload from PAOP.[84,85]

In the absence of marked tachycardia or pulmonary vascular disease, pulmonary artery diastolic pressure is equivalent to PAOP with the PA diastolic pressure exceeding the PAOP by no more than 5 mm Hg. In this case both reflect mean left ventricular filling pressure. By comparing pulmonary artery diastolic pressure with mean PAOP, it can be determined whether pulmonary vascular disease (with elevated pulmonary vascular resistance) is present and whether pulmonary artery diastolic pressure will reliably reflect mean left ventricular filling pressure. If the pulmonary artery diastolic pressure and the PAOP differ by less than 5 mm Hg, the pulmonary artery diastolic pressure may be used to monitor mean left ventricular diastolic pressure. This may be especially important when the balloon ceases to function and PAOP can no longer be obtained. Unfortunately, increased pulmonary vascular resistance is common among the critically ill, and this approximation frequently cannot be used.

In the presence of acute mitral regurgitation with the transmission of the large V wave into the pulmonary capillary and pulmonary arterial bed (Fig 15), mean PAOP pressure may exceed pulmonary artery diastolic pressure.[86] However, this would be detected by the presence of a large V wave on the downslope of the pulmonary artery pressure tracing or on the PAOP tracing. In this circumstance, the Z point (the pressure immediately after the A wave) will correlate best with left atrial pressure.[87] If PAOP exceeds PA diastolic pressure and a large V wave is absent, care must be taken to determine that one is actually measuring PAOP pressure rather than mean or damped pulmonary artery pressure (Fig 16) or a pseudo-occlusive pressure (Fig 22).

Central venous or right atrial pressure can be measured by inserting a catheter into the superior vena cava or right atrium. Before the advent of pulmonary artery flotation catheters, central venous pressure frequently was used to estimate left ventricular filling pressures. However, Forrester et al[88] showed that in patients with acute myocardial infarction, central venous pressure does not reflect left ventricular filling pressure. The level of central venous pressure correlates poorly with both the level of PAOP and radiological evidence of left ventricular failure. Furthermore, directional changes in central venous pressure are often of no value in following the results of acute blood volume manipulation. Several factors increase central venous pressure.[89] The major determinants are pumping effectiveness of the right heart (central venous pressure is elevated with right ventricular failure) and increased venous return caused by either decreased resistance to blood flow from the arteries to the veins or an increased ratio of blood volume to vascular blood-holding capacity. Elevation of pressures outside the myocardium, such as cardiac tamponade, positive-pressure breathing, pneumothorax, or obstructive pulmonary disease, increases central venous pressure as well.

In the presence of normal right heart function, acute deterioration of left ventricular function will not be reflected by a change in the central venous pressure. In critically ill patients there may be no correlation between central venous pressure and PAOP: PAOP may change while central venous pressure remains unchanged or moves in the opposite direction. This suggests that there may be discrepancies in function between the right and left sides of the heart in such patients.[90-92]

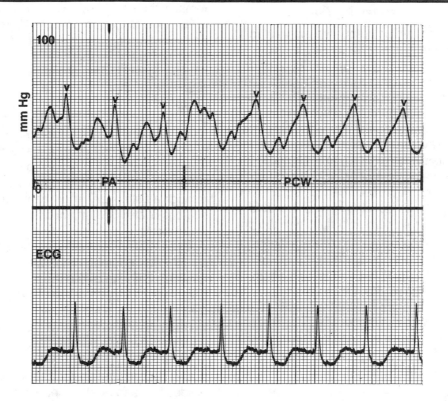

Fig 15. V waves in acute mitral regurgitation. V wave can be seen immediately following systolic pulmonary artery (PA) waveform but is more prominent on PAOP (PCW) waveform. The second wave in PA tracing can be identified as V wave; it peaks at same time, following R wave of ECG (0.4 second), as V wave on wedge tracing. Mean PAOP is higher than PA diastolic pressure.

There are limitations to the use of chest radiographs in predicting the hemodynamic status of patients with acute myocardial infarction.[93,94] There is a good correlation between the level of PAOP and the development of interstitial and alveolar pulmonary edema, both occurring as PAOP rises above 20 to 25 mm Hg (an exception is dilated cardiomyopathy). However, there may be a significant delay of up to 12 hours between the onset of elevation of the occlusive pressure and clinical and radiological evidence of pulmonary edema. There may also be a signifi-

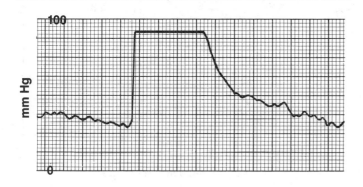

Fig 16. Damped pulmonary artery pressure tracing and damped square wave response during rapid flushing with continuous flush system.

cant lag between the lowering of occlusive pressure and the clearing of pulmonary edema on x-ray film. This lag may persist as long as 4 days. These delays in appearance and clearing of pulmonary edema on chest x-ray films are probably related to the fact that during the acute phase of myocardial infarction the hemodynamics change rapidly. It may take several hours for enough edema fluid to accumulate to be visible on chest x-ray film and several days for the fluid to be resorbed.[93,94]

Even the clinical examination may fail to separate patients whose PAOP is high from those whose occlusive pressure is low. In one study, 39% of patients who developed hypotension during the course of acute myocardial infarction were found to have low PAOP.[95] Yet a third of these patients with low occlusive pressure had third heart sounds on physical examination, and two thirds had abnormal pulmonary findings on chest x-ray film, including pulmonary vascular redistribution and frank pulmonary edema. Since the therapy in these patients was to expand the blood volume, treatment directed toward pulmonary edema based on the findings of the clinical examination would have been inappropriate. Because of the difficulty in estimating the PAOP even under stable circumstances, in the unstable situation, especially when rapidly activating vasoactive agents are being used, serial measurement of the PAOP is essential.

The Need for Measuring Cardiac Output

Extreme reductions of cardiac output are manifested by signs of tissue hypoperfusion; hypotension may or may not be present. However, significant reduction of cardiac output may occur without these clinical findings and with the reading of a normal blood pressure. Blood pressure is the product of cardiac output and systemic vascular resistance; as cardiac output falls, blood pressure may be maintained by an elevation of systemic vascular resistance. In some patients systemic vascular resistance becomes markedly elevated so that blood pressure is high despite a significantly decreased cardiac output. On the other hand, a patient may develop hypotension and still have a markedly elevated cardiac output, with the primary defect being a fall in systemic vascular resistance. Only by knowing left ventricular filling pressure, cardiac output, and calculated systemic vascular resistance can one rationally develop a therapeutic program.

The mixed venous O_2 content is commonly used to follow changes in cardiac output. According to the Fick principle, cardiac output (CO) is equal to oxygen consumption (VO_2) divided by the arteriovenous oxygen content difference [$C(a-v)O_2$].

$$CO = \frac{VO_2}{C(a-v)O_2}$$

As long as oxygen consumption and the arterial oxygen content remain constant, the level of mixed venous oxygen content may accurately reflect the arteriovenous oxygen content difference and, hence, cardiac output. However, there may be conditions other than changes in cardiac output that alter the mixed venous oxygen content.

The oxygen content of blood is primarily a function of the hemoglobin concentration and oxygen saturation. With depression of either the hemoglobin or the oxygen saturation of arterial blood, arterial oxygen content will be reduced. If oxygen consumption and cardiac output are stable according to the Fick relationship, arteriovenous oxygen content difference must also remain constant. Yet mixed venous oxygen content will be lower in this situation as well, independent of changes in cardiac output. For example, if arterial oxygen content (Cao_2) is reduced from 20 to 15 vol%, and $C(a-v)O_2$, cardiac output, and oxygen consumption remain the same, mixed venous content (C_vO_2) will decrease by 5 vol% as well. Thus, in the absence of a change in cardiac output (or oxygen consumption), the fall in C_vO_2 would suggest that cardiac output had fallen when in fact the only change may have been due to a fall in arterial oxygen content, ie, a change due to a decrease in either hemoglobin or oxygen saturation.

On the other hand, patients may have changes in oxygen consumption caused by fever, seizures, shivering, or agitation as well as by excessive circulating catecholamines. According to the Fick equation, if cardiac output

remains the same and oxygen consumption increases, arteriovenous oxygen content difference must increase and mixed venous oxygen content will fall. In conclusion, while simply following the mixed venous oxygen content may be helpful, it may also give misleading information regarding cardiac output.

Use of central venous oxygen content instead of mixed venous oxygen content in critically ill patients with shock or heart failure also introduces significant error, since there is a poor correlation in these patients between the level of mixed venous oxygen content and central venous oxygen content.[96,97] Obtaining mixed venous blood through a pulmonary artery catheter eliminates most sources of error that might arise, unless a left-to-right shunt exists.

If the goal of fluid resuscitation is to achieve an adequate cardiac output, PAOP alone cannot be considered a reliable guide to define the end point of resuscitation, and cardiac output must be measured. Nevertheless, the measurement of PAOP is important because it will detect the early onset of congestive heart failure or fluid overload[98-100] and guide the determination of optimal fluid administration. A ventricular function curve can be drawn during volume loading if stroke work index (cardiac output divided by heart rate) is measured at different levels of PAOP (Fig 17). The occlusive pressure that provides the best stroke volume then can be determined ("optimal filling pressure").[101,102]

One other pitfall must be described. The thermodilution technique measures the output of the right side of the heart, which is normally equal to that of the left. However, in the presence of an intracardiac shunt, right ventricular output does not equal left ventricular output; considerable error is introduced in assuming that thermodilution car-

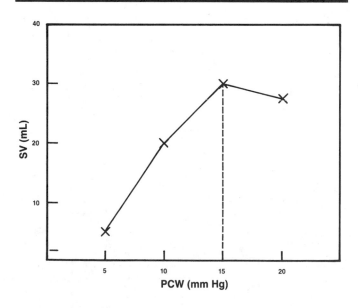

Fig 17. Ventricular function curve. Optimal filling pressure (dotted line) is PAOP (PCW) that produces highest stroke volume (SV).

diac output reflects systemic flow. Fortunately one can determine the fraction of left-to-right or right-to-left shunt according to standard formulas and can correct the value for thermodilution cardiac output with this fraction to obtain systemic cardiac output.[76]

The Need for Measuring Intrapulmonary Shunt (Q_s/Q_t)

The difference between the calculated alveolar oxygen tension and the measured arterial oxygen tension ($P_{AO_2} - P_{aO_2}$) has been commonly used as an indicator of the magnitude of venous mixture and intrapulmonary shunting. Only if mixed venous oxygen content is normal will the alveolar arterial oxygen tension difference correlate with intrapulmonary shunt. In critically ill patients, mixed venous oxygen content cannot be assumed to be normal, and the alveolar-arterial oxygen difference may reflect changes in mixed venous oxygen content rather than changes in intrapulmonary shunt.

The mixture that is pumped from the left ventricle is blood that is fully oxygenated as it passes through ventilated alveoli and mixed venous blood that bypasses ventilated alveoli through right-to-left shunts (Fig 18). Any condition that increases intrapulmonary shunting will lower the arterial oxygen content and thereby increase the $P_{AO_2} - P_{aO_2}$.

Approximately 5% of right ventricular output is normally shunted from right to left through the lungs. If mixed venous blood is markedly desaturated with a low oxygen content, even moderate amounts of this very desaturated

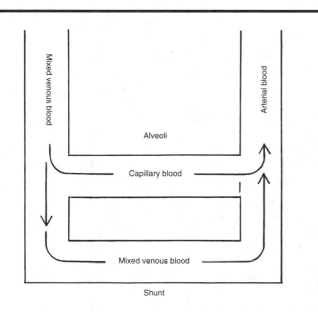

Fig 18. Mixed venous blood perfusing functioning alveolar units equilibrates with alveolar oxygen (capillary blood), but mixed venous blood that passes through intrapulmonary shunts is unchanged (mixed venous blood). Arterial blood is mixture of capillary blood and shunted mixed venous blood. Oxygen tension and content of arterial blood are therefore determined by both volume (quantity) and oxygen content (quality) of capillary blood and shunt blood.

blood passing through normal anatomic shunts (or slightly increased physiological shunts) will contaminate fully oxygenated blood and lower the arterial oxygen content. This will also cause a widened alveolar-arterial oxygen difference. If one assumes that the widened $P_{AO_2} - P_{aO_2}$ is due to a large right-to-left intrapulmonary shunt when actually it is due to mixed venous blood with a markedly lowered oxygen content bypassing alveoli through normal or slightly increased shunts, therapy directed toward intrapulmonary shunting (such as PEEP) would be inappropriate and perhaps deleterious. Therefore, if it is necessary to know the magnitude of the intrapulmonary shunt for optimal therapy, it must be calculated. For the calculation, mixed venous oxygen content must be measured. Using an assumed arteriovenous oxygen content difference to determine the mixed venous oxygen content without actual measurement should be avoided since it will introduce a significant error in the shunt calculation.[103]

Technique

The following discussion includes a description of the catheter itself, the technique of insertion, and pitfalls and complications of pulmonary artery catheterization.

Description of the Pulmonary Artery Catheter

Both 5F and 7F radiopaque pulmonary artery catheters are available, but the standard thermodilution catheter for adults is made only in 7F size. This thermodilution catheter is 100 cm long and is marked with black rings at 10-cm intervals measured from the tip. It contains three lumens and a wire. The distal lumen terminates at the tip of the catheter and is used for measuring pulmonary artery pressure and PAOP and for blood sampling. A proximal lumen terminates approximately 30 cm from the tip of the catheter and is used for injecting the thermal bolus into the right atrium for thermodilution cardiac output, for measuring right atrial or central venous pressure, for fluid and drug administration, and for blood sampling. A third lumen terminates in a balloon near the catheter tip. The balloon is inflated with 1.25 to 1.50 mL air. This distention facilitates advancement of the catheter during insertion and allows measurement of PAOP once the catheter is in the pulmonary artery. The wire terminates in a thermistor bead 3.5 to 4.0 cm proximal to the tip and provides electrical connections between the thermistor and the cardiac output computer. This thermistor allows continuous measurement of pulmonary artery blood temperature (body core temperature) as well as measurement of cardiac output by thermodilution. Many of the catheters require a specific computer for determining cardiac output by thermodilution, although some function with cardiac output computers of different manufacturers. Catheters made by different manufacturers may vary slightly, and the reader is advised to consult the package insert for the catheter being used.

Recently 7.5F catheters have become available with either an additional right atrial lumen for fluid administration or a right ventricular lumen for fluid administration, pressure monitoring, or passing a probe for pacing the right ventricle.

Equipment Needed for Insertion

The following equipment is needed for catheterization:

1. Pulmonary artery catheter
2. Two three-way stopcocks to connect to the proximal right atrial and the distal pulmonary arterial ports
3. Pressure monitoring lines to be connected to the transducer
4. Syringe for balloon inflation
5. Equipment for percutaneous catheter sheath insertion or cutdown
6. Sterile gowns, drapes, gloves, mask, and hair cover
7. Transducer/oscilloscope equipment

Preparation

If the patient is on mechanical ventilation before catheter insertion, the ventilatory settings and alarms should be checked, the connecting tubing emptied of water, and the trachea suctioned. Since insertion of the pulmonary artery catheter may cause cardiac arrhythmias, an IV line must be in place. Lidocaine, atropine, and a defibrillator must be available at the bedside, and the patient should be monitored continuously with an ECG. The transducer and connecting tubing should be set up, the transducer leveled, and the electrical equipment tested, zeroed, and calibrated before the catheter is inserted.

Careful preparation of the area of insertion with povidone-iodine solution, as for any other surgical procedure, should be performed. Since the catheter may remain in the patient for several days, strict attention to aseptic technique during insertion is vital to minimizing later infection. The operator and assistants should be fully gowned and should wear hair covers, face masks, and sterile gloves. In addition, once the area of insertion is adequately prepared with antiseptic solution, the largest possible area should be draped. This generally includes most of the bed on which the patient is lying. Such meticulous preparation allows the operator to have a large sterile area on which to keep all equipment and to test the catheter. It also minimizes the chance of contamination of the long, coiled catheter during insertion.

Site of Insertion

The pulmonary artery catheter may be inserted percutaneously via an insertion sheath through either the internal jugular vein, the subclavian vein, or the femoral vein. It can also be inserted through a cutdown into a median basilic vein in the antecubital fossa. The choice of site of insertion depends on the skill and preference of the operator as well as the urgency of the situation. As a rule,

percutaneous catheter insertion can be performed in less time than venous cutdown. However, the use of the venous cutdown avoids the hazards of pneumothorax and hemorrhage that exist with internal jugular or subclavian insertions. The major difficulty with insertion of the catheter through a cutdown in the antecubital fossa is that the catheter tends to become dislodged more easily with motion of the arm, requiring the patient's arm to be restrained. Venous cutdowns have been advocated by some for cardiovascular patients who have just received a thrombolytic agent.[104]

If the catheter is inserted through the femoral vein, it has to traverse a long distance before arriving at the right heart, and it tends to become deflected by the various veins entering the inferior vena cava. In addition, the femoral approach may place the patient at greater risk for catheter-related infection. If the femoral approach is used, careful skin preparation and attention to aseptic technique should minimize the risk of infection, as with other sites of insertion.

Testing of the Catheter Before Insertion

Once the insertion site has been prepared and the patient and the bed are draped, the catheter should be removed from its container, using sterile technique. With some cardiac output computers, the thermistor can be tested by connecting the catheter connector cable from the cardiac output computer to the thermistor attachment at the end of the catheter. Either the ambient room temperature will be displayed on the computer or an indicator for thermistor continuity will appear. Since the products of various manufacturers differ, the operator must be familiar with his or her own equipment.

The balloon is tested by inflating it to the recommended inflation volume. For general purposes, testing should be with air, but if there is a possibility of right-to-left shunt within the heart, carbon dioxide should be used. Never use liquid for balloon inflation. To be certain there are no leaks in the balloon, it can be inflated under water. If air bubbles appear around the balloon, the catheter should be discarded. A three-way stopcock should be attached to both the right atrial or CvP (proximal) and pulmonary artery (distal) lumen, and pressure monitoring lines attached to the stopcocks and to the transducers. Both lumens should be flushed with sterile saline solution containing 2 to 4 U of heparin per milliliter so that fluid remains in the catheter and the lumens are free of air bubbles.

Inserting the Catheter

Several principles should be followed in catheter insertion. To avoid damage to the catheter or the balloon when inserting it through a cutdown, use a vessel dilator or disposable vein guide. Never use forceps on the catheter. To avoid damaging the balloon during percutaneous insertions through a catheter introducer, use an 8F catheter sheath for the 7F pulmonary artery catheter. Some manufacturers, however, provide catheters with a tapered tip that can be passed through an introducer that is the same French size as the catheter. Consult the specific instructions for each catheter. During insertion the balloon should be fully inflated when the catheter is in the right ventricle; this will minimize ventricular irritability. Do not exceed the recommended volume for balloon inflation because balloon rupture can result. Always deflate the balloon before withdrawing the catheter to avoid damage to intracardiac structures.

To determine the distance of insertion before reaching the level of the superior vena cava and the right atrium, use surface markers as illustrated in Fig 16, chapter 11. The distance from the tip of the catheter to the point of skin insertion can be noted using the markers on the catheter for every 10-cm length. Generally if the catheter is inserted from the internal jugular or the subclavian vein, it should be in the right atrium after about 15 to 20 cm. If the catheter is inserted from the arm, the right atrium should be reached after advancing the catheter approximately 40 cm if from the right antecubital fossa and 50 cm if from the left.

Introduce the catheter by cutdown or percutaneously through a suitable sheath. As the catheter approaches the central circulation either from above or from below, it may be helpful to partially inflate the balloon with approximately half the recommended volume to facilitate its passage.

While monitoring the pressure waveform from the distal lumen, gently advance the catheter into the vena cava and the right atrium. Once the catheter is in the right atrium, inflate the balloon to its full volume. With continuous waveform monitoring, advance the catheter carefully through the right atrium into the right ventricle, into the pulmonary artery, and to the pulmonary artery wedge position (Fig 19).

When the catheter is in the vena cava, the waveform is usually relatively damped. If the patient is asked to cough, there should be an abrupt increase in pressure, indicating that the catheter tip is within the veins of the thorax. When the catheter enters the right atrium, the amplitude of the waveform should be unchanged, but venous waves should still be recognized. As the catheter passes the tricuspid valve and enters the right ventricle, there is an abrupt increase in systolic pressure that falls rapidly toward zero and then plateaus before the next abrupt rise with systole. The diastolic waveform in the right ventricle looks like a square root sign. When the catheter enters the pulmonary artery, the systolic pressure remains the same (in the absence of obstruction at the pulmonic valve), but the waveform is that of an arterial pressure with a dicrotic notch and a gradual fall during diastole before the next abrupt upstroke. The diastolic pressure is higher in the pulmonary artery than in the right ventricle. When the catheter reaches the occlusive position, the waveform should again become damped with the appearance of a and V waves; the mean PAOP should be equal to or less than pulmonary artery diastolic pressure. Once the proper position is reached, the balloon should be deflated, at which time the waveform should be equal to or less than pulmonary artery diastolic pressure. When the balloon is deflated, the waveform should abruptly change from that of the occlusive pressure to that of the pulmonary artery.

The following are criteria to confirm proper position:

1. The ability to flush the catheter before inflating the balloon, which excludes the possibility of catheter obstruction
2. The disappearance of the typical pulmonary artery pressure tracing when the balloon is inflated and its reappearance promptly after deflation
3. The presence of a PAOP lower than or equal to pulmonary artery diastolic pressure[105]
4. Oxygen tension or saturation of blood drawn from the occlusive position greater than or equal to that of systemic arterial blood

In the average-sized adult, if the catheter is inserted from the internal jugular or the subclavian vein, the pulmonary artery should be entered after about 50 cm of the catheter has been inserted; if from the arm or the femoral vein, the pulmonary artery should be entered after about 70 cm of catheter has been inserted. Insertion of the catheter beyond this length without reaching the

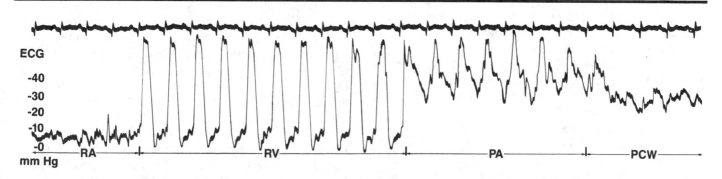

Fig 19. Pressure waveforms recorded as pulmonary artery catheter is advanced through right atrium (RA) and right ventricle (RV) into pulmonary artery (PA) and to PAOP (PCW) position.

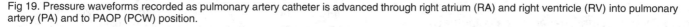

pulmonary artery suggests that the catheter is coiling up either in the right atrium or the right ventricle. If the pulmonary artery is not entered, deflate the balloon and withdraw the catheter back to the right atrium. Since the 7F catheter has a preformed curve to the tip, it is important to insert the catheter with the curve pointing in such a way as to easily pass through the right atrium and the right ventricle and into the pulmonary artery.

Once the occlusive position has been reached, alternately inflate and deflate the balloon and position the catheter so that a PAOP waveform can be obtained with full inflation of the balloon. Always inflate the balloon slowly while monitoring the waveform, and stop inflation once wedge waveform appears. Inflation beyond this point may lead to pulmonary artery rupture.

In conditions of low-output state, tricuspid regurgitation, or pulmonary hypertension, it may be difficult to pass the catheter into the pulmonary artery. On occasion, having the patient take deep breaths will facilitate the passage of the catheter; if unsuccessful, fluoroscopy may be needed.

As the catheter remains in the vascular compartment, it softens. At times it may be necessary to flush the catheter with cold solution to stiffen it and make passage easier. In addition, if several attempts at passage are unsuccessful, it may be necessary to remove and replace the catheter.

Cardiac arrhythmias that appear during insertion of the catheter usually disappear once the catheter is withdrawn from that chamber or passed through that chamber into the next. Arrhythmias most commonly occur when the catheter is in the right ventricle. When the catheter is in this position, the balloon must be inflated so that the catheter tip is completely covered, reducing the likelihood of stimulating the right ventricular endocardium and producing cardiac arrhythmias. If the arrhythmia does not cease following withdrawal of the catheter, drug therapy or countershock may have to be used. In addition, transient right bundle branch block may occur as the catheter tip passes through the right ventricle. This condition can be especially hazardous in a patient who has preexisting left bundle branch block since it may cause complete heart block.[106] In such patients it is prudent to insert a temporary transvenous pacing catheter or to establish standby transcutaneous cardiac pacing before attempting insertion of a pulmonary artery catheter. In these situations fluoroscopy is mandatory.

Once the catheter is in place in the pulmonary artery, secure the catheter with suture. If a catheter sheath introducer was used, it may have to be pulled back, although now sheaths are made with side ports and can be left in place if fluid is continuously infused via the port. Each time the catheter or sheath is manipulated and while the catheter is being secured, reconfirm that PAOP can be obtained to ensure that the catheter has not been moved. As soon as the catheter is secured, obtain a chest x-ray film to document the location of the catheter tip. This procedure will exclude the presence of pneumothorax or

other complications if the insertion was by way of the internal jugular or subclavian technique. If the catheter was inserted from the arm, immobilize the arm.

The pulmonary artery waveform must be continuously monitored so that inadvertent wedging can be recognized immediately and the catheter withdrawn. Failure to withdraw the catheter from an occlusive position may lead to pulmonary infarction.

After the catheter has been in place for some time, if the tip has slipped back toward the pulmonic valve so that occlusive pressures can no longer be obtained, do not advance the catheter. Bacteria may be introduced from either that part of the catheter outside the patient or from the skin insertion site itself. Recently special catheter sleeves have been developed that are said to allow the catheter to be repositioned aseptically. There is little data to provide reassurance that repositioning of a catheter, especially after 24 to 48 hours, can be accomplished aseptically with the sleeves.

Pitfalls[107]

Although a specific numerical value relating to either intravascular pressure or cardiac output can be obtained with hemodynamic monitoring, one must continually be wary of the error within the system. Such error can be introduced at many points — from the transducer, the connecting tubing, the catheter itself, the balloon, the location of the catheter tip within the chest, or the effects of changes in intrathoracic pressure. Several of these pitfalls will be discussed in the following section.

The Transducer

The transducer must be calibrated frequently using a mercury manometer with a sterile connector. It should be calibrated at least before each use and perhaps daily while in use. The dome must be screwed on tightly to ensure contact between the dome and the transducer diaphragm. The fluid-filled system must be completely free of air.

Zero Reference Point

The level of the right atrium is the standard zero reference point for the transducer. The level of the right atrium, or the phlebostatic axis (Fig 20), is defined as the junction between the transverse plane of the body passing through the fourth intercostal space at the lateral margin of the sternum and a frontal plane of the body passing through the midpoint of a line from the outermost point of the sternum to the outermost point of the posterior chest.[109,110] With the patient supine, this is the midaxillary line. In a position other than supine, the transducer can be zeroed at the phlebostatic level (a plane that rotates about the phlebostatic axis as the patient moves from a flat to an erect position). The phlebostatic level passes through the axis and is parallel with the horizon. If the transducer is zeroed at this phlebostatic level, there

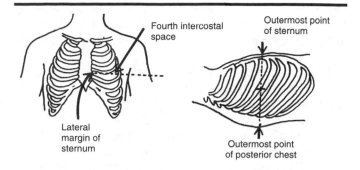

Fig 20. Level of right atrium, or phlebostatic axis, is the junction between transverse plane of body passing through fourth intercostal space at lateral margin of sternum and a frontal plane of body passing through midpoint of line from outermost point of sternum to outermost point of posterior chest. Adapted from Woods and Mansfield.[108]

should be no significant change in pressures measured with the patient being either supine or erect (Fig 21). However, a study defining the effect of body position on pulmonary artery pressure and PAOP demonstrated that there is little change in pressures when the patient is either supine or elevated to 45°; but when the patient is erect with legs dangling over the edge of the bed, there may be a slight decrease in intravascular pressures as measured at the phlebostatic axis.[108] Nevertheless, the difference in pressure between the supine position and the erect sitting position may be only 1 or 2 mm Hg.

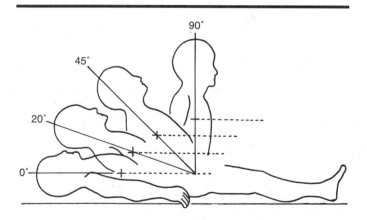

Fig 21. Phlebostatic level (. . . . .) passes through phlebostatic axis (+) and is parallel with horizon as patient moves from supine to erect sitting position. Adapted from Woods and Mansfield.[108]

Although it may not be possible to accurately compare absolute values from patient to patient using the phlebostatic axis, at least patients can serve as their own control, and changes in pressures will have an accurate reference point. The phlebostatic axis should be marked with indelible ink on each patient.

Location of the Catheter Tip Relative to the Left Atrial Level

Close approximation of left atrial pressure by PAOP requires a blood-filled segment of pulmonary vasculature to serve as an extension of the catheter system. When any part of the system distal to the catheter tip is emptied of blood, PAOP no longer reflects left atrial pressure. Whether pulmonary capillaries contain blood is a function of pulmonary artery pressure, alveolar pressure, left atrial pressure, and the hydrostatic relation of these vessels to the left atrium. Several studies have shown that pulmonary artery catheters placed below the left atrium correctly record PAOPs that are equal to left atrial pressures at all levels of PEEP. However, pulmonary artery catheters placed above the left atrium may record PAOP higher than left atrial pressure in the presence of PEEP.

In the zones of the lung where alveolar pressure exceeds both pulmonary artery and pulmonary venous pressure, the collapsible pulmonary capillaries are closed with no flow (zone 1).[111,112] In the center of the lung, where alveolar pressure is greater than pulmonary venous pressure but less than pulmonary arterial pressure, flow is determined by the difference between pulmonary arterial and alveolar pressure (zone 2). In the lower zones of the lung, all capillaries are held open because pulmonary venous pressure is higher than alveolar pressure, and flow is determined by the difference between pulmonary artery pressure and pulmonary venous pressure (zone 3).

A pulmonary artery catheter located in zones 1 or 2 will not reflect left atrial pressure. Zone 1 is without perfusion before the balloon is inflated, and the vascular segment downstream from the catheter in zone 2 will change to zone 1 as soon as the balloon is inflated. In both instances alveolar pressure exceeds pulmonary capillary wedge pressure. A catheter located in the upper or mid-zone of the lung will also detect a change in alveolar pressure transmitted to its tip with each increment of PEEP, since its initial downstream pressure is alveolar pressure.

When a catheter is referenced to atmosphere at the vertical height of the left atrium and is not in the lower zone (zone 3), the pressure recorded at the transducer level is a function of the vertical height of the column of fluid in the catheter above the left atrium and any alveolar pressure transmitted to the catheter. Lateral x-ray films must be taken to establish the position of the catheter with respect to the left atrium. If it is found to be above the left atrium, the catheter should be removed to a position below the left atrium.[113-116]

Berryhill and Benumof[117] have demonstrated in research with dogs that the discrepancy between PAOP and left atrial pressure appears to be minimized during spontaneous breathing with PEEP (so-called CPAP, or continuous positive airway pressure), even if the catheter tip is above the left atrium. This suggests that PAOP should be measured either during the spontaneous breathing phase of intermittent mandatory ventilation or during CPAP.

Balloon Problems

In one study, 15 of 16 catheters located peripherally showed eccentric inflation of the balloon; in nine of those instances, the waveform did not change on inflation of the balloon.[118] In the remaining six, the waveform became flat either without a change of pressure or with a gradual increase of pressure. One patient with an eccentric balloon inflation developed hemoptysis following repeated measurements of PAOP. Nine of the 16 balloons inflated normally following withdrawal of the catheter tip to a large branch of the pulmonary artery. In the cadaveric lung, 5 of 10 balloons showed eccentric inflation when the catheter was advanced to a smaller artery, but a normal inflation was observed when the catheter was withdrawn to the large arteries.

The ideal position of the Swan-Ganz catheter is in a large pulmonary artery from which it can advance into the occlusive position on inflation of the balloon but slip back to the previous location on deflation. When located in smaller vessels, particularly at a bifurcation, the catheter may be fixed prematurely (with only partial inflation of the balloon) before the vessel is occluded. Further inflation can cause an eccentricity in the partially inflated balloon if it expands to the less resistant area. A balloon of this type at a bifurcation may not occlude the lumen. Instead, it may force the catheter tip to impinge on a vessel wall, resulting in a loss of pulmonary artery waveform. If a continuous flush system is used, a gradual increase of pressure higher than the mean pulmonary artery pressure may be seen (so-called pseudo-occlusive pressure) in the presence of impingement of the catheter tip (Fig 22). The pressure recorded is the pressure in the flush system, not the pulmonary artery. Repeated overinflation, or forced inflation of the balloon to wedge in a smaller pulmonary artery or a vasoconstricted vessel, may rupture

the pulmonary artery, particularly when there is an eccentric inflation of the balloon. Most reports of pulmonary artery rupture are related to catheters that were in peripheral locations.

Catheters that initially are in correct position may later advance peripherally. Poor wedging of the balloon may occur after the introduction of high PEEP, high tidal volume ventilation, positional changes of the patient, coughing, or even movement of the catheter tip with contraction of the heart.[119] Distortion of surrounding lung tissue due to existing disease may also cause catheter mislocation.

In addition, forced water injection for cardiac output measurements may relocate the catheter peripherally. Catheter position should be checked daily by x-ray film to ensure an accurate wedge and to avoid perforation of the vessel. The balloon should be deflated and the catheter pulled back gradually if (1) the catheter is located peripherally, (2) a pseudo-occlusive pressure tracing is obtained when the balloon is inflated, or (3) the inflation volume necessary to wedge the balloon is significantly less than the maximum recommended. If it is pulled back rapidly, the loop of the catheter in the ventricle will tighten, which may eventually pull the catheter back farther than desired into the main pulmonary artery or even into the right ventricle.

Changes in Intraluminal Pressure With Respiration

During spontaneous breathing the pressure within the pulmonary artery (the intraluminal pressure) follows intrathoracic pressure. This is especially exaggerated during deep breathing. During deep inspiration the measured intraluminal pressure is significantly lower than

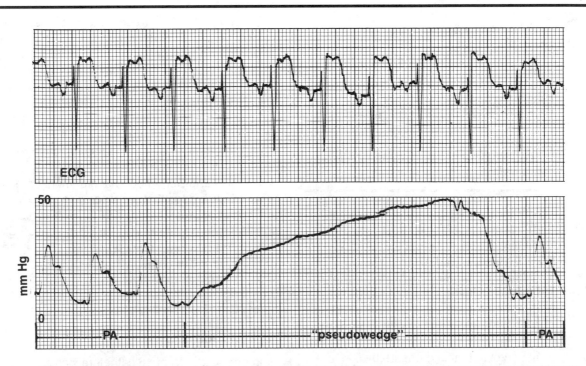

Fig 22. Pseudo-occlusive ("pseudowedge") pressure tracing recorded with inflation of balloon in presence of impingement of catheter tip.

during exhalation. If the patient is being treated with mechanical ventilation, intrathoracic pressure will become positive during the inspiratory cycle of the ventilator and falsely elevate intraluminal pressure. If the patient is receiving intermittent mandatory ventilation, the intrathoracic pressure will become subatmospheric during spontaneous inspiration, thus lowering the measured intraluminal pressure. During the inspiratory cycle of the ventilator, intrathoracic and therefore intraluminal pressures are elevated. If an electronic digital pressure read-out is used, significant error may be introduced into the reading. The electronic equipment records the highest pressure as the systolic pressure and the lowest pressure as diastolic; both may be incorrect.

Intraluminal pressure should be recorded at end-expiration in all patients, both those breathing spontaneously and those on mechanical ventilation, to eliminate the artifact of the positive-negative intrathoracic pressure swings.[120,121] This may be done either by reading the pressure from the oscilloscope or from a paper writeout. Simultaneous recording of intraluminal pressure and airway pressure may facilitate identifying the point of end-expiration (Fig 23).[121]

Intraluminal vascular pressure minus intrapleural pressure represents transmural, or effective, vascular filling pressure. Change in intraluminal vascular pressures will reflect change in transmural vascular pressures only if intrapleural pressure remains constant. The extent of airway pressure transmission to the intrapleural space will depend on airway resistance and lung and thoracic wall compliance; it may vary greatly from patient to patient. The more intrapleural pressure varies from normal, the greater the error in interpreting intraluminal pressure as a reflection of transmural or effective vascular filling pressure.[122,123]

In a patient with chronic obstructive pulmonary disease with both airway obstruction and loss of lung recoil, markedly positive intrathoracic pressures can be produced during the active process of expiration, and intraluminal vascular pressures recorded as mean or average can be elevated because of the addition of this positive intrathoracic pressure.[124] Similarly, patients treated with PEEP will have raised intraluminal vascular pressures, yet transmural filling pressure may remain unchanged or actually decrease.

Intrapleural pressure can be measured either by an intrapleural catheter[122,123] or by an esophageal balloon.[125] The intrapleural catheter probably gives a more accurate measurement of intrapleural pressure, but during insertion there is always the hazard of pneumothorax. Supine esophageal pressure reflects intrathoracic pressure with reasonable accuracy if there is proper balloon design and use, although pressures in the supine position may be higher than in the upright position, presumably due to the weight of the contents of the mediastinum.[126,127]

Transmural or effective vascular filling pressure is equal to intraluminal vascular pressure minus intrapleural or intraesophageal pressure. A considerable number of patients with acute respiratory failure being treated with mechanical ventilation and PEEP have elevated

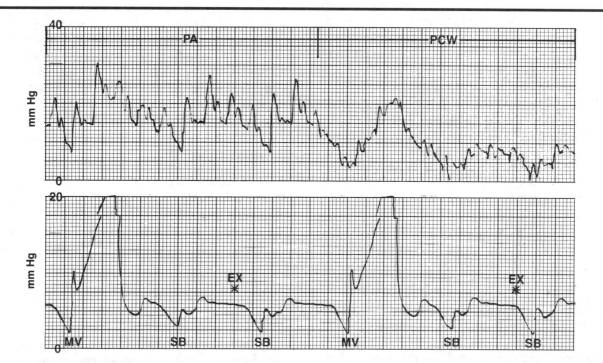

Fig 23. Changes in pulmonary artery (PA) and PAOP (PCW) pressure induced by changes in intrathoracic pressure during both spontaneous breathing (SB) and intermittent mandatory ventilation (MV). To eliminate artifact, intraluminal pressures should be recorded at end-expiration (EX). Upper tracing is intraluminal pressure; lower tracing is airway pressure recorded simultaneously (with 7.5 mm Hg or 10 cm H_2O positive end-expiratory pressure).

intraluminal filling pressure, often exceeding 20 mm Hg. However, by measuring intrapleural pressure and by calculating the transmural pressure, one may find an actual decrease in cardiac filling pressure, necessitating transfusion in those patients. On the other hand, patients who have decreased lung compliance may not have intrapleural pressure elevated significantly by PEEP; in these patients, elevated intraluminal pressure reflects increased filling pressure, indicating intravascular hypervolemia, congestive heart failure, or both. Despite similar intraluminal vascular pressure in these two groups of patients, appropriate therapy in these extremes is quite different.[122,123] In the patient with chronic obstructive pulmonary disease who exhibits large swings in intrathoracic pressure with spontaneous breathing, transmural pressure is more useful as an estimation of left ventricular function or pulmonary venous hypertension.[124,128]

In a study designed to determine whether there were significant changes in intravascular pressure measured both on and off PEEP, a group of patients with a variety of illnesses (including postoperative complications, pulmonary disease, neurological disease, and cardiovascular disease) had PAOP recorded.[129] The patients were then disconnected from the ventilator for 10 to 15 seconds. No significant change was noted in PAOP on and off the ventilator even with PEEP. However, in 21% of the patients there was a delayed progressive elevation of PAOP throughout the recording. This was observed in the setting of underlying heart disease, presumably reflecting the higher filling pressures required by the failing left ventricle to accommodate the increased venous return that resulted from the restoration of intrathoracic pressures to atmospheric levels.[130] Results of the study suggested that it is not necessary to discontinue PEEP or mechanical ventilation to record PAOP.[129] However, in another study, a group of patients was investigated who had acute respiratory failure requiring PEEP ranging from 5 to 25 cm H_2O. It was demonstrated that for every 5 cm of water increase in PEEP, PAOP increased by 1 mm Hg. Beyond 25 cm of PEEP, the correlation decreased significantly.[131]

Whether PEEP raises intraluminal vascular pressure depends on pulmonary compliance. In the patient with severe respiratory failure with markedly decreased pulmonary compliance, PAOP may not differ much on and off PEEP. On the other hand, the patient with highly compliant lungs will have a marked increase in intraluminal PAOP as PEEP is increased. It may be appropriate to define the alteration in pressure caused by PEEP by measuring PAOP with PEEP, then momentarily disconnecting PEEP to determine the change in PAOP. The patients who show a marked disparity between pressures recorded on and off PEEP may best be managed with an esophageal balloon or an intrapleural catheter to accurately measure effective vascular filling pressure.[122,125]

In the patient treated with PEEP for respiratory failure, even if transmural or effective vascular PAOP is determined by measuring intrapleural pressure, one cannot be certain that this reflects left ventricular preload. Although left ventricular diastolic pressure and PAOP are commonly used to reflect left ventricular preload, preload is defined as left ventricular end-diastolic volume or fiber length. In the presence of acute respiratory failure and high PEEP, pulmonary vascular resistance may be elevated. This leads to right ventricular dilatation, which compresses the left ventricle within the rigid pericardium and alters the pressure-volume relationships (compliance) of the left ventricle. Serial PAOP measurements that become elevated over the course of time may give the misleading impression of left ventricular failure when in fact left ventricular diastolic volume or preload is actually decreased because of the decrease in left ventricular compliance.[132-135]

Errors in Sampling Blood From the Pulmonary Artery

Ability to obtain true mixed venous blood from the pulmonary artery depends on the position of the catheter, the flow past the catheter from the more proximal pulmonary artery, the relative resistance to the flow from the pulmonary capillary bed, and the proximity of the tip of the catheter to the gas exchange area. Rapid withdrawal rates of blood from the distal tip of the pulmonary artery catheter may draw in oxygenated blood from the capillary bed and cause falsely elevated mixed venous PO_2 values. However, at withdrawal rates of 3 mL/min, results of one study showed no contamination of pulmonary arterial blood with pulmonary capillary blood.[98] To define whether pulmonary arterial blood is contaminated with pulmonary capillary blood, the pulmonary venous CO_2 is measured after ventilation has been stable for more than 10 minutes. If the mixed venous PCO_2 is equal to or lower than a simultaneous arterial PCO_2, it suggests contamination of pulmonary arterial blood by the pulmonary capillary blood. Nevertheless, blood drawn from atelectatic areas of the lung would not be subject to this artifact since equilibrium with alveolar gas is prevented.[136]

Complications

Complications of pulmonary artery catheterization include pulmonary vascular damage (thrombosis, hemorrhage, and pulmonary infarction), entanglement or damage to intracardiac structures, cardiac arrhythmias, endocarditis and sepsis, catheter fracture, balloon malfunction, misplacement of catheters outside the right heart, and electrical hazards. Some of these complications will be discussed in the following section.

Thrombotic Complications

Thrombosis may develop around the catheter and occlude any of the veins through which the catheter has been inserted.[137,138] Heparin bonding of the catheter may reduce the incidence of thrombosis.[139] In a patient who has a pulmonary artery catheter inserted via an antecubital cutdown or percutaneously via the subclavian or internal jugular veins, the development of unilateral upper extremity edema or unilateral neck pain and venous distention suggests deep venous thrombosis of the upper extremity and possibly the superior vena cava.[137]

Pulmonary infarction may occur from thrombus developing around the catheter (either from its tip or more proximally), with emboli passing to the pulmonary circulation, by embolization of thrombus that has formed within the catheter, or by catheter occlusion of a branch of the pulmonary artery.[140] The incidence of thrombus forming about the pulmonary artery catheter with subsequent pulmonary embolization is increased in patients with disseminated intravascular coagulation,[141] decreased cardiac output, hypotension, and congestive heart failure.[141-143]

Several observations may suggest obstruction of the pulmonary vasculature by thrombosis or embolism. Damping of the pressure tracings with only intermittent patency of the catheter present after flushing with saline solution may be observed even with thrombus or embolus restricted to the vascular segment containing the catheter. Manifestations of more extensive vascular obstruction may include falling systemic blood pressure, decreased urine output, and the development of hypercapnia while minute ventilation remains constant (indicating an increase in dead space ventilation); widening of the alveolar-arterial oxygen tension difference; an increase in intrapulmonary shunt; and a shift in the electrical axis of the ECG toward the right.[141]

Persistent wedging of the pulmonary artery catheter may in itself produce pulmonary infarction or may predispose to in situ thrombosis. Wedging may occur because of the tendency of the catheter to advance into the lung owing to the rhythmic contractions of the heart and the pulsatile propelling force of the blood flow. The loop in the right side of the heart tends to become smaller, causing the end of the catheter to be propelled into narrower pulmonary artery branches, especially during the first 12 hours of catheterization. Persistent inflation of the balloon can occur even though the stopcock is open if the air lumen of the catheter is on the inside of a moderate bend that traps air beyond that point, presumably by pinching off the air lumen, leaving the balloon filled. To prevent pulmonary infarction from persistent wedging of the catheter, the following measures should be taken:

- Since the catheter loop tends to tighten and the tip migrates into the distal pulmonary artery with time (especially during the first 24 hours), the pulmonary artery waveform should be monitored continuously.
- Frequent chest x-ray films should be obtained with attention to the position of the catheter tip and to the possibility of air within the balloon.

If a PAOP is obtained with less than the recommended inflation volume on subsequent balloon inflations, the catheter has probably advanced too far and should be partially withdrawn. A constant infusion of heparinized saline solution should be maintained at all times.[140]

A study by Hoar et al[144] has demonstrated that thrombus may form in the central circulation around pulmonary artery catheters in most, if not all, patients. Pulmonary artery catheters that had been inserted percutaneously via the internal jugular vein preoperatively into patients undergoing cardiac surgery were examined through a right atriotomy approximately 2 hours after insertion. All were found to have thrombus extending from the tip of the catheter along the shaft of the catheter. Each patient had a normal coagulation profile. In all patients the introducer and the catheter were filled with heparinized saline solution before introduction, and the catheters were rapidly placed into the pulmonary artery. There was no statistical correlation between thrombus size and the hemodynamic status of the patient or the duration of catheter insertion.

Pulmonary Hemorrhage

Pulmonary hemorrhage may occur either as a result of pulmonary infarction or from direct damage to the pulmonary artery, especially in the presence of pulmonary hypertension. The elevated pulmonary artery pressure may force the tip of the catheter (with the balloon inflated) peripherally into a small branch of the pulmonary artery. The pressure gradient across the segment of the pulmonary artery may then force the tip through the vessel wall. Therefore, in patients with pulmonary hypertension, PAOP measurement should be approached with caution, and length of time in the wedge position should be kept at a minimum.[145,146]

Knotting and Entanglement or Damage to Intracardiac Structures

If the pulmonary artery catheter is withdrawn with the balloon inflated, injury to either the pulmonic or the tricuspid valvular apparatus may follow.[147] Not only has rupture of the chordae tendineae of the tricuspid valve been reported,[147] but the catheter may become looped around the papillary muscle of the tricuspid valve so that removal is impossible.[148] Finally, a knot may form in the distal catheter.[149] To avoid damage to valvular structures during withdrawal, the balloon should be deflated. The incidence of knotting and coiling of the catheter is probably increased with the smaller 5F catheter. Partially inflating the balloon when the catheter tip reaches the subclavian vein or the superior vena cava during insertion may prevent coiling of the catheter in the right atrium or the right ventricle. If when attempting to remove the catheter there is resistance to withdrawal, the attempt should be interrupted and a chest x-ray film obtained to exclude the possibility of knotting or entanglement of the catheter within the heart.

Cardiac Arrhythmias

Atrial and ventricular arrhythmias are common during transit of the catheter through the right side of the heart.[150-152] Tachyarrhythmias may persist even after the catheter is removed. Arrhythmias are usually caused by the bare tip of the catheter impinging upon the endocardium. This possibility can be minimized by making certain that the balloon is fully inflated so that the tip of the catheter is covered. Right bundle branch block can occur during passage of the catheter through the right heart. In a patient with preexisting left bundle branch block, this condition can lead to complete heart block. In a patient with left bundle branch block, a transvenous pacing catheter should be placed before inserting a pulmonary artery catheter,[106] or a pulmonary artery catheter with pacing capabilities should be used.

Endocarditis

Septic endocarditis of the right side of the heart due to prolonged pulmonary artery catheterization occurs rarely. However, aseptic endocarditis and thrombotic endocardial vegetations involving the right side of the heart occur in approximately 30% of autopsied patients who have had a pulmonary artery catheter in place. These aseptic vegetations may be of significance in providing a nidus for subsequent sepsis as well as a source of pulmonary emboli. Both septic and aseptic endocarditis may be more common in burn patients.[153-157]

Sepsis

Frequent manipulations of the pulmonary artery catheter, as well as leaving the pulmonary catheter in place for more than 3 days, increase the incidence of positive blood cultures drawn through the pulmonary artery catheter and positive cultures from catheter tips.[152,158,159]

Fracture of Catheter

There is one report of fracture of a pulmonary artery catheter 0.5 cm proximal to the right atrial opening.[160] This catheter was inserted via a cutdown from the right antecubital fossa; difficulty was experienced in passing the catheter. An acceptable waveform was never obtained. When the catheter was withdrawn, the distal point of the catheter beyond the fracture was attached to the proximal part by only the wires leading to the thermistor.

Balloon Rupture

The balloon may be defective before insertion, it may be damaged during insertion, or balloon rupture may occur while the catheter is in use. Several recommendations for balloon care have been published in *Health Devices*.[161] Since excessive storage temperatures may cause the latex balloons to rupture, the catheters should be stored in well-ventilated areas (away from direct sunlight, nearby heat sources, or chemical fumes) at temperatures no higher than 25°C. An air-filled balloon-tipped catheter should not be used in a patient with an intracardiac right-to-left shunt because systemic air embolism will occur if the balloon ruptures. Use carbon dioxide for balloon inflation in this situation. Test the balloon before catheterization by submerging it in sterile water and inflating it with air. Leave the catheters in the original packages until needed and remove them carefully to avoid damage to the balloons. Use care during insertion. Do not exceed maximum inflation volumes. Monitor the pulmonary artery waveform and stop inflation when proper wedging is achieved. The balloon should resist inflation, and the syringe plunger should spring back when released. Failure to wedge the device and the absence of inflation resistance indicate balloon rupture, distention of the pulmonary artery, or displacement of the catheter tip back into the main pulmonary artery or right ventricle.

If balloon rupture is suspected, aspirate into the syringe the same gas volume used for inflation; disconnect the syringe and leave the stopcock open to vent the balloon. If the balloon is broken, a few drops of blood may appear at the inflation port. Remove the catheter immediately because fragments from deteriorating latex form emboli.

Complications Relating to Insertion

Any complications described in chapter 11 may occur during placement of a pulmonary artery catheter percutaneously into a central vein. Pneumothorax may occur during subclavian venipuncture, and the carotid artery may be entered during internal jugular venipuncture. Even inadvertent placement of the pulmonary artery catheter into the right pleural space has been reported.[162] Injury to nerve or artery may occur during cutdown.

Arterial Puncture

Arterial puncture is indicated to obtain a specimen of arterial blood for various laboratory determinations such as arterial gas levels or lactate.[163,164] If frequent specimens are required or continuous pressure monitoring is indicated, an indwelling arterial line should be used as described earlier in this chapter.

The sites commonly used for arterial puncture are the radial artery, the brachial artery, and the femoral artery.

Equipment Needed

The following equipment and supplies are needed for arterial puncture:

1. 3- to 5-mL sterile syringe (glass or plastic)
2. 25-gauge, ⅝-inch (1.6 cm) needle for radial, brachial, and femoral puncture, *or*
3. 22-gauge, 1½-inch (3.8 cm) needle for femoral puncture in obese patients
4. Plug for syringe or rubber stopper for end of needle
5. Heparin —1000 U/mL
6. Povidone-iodine or 70% isopropyl alcohol for skin cleansing
7. 1% lidocaine without epinephrine

8. 3-mL syringe—25-gauge, ⅝-inch (1.6 cm) needle for lidocaine

9. Container of crushed ice (plastic bag, cup, emesis basin, etc)

Technique

The steps in arterial puncture are as follows:

1. Fill the syringe for drawing arterial specimen with a small amount of heparin. If the syringe is glass, rinse the barrel with heparin and eject the residue from the syringe with the needle pointing upward. Push the plunger home to expel the air and leave only the dead space of the needle and the syringe filled with heparin. If a plastic syringe is used, the syringe does not need to be rinsed, since heparin does not adhere to the wall of the plastic syringe. However, it is still essential to discard the excess heparin and air, leaving only the dead space filled.

2. For radial artery puncture: Extend the wrist as for insertion of an arterial line; the site of puncture should be ½ to 1 inch (1.3 to 2.5 cm) proximal to the wrist crease.

3. For brachial artery puncture: The arm should be extended at the elbow and supinated (palm up); the site of puncture should be slightly above the elbow crease.

4. For femoral artery puncture: The patient should be supine with the legs straight; the puncture should be made distal to the inguinal ligament at the level of the inguinal crease.

5. Wear sterile gloves for optimal asepsis.

6. Cleanse the skin with povidone-iodine or alcohol.

7. Palpate the artery selected. It is usually best to place two or three fingers along the course of the artery, both to locate its position and direction and to immobilize it.

8. Inject lidocaine to raise a skin wheal at the puncture site (optional).

9. Insert the needle for radial (Fig 24) or brachial (Fig 25) artery puncture through the skin wheal at an angle of about 45° to 60° and direct it slowly toward the pulsation. For femoral artery puncture (Fig 26), insert the needle at a 90° angle. Occasionally penetration into the artery can be sensed, but usually puncture is detected by blood slowly entering the syringe as a result of arterial pressure. This occurs most easily with a glass syringe. If a plastic syringe is used, gentle aspiration may be required. If blood is not obtained during insertion, slowly withdraw the needle and stop once blood appears. If no blood appears, withdraw the needle altogether and start again.

10. Obtain 2 to 3 mL of blood and remove the needle from the artery while applying pressure to the site.

11. Pressure should be maintained at the puncture site for at least 5 to 10 minutes, longer if the patient has a coagulopathy or is hypertensive.

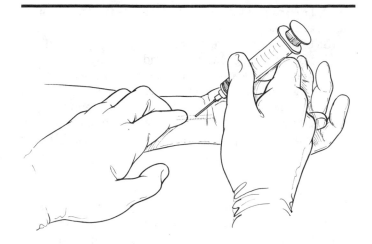

Fig 24. Radial artery puncture.

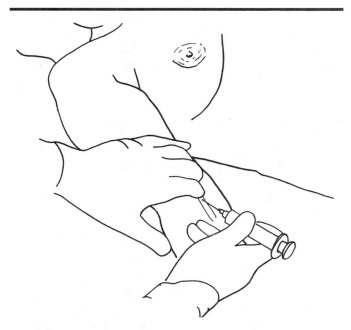

Fig 25. Brachial artery puncture.

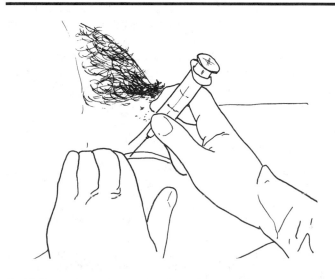

Fig 26. Femoral artery puncture.

12. Hold the syringe vertically (needle tip upright) and expel any air bubbles.
13. Either remove the needle from the syringe and apply a rubber cap to the end of the syringe, or leave the needle attached and apply the needle cover, or plug the tip into a rubber stopper.
14. Roll the syringe four to five times between the palms of the hands to mix blood with heparin.
15. Place the syringe in ice, and transport it immediately to the laboratory.

Complications

The major complication of arterial puncture is a hematoma. This generally can be prevented or minimized by using a 25-gauge needle and applying pressure for at least 5 to 10 minutes after the puncture has been completed. Thrombosis of the artery may occur after repeated punctures, as mentioned in part I. Infection is a possible but uncommon complication. Injury to an adjacent nerve may occur with attempts at puncturing the femoral or brachial arteries.

Pitfalls

Since heparin has a low P_{CO_2} and an acidic pH, more heparin in the syringe than needed to fill the dead space will lower the P_{CO_2} and pH of the arterial blood.[165]

Blood gas samples should be analyzed as soon as possible and should be placed in ice for even short delays. The blood sample must be adequately submerged in the ice or ice water. Since blood metabolism occurs in the syringe, the P_{O_2} and the pH decrease and the P_{CO_2} increases. Therefore, unless arterial blood samples are analyzed immediately after they are drawn, they should be immersed in ice.[165,166]

A small amount of air in the syringe may markedly lower P_{CO_2} since air contains negligible carbon dioxide. The direction of change in P_{O_2} depends on whether arterial P_{O_2} initially was lower or greater than ambient oxygen tension.

Vacutainers, even though nitrogen-filled, should not be used for drawing arterial blood gas specimens since they contain measurable amounts of oxygen and will alter arterial P_{O_2} significantly.[167]

References

1. Cohn JN. Blood pressure measurement in shock: mechanism of inaccuracy in auscultatory and palpatory methods. *JAMA*. 1967; 199:118-122.
2. Harrington DP. Disparities between direct and indirect arterial systolic blood pressure measurements. *Cardiovasc Pulmonary Tech*. 1978;6:40.
3. Hamilton WF, Dow P. An experimental study of standing waves in pulse propagated through the aorta. *Am J Physiol*. 1939;125:48-59.
4. Remington JW. Contour changes of the aortic pulse during propagation. *Am J Physiol*. 1960;199:331-334.
5. Nutter DO. Measuring and recording systemic blood pressure. In: Hurst JW, Logue RB, Schlant RC, Wenger NK, eds. *The Heart, Arteries, and Veins*. 4th ed. New York, NY: McGraw-Hill Book Co Inc; 1978:217-226.
6. Evaluation: physiological pressure transducers. *Health Devices*. 1979; 8:199-204.
7. Civetta JM. Invasive catheterization. In: Shoemaker WC, Thompson WL, eds. *Critical Care, State of the Art*. Fullerton, Calif: The Society of Critical Care Medicine; 1980;1(chap B):18-21.
8. Waltemath CL, Preuss DD. Determination of blood pressure in low-flow states by the Doppler technique. *Anesthesiology*. 1971;34: 77-79.
9. Kazamias TM, Gander MP, Franklin DL, Ross J Jr. Blood pressure measurement with Doppler ultrasonic flowmeter. *J Appl Physiol*. 1971;30:585-588.
10. Harken AH, Smith RM. Aortic pressure versus Doppler-measured peripheral arterial pressure. *Anesthesiology*. 1973;38:184-186.
11. Paulus DA. Noninvasive blood pressure measurement. *Med Instrum*. 1981;15:91-94.
12. Van Bergen FH, Weatherhead DS, Treloar EF, et al. Comparison of indirect and direct methods of measuring arterial blood pressure. *Circulation*. 1954;10:481-490.
13. Berliner K, Fujiy H, Ho Lee D, Yildiz M, Garnier B. The accuracy of blood pressure determinations: a comparison of direct and indirect measurements. *Cardiologia*. 1960;37:118-128.
14. Lowry RL, Lichti EL, Eggers GW Jr. The Doppler: an aid in monitoring blood pressure during anesthesia. *Anesth Analg*. 1973;52:531-535.
15. Geddes LA, Whistler SJ. The error in indirect blood pressure measurement with the incorrect size of cuff. *Am Heart J*. 1978;96:4-8.
16. Venus B, Mathru M, Smith RA, Pham CG. Direct versus indirect blood pressure measurements in critically ill patients. *Heart Lung*. 1985;14:228-231.
17. Johnson CJ, Kerr JH. Automatic blood pressure monitors: a clinical evaluation of five models in adults. *Anaesthesia*. 1985;40:471-478.
18. Bjork L, Enghoff E, Grenvik A, Hallen A, Hogstrom S, Nordgren L, Pongracz G von. Local circulatory changes following brachial artery catheterization. *Vasc Dis*. 1965;2:283-292.
19. Bedford RF, Wollman H. Complications of percutaneous radial-artery cannulation: an objective prospective study in man. *Anesthesiology*. 1973;38:228-236.
20. Mandel MA, Dauchot PJ. Radial artery cannulation in 1000 patients: precautions and complications. *J Hand Surg [Am]*. 1977;2:482-485.
21. Palm T. Evaluation of peripheral arterial pressure on the thumb following radial artery cannulation. *Br J Anaesth*. 1977;49:819-824.
22. Little JM, Clarke B, Shanks C. Effects of radial artery cannulation. *Med J Aust*. 1975;2:791-793.
23. Ersoz CJ, Hedden M, Lain L. Prolonged femoral arterial catheterization for intensive care. *Anesth Analg*. 1970;49:160-164.
24. Gurman GM, Kriemerman S. Cannulation of big arteries in critically ill patients. *Crit Care Med*. 1985;13:217-220.
25. Bedford RF. Radial arterial function following percutaneous cannulation with 18- and 20-gauge catheters. *Anesthesiology*. 1977;47: 37-39.
26. Downs JB, Rackstein AD, Klein EF Jr, Hawkins IF Jr. Hazards of radial-artery catheterization. *Anesthesiology*. 1973;38:283-286.
27. Davis FM. Radial artery cannulation: influence of catheter size and material on arterial occlusion. *Anaesth Intensive Care*. 1978;6: 49-53.
28. Downs JB, Chapman RL Jr, Hawkins IF Jr. Prolonged radial-artery catheterization: an evaluation of heparinized catheters and continuous irrigation. *Arch Surg*. 1974;108:671-673.
29. Arthurs GJ. Case report: digital ischemia following radial artery cannulation. *Anaesth Intensive Care*. 1978;6:54-55.
30. Shinebourne E, Pfitzner J. Continuous flushing device for indwelling arterial and venous cannulae. *Br J Hosp Med*. 1973;9(suppl):64.
31. Gardner RM, Bond EL, Clark JS. Safety and efficacy of continuous flush systems for arterial and pulmonary artery catheters. *Ann Thorac Surg*. 1977;23:534-538.
32. Gardner RM, Warner HR, Toronto AF, Gaisford WD. Catheter-flush system for continuous monitoring of central arterial pulse waveform. *J Appl Physiol*. 1970;29:911-913.
33. Band JD, Maki DG. Infections caused by arterial catheters used for hemodynamic monitoring. *Am J Med*. 1979;67:735-741.

34. Gardner RM, Schwartz R, Wong HC, Burke JP. Percutaneous indwelling radial-artery catheters for monitoring cardiovascular function: prospective study of the risk of thrombosis and infection. *N Engl J Med.* 1974;290:1227-1231.
35. Grant JCB. *An Atlas of Anatomy.* 6th ed. Baltimore, Md: Williams & Wilkins Co; 1972:224-258.
36. Mortensen JD. Clinical sequelae from arterial needle puncture, cannulation, and incision. *Circulation.* 1967;35:1118-1123.
37. Bolasny BL, Killen DA. Surgical management of arterial injuries second to angiography. *Ann Surg.* 1971;174:962-964.
38. Shah A, Gnoj J, Fisher VJ. Complications of selective coronary arteriography by the Judkins technique and their prevention. *Am Heart J.* 1975;90:353-359.
39. Colvin MP, Curran JP, Jarvis D, O'Shea PJ. Femoral artery pressure monitoring: use of the Seldinger technique. *Anaesthesia.* 1977;32:451-455.
40. Christian CM II, Naraghi M. A complication of femoral arterial cannulation in a patient undergoing cardiopulmonary bypass. *Anesthesiology.* 1978;49:436-437.
41. Katz AM, Birnbaum M, Moylan J, Pellett J. Gangrene of the hand and forearm: a complication of radial artery cannulation. *Crit Care Med.* 1974;2:270-272.
42. Williams CD, Cunningham JN. Percutaneous cannulation of the femoral artery for monitoring. *Surg Gynecol Obstet.* 1975;141:773-774.
43. Morris T, Bouhoutsos J. The dangers of femoral artery puncture and catheterization. *Am Heart J.* 1975;89:260-261.
44. Grant JC. *An Atlas of Anatomy.* 6th ed. Baltimore, Md: Williams & Wilkins Co; 1972:1-79.
45. De Angelis J. Axillary arterial monitoring. *Crit Care Med.* 1976;4:205-206.
46. Adler DC, Bryan-Brown CW. Use of the axillary artery for intravascular monitoring. *Crit Care Med.* 1973;1:148-150.
47. Bryan-Brown CW, Kwun KB, Lumb PD, Pia RL, Azer S. The axillary artery catheter. *Heart Lung.* 1983;12:492-497.
48. Barnes RW, Foster EJ, Janssen GA, Boutros AR. Safety of brachial arterial catheters as monitors in the intensive care unit: a prospective evaluation with the Doppler ultrasonic velocity detector. *Anesthesiology.* 1976;44:260-264.
49. Macon WL IV, Futrell JW. Median-nerve neuropathy after percutaneous puncture of the brachial artery in patients receiving anticoagulants. *N Engl J Med.* 1973;288:1396.
50. Mozersky DJ, Buckley CJ, Hagood CO Jr, Capps WF Jr, Dannemiller FJ Jr. Ultrasonic evaluation of the palmar circulation: a useful adjunct to radial artery cannulation. *Am J Surg.* 1973;126:810-812.
51. Crossland SG, Neviaser RJ. Complications of radial artery catheterization. *Hand.* 1977;9:287-290.
52. Ryan JF, Raines J, Dalton BC, Mathieu A. Arterial dynamics of radial artery cannulation. *Anesth Analg.* 1973;52:1017-1025.
53. Allen EV. Thromboangiitis obliterans: methods of diagnosis of chronic occlusive arterial lesions distal to the wrist with illustrative cases. *Am J Med Sci.* 1929;178:237-244.
54. Kamienski RW, Barnes RW. Critique of the Allen test for continuity of the palmar arch assessed by Doppler ultrasound. *Surg Gynecol Obstet.* 1976;142:861-864.
55. Brodsky JB. A simple method to determine patency of the ulnar artery intraoperatively prior to radial-artery cannulation. *Anesthesiology.* 1975;42:626-627.
56. Brown AE, Sweeney DB, Lumley J. Percutaneous radial artery cannulation. *Anesthesia.* 1969;24:532-536.
57. Slogoff S, Keats AS, Arlund C. On the safety of radial artery cannulation. *Anesthesiology.* 1983;59:42-47.
58. Weiss BM, Galliker RI. Complications during and following radial artery cannulation: a prospective study. *Intensive Care Med.* 1986;12:424-428.
59. Dalton B, Laver MB. Vasospasm with an indwelling radial artery cannula. *Anesthesiology.* 1971;34:194-197.
60. Cohn JN. Central venous pressure as a guide to volume expansion. *Ann Intern Med.* 1967;66:1283-1287.
61. Lowenstein E, Little JW III, Lo HH. Prevention of cerebral embolization from flushing radial-artery cannulas. *N Engl J Med.* 1971;285:1414-1415.
62. Meguid M, Bevilacqua R. Management of arterial cannulas. *N Engl J Med.* 1972;286:376.
63. Wyatt R, Glaves I, Cooper DJ. Proximal skin necrosis after radial-artery cannulation. *Lancet.* 1974;1:1135-1138.
64. Johnson RW. A complication of radial-artery cannulation. *Anesthesiology.* 1974;40:598-600.
65. Mathieu A, Dalton B, Fischer JE, Kumar A. Expanding aneurysm of the radial artery after frequent puncture. *Anesthesiology.* 1973;38:401-403.
66. Barnhorst DA, Barner HB. Prevalence of congenitally absent pedal pulses. *N Engl J Med.* 1968;278:264-265.
67. Johnstone RE, Greenhow DE. Catheterization of the dorsalis pedis artery. *Anesthesiology.* 1973;39:654-655.
68. Huber JF. The arterial network supplying the dorsum of the foot. *Anat Rec.* 1941;80:373-391.
69. Grant JC. *An Atlas of Anatomy.* 6th ed. Baltimore, Md: Williams & Wilkins Co; 1972:306-326.
70. Youngberg JA, Miller ED Jr. Evaluation of percutaneous cannulations of the dorsalis pedis artery. *Anesthesiology.* 1976;44:80-83.
71. Swan HJ, Ganz W, Forrester J, Marcus H, Diamond G, Chonette D. Catheterization of the heart in man with use of a flow-directed balloon-tipped catheter. *N Engl J Med.* 1970;283:447-451.
72. Ganz W, Swan HJ. Measurement of blood flow by thermodilution. *Am J Cardiol.* 1972;29:241-246.
73. Ganz W, Donoso R, Marcus HS, Forrester JS, Swan HJ. A new technique for measurement of cardiac output by thermodilution in man. *Am J Cardiol.* 1971;27:392-396.
74. Forrester JS, Ganz W, Diamond G, McHugh T, Chonette DW, Swan HJ. Thermodilution cardiac output determination with a single flow-directed catheter. *Am Heart J.* 1972;83:306-311.
75. Alpert JS, Dexter L. Blood flow measurement: the cardiac output. In: Grossman W, ed. *Cardiac Catheterization and Angiography.* Philadelphia, Pa: Lea & Febiger; 1974:61-71.
76. Franch RH. Cardiac catheterization. In: Hurst JW, Logue RB, Schlant RC, Wenger NK, eds. *The Heart, Arteries, and Veins.* 4th ed. New York, NY: McGraw-Hill Book Co Inc; 1978:479-501.
77. Forrester JS, Diamond G, Chatterjee K, Swan HJ. Medical therapy of acute myocardial infarction by application of hemodynamic subsets. *N Engl J Med.* 1976;295:1356-1362,1404-1413.
78. Meister SG, Helfant RH. Rapid bedside differentiation of ruptured interventricular septum from acute mitral insufficiency. *N Engl J Med.* 1972;287:1024-1025.
79. Swan HJ. Second annual SCCM lecture. The role of hemodynamic monitoring in the management of the critically ill. *Crit Care Med.* 1975;3:83-89.
80. Swan HJC. What is the role of invasive monitoring procedures in the management of the critically ill? In: Corday E, ed. *Controversies in Cardiology.* Philadelphia, Pa: FA Davis Co; 1977;8(No. 1). Cardiovascular Clinics Series.
81. Walston A II, Kendall ME. Comparison of pulmonary wedge and left atrial pressure in man. *Am Heart J.* 1973;86:159-164.
82. Falicov RE, Resnekov L. Relationship of the pulmonary artery end-diastolic pressure to the left ventricular end-diastolic and mean filling pressures in patients with and without left ventricular dysfunction. *Circulation.* 1970;42:65-73.
83. Fisher ML, De Felice CE, Parisi AF. Assessing left ventricular filling pressure with flow-directed (Swan-Ganz) catheters: detection of sudden changes in patients with left ventricular dysfunction. *Chest.* 1975;68: 542-547.
84. Sibbald WJ, Driedger AA, Myers ML, Short AI, Wells GA. Biventricular function in the adult respiratory distress syndrome. *Chest.* 1983;84:126-134.
85. Raper R, Sibbald WJ. Misled by the wedge? the Swan-Ganz catheter and left ventricular preload. *Chest.* 1986;89:427-434.
86. Carley JE, Wong BY, Pugh DM, Dunn M. Clinical significance of the V wave in the main pulmonary artery. *Am J Cardiol.* 1977;39:982-985.
87. Braunwald E, Fishman AP, Cournand A. Time relationship of dynamic events in the cardiac chambers, pulmonary artery and aorta in man. *Circ Res.* 1956;4:100-107.
88. Forrester JS, Diamond G, McHugh TJ, Swan HJ. Filling pressures in the right and left sides of the heart in acute myocardial infarction: a reappraisal of central-venous-pressure monitoring. *N Engl J Med.* 1971; 285:190-193.
89. Guyton AC, Jones CE. Central venous pressure: physiological significance and clinical implications. *Am Heart J.* 1973;86:431-437.
90. Civetta JM, Gabel JC. Flow directed-pulmonary artery catheterization in surgical patients: indications and modifications of technic. *Ann Surg.* 1972;753-756.

91. Rice CL, Hobelman CF, John DA, Smith DE, Malley JD, Cammack BF, James DR, Peters RM, Virgilio RW. Central venous pressure or pulmonary capillary wedge pressure as the determinant of fluid replacement in aortic surgery. *Surgery.* 1978;84:437-440.

92. Risk C, Rudo N, Falltrick R, Feeley T, Don HF. Comparison of right atrial and pulmonary capillary wedge pressures. *Crit Care Med.* 1978;6:172-175.

93. Kostuk W, Barr JW, Simon AL, Ross J Jr. Correlations between the chest film and hemodynamics in acute myocardial infarction. *Circulation.* 1973;48:624-632.

94. McHugh TJ, Forrester JS, Adler L, Zion D, Swan HJ. Pulmonary vascular congestion in acute myocardial infarction: hemodynamic and radiologic correlations. *Ann Intern Med.* 1972;76:29-33.

95. Carabello B, Cohn PF, Alpert JS. Hemodynamic monitoring in patients with hypotension after myocardial infarction: the role of the medical center in relation to the community hospital. *Chest.* 1978;74:5-9.

96. Lee J, Wright F, Barber R, Stanley L. Central venous oxygen saturation in shock: a study in man. *Anesthesiology.* 1972;36:472-478.

97. Scheinman MM, Brown MA, Rapaport E. Critical assessment of use of central venous oxygen saturation as a mirror of mixed venous oxygen in severely ill cardiac patients. *Circulation.* 1969;40:165-172.

98. Crexells C, Chatterjee K, Forrester JS, Dikshit K, Swan HJ. Optimal level of filling pressure in the left side of the heart in acute myocardial infarction. *N Engl J Med.* 1973;289:1263-1266.

99. Russell RO Jr, Rackley CE, Pombo J, Hunt D, Potanin C, Dodge HT. Effects of increasing left ventricular filling pressure in patients with acute myocardial infarction. *J Clin Invest.* 1970;49:1539-1550.

100. Shah DM, Browner BD, Dutton RE, Newell JC, Powers SR Jr. Cardiac output and pulmonary wedge pressure: use for evaluation of fluid replacement in trauma patients. *Arch Surg.* 1977;112:1161-1168.

101. Weisel RD, Vito L, Dennis RC, Berger RL, Hechtman HB. Clinical applications of thermodilution cardiac output determinations. *Am J Surg.* 1975;129:449-454.

102. Malin CG, Schwartz S. Starling curves as a guide to fluid management in the critically ill. *Heart Lung.* 1975;4:588-592.

103. Horovitz JH, Carrico CJ, Shires GT. Venous sampling sites for pulmonary shunt determinations in the injured patient. *J Trauma.* 1971;11:911-914.

104. Standards and guidelines for cardiopulmonary resuscitation (CPR) and emergency cardiac care (ECC). *JAMA.* 1986;255:2905-2989.

105. Suter PM, Lindauer JM, Fairley HB, Schlobohm RM. Errors in data derived from pulmonary artery blood gas values. *Crit Care Med.* 1975;3:175-181.

106. Abernathy WS. Complete heart block caused by the Swan-Ganz catheter. *Chest.* 1974;65:349.

107. Pace NL. A critique of flow-directed pulmonary arterial catheterization. *Anesthesiology.* 1977;47:455-465.

108. Woods SL, Mansfield LW. Effect of body position upon pulmonary artery and pulmonary capillary wedge pressures in noncritically ill patients. *Heart Lung.* 1976;5:83-90.

109. Winsor T, Burch GE. Phlebostatic axis and phlebostatic level: reference levels for venous pressure measurements in man. *Proc Soc Exp Biol.* 1945; 58:165-169.

110. Winsor T, Burch GE. Use of the phlebomanometer: normal venous pressure values and a study of certain clinical aspects of venous hypertension in man. *Am Heart J.* 1946;31:387-406.

111. West JB, Dollery CT, Naimark A. Distribution of blood flow in isolated lung: relation to vascular and alveolar pressures. *J Appl Physiol.* 1964;19:713-724.

112. West JB, Dollery CT. Distribution of blood flow and the pressure-flow relations of the whole lung. *J Appl Physiol.* 1965;20:175-183.

113. Tooker J, Huseby J, Butler J. The effect of Swan-Ganz catheter height on the wedge pressure-left atrial pressure relationships in edema during positive-pressure ventilation. *Am Rev Respir Dis.* 1978;117:721-725.

114. Roy R, Powers SR, Feustel PJ, Dutton RE. Pulmonary wedge catheterization during positive end-expiratory pressure ventilation in the dog. *Anesthesiology.* 1977;46:385-390.

115. Benumof JL, Saidman LF, Arkin DB, Diamant M. Where pulmonary arterial catheters go: intrathoracic distribution. *Anesthesiology.* 1977;46:336-338.

116. Kane PB, Askanazi J, Neville JF Jr, Mon RL, Hanson EL, Webb WR. Artifacts in the measurement of pulmonary artery wedge pressure. *Crit Care Med.* 1978;6:36-38.

117. Berryhill RE, Benumof JL. PEEP-induced discrepancy between pulmonary arterial wedge pressure and left atrial pressure: the effects of controlled vs. spontaneous ventilation and compliant vs. noncompliant lungs in the dog. *Anesthesiology.* 1979;51:303-308.

118. Shin B, Ayella RJ, McAslan TC. Pitfalls of Swan-Ganz catheterization. *Crit Care Med.* 1977;5:125-127.

119. Shin B, McAslan TC, Ayella RJ. Problems with measurement using the Swan-Ganz catheter. *Anesthesiology.* 1975;43:474-476.

120. Gooding JM, Laws HL. Interpretation of pulmonary capillary wedge pressure during different modes of ventilation. *Resp Care.* 1977;22:161.

121. Berryhill RE, Benumof JL, Rauscher LA. Pulmonary vascular pressure reading at the end of exhalation. *Anesthesiology.* 1978;49:365-368.

122. Qvist J, Pontoppidan H, Wilson RS, Lowenstein E, Laver MB. Hemodynamic responses to mechanical ventilation with PEEP: the effect of hypervolemia. *Anesthesiology.* 1975;42:45-55.

123. Downs JB. A technique for direct measurement of intrapleural pressure. *Crit Care Med.* 1976;4:207-210.

124. Rice DL, Awe RJ, Gaasch WH, Alexander JK, Jenkins DE. Wedge pressure measurement in obstructive pulmonary disease. *Chest.* 1974;66:628-632.

125. Milic-Emili J, Mead J, Turner JM, et al. Improved technique for estimating pleural pressure from esophageal balloons. *J Appl Physiol.* 1964;19:207-211.

126. Ferris BG Jr, Mead J, Frank NR. Effect of body position on esophageal pressure and measurement of pulmonary compliance. *J Appl Physiol.* 1959;14: 321-324.

127. Knowles JH, Hong SK, Rahn H. Possible errors using esophageal balloon in determination of pressure-volume characteristics of the lung and thoracic cage. *J Appl Physiol.* 1959;14:525-530.

128. Bahler RC, Chester EH, Belman MJ, Baum GL. Multidisciplinary treatment of chronic pulmonary insufficiency, 4: the influence of intrathoracic pressure variations on increases in pulmonary vascular pressure during exercise in patients with chronic obstructive pulmonary disease. *Chest.* 1977;72:703-708.

129. Davison R, Parker M, Harrison RA. The validity of determinations of pulmonary wedge pressure during mechanical ventilation. *Chest.* 1978;73:352-355.

130. Beach T, Millen E, Grenvik A. Hemodynamic response to discontinuance of mechanical ventilation. *Crit Care Med.* 1973;1:85-90.

131. Kirby RR, Civetta JM, Gallagher TJ, et al. The effect of PEEP upon pulmonary capillary pressures (PCWP). American Society of Anesthesiologists Annual Refresher Course Lecture; 1976; 229-230.

132. Pontoppidan H, Wilson RS, Rie MA, Schneider RC. Respiratory intensive care. *Anesthesiology.* 1977;47:96-116.

133. Scharf SM, Brown R, Saunders N, Green LH, Ingram RH Jr. Changes in canine left ventricular size and configuration with positive end-expiratory pressure. *Circ Res.* 1979;44:672-678.

134. Laver MB, Strauss HW, Pohost GM. Herbert Shubin Memorial Lecture. Right and left ventricular geometry: adjustments during acute respiratory failure. *Crit Care Med.* 1979;7:509-519.

135. Jardin F, Farcot JC, Boisante L, Curien N, Margairaz A, Bourdarias JP. Influence of positive end-expiratory pressure on left ventricular performance. *N Engl J Med.* 1981;304:387-392.

136. Shapiro HM, Smith G, Pribble AH, Murray JA, Cheney FW Jr. Errors in sampling pulmonary arterial blood with a Swan-Ganz catheter. *Anesthesiology.* 1974;40:291-295.

137. Dye LE, Segall PH, Russell RO Jr, Mantle JA, Rogers WJ, Rackley CE. Deep venous thrombosis of the upper extremity associated with use of the Swan-Ganz catheter. *Chest.* 1978;73:673-675.

138. Chastre J, Cornud F, Bouchama A, Viau F, Benacerraf R, Gibert C. Thrombosis as a complication of pulmonary-artery catheterization via the internal jugular vein: prospective evaluation by phlebography. *N Engl J Med.* 1982;306:278-281.

139. Hoar PF, Wilson RM, Mangano DT, Avery GJ II, Szarnicki RJ, Hill JD. Heparin bonding reduces thrombogenicity of pulmonary-artery catheters. *N Engl J Med.* 1981;305:993-995.

140. Foote GA, Schabel SI, Hodges M. Pulmonary complications of the flow-directed balloon-tipped catheter. *N Engl J Med.* 1974;290:927-931.

141. Yorra FH, Oblath R, Jaffe H, Simmons DH, Levy SE. Massive thrombosis associated with use of the Swan-Ganz catheter. *Chest.* 1974;65:682-684.

142. Goodman DJ, Rider AK, Billingham ME, Schroeder JS. Thromboembolic complications with the indwelling balloon-tipped pulmonary arterial catheter. *N Engl J Med.* 1974;291:777.

143. Colvin MP, Savege TM, Lewis CT. Pulmonary damage from a Swan-Ganz catheter. *Br J Anaesth.* 1975;47:1107-1110.

144. Hoar PF, Stone JG, Wicks AE, Edie RN, Scholes JV. Thrombogenesis associated with Swan-Ganz catheters. *Anesthesiology.* 1978;48:445-447.

145. Page DW, Teres D, Hartshorn JW. Fatal hemorrhage from Swan-Ganz catheter. *N Engl J Med.* 1974;291:260. Letter.

146. Lapin ES, Murray JA. Hemoptysis with flow-directed cardiac catheterization. *JAMA.* 1972;220:1246.

147. Smith WR, Glauser FL, Jemison P. Ruptured chordae of the tri-cuspid valve: the consequence of flow-directed Swan-Ganz catheterization. *Chest.* 1976;70:790-792.

148. Schwartz KV, Garcia FG. Entanglement of Swan-Ganz catheter around an intracardiac structure. *JAMA.* 1977;237:1198-1199. Letter.

149. Daum S, Schapira M. Intracardiac knot formation in a Swan-Ganz catheter. *Anesth Analg.* 1973;52:862-863.

150. Geha DG, Davis NJ, Lappas DG. Persistent atrial arrhythmias associated with placement of a Swan-Ganz catheter. *Anesthesiology.* 1973;39:651-653.

151. Sprung CL, Jacobs LJ, Caralis PV, Karpf M. Ventricular arrhythmias during Swan-Ganz catheterization of the critically ill. *Chest.* 1981;79:413-415.

152. Damen J, Bolton D. A prospective analysis of 1400 pulmonary artery catheterizations in patients undergoing cardiac surgery. *Acta Anaesthesiol Scand.* 1986;30:386-392.

153. Pace NL, Horton W. Indwelling pulmonary artery catheters: their relationship to aseptic thrombotic endocardial vegetations. *JAMA.* 1975;233:893-894.

154. Greene JF Jr, Fitzwater JE, Clemmer TP. Septic endocarditis and indwelling pulmonary artery catheters. *JAMA.* 1975;233:891-892.

155. Ehrie M, Morgan AP, Moore FD, O'Connor NE. Endocarditis with the indwelling balloon-tipped pulmonary artery catheter in burn patients. *J Trauma.* 1978;18:664-666.

156. Sasaki TM, Panke TW, Dorethy JF, Lindberg RB, Pruitt BA. The relationship of central venous and pulmonary artery catheter position to acute right-sided endocarditis in severe thermal injury. *J Trauma.* 1979;19:740-743.

157. Ducatman BS, McMichan JC, Edwards WD. Catheter-induced lesions of the right side of the heart: a one-year prospective study of 141 autopsies. *JAMA.* 1985;253:791-795.

158. Applefeld JJ, Caruthers TE, Reno DJ, Civetta JM. Assessment of the sterility of long-term cardiac catheterization using the thermo-dilution Swan-Ganz catheter. *Chest.* 1978;74:377-380.

159. Prachar H, Dittel M, Jobst C, Kiss E, Machacek E, Nobis H, Spiel R. Bacterial contamination of pulmonary artery catheters. *Intensive Care Med.* 1978;4:79-82.

160. Parulkar DS, Grundy EM, Bennett EJ. Fracture of a float catheter: a case report. *Br J Anaesth.* 1978;50:201-203.

161. Latex balloons on wedge-pressure catheters. *Health Devices.* 1977;6:123-124.

162. Carlon GC, Howland WS, Kahn RC, Turnbull AD, Makowsky M. Unusual complications during pulmonary artery catheterization. *Crit Care Med.* 1978;6:364-365.

163. Petty TL, Bigelow DB, Levine BE. The simplicity and safety of arterial puncture. *JAMA.* 1966;195:693-695.

164. Sackner MA, Avery WG, Sokolowski J. Arterial punctures by nurses. *Chest.* 1971;59:97-98.

165. Bageant RA. Variations in arterial blood gas measurements due to sampling techniques. *Resp Care.* 1975;20:565-570.

166. Kemp GL. Questions and answers: arterial blood samples should be stored in ice for gas analysis. *JAMA.* 1973;223:696.

167. Lang GE, Mueller RG, Hunt PK. Possible error resulting from use of 'Nitrogen-filled' Vacutainers for blood-gas determinations. *Clin Chem.* 1973;19:559-563.

Credit is given to Peter Miniscalco for artwork and photography.

Invasive Therapeutic Techniques

Chapter 13

The ACLS provider course presents three invasive therapeutic techniques: pericardiocentesis, intracardiac injections, and relief of tension pneumothorax.

Pericardiocentesis

Pericardiocentesis, or needle aspiration of fluid from the pericardium, is indicated to obtain fluid for diagnostic study, obtain information regarding the physiological mechanism of venous pressure elevation, and relieve cardiac tamponade.[1] This section describes the pathophysiology of cardiac tamponade, the clinical diagnosis of tamponade, and the technique of pericardiocentesis.

Anatomy of the Pericardium[2]

The pericardium encloses the heart and the first few centimeters of the great vessels in a serous sac lined by mesothelial cells. The visceral pericardium lies close to the heart surface as the epicardium. The pericardial sac normally contains up to 50 mL of fluid with similar or the same composition as serum. In the adipose tissue beneath the visceral pericardium and on the mediastinal aspect of the parietal pericardium are arteries, veins, lymphatics, and nerves. The pericardium reacts to injury by exuding fluid, fibrin, or cells.

Cardiac Tamponade

Pathophysiology

In cardiac tamponade ventricular diastolic filling is impaired. This occurs because of increased pressure from accumulation of fluid within the pericardial sac.[3-6] Tamponade is most commonly related to one of three causes: (1) trauma, which may be direct or indirect, penetrating or nonpenetrating; (2) infection; and (3) neoplastic disease.[7] Myocardial rupture following acute myocardial infarction, uremia, and collagen-vascular diseases are also important causes of tamponade. Iatrogenic cardiac tamponade may follow cardiac surgery, CPR, or perforation of the heart by a vascular catheter or transvenous pacemaker, or it may be due to radiation or drug reactions, such as to hydralazine or procainamide.[8]

As fluid is added to the pericardial space, the rate of rise of the pressure within the pericardial space depends on several factors. With acute increases in fluid, as little as 200 mL may produce a marked rise in intrapericardial pressure. This explains why the removal of only small amounts of fluid may be followed by a dramatic decrease in intrapericardial pressure and improvement of the patient. However, with slow accumulation of pericardial fluid over weeks or months, there is a gradual stretching of the pericardium, with an increase in its compliance.

More than 2 L of fluid may then accumulate without a severe rise in intrapericardial pressure.

Hypovolemia may mask the usual clinical manifestations of cardiac tamponade, including jugular venous distention. The dynamics of tamponade may become apparent in some patients only after volume administration. While hypervolemia can accentuate the clinical manifestations of tamponade, cardiac output can be enhanced temporarily by the initial increase in ventricular filling pressure that accompanies volume loading and results in a transient increase in stroke volume.[1]

Diagnostic Considerations[1,3-9]

Pulsus paradoxus, defined as a decline greater than 10 mm Hg in systolic arterial pressure with normal inspiration, is usually present with tamponade. However, considerable effusion may exist without pulsus paradoxus, especially if such effusion complicates left ventricular dysfunction manifested by high left ventricular diastolic pressure, atrial septal defect, aortic insufficiency, positive-pressure breathing, or pulmonary arterial obstruction.[10-12] The term *pulsus paradoxus* is a misnomer in that the decrease in arterial pressure during inspiration is merely an exaggeration of a normal phenomenon. Without tamponade there is a normal inspiratory decline in systolic pressure of less than 10 mm Hg that is due both to the transmission of the inspiratory decline in intrathoracic pressure to the heart and aorta and to the delay in transit through the lungs of the normal inspiratory increase of right ventricular stroke volume. In the presence of cardiac tamponade there is a normal decrease in intrapericardial pressure with inspiration and a normal increase in right ventricular filling. However, because of competition of the ventricles for space within the distended and restricted pericardial sac and a shift of the ventricular septum to the left, there is selective impairment of left ventricular filling and a decrease in left ventricular stroke volume. There is also increased capacity of the pulmonary veins since there is a greater fall in pulmonary venous pressure than in intrapericardial pressure; this also leads to reduced left ventricular filling.

Echocardiography may be used not only to document the presence of pericardial effusion but also to show evidence of cardiac tamponade.[13-16] In the presence of tamponade, there is right ventricular compression evidenced by a markedly reduced end-expiratory, end-diastolic dimension due to a sudden increase in anterior motion of the interventricular septum toward the right rather than the left ventricular cavity. Right ventricular compression disappears following pericardiocentesis and is not present with pericardial effusion without tamponade.

As the rise in pericardial pressure becomes severe, stroke volume decreases and systemic vascular resistance increases, resulting in a fall in systolic pressure, a rise in diastolic pressure, and a narrowing of the arterial pulse pressure. However, hypotension in the presence of tamponade is usually a late finding.

The electrocardiogram (ECG) often shows low voltage and nonspecific ST-T wave abnormalities. Electric alternans, a beat-to-beat change in the axis of the ECG that is due to a swinging motion of the heart within the pericardial effusion, may be present. Total alternans, which involves the P wave as well as the QRS, may be more specific for pericardial effusion.[17] Electromechanical dissociation also may be a manifestation of cardiac tamponade.

Treatment[1,3-6,18]

The specific therapy for cardiac tamponade is drainage of the pericardial fluid. However, until drainage can be performed, the following measures may be helpful.

Volume infusion increases stroke volume in cardiac tamponade by increasing ventricular filling pressure. Rapid intravenous (IV) administration of fluid will provide temporary hemodynamic support for the patient with acute tamponade. The first 500 mL of fluid should be given over a 10-minute period, followed by 100 to 500 mL/h thereafter, according to the patient's response to the initial volume load. The administration of fluid volume appears most beneficial with an acute tamponade[19] but is of limited value when tamponade follows a subacute or chronic pericardial effusion.[20]

Description of Pericardiocentesis

Decompression of a pericardial effusion producing cardiac tamponade is always indicated. Surgical decompression is preferred. Needle pericardiocentesis is indicated when cardiac tamponade represents an immediate threat to life, ie, when it produces increasingly severe hemodynamic impairment. In general, pericardiocentesis should be performed in any patient with acute tamponade and respiratory distress, progressive hypotension with jugular venous distention, or other signs of circulatory compromise. Open drainage is safer and more effective. Procedures include subxiphoid pericardiotomy, which not only allows for drainage of pericardial fluid but also permits a biopsy specimen that is especially helpful for the diagnosis of granulomatous and lymphomatous invasion of the pericardium; parietal pericardiectomy (pericardial window) via a left thoracotomy, which provides for continuing drainage of fluid and thereby prevents recurrence; and visceral pericardiectomy, which is necessary for effusive constrictive pericarditis and constrictive pericarditis.[2,21] If time and resources permit, most cardiologists now drain pericardial effusions in the catheterization laboratory using fluoroscopy, echocardiography, and flexible catheters introduced by the Seldinger technique.

Needle pericardiocentesis should be performed only by a skilled and experienced physician. It is optimally performed in the presence of large amounts of pericardial fluid. When time permits, pericardial fluid is best documented and localized by echocardiography. During pericardiocentesis the patient's ECG should be continuously monitored, and ideally, invasive hemodynamic monitoring should be used as well. Full resuscitative equipment, as well as personnel experienced in its use, must be available. Different approaches have been advocated.[18] Some echocardiographic[22,23] and autopsy[24] data suggest that the left fifth intercostal approach (Fig 1) may be optimal.

The following technique should be used when the resources of a fully equipped catheterization laboratory are not immediately available. Ideally the ECG V lead should be connected to the needle with a sterile alligator clip with care to ensure that the patient limb leads are attached. If ST-segment elevation occurs as the needle is advanced, ventricular contact is suggested; if PR-segment elevation occurs, atrial contact is suggested. Elevation of both ST and PR segments may also indicate pericardial contact with no intervening fluid within the pericardial sac. However, these are signs indicating need for withdrawal of the needle. Other signs of epicardial contact include atrial and ventricular arrhythmias and atrioventricular conduction abnormalities. Monitoring the ECG from the pericardiocentesis needle may prevent entry of the needle into the pericardium when there is no cushioning layer of fluid present. It also immediately signals entry of the needle into the myocardium, allowing the operator to withdraw the needle and minimize any myocardial or coronary artery laceration. If blood or fluid is obtained without the appearance of ST- or PR-segment shift or cardiac arrhythmias, this is an indication that the fluid was obtained from the pericardial sac rather than the cardiac chamber. However, in the presence of myocardial scarring due to old transmural infarction or infiltrative

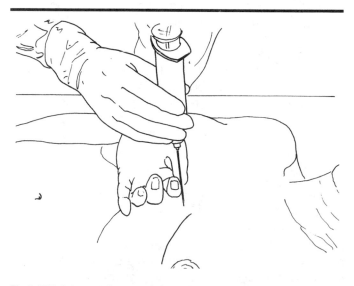

Fig 1. Fifth intercostal approach for pericardiocentesis.

myocardial disease, the needle may enter an electrically silent area of the myocardium and not produce PR- or ST-segment elevation or cardiac arrhythmias.[25-27]

If immediate pericardiocentesis is necessary to sustain the life of the patient, an alternative approach is to use the Seldinger technique with a thin scout needle to locate the pericardial space. Once the pericardial space is entered, the guidewire is passed and used to facilitate placement of a large-bore catheter into the space.

Equipment Needed

1. A short-bevel, large-bore needle at least 16 gauge and 9 cm long (a Seldinger catheter set for central venous lines may also be used)
2. A 30- or 50-mL syringe
3. Sterile alligator connector to ECG V lead
4. Povidone-iodine solution for skin preparation
5. Syringe with small-bore needle and 1% lidocaine without epinephrine for local anesthetic
6. Sterile gloves and sterile drapes; ideally, sterile gowns and face masks

Technique (Fig 1)

1. Have the patient in a supine position or with the upper torso elevated 20° to 30°.
2. Prepare the anterior midthorax with povidone-iodine solution.
3. If the patient is conscious or responsive to pain, infiltrate the skin and subcutaneous tissues immediately to the left of the sternum in the fifth intercostal space with 1% lidocaine without epinephrine. A small skin incision with a scalpel blade will facilitate entry of the large-bore needle.
4. Attach the large-bore needle to the syringe and connect the alligator clamp with ECG V lead to the needle. Insert the large-bore needle attached to the syringe perpendicular to the frontal plane. Aspiration should be continuous. As the needle is advanced beneath the skin, the resistance of the taut pericardium may be felt, and entry into the pericardial space may produce a distinct "giving" sensation. Contact of the needle against the epicardium may be accompanied by a scratching sensation or by PR- and ST-segment elevation if the ECG V lead is connected to the pericardiocentesis needle as described above.
5. If grossly bloody fluid is obtained, it should not clot if from the pericardial space. A spun hematocrit may also denote a difference between venous and bloody pericardial fluids.

It may be advantageous to insert a catheter into the pericardial space. This avoids the potential epicardial or coronary artery injury that might be produced by the sharp tip of a needle. It also allows for continuous drainage of fluid from the pericardial space. As noted above, use of a Seldinger (guidewire) system is useful for this indication. Use of the wire allows a larger catheter to be passed into the pericardial space than can be inserted through a needle.[28]

Alternative Approach[18]

Some clinicians prefer the xiphisternal or subxiphoid approach for pericardiocentesis (Fig 2). This technique is performed like the fifth intercostal approach, although the needle is inserted between the xiphoid process and the left costal margin at a 30° to 45° angle to the skin. The heart is located between the neck and left shoulder when the needle is directed in the coronal plane.

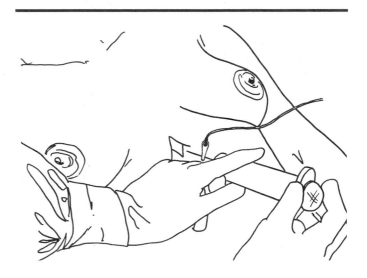

Fig 2. Subxiphoid approach for pericardiocentesis.

Hazards[7,18,21,29,30]

Significant risks accompany pericardiocentesis. Cardiac arrhythmias, including ventricular fibrillation and asystole, may occur. Puncture or laceration of the cardiac chambers or the coronary arteries is a possibility. Air may be inadvertently injected into the cardiac chambers if a catheter or needle placed into a cardiac chamber is left open to air. Hemothorax, pneumothorax, or both may occur. Hemorrhage from myocardial or coronary artery puncture or laceration following pericardiocentesis may in itself produce cardiac tamponade, especially in the patient with thrombocytopenia or if thrombolytic therapy has been used.

Intracardiac Injections

Intracardiac injections are not recommended. However, in desperate clinical situations when an IV cannot be started or an endotracheal tube placed, intracardiac injections can be used to administer epinephrine to treat ventricular fibrillation, asystole, or PEA.[31-33] Anecdotal data suggest that intracardiac epinephrine may have been effective in restoring cardiac contractions in asystole or electromechanical dissociation when IV epinephrine was ineffective. Whether the needle stick or the drug itself was effective has not been resolved. Regardless, IV and endotracheal routes should always be attempted initially.

Equipment Needed

Equipment for intracardiac injections should include the following:

1. Povidone-iodine solution for skin sterilization
2. A 19-gauge, 3½-inch ($\approx$ 9-cm) needle attached to a syringe filled with the drug to be injected
3. Sterile gloves to be worn for optimal asepsis

Technique

As with pericardiocentesis, the parasternal and subxiphoid approaches are preferred. The steps in the process of intracardiac injections are as follows:

1. Place the patient in a supine position.
2. Cleanse the area of insertion with povidone-iodine solution.
3. Insert the needle using one of the sites and approaches previously described for pericardiocentesis.
4. Maintain suction on the syringe and stop once blood appears. If no blood appears when the needle is fully advanced, continue maintaining suction and slowly withdraw the needle. If no blood appears, withdraw the needle altogether and repeat the attempt.
5. When brisk filling of the syringe occurs, the needle is inside the ventricular cavity. The medication can now be injected.

Complications[31-33]

The major hazard of an intracardiac injection is the need to interrupt CPR during injection. Although uncommon, complications may follow intracardiac injection — pneumothorax, pneumopericardium, hemopericardium (with or without tamponade), myocardial laceration, coronary artery laceration, internal mammary artery laceration, and intramyocardial injection.

Tension Pneumothorax

Intrapleural pressure is normally subatmospheric throughout the respiratory cycle. Because of elastic recoil of the lung, the intra-alveolar pressure is at all times greater than intrapleural pressure. Thus transpulmonary pressure, which is alveolar pressure minus intrapleural pressure, is always positive.[34,35] The transpulmonary pressure gradient is markedly increased during coughing, breathing against an airway obstruction, and positive-pressure ventilation.

If a break occurs in the alveolar-pleural barrier, air enters the pleural space, and the elasticity of the lung causes it to collapse. This condition is called a *pneumothorax*. As long as the transpulmonary gradient is maintained, the air leak will continue. Lung collapse ceases when either the communication is sealed or intra-alveolar and intrapleural pressures become equal.[34-37]

Causes of Pneumothorax

There are four general causes of pneumothorax[38]:

Group 1: Alveoli become overdistended and rupture.

Group 2: The facial planes of the neck are injured by being either incised at operation or lacerated by trauma, allowing entry of air into the mediastinum, producing mediastinal emphysema.

Group 3: There is a direct connection of the distal airway to the pleural space. High airway pressure from either positive-pressure ventilation or coughing may cause rupture of a bleb on the surface of the lung. Fractured ribs caused by nonpenetrating injuries to the chest wall may puncture both the parietal and visceral pleura and tear the underlying lung, or a needle introduced through the chest wall into the pleural space may tear the lung; the tear may be inapparent until positive pressure is applied to the airway. Each of these produces a pneumothorax.

Group 4: Breaks in the parietal pleura can connect the pleural space with an extrathoracic source of air, producing pneumothorax. Causes include traumatic esophageal pleural fistulas, emergency tracheostomy, thoracotomy, diaphragmatic tears (both traumatic and during abdominal operations), or a needle in the pleural space that is open to air, such as during thoracentesis.

Causes of Tension Pneumothorax

Air under pressure in the pleural space is referred to as a tension pneumothorax. A simple pneumothorax may be converted to a tension pneumothorax if there is a ball-valve mechanism at the site of the leak that permits air to enter but not to leave the pleural space; at each inspiration the volume of gas in the pleural space increases, and the pressure becomes markedly elevated during exhalation.[34,37] If positive pressure is applied to the airway, such as during positive-pressure ventilation or coughing,[39,40] intra-alveolar pressure becomes markedly elevated, air leak increases, and air under pressure rapidly accumulates in the pleural space.[40]

Direct causes of a tension pneumothorax include (1) barotrauma from positive-pressure ventilation alone (especially with positive end-expiratory pressure) and with endobronchial intubation and (2) malfunctioning exhalation valves on bag-valve–mask units,[41,42] ventilators, or anesthesia machines,[43] especially with preexisting chronic obstructive pulmonary disease, acute necrotizing pneumonitis, or pulmonary infarction.[44-48] Tension pneumothorax has also been reported following fiberoptic bronchoscopy with closed lung biopsy[49] and with pneumoperitoneum.[36,37,40,50,51]

Clinical Manifestations

In this syndrome the spontaneously breathing patient experiences dyspnea and may complain of chest pain. Examination reveals tachypnea, tachycardia, and distended neck veins with florid facies. The patient may be hypertensive initially, with hypotension a later finding. Compared with the contralateral side, the hemithorax under tension may be more prominent and hyperresonant with diminished breath sounds; wheezing may be audible.[36] The trachea may be deviated contralaterally. However, significant tension pneumothorax may be present without these typical physical findings.

In the patient being treated with positive-pressure ventilation, an increase in peak pressure is needed to deliver the tidal volume because of increased pleural pressure; there is a diminution of expiratory volume because the air leaks from the lungs. There may be increased end-expiratory pressure even with the discontinuation of positive end-expiratory pressure.[40,52]

If a pulmonary artery catheter is in position, a sudden increase in pulmonary artery pressure will be noted, presumably due to both the compressive effect of the pneumothorax and hypoxic pulmonary arterial vasoconstriction.[53] The ECG may show a rightward shift in the mean frontal axis, a diminution in precordial voltage, and precordial T-wave inversion. Hypoxemia, caused both by intrapulmonary shunting and decreased cardiac output, may be present.

A chest x-ray film generally will show the ipsilateral lung collapsed toward the hilum.[36,37] However, there may be localized tension pneumothorax with various degrees of lung collapse if there is coexistent pulmonary or pleural disease. The trachea and the heart are usually displaced contralaterally, whereas the ipsilateral intercostal spaces are widened and the hemidiaphragm is pushed downward. The hemidiaphragm may be inverted if the pneumothorax occurs on the left side, but this effect is prevented on the right side by the liver.

Treatment

Since a *tension* pneumothorax may produce cardiovascular collapse and cardiac arrest, emergency relief of pressure must be accomplished as soon as the clinical diagnosis is apparent. This may allow little time for x-ray film confirmation. A diagnostic needle tap with a large-bore needle should be performed in the second or third anterior intercostal space. Since the internal mammary artery parallels the sternum approximately the breadth of one or two fingers from its edge, the needle is best inserted in the midclavicular line to avoid serious bleeding from this vessel. In addition, the needle should be inserted over the top of a rib to avoid the intercostal artery and vein that run on the lower border of each rib.

In the presence of cardiovascular collapse from a tension pneumothorax, simply inserting a catheter-over-needle device into the chest, removing the needle, and leaving the catheter open to the air is appropriate. Air escaping through the needle with a hissing noise is proof of tension pneumothorax. Although this maneuver technically produces a pneumothorax in itself, an external *open* pneumothorax is less likely to be lethal than an internal closed valve-like tension pneumothorax. With open pneumothorax, positive-pressure ventilation or spontaneous exhalation against resistance can reexpand the lung.

Equipment Needed

1. Povidone-iodine solution for skin preparation
2. A 14-gauge catheter-over-needle device

Technique

1. Cleanse the overlying skin with povidone-iodine solution.
2. Insert the 14-gauge catheter-over-needle device into the second intercostal space in the midclavicular line just above the top of the third rib. Entry into the pleural space and confirmation of air under tension will be evident by hearing the escape of air through the open needle.
3. Remove the needle and leave the catheter in the pleural space open to atmospheric air.
4. As soon as possible, perform tube thoracostomy with underwater seal drainage for definitive treatment.

Complications of Treatment

The most common complication is due to misdiagnosis. If a pneumothorax is present but not under tension, inserting the needle will convert it from a closed pneumothorax to an open pneumothorax. If there is no pneumothorax, insertion of a needle open to the atmosphere will produce a pneumothorax. This can be easily treated with a tube thoracostomy.

Insertion of either a steel needle or a Teflon catheter may lacerate the lung and produce a significant pulmonary injury or hemothorax. If the needle is inserted adjacent to the sternum, the internal mammary artery may be punctured. If the needle is inserted at the lower margin of the rib, the intercostal vessels may be lacerated. Either event may lead to significant hemothorax. Also, the catheter may become kinked or displaced, permitting a closed pneumothorax to reaccumulate. Since simple needle placement will not expand most pneumothoraces, chest tube placement and application of negative pressure should follow needle placement as soon as possible.

References

1. Hancock EW. Management of pericardial disease. *Mod Concepts Cardiovasc Dis*. 1979;48:1-6.
2. Roberts WC, Spray TL. Pericardial heart disease: a study of its causes, consequences, and morphologic features. In: Spodick D, ed. *Pericardial Diseases*. Philadelphia, Pa: FA Davis Co; 1976;7(No. 3):11-65. Cardiovascular Clinics series.

3. Fowler NO. Physiology of cardiac tamponade and pulsus paradoxus, II: physiological, circulatory, and pharmacological responses in cardiac tamponade. *Mod Concepts Cardiovasc Dis.* 1978; 47:115-118.

4. Shabetai R. The pathophysiology of cardiac tamponade and constriction. In: Spodick D, ed. *Pericardial Diseases.* Philadelphia, Pa: FA Davis Co; 1976;7(No. 3):67-89. Cardiovascular Clinics series.

5. Shabetai R, Fowler NO, Guntheroth WG. The hemodynamics of cardiac tamponade and constrictive pericarditis. *Am J Cardiol.* 1970;26:480-489.

6. Fowler NO. Physiology of cardiac tamponade and pulsus paradoxus, I: mechanisms of pulsus paradoxus in cardiac tamponade. *Mod Concepts Cardiovasc Dis.* 1978;47:109-113.

7. Fowler NO. The recognition and management of pericardial disease and its complications. In: Hurst JW, Logue RB, Schlant RC, Wenger NK, eds. *The Heart, Arteries, and Veins.* 4th ed. New York, NY: McGraw-Hill Book Co Inc; 1978:1640-1659.

8. Spodick DH. The pericardium: structure, function, and disease spectrum. In: Spodick DH, ed. *Pericardial Diseases.* Philadelphia, Pa: FA Davis Co; 1976;7(No. 3):1-10. Cardiovascular Clinics series.

9. Beck CS. Two cardiac compression triads. *JAMA.* 1935;104: 714-716.

10. Reddy PS, Curtiss EI, O'Toole JD, Shaver JA. Cardiac tamponade: hemodynamic observations in man. *Circulation.* 1978;58:265-272.

11. Shabetai R. The pericardium: an essay on some recent developments. *Am J Cardiol.* 1978;42:1036-1043.

12. Fowler NO. Cardiac tamponade: a clinical or an echocardiographic diagnosis? *Circulation.* 1993;87:1738-1741.

13. Cosio FG, Martinez JP, Serrano CM, de la Calada CS, Alcaine CC. Abnormal septal motion in cardiac tamponade with pulsus paradoxus: echocardiographic and hemodynamic observations. *Chest.* 1977;71:787-788.

14. Settle HP, Adolph RJ, Fowler NO, Engel P, Agruss NS, Levenson NI. Echocardiographic study of cardiac tamponade. *Circulation.* 1977;56:951-959.

15. Schiller NB, Botvinick EH. Right ventricular compression as a sign of cardiac tamponade: an analysis of echocardiographic ventricular dimensions and their clinical implications. *Circulation.* 1977;56: 774-779.

16. Armstrong WF, Schilt BF, Helper DJ, Dillon JC, Feigenbaum H. Diastolic collapse of the right ventricle with cardiac tamponade: an echocardiographic study. *Circulation.* 1982;65:1491-1496.

17. Usher BW, Popp RL. Electrical alternans: mechanism in pericardial effusion. *Am Heart J.* 1972;83:459-463.

18. Callaham ML. Pericardiocentesis. In: Roberts JR, Hedges JR, eds. *Clinical Procedures in Emergency Medicine.* 2nd ed. Philadelphia, Pa: WB Saunders Co; 1991:210-228.

19. Cooper FW Jr, Stead EA Jr, Warren JV. Beneficial effect of intravenous infusions in acute pericardial tamponade. *Ann Surg.* 1944;120:822-825.

20. Kerber RE, Gascho JA, Litchfield R, Wolfson P, Ott D, Pandian NG. Hemodynamic effects of volume expansion and nitroprusside compared with pericardiocentesis in patients with acute cardiac tamponade. *N Engl J Med.* 1982;307:929-931.

21. Kilpatrick ZM, Chapman CB. On pericardiocentesis. *Am J Cardiol.* 1965;16:722-728.

22. Callahan JA, Seward JB, Nishimura RA, Miller FA Jr, Reeder GS, Shub C, Callahan MJ, Schattenberg TT, Tajik AJ. Two-dimensional echocardiographically guided pericardiocentesis: experience in 117 consecutive patients. *Am J Cardiol.* 1985;55:476-479.

23. Clarke DP, Cosgrove DO. Real-time ultrasound scanning in the planning and guidance of pericardiocentesis. *Clin Radiol.* 1987;38: 119-122.

24. Brown CG, Gurley HT, Hutchins GM, MacKenzie EJ, White JD. Injuries associated with percutaneous placement of transthoracic pacemakers. *Ann Emerg Med.* 1985;14:223-228.

25. Bishop LH Jr, Estes EH Jr, McIntosh HD. The electrocardiogram as a safeguard in pericardiocentesis. *JAMA.* 1956;162:264-265.

26. Sobol SM, Thomas HM Jr, Evans RW. Myocardial laceration not demonstrated by continuous electrocardiographic monitoring occurring during pericardiocentesis. *N Engl J Med.* 1975;292: 1222-1223.

27. Kerber RE, Ridges JD, Harrison DC. Electrocardiographic indications of atrial puncture during pericardiocentesis. *N Engl J Med.* 1970;282:1142-1143.

28. Wei JY, Taylor GJ, Achuff SC. Recurrent cardiac tamponade and large pericardial effusions: management with an indwelling pericardial catheter. *Am J Cardiol.* 1978;42:281-282.

29. Krikorian JG, Hancock EW. Pericardiocentesis. *Am J Med.* 1978;65:808-814.

30. Wong B, Murphy J, Chang CJ, Hassenein K, Dunn M. The risk of pericardiocentesis. *Am J Cardiol.* 1979;44:1110-1114.

31. Amey BD, Harrison EE, Straub EJ, McLeod M. Paramedic use of intracardiac medications in prehospital sudden cardiac death. *J Am Coll Emerg Phys.* 1978;7:130-134.

32. Davison R, Barresi V, Parker M, Meyers SN, Talano JV. Intracardiac injections during cardiopulmonary resuscitation: a low-risk procedure. *JAMA.* 1980;244:1110-1111.

33. Frolich TG, Davison R. Intracardiac injections. In: Roberts JR, Hedges JR, eds. *Clinical Procedures in Emergency Medicine.* 2nd ed. Philadelphia, Pa: WB Saunders Co; 1991:377-382.

34. Killen DA, Gobbel WG. *Spontaneous Pneumothorax.* Boston, Mass: Little Brown & Co; 1968.

35. Comroe JH. *Physiology of Respiration.* Chicago, Ill: Yearbook Medical Publishers; 1974:102.

36. Teplick SK, Clark RE. Various faces of tension pneumothorax. *Postgrad Med.* 1974;56:87-92.

37. Fraser RG, Pare JAP. *Diagnosis of Diseases of the Chest.* 2nd ed. Philadelphia, Pa: WB Saunders Co; 1977;1:598-600.

38. Martin JT, Patrick RT. Pneumothorax: its significance to the anesthesiologist. *Anesth Analg.* 1960;39:420-429.

39. Macklin CC. Transport of air along sheaths of pulmonic blood vessels from alveoli to mediastinum: clinical implications. *Arch Intern Med.* 1939;64:913-926.

40. Safar P. Blunt chest injuries. In: Weil MH, Henning RJ, eds. *The Handbook of Critical Care Medicine.* New York, NY: EM Brooks; 1979:93-103.

41. Klick JM, Bushnell LS, Bancroft ML. Barotrauma, a potential hazard of manual resuscitators. *Anesthesiology.* 1978;49:363-365.

42. Wisborg K, Jacobsen E. Functional disorders of Ruben and ambu-E valves after dismantling and cleaning. *Anesthesiology.* 1975;42: 633-634.

43. Dean HN, Parsons DE, Raphaely RC. Case report: bilateral tension pneumothorax from mechanical failure of anesthesia machine due to misplaced expiratory valve. *Anesth Analg.* 1971;50:195-198.

44. Mundth ED, Foley FD, Austen WG. Pneumothorax as a complication of pulmonary infarct in patients on positive pressure respiratory assistance. *J Thorac Cardiovasc Surg.* 1965;50:555-560.

45. Rohlfing BM, Webb WR, Schlobohm RM. Ventilator-related extra-alveolar air in adults. *Radiology.* 1976;121:25-31.

46. Kumar A, Pontoppidan H, Falke KJ, Wilson RS, Laver MB. Pulmonary barotrauma during mechanical ventilation. *Crit Care Med.* 1973;1:181-186.

47. Zwillich CW, Pierson DJ, Creagh CE, Sutton FD, Schatz E, Petty TL. Complications of assisted ventilation: a prospective study of 354 consecutive episodes. *Am J Med.* 1974;57:161-170.

48. Powner DJ, Snyder JV, Morris CW, Grenvik A. Retroperitoneal air dissection associated with mechanical ventilation. *Chest.* 1976;69: 739-742.

49. Stalker R, Ward RL. Hazards of fiberoptic bronchoscopy. *BMJ.* 1979;1:553. Letter.

50. Stutz FH. Bilateral tension pneumothorax after pneumoperitoneum: a case report. *Mil Med.* 1971;136:894-895.

51. Nayak IN, Lawrence D. Tension pneumothorax from a perforated gastric ulcer. *Br J Surg.* 1976;63:245-247.

52. Estafanous FG, Viljoen JF, Barsoum KN. Diagnosis of pneumothorax complicating mechanical ventilation. *Anesth Analg.* 1975; 54:730-735.

53. McLoud TC, Barash PG, Ravin CE, Mandel SD. Elevation of pulmonary artery pressure as a sign of pulmonary barotrauma (pneumothorax). *Crit Care Med.* 1978;6:81-84.

Credit is given to Peter Miniscalco for artwork.

Cerebral Resuscitation: Treatment of the Brain After Cardiac Resuscitation

Chapter 14

Pathophysiology

The human brain is a complex organ. It consists of some 10 billion neurons, each with multiple axonal and dendritic connections to other cells, totaling an estimated 500 trillion synapses. Although the brain represents only 2% of body weight, because of its high metabolic activity it receives 15% of the body's cardiac output and accounts for 20% of the body's oxygen use. Although no mechanical and little secretory work is performed, energy expenditures include the synthesis of cellular constituents (eg, an estimated 2000 mitochondria are reproduced each day by each cell) and neurotransmitter substances as well as the axoplasmic transport of these substances and the transmembrane pumping of ions.

During cardiac arrest the brain converts to anaerobic metabolism. This energy production is inadequate to supply the high metabolic needs of the brain. Thus, during total circulatory arrest, brain function quickly deteriorates as the brain "turns itself off." This "turning off" may occur in a progressive stepwise fashion if perfusion and oxygen delivery are compromised gradually (Table 1).

Table 1. Correlation of Progressive Deterioration of Cerebral Blood Flow and Tissue Oxygenation With Resultant Effects on Brain

CBF (mL/100 g/min)	Effect on Central Nervous System	Po_2 (mm Hg)
50	**Normal**	100
30-40	Depression of electroencephalogram	
20-30	Anaerobic metabolism	40
15-20	Adenosine triphosphate depletion, coma	25
8-10	**Viability threshold**	12
	K+ leak	
	Membrane depolarization	
Trickle	Continued electrolyte flux	
	Continued anaerobic metabolism/ lactate production	
	Worsened acidosis	
0	Metabolism ceases	
	Electrolyte flux ceases	

CBF indicates cerebral blood flow.

With the onset of cardiac arrest, people quickly lose consciousness, usually within 15 seconds. By the end of 1 minute, brain stem function ceases, respirations become agonal, and pupils are fixed or dilated. This clinical picture corresponds to the biochemical changes of oxygen depletion that occur over 15 seconds. In these 15 seconds the patient loses consciousness. Glucose and adenosine triphosphate are exhausted within 4 to 5 minutes.

While irreversible brain damage is commonly believed to occur after 4 to 6 minutes of cardiac arrest,[1] current evidence suggests that neurons are more resistant to ischemia than was previously thought.[2,3] Even after as many as 60 minutes of complete ischemia (without reperfusion), neurons maintain some electrical and biochemical activity.[4,5]

Reperfusion of the brain after cardiac arrest produces additional brain damage. This "postresuscitation syndrome" includes variable but persistent hypoperfusion thought to be caused by vasoconstriction, decreased red blood cell deformability, platelet aggregation, pericapillary cellular edema, and abnormal calcium ion fluxes. Increased intracranial pressure has not been implicated.[6-10] The inability to regain cerebral blood flow after a significant period of flow interruption has also been called the "no-reflow phenomenon."[11,12] It may last for 18 to 24 hours. Following this, regional cerebral blood flow may improve, leading to functional recovery, or decline, leading to progressive ischemic damage and cell death.[11,13]

Also implicated in the postresuscitation syndrome are the effects of ischemia-induced intracellular calcium overload. Calcium overload is hypothesized to precipitate vasospasm, uncouple oxidative phosphorylation, destroy cellular membranes, and produce a wide variety of toxic chemicals, including prostaglandins, leukotrienes, and free radicals.[14,15] Although the unfolding story of the pathophysiology of the postresuscitation syndrome reveals previously unknown mechanisms of tissue damage, there are also reasons for increasing optimism. First, neurons have recently been demonstrated to be more resistant to ischemia than was previously believed. Second, the secondary mechanisms of tissue injury occur during postischemic reperfusion. Consequently, interventions can be used to mitigate this tissue injury. Increasing numbers of potentially beneficial agents are being identified in the continuing search for effective therapies for resuscitation of the brain.

Both the brain and noncerebral organs must be supported during the postischemic period. Table 2 presents brain-oriented intensive care for survivors of cardiac arrest.

Table 2. General Brain-Oriented Intensive Care

Normotension throughout coma (eg, mean arterial pressure, 90-100 mm Hg or normal systolic level for patient): titrated fluids and vasopressors as needed

Moderate hyperventilation (arterial P_{CO_2}, 30-35 mm Hg)

Moderate hyperoxia (arterial P_{CO_2}, > 100 mm Hg): titrated F_{IO_2}; least positive end-expiratory pressure (PEEP) possible

Arterial pH 7.3-7.5

Immobilization (neuromuscular paralysis) as needed

Sedation (morphine or diazepam) as needed

Anticonvulsants (eg, diazepam, phenytoin, or barbiturates) as needed

Normalization of blood chemistry (hematocrit, electrolytes, osmolality, and glucose)

Osmotherapy (mannitol or glycerol) as needed for monitored intracranial pressure elevation or secondary neurological deterioration

Normothermia

Nutritional support started by 48 hours

Brain-Oriented Treatment of the Patient After Resuscitation From Cardiac Arrest

Noncerebral Organ Systems After Cardiac Arrest

Perfusion Pressures

Maintenance of adequate cerebral perfusion pressure (ie, normal to high normal standard range as determined by the individual patient's baseline prearrest blood pressure) is a mainstay of treatment. Normally cerebral blood flow is autoregulated, so flow is independent of perfusion pressure over a wide range of blood pressures (between approximately 50 and 150 mm Hg mean arterial pressure). During ischemia, however, accumulation of tissue metabolites and abnormal calcium ion fluxes cause autoregulation to be compromised (false autoregulation) if not lost.[16] Perfusion of ischemic tissue then becomes dependent on arterial pressure. The occurrence of postischemic hypotension can cause severe compromise of cerebral blood flow and result in significant additional brain damage.[17] Therefore, following restoration of spontaneous circulation, arterial pressure should be rapidly normalized, using intravascular volume administration and vasopressors.[18]

In experimental studies a transient period of vasopressor-induced moderate hypertension improved postischemic brain reperfusion and neurological recovery.[19-22] Such transient hypertensive reperfusion may occur after CPR because of epinephrine loading during resuscitation.

Oxygenation

Adequate tissue oxygenation is necessary to preserve cellular function and to allow postischemic reparative processes to occur. Moderate hyperoxia (P_{O_2} greater than 100 mm Hg) should be maintained. This prevents transient pulmonary problems from causing a significant deterioration of oxygenation in already compromised tissues. Adequate arterial P_{O_2} levels should be maintained using the lowest F_{IO_2} possible with carefully titrated positive end-expiratory pressure (PEEP). Some controversy exists concerning a possible role of high arterial oxygen levels in the generation of postischemic, reperfusion-induced free radicals. These concerns are speculative and should not affect current clinical practice.

Hyperventilation

By lowering intracranial blood volume through cerebral vasoconstriction, passive hyperventilation can effectively lower intracranial pressure (in patients in whom it is elevated). This may result in improved cerebral perfusion. Although cytotoxic cellular edema occurs after ischemic brain insults,[23-25] it does not usually accumulate enough to cause continued elevation of intracranial pressure following cardiac arrest.[6-10] Thus, if hyperventilation is beneficial after cardiac arrest, it is not through this mechanism.

Hyperventilation may correct postischemic tissue acidosis and helps excretion of the carbon dioxide load generated from bicarbonate administration during CPR. As hyperventilation continues, however, cerebrospinal fluid and renal ion transport mechanisms attempt to compensate.[26] After approximately 4 hours, the effectiveness of hyperventilation may decline.[27] Passive hyperventilation is of unproven value for the comatose cardiac arrest survivor,[24,27] with the possible exception of benefit for the hypothesized vasogenic edema and intracranial hypertension of late secondary neurological deterioration (24 hours or more after insult).

Correction of Acidosis

Severe tissue lactic acidosis limits cell survival after brain ischemia.[16,28] Experimental data strongly suggest that therapeutic measures aimed at preventing or ameliorating tissue acidosis are of significant clinical benefit.[28] Accumulation of metabolic acids during ischemia is in part compensated by a decrease in P_{CO_2}; however, respiratory compensation for a metabolic acid load is limited.[28] Unfortunately correction of intracellular acidosis remains a clinical challenge.

Temperature Control

Cerebral metabolic rate increases about 8% per degree centigrade of body temperature elevation. The regional cerebral metabolic rate determines the regional blood flow requirements. Thus elevation of temperature above normal can create significant imbalance between oxygen supply and demand, and it should be aggressively treated in the postischemic period.

Hypothermia, on the other hand, is an effective method of suppression of cerebral metabolic activity. Although widely used during cardiovascular surgery, hypothermia has significant detrimental effects that might adversely affect the post–cardiac arrest patient, including increased blood viscosity, decreased cardiac output, and increased susceptibility to infection.[29] Many reports indicate benefit after brain ischemia,[30-32] although some document detrimental effects or lack of improvement.[33,34] Recent evidence indicates that mild levels of hypothermia (eg, 34°C) are effective in mitigating postischemic brain damage without inducing detrimental side effects.[35,36]

The delayed hypermetabolism believed to occur after normothermic cardiac arrest, with its attendant potential imbalance of cerebral oxygen supply and demand, also suggests a possible clinical role for induced hypothermia.[16,37] Clinical investigation seems indicated, but at present therapeutic hypothermia cannot be recommended for routine clinical use after cardiac arrest.

Other Biochemical Parameters

Alteration of hematocrit (hemodilution). The balance between improving blood flow by reducing viscosity with hemodilution and the associated compromise of oxygen-carrying capacity has not been resolved.

Glucose. Continued supply of glucose to ischemic tissues, either through high pre–cardiac arrest tissue stores or because of continued trickle blood flow, allows continued anaerobic metabolism. This results in excessive lactate production. As a result, tissue lactic acidosis becomes more severe, exacerbating tissue damage. Although high preischemic blood glucose levels can exacerbate brain damage, adequate nutritional support and at least normal blood glucose levels should be maintained after resuscitation to supply needed metabolic substrates for tissue repair.[38,39]

Immobilization/Sedation

The comatose brain can respond to external stimuli, such as physical examination and airway suctioning, and this can increase cerebral metabolism. This elevated regional brain metabolism requires increased regional cerebral blood flow at a time when the oxygen demand-perfusion rates may be precariously balanced. Protection from afferent sensory stimuli with administration of titrated doses of sedative-anesthetic drugs and muscle relaxants may prevent oxygen supply-demand imbalance and improve the chances for neuronal recovery.

Anticonvulsant Therapy

Seizure activity can increase brain metabolism by 300% to 400%.[40] This extreme increase in metabolic demand may tip the tissue oxygen supply-demand balance unfavorably with catastrophic neurological consequences. Conflicting evidence about the effects of postischemic seizures on neurological recovery has been reported. Some report exacerbation of postischemic brain damage,[41-43] whereas others report no effect on neurological recovery.[44-46] Although there is disagreement about the prophylactic use of anticonvulsant drugs, ie, treatment before a seizure occurs, there is general agreement that

a postischemic seizure should be quickly and effectively treated. Commonly used drugs include barbiturates, phenytoin, and diazepam.

Corticosteroids

Although corticosteroids are commonly administered to patients with intracranial pathology of any cause, their value is largely unproved. Evidence does support a benefit in patients with intracranial tumor-related cerebral edema,[47] but there is no benefit in patients with other types of cerebral pathology.[48,49]

Brain-Specific Therapies After Cardiac Arrest

Researchers are investigating brain resuscitation measures specifically aimed at reversing the secondary postreperfusion pathophysiology that occurs after prolonged cardiac arrest. Among the first to look promising in studies of laboratory animals were the barbiturates. However, a randomized clinical trial of thiopental loading after cardiac arrest did not indicate benefit in humans.[44] On the basis of this study, high-dose thiopental loading cannot be recommended for routine clinical use after cardiac arrest. Nonetheless, for specific therapeutic effects in, eg, sedation, anticonvulsant therapy, or intracranial pressure reduction, barbiturates can be safely administered to patients resuscitated from cardiac arrest.

Calcium Entry Blocking Drugs

In the wake of the unfolding theory of calcium-related pathophysiology of brain ischemia, investigators have been examining the potential usefulness of these drugs after circulatory arrest. With the support of the National Institutes of Health, 20 hospitals in eight countries tested the effects of lidoflazine, an investigational calcium entry blocker, on neurological recovery in comatose cardiac arrest survivors. No differences in outcomes between patients treated with lidoflazine or standard therapy were found.[50] Clinical trials of nimodipine[51] and flunarizine similarly did not show benefit of treatment. No drug of this type has yet proved beneficial for clinical treatment of post–cardiac arrest brain damage.

Other Experimental Modalities

A number of experimental brain resuscitation therapies of varying potential promise, eg, prostaglandin synthesis inhibitors, free radical scavengers, free iron chelators, excitatory amino acid receptor blockers, and combinations of these therapies, are still awaiting definitive investigation. None is yet ready for clinical use.

Summary

Rapidly expanding knowledge about the pathophysiology of postischemic encephalopathy is leading to new avenues of research for developing effective therapies for brain resuscitation. Experimental work suggests many promising therapies. Unfortunately, varying animal models and research protocols make comparison and synthesis of experimental results difficult. Currently no single drug or therapeutic modality has conclusively proved to be of benefit after global brain ischemia. The most effective therapeutic regimen available is meticulous adherence to a standard, brain-oriented therapeutic protocol, such as previously described in this chapter.

Adapted from Abramson NS. Brain resuscitation after cardiac arrest. In: Rosen P, ed. *Emergency Medicine: Concepts and Clinical Practice*. St Louis, Mo: Mosby Year Book Co; 1992.

References

1. Weinberger LM, Gibbon MH, Gibbon JH Jr. Temporary arrest of circulation to central nervous system: physiologic effects. *Arch Neurol Psych*. 1940;43:615-634.
2. Neely WA, Youmans JR. Anoxia of canine brain without damage. *JAMA*. 1963;183:1085-1087.
3. Rehncrona S, Mela L, Siesjo BK. Recovery of brain mitochondrial function in the rat after complete and incomplete cerebral ischemia. *Stroke*. 1979;10:437-446.
4. Hossmann KA, Zimmermann V. Resuscitation of the monkey brain after 1 hour complete ischemia. I: physiological and morphological observations. *Brain Res*. 1974;81:59-74.
5. Kleihues P, Hossmann KA, Pegg AE, Kobayashi K, Zimmermann V. Resuscitation of the monkey brain after one hour complete ischemia. III: indications of metabolic recovery. *Brain Res*. 1975; 95:61-73.
6. Graham DI. The pathology of brain ischaemia and possibilities for therapeutic intervention. *Br J Anaesth*. 1985;57:3-17.
7. Snyder JV, Nemoto EM, Carroll RG, Safar P. Global ischemia in dogs: intracranial pressures, brain blood flow and metabolism. *Stroke*. 1975;6:21-27.
8. Vaagenes P, Cantadore R, Safar P, et al. Amelioration of brain damage by lidoflazine after prolonged ventricular fibrillation cardiac arrest in dogs. *Crit Care Med*. 1984;12:846-855.
9. Miller CL, Lampard DG, Alexander K, Brown WA. Local cerebral blood flow following transient cerebral ischemia, part 1: onset of impaired reperfusion within the first hour following global ischemia. *Stroke*. 1980;11:534-541.
10. Jackson DL, Dole WP. Total cerebral ischemia: a new model system for the study of post-cardiac arrest brain damage. *Stroke*. 1979;10:38-43.
11. Obrenovitch TP, Hallenbeck JM. Platelet accumulation in regions of low blood flow during the postischemic period. *Stroke*. 1985;16: 224-234.
12. Rogers MC, Kirsch JR. Current concepts in brain resuscitation. *JAMA*. 1989;261:3143-3147.
13. Hossmann V, Hossmann KA, Takagi S. Effect of intravascular platelet aggregation on blood recirculation following prolonged ischemia of the cat brain. *J Neurol*. 1980;222:159-170.
14. Siesjo BK. Cell damage in the brain: a speculative synthesis. *J Cereb Blood Flow Metab*. 1981;1:155-185.
15. McCord JM. Oxygen-derived free radicals in postischemic tissue injury. *N Engl J Med*. 1985;312:159-163.
16. Siesjo BK. Cerebral circulation and metabolism. *J Neurosurg*. 1984;60:883-908.
17. Cantu RC, Ames A III, DiGiacinto G, Dixon J. Hypotension: a major factor limiting recovery from cerebral ischemia. *J Surg Res*. 1969; 9:525-529.
18. Thompson RG, Hallstrom AP, Cobb LA. Bystander-initiated cardiopulmonary resuscitation in the management of ventricular fibrillation. *Ann Intern Med*. 1979;90:737-740.
19. Safar P. Recent advances in cardiopulmonary-cerebral resuscitation: a review. *Ann Emerg Med*. 1984;13(pt 2):856-862.
20. Nemoto EM, Erdmann W, Strong E, Rao GR, Moossy J. Regional brain Po_2 after global ischemia in monkeys: evidence for regional differences in critical perfusion pressures. *Stroke*. 1979;10:44-52.
21. Wise G, Sutter R, Burkholder J. The treatment of brain ischemia with vasopressor drugs. *Stroke*. 1972;3:135-140.
22. Sterz F, Leonov Y, Safar P, Radovsky A, Tisherman SA, Oku K. Hypertension with or without hemodilution after cardiac arrest in dogs. *Stroke*. 1990;21:1178-1184.
23. Symon L. Flow thresholds in brain ischaemia and the effects of drugs. *Br J Anaesth*. 1985;57:34-43.
24. Klatzo I. Brain oedema following brain ischaemia and the influence of therapy. *Br J Anaesth*. 1985;57:18-22.
25. Weil MH, Ruiz CE, Michaels S, Rackow EC. Acid-base determinants of survival after cardiopulmonary resuscitation. *Crit Care Med*. 1985;13:888-892.
26. Plum F, Siesjo BK. Recent advances in CSF physiology. *Anesthesiology*. 1975;42:708-730.
27. Shapiro HM. Brain protection: fact or fancy. In: Shoemaker WC, ed. *Critical Care: State of the Art*. Fullerton, Calif: Society of Critical Care Medicine; 1985;6.
28. Rehncrona S. Brain acidosis. *Ann Emerg Med*. 1985;14:770-776.
29. Steen PA, Soule EH, Michenfelder JD. Detrimental effect of prolonged hypothermia in cats and monkeys with and without regional cerebral ischemia. *Stroke*. 1979;10:522-529.
30. Rosomoff HL. Hypothermia and cerebral vascular lesions, 1: experimental interruption of the middle cerebral artery during hypothermia. *J Neurosurg*. 1956;13:332-343.
31. Frost EA. Brain preservation. *Anesth Analg*. 1981;60:821-832.
32. Leonov Y, Sterz F, Safar P, et al. Mild cerebral hypothermia during and after cardiac arrest improves neurologic outcome in dogs. *J Cereb Blood Flow Metab*. 1990;10:57-70.
33. Steen PA, Milde JH, Michenfelder JD. The detrimental effects of prolonged hypothermia and rewarming in the dog. *Anesthesiology*. 1980;52:224-230.
34. Selman WR, Spetzler RF. Therapeutics for focal cerebral ischemia. *Neurosurgery*. 1980;6:446-452.
35. Weinrauch V, Safar P, Tisherman S, Kuboyama K, Radovsky A. Beneficial effect of mild hypothermia and detrimental effect of deep hypothermia after cardiac arrest in dogs. *Stroke*. 1992;23: 1454-1462.
36. Sterz F, Safar P, Tisherman S, Radovsky A, Kuboyama K, Oku K. Mild hypothermic cardiopulmonary resuscitation improves outcome after prolonged cardiac arrest in dogs. *Crit Care Med*. 1991;19: 379-389.
37. Raichle ME. The pathophysiology of brain ischemia. *Ann Neurol*. 1983;13:2-10.
38. Myers RE. Lactic acid accumulation as a cause of brain edema and cerebral necrosis resulting from oxygen deprivation. In: Guilleminault C, Korobkin R, eds. *Advances in Perinatal Neurology*. New York, NY: SP Medical & Scientific Books; 1979.
39. Pulsinelli WA, Waldman S, Rawlinson D, Plum F. Moderate hyperglycemia augments ischemic brain damage: a neuropathologic study in the rat. *Neurology*. 1982;32:1239-1246.
40. Siesjö BK. *Brain Energy Metabolism*. New York, NY: John Wiley & Sons Inc; 1978.
41. Hossmann KA, Kleihues P. Reversibility of ischemic brain damage. *Arch Neurol*. 1973;29:375-384.
42. Todd MM, Chadwick HS, Shapiro HM, Dunlop BJ, Marshall LF, Dueck R. The neurologic effects of thiopental therapy following experimental cardiac arrest in cats. *Anesthesiology*. 1982;57:76-86.
43. Gisvold SE, Safar P, Hendrickx HH, Rao G, Moossy J, Alexander H. Thiopental treatment after global brain ischemia in pigtailed monkeys. *Anesthesiology*. 1984;60:88-96.
44. Randomized clinical study of thiopental loading in comatose survivors of cardiac arrest: Brain Resuscitation Clinical Trial I Study Group. *N Engl J Med*. 1986;314:397-403.
45. Snyder BD, Hauser WA, Loewenson RB, Leppik IE, Ramirez-Lassepas M, Gumnit RJ. Neurologic prognosis after cardiopulmonary arrest, III: seizure activity. *Neurology*. 1980;30:1292-1297.
46. Levy DE, Caronna JJ, Singer BH, Lapinski RH, Frydman H, Plum F. Predicting outcome from hypoxic-ischemic coma. *JAMA*. 1985;253:1420-1426.
47. Galich JH, French LA. Use of dexamethasone in the treatment of cerebral edema resulting from brain tumors and brain surgery. *Am Pract Dig*. 1961;12:169-174.

48. Fishman RA. Steroids in the treatment of brain edema. *N Engl J Med.* 1982;306:359-360.

49. Jastremski M, Sutton-Tyrrell K, Vaagenes P, Abramson N, Heiselman D, Safar P. Glucocorticoid treatment does not improve neurological recovery following cardiac arrest: Brain Resuscitation Clinical Trial I Study Group. *JAMA.* 1989;262:3427-3430.

50. A randomized clinical study of a calcium-entry blocker (lidoflazine) in the treatment of comatose survivors of cardiac arrest: Brain Resuscitation Clinical Trial II Study Group. *N Engl J Med.* 1991;324:1225-1231.

51. Roine RO, Kaste M, Kinnunen A, Nikki P, Sarna S, Kajaste S. Nimodipine after resuscitation from out-of-hospital ventricular fibrillation: a placebo-controlled, double-blind, randomized trial. *JAMA.* 1990;264:3171-3177.

Cardiopulmonary resuscitation (CPR) and emergency cardiac care (ECC) have the same goals as all other medical interventions — to preserve life, restore health, relieve suffering, and limit disability. An additional goal unique to CPR is the reversal of "clinical death." However, in providing CPR these goals are often not achieved. Moreover, the provision of resuscitation may conflict with a patient's own desires and requests or may not be in the patient's best interest.[1] Like other medical therapies, CPR and ECC have specific indications and contraindications. In certain circumstances CPR can be predicted to be unsuccessful and may be considered futile. In certain instances CPR may not be a wise or just use of limited medical resources. However, concern about costs associated with prolonged intensive care should not preclude emergency resuscitative attempts. The purpose of this section is to guide ECC providers in making difficult decisions about starting and stopping CPR and ECC. These are guidelines only. Each decision must be individualized and made with compassion and reason.

Competent and informed patients have a moral and legal right to consent to or refuse recommended medical interventions, including CPR.[2-7] The right to refuse medical treatment does not depend on the presence or absence of terminal illness, the agreement of family members, or the approval of physicians or hospital administrators. Under ideal circumstances adult patients are presumed to be competent unless a court has declared them incompetent to make medical decisions.[8] In practice, physicians often determine whether patients can make informed decisions about their medical care. To have this decision-making capacity, patients must be able to understand basic information about their condition and prognosis, the nature of the proposed intervention, the alternatives, the risks and benefits, and the consequences. In addition, the patient must be able to deliberate and choose among alternatives. In cases of doubt, the patient should be regarded as competent. When decision-making capacity is temporarily impaired by such factors as concurrent illness, medications, or depression, treatment of these conditions may restore that capacity.

If the patient cannot make an informed decision about CPR, the attending physician should consider the patient's advance directives or decisions by appropriate surrogates, as well as the likely response to CPR.

Ethical Principles and Guidelines

Advance Directives and Surrogate Decision Making

By using advance directives, competent patients indicate what interventions they would refuse or accept if they were to lose the capacity to make decisions about their care.[9,10] Following the advance directives of patients who have lost their decision-making capacity respects their autonomy, individuality, and self-determination as well as the law.[1,3,4,7]

Advance directives include conversations, written directives, living wills, and durable powers of attorney for health care. Conversations the patient had with relatives, friends, or physicians while still competent are the most common form of advance directives. However, the courts consider written advance directives more trustworthy.

Living wills constitute clear and convincing evidence of a patient's wishes, and in most states living wills are legally enforceable. In living wills, patients direct their physicians in the provision of medical care if the patients become terminally ill and are incapable of making decisions.

The durable power of attorney for health care allows a competent patient to designate a surrogate, typically a relative or close friend, to make medical decisions if the patient loses decision-making capacity.[11] The surrogate (also referred to as the healthcare agent or proxy) should base decisions on the previously expressed preferences of the patient if they are known or in the patient's best interest if the patient's values are not known. Unlike the living will, the durable power of attorney for health care applies to all situations in which the patient is incapable of making medical decisions, not only terminal illness. Appointing a surrogate, together with providing a statement of preferences regarding life-sustaining treatment, is the preferred way for a patient to provide written advance directives.

Physicians should encourage patients to provide advance directives and should make forms readily available.[12] Physicians need to know the requirements in their states, for example, about witnesses or notarization. In discussions with patients, physicians can ensure that advance directives are informed, specific, and up-to-date.[12,13]

When patients lack the capacity to make informed decisions, a surrogate, informed and advised by the attending physician, should be identified to make medical decisions for the patient. In some instances, the patient while still competent will have selected a surrogate by executing a durable power of attorney for health care. When the patient has not selected a proxy, state law may dictate the order in which relatives should be asked to serve as surrogates.[7,14] Physicians can ask the courts to appoint surrogates for patients lacking decision-making capacity. However, legal proceedings may result in long delays or superficial review of the case, even when expedited procedures are used. In practice, the physician and the family often select the appropriate surrogate. The person chosen for that role should be someone who knows the patient's value system and respects its values and will act in the patient's best interest. Generally the appropriate surrogate is a relative or close friend, or the parents if the patient is a child.

In pediatric patients, respect for the principles of autonomy and self-determination requires that children be included in decision making consistent with their neurological status and level of maturity. There is legal precedent for participation by mature adolescents in personal decisions concerning CPR.[15]

Some patients with impaired decision-making capacity have no family members or close friends who can make decisions on their behalf. Decisions for such patients may present serious ethical dilemmas. In clinical practice, decisions for such patients are commonly made without resorting to the courts. It is desirable but not always possible for the attending physician to ask someone who is not directly involved in the patient's care to consult on the case. Such consultation helps to ensure that hidden assumptions and value judgments are made explicit, that the personal values of the caregivers are not projected onto the patient, that all points of view and alternatives are considered, and that the decision is made thoughtfully. Review by the hospital ethics committee, an ethics consultant, or another physician can be useful.

Futility

Physicians should not be obligated to provide futile therapy when asked to do so by patients or surrogates.[2,16-18] While this general rule seems obvious, it may be difficult to define futility in a particular case. People often use the term *futile* in very different ways, and unilateral decisions by physicians to withhold or terminate resuscitation are justified only when it is futile in a strict sense.[16,19] Medical futility justifies unilateral decisions by physicians to withhold or terminate resuscitation under the following circumstances:

1. Appropriate basic life support (BLS) and advanced life support (ALS) have already been attempted without restoration of circulation and breathing.
2. No physiological benefit from BLS and ALS can be expected because a patient's vital functions are deteriorating despite maximum therapy. For example, CPR would not restore circulation in a patient who suffered a cardiac arrest despite optimal treatment for progressive septic or cardiogenic shock.
3. No survivors after CPR have been reported under the given circumstances in well-designed studies. For example, when CPR has been attempted in patients with metastatic cancer, several large series have reported that no patients survived to hospital discharge.[20]

In these strictly defined situations, the decision to stop or withhold resuscitation is appropriately a medical judgment.[18,21] Patients (or surrogates of incompetent patients) should be informed of the no-CPR order but not offered the choice of CPR.

The term *futility*, however, is also used in less strict and less objective ways that do not justify unilateral decisions by physicians to withhold CPR.[16,19] Some physicians regard CPR as "futile" when important goals of care cannot be achieved, although other significant goals might be. For example, for a young patient in a persistent vegetative state, CPR in the case of cardiopulmonary arrest would not restore cerebral function, although it might restore circulation and allow long-term survival. Another looser meaning of futility is that the reported survival rate after CPR is low but not 0%. In calling CPR futile in these circumstances, physicians make value judgments about which goals of treatment and what probability of success are worthwhile. Physicians need to appreciate that in these situations their role is to initiate discussions with patients or their surrogates and to provide information and advice but not to be the sole decision makers.

Allocation of Resources

Recent ethical deliberations have arisen out of concern for overtreatment of patients with a poor prognosis; however, a major consideration should be the lack of consistent access to and quality of ECC and other medical services. Efforts should continue to be devoted to decreasing response times and improving CPR performance through all links in the chain of survival. Justice dictates that a certain level of emergency care should be provided to all citizens and that resources should be justly allocated to ensure some degree of equitable distribution of medical resources to all citizens. Physicians must play a major role in determining how to derive maximum benefit from available medical resources. However, when making individual treatment decisions for a patient, the physician should maintain a position of advocacy for that patient's best interest. When resources are inadequate to meet immediate patient care needs, rationing (ie, triage) of medical services occurs. Rationing, the distribution of a scarce resource, should be based on ethically oriented criteria.

No-CPR Orders

Most patients want to discuss the no-CPR or do-not-resuscitate (DNR) decision with their physicians. Physicians, however, often hesitate to initiate the discussions, fearing that such discussions would harm some patients by provoking severe anxiety or undermining hope, even though there is little evidence to support this. On a practical level, busy physicians may think they do not have time to discuss CPR in a meaningful way with patients.

Often physicians discuss CPR only with patients whom they consider at risk for cardiopulmonary arrest.[22] Typically the possibility of cardiopulmonary arrest becomes clear as a patient's condition worsens. At that point the patient often is no longer capable of making decisions,[19] although often the patient was capable of doing so on admission to the hospital.[22] Targeting sicker patients reinforces the belief that discussion of no-CPR or DNR orders signifies a bleak prognosis. Selective discussions may also be inequitable. Physicians discuss no-CPR orders more frequently with patients who have acquired immunodeficiency syndrome (AIDS) or cancer than with patients who have coronary artery disease, cirrhosis, and other diseases with a similarly poor prognosis.[23] For these reasons, physicians must consider taking the initiative in discussing CPR with all adults admitted for medical and surgical care or with their surrogates.

To allow patients or surrogates to make informed decisions, physicians need to disclose pertinent information about the patient's condition and prognosis, the nature of CPR, the likely outcome, the risk, and the alternative of certain death. Patients need to understand that CPR is often unsuccessful. About 15% of hospitalized patients on general medical or surgical floors in whom CPR is attempted survive.[22,24-26] Terminally ill patients may fear abandonment and pain more than death. In discussions with such patients, physicians need to emphasize their plans to control pain, provide comfort, and see the patient regularly, even if resuscitation is withheld.

All medical decision making, including choices about CPR, begins with the physician's recommendation based on medical judgment, which is then communicated to patients or their surrogates or parents when they are asked to give their informed consent. Patients and their surrogates have a right to choose from among medically appropriate options based on their assessment of the relative benefits and burdens of the proposed intervention. This right to choose does not imply the right to demand care beyond appropriate options based on medical judgment and accepted standards of care, nor are physicians required to provide care in ways that in their personal judgment violate the principles of medical ethics. Physicians may choose to transfer care in such cases to other providers. There may be circumstances when conflicts of interest may lead parents to decisions not in the best interest of the infant or child. If patients or their surrogates or parents and physicians cannot agree on a course of action, steps should be taken to resolve the differences of opinion by involving consultants, ethics committees, or — as a last resort in pediatric cases — state child protection agencies.

A growing number of children with chronic and potentially life-threatening conditions live in foster care environments under state jurisdiction. Existing ambiguities about the scope of decision-making authority vested in custodial guardians, especially decisions about CPR and prolonged life support, need to be clarified.

Decisions to limit resuscitative efforts should be communicated to all professionals involved in the care of the adult or child in the context of an overall plan for patient care. Such interactions provide a wider information base,

ensure that the staff is fully informed, and offer an opportunity for conflicts to be aired.

Unlike other medical interventions, CPR is initiated without a physician's order, under the theory of implied consent for emergency treatment. However, a physician's order is required to withhold CPR.[25]

DNR or no-CPR orders represent one aspect of a patient treatment plan, ie, not to attempt CPR, and carry no inherent implications for limitations of other forms of treatment. Other aspects of the treatment plan should be separately documented and communicated. Admission to an intensive care unit for necessary care best provided in that facility is not necessarily inconsistent with a decision not to attempt CPR in the event of an arrest.[27]

The commonly used term *do not resuscitate* may be misleading. It suggests that healthcare workers could resuscitate a patient if they tried to do so, but this often is not the case. The term *do not attempt resuscitation* (DNAR) may more clearly connote that success at resuscitation is often not achieved. The scope of a DNR order may also be ambiguous. Even though CPR will be withheld, it may be appropriate to provide interventions such as fluids, nutrition, oxygen, antiarrhythmic agents, or vasopressors. The order *no CPR* may more effectively communicate the intended meaning that "in the event of an acute cardiac arrest, no CPR measures will be instituted or continued." Each of these terms — *DNR, DNAR,* and *no CPR* — is currently in use, and local custom will determine the preferred term. The term *no CPR* will be used throughout the remainder of this chapter.

No-CPR orders should be reviewed before surgery to determine their applicability in the operating room and postoperative recovery room.[28-30] They should be reviewed by the anesthesiologist, attending physician, and patient or surrogate to determine how they should apply to events that may occur during the intraoperative or immediate postoperative period. The result of that review may be a suspension or continuance of the no-CPR order through the perioperative period.[29]

Initiating and Discontinuing Resuscitation in the Prehospital Setting

When a person has suffered a cardiac or respiratory arrest, there is a strong presumption for initiation of CPR in the prehospital, hospital, and delivery room settings. Except in narrowly defined circumstances, citizen first responders are urged and professional first responders are expected always to attempt BLS and ACLS. Exceptions to this rule in the prehospital setting are the presence of obvious clinical signs of death, cases where attempts would place the rescuer at significant risk of physical injury, or cases where there is documentation or another reliable reason to believe that CPR is not indicated, wanted, or in the patient's best interest. Unwitnessed deaths in the presence of known serious, chronic, debilitating disease or in the terminal state of a fatal illness may be a reliable criterion in some settings to believe that CPR is not indicated. CPR is not indicated for traumatic arrests with extended response or transport times after a patent airway is ensured. In the past, debate has centered on the question of whether to initiate CPR when "irreversible brain damage" or "brain death" is suspected. Neither of these conditions can be reliably assessed in the prehospital setting. Thus, anticipated neurological status should not be used as a criterion to withhold CPR.

Emergency medical services (EMS) protocols should have provisions to identify adults and children who have no-CPR orders.[31,32] This could be done with a formal order sheet, identification cards, bracelets, or some other mechanism.

In certain cases it may be difficult to determine if resuscitation should be started. For example, despite the presence of a no-CPR order, family members, surrogates, or the patient's physician may request that CPR be initiated. If there is reasonable doubt or substantive reason to believe the no-CPR order is invalid, CPR should be initiated. If evidence later indicates that no resuscitation is the patient's clearly expressed wish, CPR or other life support can be discontinued.

No-CPR orders should not be confused with advance directives or living wills, which are requests by individuals to direct their medical care should they lose decision-making capacity. Advance directives and living wills require interpretation by a physician and need to be formulated into a treatment plan, including specific orders (no CPR), consistent with the patient's wishes. The existence of a living will does not necessarily indicate that a patient is foregoing aggressive medical care or CPR.

Interpreting living wills and identifying proxies in the prehospital setting are fraught with difficulty, requiring the rescuer to interpret a legal document at the time of a medical emergency. A number of EMS systems are developing methods to ensure that no-CPR orders can be honored in the prehospital setting. This practice should be encouraged. Unless there are such policies in place authorizing the withholding of emergency treatment, first responders, emergency medical technicians, and paramedics should treat patients according to standard protocols and provide any advance directives to the physician responsible for subsequent treatment. Family members may be concerned that emergency medical personnel are not honoring the advance directives. However, EMS responders must sensitively and emphatically convey their responsibility to initiate treatment and await physician direction regarding advance directives or requests in a living will. Treatments initiated by EMS personnel should be discontinued in the emergency department or hospital if there is evidence that they are not wanted by the patient, not in the patient's best interest, or not medically indicated.

Rescuers who initiate BLS should continue until one of the following occurs:
1. Effective spontaneous circulation and ventilation have been restored.
2. Care is transferred to emergency medical responders or another trained person who continues BLS.
3. Care is transferred to ALS emergency medical personnel.
4. Care is transferred to a physician who determines that resuscitation should be discontinued.
5. Reliable criteria for the determination of death are recognized.
6. The rescuer is too exhausted to continue resuscitation, environmental hazards endanger the rescuer, or continued resuscitation would jeopardize the lives of others.
7. A valid no-CPR order is presented to the rescuers. Ethically and legally there is no distinction between discontinuing CPR and not starting it in the first place.

There is ongoing debate about the efficacy of BLS beyond 30 minutes. Rescuers in a remote environment and some BLS ambulance services may have prolonged transport times before ALS can be instituted, making them unavailable for other calls. The risk of vehicular accidents during high-speed emergency transport must be weighed against the likelihood of successful resuscitation after prolonged BLS resuscitative efforts. State or local EMS authorities should be encouraged to develop protocols for initiation and withdrawal of BLS in areas where ALS is not readily available, taking into account local circumstances, resources, and risk to rescuers. Since defibrillators are now recommended as standard equipment on all ambulances, the absence of a "shockable" rhythm on the defibrillator after an adequate trial of CPR can be an additional criterion for withdrawing BLS.

Resuscitation may be discontinued in the prehospital setting when the patient is nonresuscitable after an adequate trial of ACLS. This determination should be made by EMS authorities and ambulance medical directors, who should generally ensure that (1) endotracheal intubation has been successfully accomplished, (2) intravenous access has been achieved and rhythm-appropriate medications and countershocks for ventricular fibrillation have been administered according to ACLS protocols, and (3) persistent asystole or agonal electrocardiographic patterns are present and no reversible causes are identified. The interval since cardiac arrest should be considered, but no specific duration of time predicts unsuccessful resuscitation. Studies have shown that rapid transport for in-hospital resuscitation after unsuccessful prehospital ACLS rarely if ever results in survival to hospital discharge and that the costs and risks associated with high-speed transport may outweigh the extremely small likelihood of benefit.[33-35] Physician ambulance medical directors remain ultimately responsible for determination of death, and pronouncement of death in the field should have the concurrence of on-line medical control.[36] Although duration of resuscitation and the patient's age influence the success of resuscitation, by themselves they are not accurate predictors of outcome. Return of spontaneous circulation for even a brief period is a positive prognostic sign and warrants consideration of transport to a hospital. Transport may also be warranted in special circumstances such as profound hypothermia.

In EMS systems where resuscitation is discontinued in the prehospital setting, mechanisms should be established for the pronouncement of death and appropriate disposition of the body by means other than EMS vehicles. EMS providers must be trained to deal sensitively with family and others present, and the involvement of a member of the clergy or a social worker should be considered.

Ambulance and rescue personnel commonly encounter terminally ill patients in private homes, often in hospice programs. These patients may require treatment for acute medical illness or traumatic injuries, measures to relieve suffering, or simply ambulance transportation to a medical facility. Use of 911 telephone numbers and the emergency system may or may not be appropriate. Comprehensive policies should be adopted by local or state EMS authorities to allow persons to decline an attempt at resuscitation but still have access to other emergency medical treatments and ambulance transportation. A legally valid, widely recognized form or other method of identification should be available for presentation to prehospital personnel when they are called to the scene of a patient with a no-CPR order.

Personal physicians should initiate predeath planning for patients entering the terminal stages of illness. Physicians must be knowledgeable about state laws related to death certification, pronouncement of death, the role of the coroner and police, and disposition of bodies.[37] They may not realize that no-CPR orders written in the hospital may not be transferable to outside the hospital setting.[37,38] Failure to address these issues may result in unnecessary conflict.[39]

Many patients prefer to die at home, surrounded by friends and loved ones. The hospice movement and many societies for specific diseases (eg, multiple sclerosis, AIDS, and muscular dystrophy) provide excellent models for planning an expected death at home and for answering questions from physicians and families.[40] Physicians, patients, and family members together should discuss measures of comfort, pain control, terminal support, and hygiene; when (and when not) to call 911; use of a local hospice; and when and how to contact the personal physician. Funeral plans, disposition of the body, psychological concerns surrounding death and dying, and availability of counseling services and ministerial support should be discussed. Such knowledge and discussions will reduce and even eliminate many of the ethical and medicolegal issues related to CPR.

Nursing home facilities should develop and implement institutional guidelines for providing CPR to their residents. A nursing home should be considered a prehospital setting, and residents should be provided with 911 emergency service if medically indicated. Advance directives and living wills should be considered when developing treatment plans for residents lacking decision-making capacity. The treatment plans should include specific orders (DNR/DNAR/no CPR) to limit emergency care, if this accords with the patient's request. Physician orders and treatment plans to limit ECC should be provided to EMS personnel and transferred with the patient from the long-term care facility to the hospital.

Organ and Tissue Donation

The AHA supports efforts to answer the national need for increased organ and tissue donation. EMS agencies should consider prospectively contacting the organ procurement organization in their region about the need for tissue from donors pronounced dead in the field. Permission must be obtained from next of kin for organ and tissue donation. Federal guidelines for organ and tissue procurement in hospitals should be consulted.[41] Although this is an area of considerable sensitivity, EMS medical directors and prehospital providers should be alert to clinical situations where organ procurement may be appropriate. The appropriateness of initiating life support on a dying patient solely for organ procurement requires further public discussion.

Ethics of Practicing Intubation Skills

The public and healthcare professionals share an important interest in developing and maintaining a high level of technical skill in rescuers. Providing healthcare professionals with a closely supervised intubation practice using the newly deceased, especially small infants, is a common teaching method. This practice is ethically justifiable in that it is nonmutilating, brief, beneficial to others, and an effective teaching technique.[42,43] However, the sensibilities of family and staff should be compassionately respected and consent obtained whenever practical.

Resuscitation and Life Support in the Hospital

Hospitalized patients should periodically have an evaluation to determine the "appropriate level of care." The levels to consider are (1) aggressive emergency resuscitation; (2) intensive care monitoring and life support (prolonged life support); (3) general medical care, including medication, surgery, artificial nutrition, and hydration; (4) general nursing care; and (5) terminal care. Selection of the appropriate level of care is a medical decision made in accordance with an informed patient's or surrogate's consent.

Initiating Resuscitation in Hospitals

Prompt institution of CPR is indicated in hospitalized patients outside the intensive care unit (ICU) who develop airway obstruction, apnea, or pulselessness. Resuscitative efforts should be withheld when there is a no-CPR order; when, in the judgment of the physician, such efforts cannot restore and sustain cardiopulmonary function; or when widely accepted scientific data indicate there is no likelihood of survival. This prediction should be based on several credible published studies of sufficient numbers with 100% no-survival rate. The patient, surrogate, or family should be informed of the decision to withhold CPR. CPR may be discontinued after an adequate trial of ACLS or a valid no-CPR order is presented.

In the hospital or delivery room, CPR may be discontinued after a full trial according to accepted clinical protocols. Sufficient data have not yet accumulated to support a recommendation on the appropriate duration of CPR efforts in children before discontinuance. There is evidence that infants resuscitated in the delivery room whose Apgar scores remain 0 after 10 minutes will not survive.[44]

In the delivery room, resuscitation may be withheld from infants judged to be not resuscitable at birth[45] or with imminently fatal malformations. In pediatric cases in general, parents should share in the decision making whenever possible. When the potential need for CPR can be anticipated, early discussion and preplanning promote shared decision making. Physicians must discuss with parents their determination that a CPR attempt would be futile and should be withheld. The general presumption in favor of initiating attempts at resuscitation provides an important opportunity to gather and document clinical and other data to support a decision about continuing or withdrawing those efforts.

If cardiac arrest occurs in an ICU or critical care unit (CCU), the interval from arrest to restoration of spontaneous circulation should be extremely short because of close monitoring by personnel and immediate attempts to reverse the arrest.[46,47] In ICUs and CCUs every possible effort should be made to minimize the likelihood of accidental airway obstruction, hypoventilation, or pulselessness by recognizing problems with tubes or ventilators and by promptly evaluating arrhythmias. Admitting patients with no-CPR orders to ICUs and CCUs may be appropriate when care outside the ICU or CCU is difficult or impossible for logistic reasons or when a temporary and potentially reversible problem develops in a patient with an underlying irreversible illness.[27] The appropriateness of resuscitative efforts for the patient in the ICU or CCU should be reviewed regularly and modified as the patient's condition changes.

Withdrawal of Life Support

Although withdrawal of life support may be a more emotionally complex decision for family and staff, withholding and withdrawing are ethically the same. Decisions to withhold or withdraw life support are justifiable in the final stages of terminal illness when the patient, adult or child, will remain permanently unconscious, when the burden to the patient of continued treatment would exceed any benefits, or when widely accepted scientific data suggest that the chances for successful resuscitation are remote. Caution must be exercised in determining the prognosis of infants with neurological impairment.

Brain death cannot be determined during emergency resuscitative attempts. Determination of brain death must be governed by nationally accepted guidelines.[48] Care providers should not forget the need for organ donation, which the AHA encourages. Once a patient is determined to be brain dead, life-sustaining treatment should be withdrawn unless consent for cadaveric organ donation has been given. If such consent has been given, previous no-CPR orders should be rescinded until organs have been procured.

In children the clinical criteria for brain death are in most circumstances the same as in adults. However, determination of brain death should not be made until at least 7 days of age.[49,50] It is recommended that hospitals develop policies and guidelines for the determination of death by brain death criteria that reflect current consensus and address areas of controversy.

Persistent vegetative state is the irreversible cessation of the integrating function of the cerebral cortex while brainstem function remains intact.[48] After cardiac arrest and restoration of spontaneous circulation by CPR, some patients may not regain consciousness. The prognosis for adults in persistent vegetative state following cardiac arrest can be predicted with high accuracy after 3 to 7 days.[51] Withdrawal of life support, including artificially administered nutrition and hydration, is ethically permissible under these circumstances, in accordance with the previously discussed guidelines for making decisions for patients who lack decision-making capacity.[52-55]

The conscious or unconscious patient in the terminal state of an incurable disease for whom terminal care is determined to be appropriate should have care that ensures comfort and dignity.[6] Care should be provided to minimize the suffering associated with pain, dyspnea, delirium, convulsions, and other terminal complications. For such patients it is ethical to gradually increase the dosage of narcotics and sedatives to relieve pain and other symptoms, even to dosages that might also shorten the patient's life.[54,55]

Hospital No-CPR Policies

Hospitals must have written policies for no-CPR orders, as the Joint Commission on the Accreditation of Healthcare Organizations requires. These policies need to be reviewed periodically to reflect developments in medical technology, changes in guidelines for ECC and ALS, or changes in the law.

The attending physician should write no-CPR orders in the patient's chart. The rationale for the no-CPR order and other specific limits to care should be documented in the progress notes. Oral no-CPR orders may be misunderstood and may place nurses and other healthcare workers in legal and ethical jeopardy. If the attending physician is not physically present, nurses may accept a no-CPR order over the telephone, with the understanding that the physician will sign the order promptly. No-CPR orders should be reviewed periodically, particularly if the patient's condition changes.

"Show codes" or "slow codes" appear to provide CPR while not actually doing so or while doing so in a way that is known to be ineffective. Slow codes, particularly when done to deceive the relatives and friends of a patient, compromise the ethical integrity of healthcare professionals and undermine the physician-patient or nurse-patient relationship. Such codes should not be done.

Orders to limit resuscitative efforts, such as to withhold defibrillation or endotracheal intubation, are appropriate in some circumstances. For example, an informed patient or surrogate may want only limited resuscitative efforts, realizing that this may decrease the chances of successful resuscitation.

A no-CPR order means only that CPR will not be initiated. It does not mean that other care should be limited. These orders should not lead to abandonment of patients or denial of appropriate medical and nursing care. They do not constitute "giving up." The same reasons that make CPR inappropriate, however, may also render other treatments unsuitable. After a no-CPR order is written, the attending physician should clarify plans for further care with nurses, consultants, and house staff, as well as with the patient or surrogate. For many patients, interventions for diagnosis or treatment remain appropriate after a no-CPR order is written. In CCUs it is important to clarify how to respond to physiological abnormalities, such as arrhythmia or hypotension, that could lead to cardiopulmonary arrest if not treated. Basic nursing care, such as oral hygiene, skin care, and patient positioning, and measures to relieve pain and other symptoms should be continued.

Role of Hospital Ethics Committees

Hospitals are now required to have advisers such as ethics committees and bioethicists who can respond to requests for resolution of ethical questions. Ethics committees traditionally have been consultative and advisory and have been effective in organizing educational programs and developing hospital policies and guidelines. There is considerable variability among hospitals with respect to committee responsibilities, authority, membership, access, and procedural protocols, and hospitals should develop explicit statements on these issues.

Legal Considerations in CPR and ECC

The ethical and legal aspects of CPR and ECC can be conceptualized in terms of two periods. From the national implementation of CPR after the first national conference on CPR in 1973 until 1990, many physicians were greatly concerned with malpractice liability for withholding or withdrawing CPR. The second period was initiated in 1990 by the US Supreme Court decision in the *Cruzan* case and the passage of the Patient Self-Determination Act.[13] In the *Cruzan* case the court assumed that competent patients have a constitutionally protected liberty interest to refuse unwanted medical treatment. The ruling permitted states to adopt procedural requirements for withholding life-sustaining treatment. The *Cruzan* decision, together with the Patient Self-Determination Act, shifted the discussion to how to support the right of patients to make decisions about their medical care and to make advance directives more effective. Physicians need to take responsibility for maximizing the benefits of advance directives and the Patient Self-Determination Act while minimizing undesirable outcomes.

The Patient Self-Determination Act, effective December 1, 1991, was intended to encourage discussion about advance directives.[13] This act applies to hospitals, home health agencies, skilled nursing facilities, hospices, and health maintenance organizations that participate in Medicaid and Medicare. Such providers must establish written policies and procedures to inform all adult patients of their rights "to make decisions concerning medical care, including the right to accept or refuse medical or surgical treatment and the right to formulate an advance directive." This information must be provided at the time of admission to the hospital or nursing home, at the time treatment is provided by the home health agency, or at the time of enrollment in a health maintenance organization. These institutions or agencies must document in the medical record the existence of an advance directive and must respect such directives to the fullest extent possible under state law. Physicians should take advantage of these requirements of the act to talk with patients about their preferences regarding CPR in various clinical situations.

Good Samaritan laws have been expanded in a number of jurisdictions to protect from liability laypersons and health professionals who do not have a duty to respond, who are acting "in good faith," and who are not guilty of gross negligence. Such laws were intended to minimize fear of legal consequences for providing CPR, which might hinder multilevel community ECC programs.

References

1. President's Commission for the Study of Ethical Problems in Medicine and Biomedical and Behavioral Research. *Deciding to Forego Life-Sustaining Treatment.* Washington, DC: US Government Printing Office; 1983.
2. Lo B, Jonsen AR. Clinical decisions to limit treatment. *Ann Intern Med.* 1980;93:764-768.
3. Jonsen AR, Siegler M, Winslade WJ. *Clinical Ethics.* 2nd ed. New York, NY: Macmillan Publishing Co, Inc; 1986:102-109.
4. The Hastings Center. *Guidelines on the Termination of Life-Sustaining Treatment in the Care of the Dying.* Briarcliff Manor, NY: The Hastings Center; 1987.
5. Ruark JE, Raffin TA. Initiating and withdrawing life support: principles and practice in adult medicine. *N Engl J Med.* 1988;318:25-30.
6. Wanzer SH, Federman DD, Adelstein SJ, et al. The physician's responsibility toward hopelessly ill patients: a second look. *N Engl J Med.* 1989;320:844-849.
7. Weir RF, Gostin L. Decisions to abate life-sustaining treatment for nonautonomous patients: ethical standards and legal liability for physicians after Cruzan. *JAMA.* 1990;264:1846-1853.
8. Appelbaum PS, Grisso T. Assessing patients' capacities to consent to treatment. *N Engl J Med.* 1988;319:1635-1638.
9. Annas GJ. The health care proxy and the living will. *N Engl J Med.* 1991;324:1210-1213.
10. Orentlicher D. Advance medical directives: from the Office of the General Counsel. *JAMA.* 1991;263:2365-2367.
11. Steinbrook R, Lo B. Decision making for incompetent patients by designated proxy: California's new law. *N Engl J Med.* 1984;310:1598-1601.
12. Lo B, Steinbrook R. Beyond the Cruzan case: the U.S. Supreme Court and medical practice. *Ann Intern Med.* 1991;114:895-901.
13. Wolf SM, Boyle P, Callahan D, et al. Sources of concern about the Patient Self-Determination Act. *N Engl J Med.* 1991;325:1666-1671.
14. Areen J. The legal status of consent obtained from families of adult patients to withhold or withdraw treatment. *JAMA.* 1987;258:229-235.
15. *In re EG.* 549 NE2d 322 (1989).
16. Youngner SJ. Who defines futility? *JAMA.* 1988;260:2094-2095.
17. Schneiderman LJ, Jecker NS, Jonsen AR. Medical futility: its meaning and ethical implications. *Ann Intern Med.* 1990;112:949-954.
18. Tomlinson T, Brody H. Futility and the ethics of resuscitation. *JAMA.* 1990;264:1276-1280.
19. Lo B. Unanswered questions about DNR orders. *JAMA.* 1991;265:1874-1875.
20. Faber-Langendorf K. Resuscitation of patients with metastatic cancer: is a transient benefit still futile? *Arch Intern Med.* 1991;151:235-239.
21. Blackhall LJ. Must we always use CPR? *N Engl J Med.* 1987;317:1281-1285.
22. Council on Ethical and Judicial Affairs, American Medical Association. Guidelines for the appropriate use of do-not-resuscitate orders. *JAMA.* 1991;265:1868-1871.
23. Wachter RM, Luce JM, Hearst N, Lo B. Decisions about resuscitation: inequities among patients with different diseases but similar prognoses. *Ann Intern Med.* 1989;111:525-532.
24. Bedell SE, Delbanco TL, Cook EF, Epstein FH. Survival after cardiopulmonary resuscitation in the hospital. *N Engl J Med.* 1983;309:569-576.
25. Evans AL, Brody BA. The do-not-resuscitate order in teaching hospitals. *JAMA.* 1985;253:2236-2239.
26. Moss AH. Informing the patient about cardiopulmonary resuscitation: when the risks outweigh the benefits. *J Gen Intern Med.* 1989;4:349-355.
27. Edwards BS. Does the DNR patient belong in the ICU? *Crit Care Nurs Clin North Am.* 1990;2:473-480.
28. Walker RM. DNR in the OR: resuscitation as an operative risk. *JAMA.* 1991;266:2407-2412.
29. Cohen CB, Cohen PJ. Do-not-resuscitate orders in the operating room. *N Engl J Med.* 1991;325:1879-1882.
30. Truog RD. 'Do-not-resuscitate' orders during anesthesia and surgery. *Anesthesiology.* 1991;74:606-608.
31. American College of Emergency Physicians. Guidelines for 'do not resuscitate orders' in the prehospital setting. *Ann Emerg Med.* 1988;17:1106-1108.
32. Miles SH, Crimmins TJ. Orders to limit emergency treatment for an ambulance service. *JAMA.* 1985;254:525-527.
33. Gray WA, Capone RJ, Most AS. Unsuccessful emergency medical resuscitation: are continued efforts in the emergency department justified? *N Engl J Med.* 1991;325:1393-1398.
34. Kellermann AL, Staves DR, Hackman BB. In-hospital resuscitation following unsuccessful prehospital advanced cardiac life support: 'heroic efforts' or an exercise in futility? *Ann Emerg Med.* 1988;17:589-594.
35. Weaver WD. Resuscitation outside the hospital: what's lacking? *N Engl J Med.* 1991;325:1437-1439.
36. Iserson KV. Foregoing prehospital care: should ambulance staff always resuscitate? *J Med Ethics.* 1991;17:19-24.
37. Dull SM, Graves JR, Larsen MP, Cummins RO. Expected death and unwanted resuscitation in the prehospital setting. *Ann Emerg Med.* 1990;19:245. Abstract.
38. Sachs GA, Miles SH, Levin RA. Limiting resuscitation: emerging policy in the emergency medical system. *Ann Intern Med.* 1991;114:151-154.
39. Crimmins TJ. The need for a prehospital DNR system. *Prehosp Disas Med.* 1990;5:47-48.
40. Wachter RM, Luce JM, Lo B, Raffin TA. Life-sustaining treatment for patients with AIDS. *Chest.* 1989;95:647-652.
41. *56 Federal Register.* 28513-28522.
42. Orlowski JP, Kanoti GA, Mehlman MJ. The ethical dilemma of permitting the teaching and perfecting of resuscitation techniques on recently expired patients. *J Clin Ethics.* 1990;1:201-205.
43. Benfield DG, Flaksman RJ, Lin TH, Kantak AD, Kokomoor FW, Vollman JH. Teaching intubation skills using newly deceased infants. *JAMA.* 1991;265:2360-2363.
44. Jain L, Ferre C, Vidyasagar D, Nath S, Sheftel D. Cardiopulmonary resuscitation of apparently stillborn infants: survival and long-term outcome. *J Pediatr.* 1991;118:778-782.
45. Botkin JR. Delivery room decisions for tiny infants: an ethical analysis. *J Clin Ethics.* 1990;1:306-311.
46. Bircher N, Safar P. Cerebral preservation during cardiopulmonary resuscitation. *Crit Care Med.* 1985;13:185-190.
47. Safar P, Bircher NG. *Cardiopulmonary Cerebral Resuscitation: Basic and Advanced Cardiac and Trauma Life Support: An Introduction to Resuscitation Medicine.* 3rd ed. Philadelphia, Pa: WB Saunders Co; 1988.
48. Plum F, Posner JB. *The Diagnosis of Stupor and Coma.* 3rd ed. Philadelphia, Pa: FA Davis Co; 1980.
49. American Academy of Pediatrics Task Force on Brain Death in Children. Report of a special task force: guidelines for the determination of brain death in children. *Pediatrics.* 1987;80:298-300.
50. Ashwal S, Schneider S. Pediatric brain death: current perspectives. *Adv Pediatr.* 1991;38:181-202.
51. Levy DE, Caronna JJ, Singer BH, Lapinski RH, Frydman H, Plum F. Predicting outcome from hypoxic-ischemic coma. *JAMA.* 1985;253:1420-1426.
52. Position of the American Academy of Neurology on certain aspects of the care and management of the persistent vegetative state. *Neurology.* 1989;39:125-126.
53. Council on Scientific Affairs and Council on Ethical and Judicial Affairs, American Medical Association. Persistent vegetative state and the decision to withdraw or withhold life support. *JAMA.* 1990;263:426-430.
54. Wilson WC, Smedira NG, Fink C, McDowell JA, Luce JM. Ordering and administration of sedatives and analgesics during the withholding and withdrawal of life support from critically ill patients. *JAMA.* 1992;267:949-953.
55. Edwards MJ, Tolle SW. Disconnecting a ventilator at the request of a patient who knows he will then die: the doctor's anguish. *Ann Intern Med.* 1992;117:254-256.

Community Approach to ECC: Prevention and the Chain of Survival

Chapter 16

Magnitude of the Problem

Cardiovascular disease accounts for more than 930 000 deaths in the United States annually (43% of deaths from all causes)(Fig 1). This includes approximately 500 000 deaths due to coronary disease, a majority of which are sudden deaths (Table 1).[1] More than 156 000 cardiovascular deaths occur annually before the age of 65 years, and more than half of all deaths from cardiovascular disease occur in women.[2] Coronary heart disease is a major cause of morbidity and mortality in women beyond their middle to late 50s.[3] It has been estimated that almost 5 million years of potential life in people aged less than 75 years are lost annually in the United States because of cardiovascular disease (Fig 2).

Death rates from cardiovascular diseases have been declining over the past several decades[2,4] (Fig 3). From 1980 to 1990 the age-adjusted death rate from coronary heart disease fell 32.6% and from stroke, 32.4%. Advances in medical treatment and healthier lifestyles have undoubtedly played a role, but there remains much room for progress.[4] In 1990, 5.2 million people were hospitalized with a first-listed discharge diagnosis of cardiovascular disease, 2 million with a discharge diagnosis of coronary heart disease, and approximately 675 000 with a diagnosis of acute myocardial infarction (MI).[1] Forty-five percent of all heart attacks occur in people under age 65.[2] According to 1990 statistics, an estimated 6.2 million Americans have significant coronary heart disease. Many

of these people are at increased risk for sudden death or MI. Approximately two thirds of sudden deaths due to coronary disease take place outside the hospital and usually occur within 2 hours after onset of symptoms.[2,5-10] Figure 4 provides a visual display of some of these data and demonstrates the importance of early recognition and early access for ECC.

Thus, sudden death related to coronary artery disease (CAD) is the most prominent medical emergency in the United States today. It is possible that a large number of these deaths can be prevented by rapid entry into the EMS system, prompt provision of CPR, and early defibrillation.[11-16] In addition, many victims of drowning, electrocution, suffocation, and drug intoxication most likely could have been saved by the prompt initiation of CPR and early use of advanced life support (ALS). The prompt application of ALS techniques in the neonatal period

Table 1. Estimated Deaths in the United States Due to Cardiovascular Diseases, 1990

Type of Cardiovascular Disease	No. of Deaths	%
Heart attack	489 171	52.8
Stroke	144 088	15.6
High blood pressure	32 618	3.5
Rheumatic fever and rheumatic heart disease	6018	0.6
Other	254 184	27.4

From the National Center for Health Statistics and the AHA.

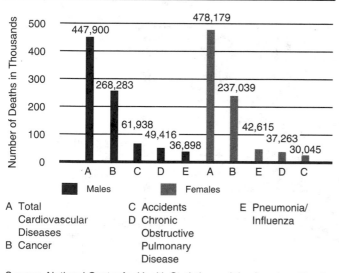

A Total Cardiovascular Diseases
B Cancer
C Accidents
D Chronic Obstructive Pulmonary Disease
E Pneumonia/Influenza

Source: National Center for Health Statistics and the American Heart Association.

Fig 1. Leading causes of death, males and females, United States, 1990 final mortality.

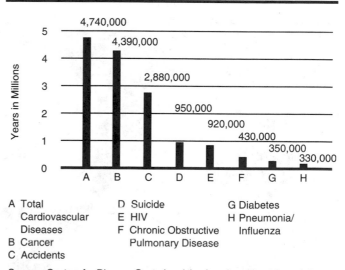

A Total Cardiovascular Diseases
B Cancer
C Accidents
D Suicide
E HIV
F Chronic Obstructive Pulmonary Disease
G Diabetes
H Pneumonia/Influenza

Source: Centers for Disease Control and the American Heart Association.

Fig 2. Estimated years of potential life lost before age 75, by cause of death, United States, 1990 estimates.

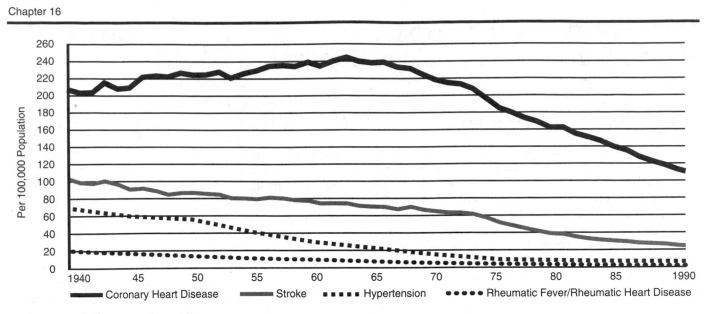

Age-Adjusted to 1940 U.S. population and to the 6th Revision ICDA.

Source: National Center for Health Statistics and the American Heart Association.

Fig 3. Age-adjusted death rates for major cardiovascular diseases, United States, 1940–1990.

promises not only to save lives but, by avoiding brain damage, also to prevent lifetimes of suffering and economic drain.

Trauma is the major cause of death and debility in the pediatric and young adult population (ages 1 to 44 years).[17-19] The emphasis on trauma prevention in the pediatric programs will educate a large segment of the lay public in injury prevention.

Prospects for the Future

Since the majority of sudden deaths caused by cardiac arrest occur before hospitalization, it is clear that the community must be recognized as "the ultimate coronary care unit."[20] The CPR-ECC programs have been and will continue to be valuable resources for teaching the community methods to control the morbidity and mortality from coronary heart disease and preventable accidents. These programs should incorporate education in primary prevention, including risk factor detection and modification and signals of impending cardiovascular events, and secondary prevention, aimed at preventing sudden cardiac death and MI in patients known to have coronary heart disease. It is clear that CAD and other forms of atherosclerotic vascular disease are supported by community nutritional patterns, prosmoking messages

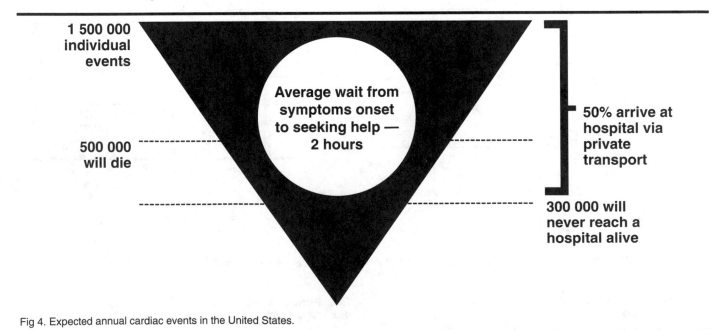

Fig 4. Expected annual cardiac events in the United States.

delivered to children, and cultural, social, and media pressures that mold unhealthy behaviors and lifestyles. Persuasive data argue in favor of aggressive community action. Educators, legislators, and business must be challenged first to declare commitment and then follow with visible, measurable actions. Optimal resources necessary for the primary prevention of atherosclerotic disease have been defined.[21]

Risk Factor Modification

Age-adjusted mortality from coronary heart disease, stroke, and other cardiovascular diseases has declined dramatically from the mid-1960s to 1989. The decline has averaged approximately 2% to 3% annually.[4,22-26] Among these declines, that of coronary heart disease mortality has had the greatest impact on life expectancy. However, it is important to recognize that as the population ages, total heart disease continues to climb.

Many factors have contributed to the decline in cardiovascular disease mortality: heightened public awareness, improved cardiovascular diagnosis and therapy, use of drugs with a cardioprotective effect by persons at high risk, improved revascularization techniques, improved and more aggressive ECC, and modification of cardiovascular risk factors in the population.

Reduction of risk factors at a young age can have the greatest impact. Nevertheless, intervention later in life must not be ignored, since preventive measures have been shown to slow the progression of and even reverse arterial disease and can be expected to reduce morbidity and mortality as well. Clearly some risk factors cannot be changed. These include heredity, gender, race, and age. Major risk factors that can be changed or modified include cigarette smoking, hypertension, elevated cholesterol levels, elevated triglyceride levels, lack of exercise, obesity, stress, and diabetes.

Patients at High Risk

Persons at high risk for cardiovascular disease because of diabetes mellitus, family history of premature cardiovascular disease, and prior MI must be made aware that their risk may be significantly increased if they have other risk factors, such as hypertension, hyperlipidemia, or cigarette smoking. Reduction of risk can be expected with regular exercise and weight control. Control or elimination of those factors amenable to change may be expected to contribute substantially to risk reduction in this group. Thus, in addition to treatment it is important that clinicians teach CPR to families of patients at high risk and stress the importance of improving risk factor status.

The following statements about atherosclerosis and risk factors should be given the broadest possible publication and promotion:

- Cardiac arrest and MI are, in the vast majority of cases, end points in the evolution of atherosclerotic arterial disease over a period of decades.

- The rate of progression of atherosclerosis is the primary determinant of the age at which MI and sudden death occur.
- The rate of progression can be significantly influenced by specific conditions and behaviors referred to as risk factors.
- Control or elimination of risk factors can be established by positive health attitudes and behaviors in the young.
- Modification of cardiovascular risk factors in adults, even those who have had an MI, can alter the rate of progression of arterial disease and reduce the incidence of major end points, ie, sudden death, MI, and stroke.
- Early recognition of cardiac symptoms and prompt intervention including CPR are everyone's responsibility, and education in these subjects should be widely available.

Millions of persons, both lay and professional, have been trained in CPR-ECC. Strong prevention messages delivered during CPR training may have as great an impact on cardiovascular mortality and morbidity as the teaching of emergency measures themselves. Many millions more need to be encouraged to obtain CPR training. Through community education and prevention, CPR training may serve as an effective means of controlling CAD. This aspect of CPR training requires more attention.

The goals of teaching the community to function as the ultimate coronary care unit include

- A lay public educated to recognize the symptoms of a possible MI and to seek prompt entry of the victim into the EMS system
- A lay public trained to support the life of the cardiac arrest victim until ACLS becomes available
- A lay public educated in the importance of early ACLS and eager to support an effective EMS system in the community
- Recognition and reduction of reversible risk factors among the population with known CAD (secondary prevention)
- A business community that measures success by the effect of its products and services on the well-being of the community
- Recognition and reduction of reversible risk factors among the population free of clinical manifestations of CAD, especially the young (primary prevention)

Efforts to accomplish these goals are already under way in many areas. Scientific knowledge of the pathogenesis of CAD and mechanisms of sudden cardiac death has greatly increased in recent years. Knowledge of the methods and importance of primary and secondary prevention of CAD is becoming more widespread. The layperson should consider learning CPR a responsibility to family, loved ones, and self.

The Responsibility to the Future

The value and cost-effectiveness of the CPR-ECC effort must continue to be monitored to justify the substantial effort and resources that volunteers and sponsoring agencies invest in it. Studies relating dollars spent to lives saved have been reported.[27-29] Such analyses are encouraged to improve CPR-ECC programs and help them reach their goal. The goal of CPR-ECC programs is to increase the number of persons reached and adequately trained, thereby increasing the number of lives saved by prevention, risk factor modification, and emergency intervention, and to do so at the most efficient cost.[30] Improving the efficacy of emergency cardiac intervention and the outcome for victims of cardiopulmonary arrest requires aggressive implementation and research.

The most important link in the CPR-ECC system in the community is the layperson. The success of ECC depends on laypersons' understanding the importance of early recognition and early activation of the EMS system and on their willingness and ability to initiate effective CPR promptly.

Lifesaving BLS at this level can be considered a public, community responsibility. The medical community, however, has the responsibility to provide leadership in educating the public and to support community education and training. Such education should include targeting higher risk populations, such as aging spouses and families of heart patients. Clinicians should accept the special challenge to recruit patients' families to become awareness experts, positive peer pressure and role models, and well-informed, well-trained interventionists.

ECC should be an integral part of a total communitywide emergency medical care system. Each system should be based on local community needs for patient care and available resources and be consistent with regional, state, and national guidelines. The success of such a system requires participation and planning to ensure operational and equipment compatibility within the system and between adjacent systems. The community must be willing to fund the program it develops, review its efficacy, and expect continuing improvement. The initial planning of a system can be done by a local advisory council on emergency services charged with assessing community needs, defining priorities, and arranging to meet those needs with available resources. Critical evaluation of operating policies, procedures, statistics, and case reports must be the continuing responsibility of the medical director. Operational activities must be evaluated against adopted protocols. Evaluation of skills of trained personnel, whether based in or out of the hospital, must be conducted on a regular schedule. Continuing education programs that prevent deterioration of necessary skills must be developed.

The ECC segment of a communitywide emergency system is best provided through a stratified system of coronary care:

- Level 1: ECC units, including basic and advanced *fixed* ECC units and basic and advanced *mobile* ECC units capable of defibrillation[31,32]
- Level 2: emergency care units, coronary care units, and intermediate care units capable of thrombolytic therapy[33,34] and intensive care
- Level 3: tertiary care centers capable of coronary revascularization and other necessary interventions

Ensuring Effectiveness of Communitywide Emergency Cardiac Care

Many clinicians, administrators, and researchers now recognize the need to improve the total ECC system to improve patient survival. An effective chain of survival is required to save victims of out-of-hospital cardiac arrest (Fig 5).[31] Communities must identify weaknesses in the ECC system, implement modifications, and optimize treatment for these critical patients.[35] Methods for achieving an effective EMS system as discussed here are Class I recommendations (definitely effective).

The central issue is whether a community's ECC system results in optimal patient survival. Achieving the optimal survival rate for out-of-hospital cardiac arrest in every community is the challenge now and in the future. However, what is optimal in one community may not be possible in all communities. Early reports of high survival in midsized cities provided the EMS prototype adopted by most communities.[36,37] The obstacles to providing care in both rural and large metropolitan areas create different challenges for EMS systems.[38] Therefore, each community will need to examine and devise its own mechanisms for achieving the goal of optimal patient survival.

Traditionally quality assurance in ECC has measured process variables. However, the emphasis of quality assurance for cardiac arrest care should be expanded to examine outcome variables in the entire ECC system.[39,40] This shift to system evaluation is necessary because a strong chain of survival is necessary for optimal outcome.[31]

The Chain of Survival

Successful survival of cardiac arrest depends on a series of critical interventions. If one of these critical actions is neglected or delayed, survival is unlikely. The AHA and others have used the term *chain of survival* to describe this sequence.[31,41] This chain has four interdependent links: early access, early basic CPR, early defibrillation, and early ACLS. The chain of survival concept underscores several principles:

- If any one link in the chain is inadequate, the result will be poor survival rates. Weakness in system components is the major explanation for variability in survival rates reported during the past 20 years.[36]

- While all links must be strong, rapid defibrillation is the single most important factor in determining survival. Unfortunately, long call-to-defibrillation intervals are common. Shorter intervals are necessary to improve survival rates.[31,35] To what degree other links contribute to optimal survival is not understood. While their positive effect is clear, we do not yet know the relative importance of bystander CPR, IV medications, or airway management, nor the importance of early versus late provision of these interventions.
- Since the chain of survival has many links, the effectiveness of a system cannot be tested by examining an individual link. Rather, the whole system must be tested. The survival rate has emerged as the "gold standard" for assessing the effectiveness of the treatment of cardiac arrest. Recently progress has been made toward providing clear methodological guide-

lines for study design, uniform terminology, and reporting of results.[36,42,43] This progress should facilitate future research on CPR and implementation of the chain of survival in each community. Evaluation of the chain of survival requires review of each link (Fig 5). (See Table 2 for definition of terms.)

The First Link: Early Access

Early access encompasses events from the patient's onset of symptoms, collapse, and the period until the arrival of EMS personnel prepared to provide care. Recognition of early warning signs, such as chest pain and shortness of breath, are key components of this link. Optimally, early access includes obtaining emergency care before the condition deteriorates into cardiac arrest. In most situations the patient is best served by calling

Table 2. Definitions and Terminology in Emergency Cardiac Care (ECC)[43]

Cardiac arrest. — Cardiac arrest is the cessation of cardiac mechanical activity. It is a clinical diagnosis, confirmed by unresponsiveness, absence of detectable pulse, and apnea (or agonal respirations).

Cardiopulmonary resuscitation (CPR). — CPR refers to attempting any of the broad range of maneuvers and techniques used to restore spontaneous circulation and respiration.

Basic CPR. — Basic CPR is the attempt to restore spontaneous circulation using the techniques of chest wall compressions and pulmonary ventilation.

Bystander CPR, layperson CPR, or citizen CPR. — These terms are synonymous; however, bystander CPR is preferred. Bystander CPR is an attempt at basic CPR provided by a person not at that moment part of the organized emergency response system.

Basic life support (BLS). — BLS is the phase of ECC that includes recognition of cardiac arrest, access to the EMS system, and basic CPR. It may also refer to the educational program in these subjects.

Advanced CPR or advanced cardiac life support (ACLS). — These terms refer to attempts at restoration of spontaneous circulation using basic CPR plus advanced airway management, endotracheal intubation, defibrillation, and intravenous medications. ACLS may also refer to the educational program that provides guidelines for these techniques.

Emergency medical services (EMS) or emergency personnel. — Persons who respond to medical emergencies in an official capacity are emergency (or EMS) personnel. The EMS system has two major functional divisions: EMS dispatchers and EMS responders.

EMS dispatchers. — EMS personnel responsible for dispatching EMS responders to the scene of a medical emergency and providing telephone instructions to bystanders at the scene while professionals are en route.

EMS responders. — EMS personnel who respond to medical emergencies by going to the scene in an emergency vehicle. They may be first responders, second responders, or third responders, depending on the EMS system. They may be trained in ACLS or BLS. All should be capable of performing defibrillation. Firefighter, first responder or emergency medical technician (EMT) usually denotes someone who has BLS training. Paramedic or EMT-P usually denotes ACLS training.

ECC system. — The ECC system refers to all aspects of ECC, including that rendered by emergency personnel. The extended ECC system also includes bystander CPR, rapid activation of the EMS system, emergency departments, intensive care units, cardiac rehabilitation, cardiac prevention programs, BLS and ACLS training programs, and citizen defibrillation.

Chain of survival. — The chain of survival is a metaphor to communicate the interdependence of a community's emergency response to cardiac arrest. This response is composed of four links: early access, early CPR, early defibrillation, and early ACLS. With a weak or missing link the result will be poor survival, despite excellence in the rest of the ECC system.

Presumed cardiac cause. — Cardiac arrest due to presumed cardiac cause is the major focus of ECC. When reporting cardiac outcome data, studies of cardiac arrest should exclude arrests due to obvious noncardiac causes. Because of practical considerations (lack of autopsy information, cost), all arrests are considered to be of cardiac cause unless an obvious noncardiac cause can be identified. Common noncardiac diagnoses that should be separated during analysis of cardiac arrest outcome include sudden infant death syndrome, drug overdose, suicide, drowning, trauma, exsanguination, and terminal states of illness.

Time intervals. — The Utstein recommendations have provided a rational nomenclature for important time intervals. Time intervals should be reported as the A-to-B interval, which represents the period that begins at time point A and ends at time point B. These are more informative than imprecise terms like "downtime" or "response time." The following terms, for example, are suggested:

911-call–to–dispatch interval. — The interval from the time the call for help is first received by the 911 center until the time the emergency vehicle leaves for the scene.

Vehicle-dispatch–to–scene interval. — The interval from when the emergency vehicle departs for the scene until EMS responders indicate the vehicle has stopped at the scene or address. This does not include the time interval until emergency personnel arrive at the patient's side or the interval until defibrillation occurs.

Vehicle-at-scene–to–patient-access interval. — The interval from when the emergency response vehicle stops moving at the scene or address until EMS responders are at the side of the patient.

Call-to-defibrillation interval. — The interval from receipt of the call at the 911 center until the patient receives the first shock.

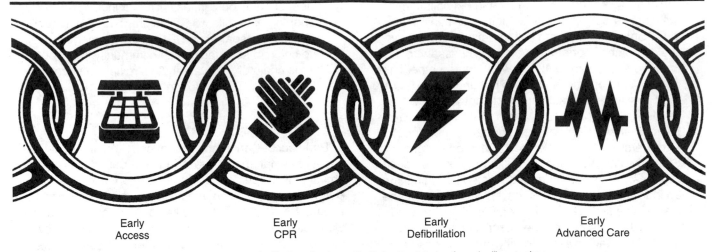

| Early Access | Early CPR | Early Defibrillation | Early Advanced Care |

Fig 5. The emergency cardiac care systems concept is displayed schematically by the "chain of survival" metaphor.

EMS support to the patient's location, avoiding the risks and delays of personal transportation.

With a cardiac arrest the major access events that must occur rapidly include

- Early identification of patient collapse by a person who can activate the EMS system
- Rapid notification (usually by telephone) of EMS dispatchers
- Rapid recognition by the dispatchers of a potential cardiac arrest
- Rapid dispatch instructions to available EMS responders (first-, second-, and third-tier EMS personnel) to guide them to the patient
- Rapid arrival of EMS responders at the address
- EMS responder arrival at the patient's side with all necessary equipment
- Identification of the arrested state

All of these must take place before defibrillation or advanced care can occur. Each event is therefore a vital part of the early access link. In most communities responsibility for these events rests with the 911 telephone system, the EMS dispatch system, and the EMS responder system.

The 911 Telephone System. In the United States, widespread use of 911 has simplified and expedited emergency assistance. Many other countries have established universal emergency telephone numbers, eg, 03 in Russia, 120 in China, and 119 in Japan. Nevertheless, many US communities lack 911 service. A recent development is the implementation of "enhanced 911" in many areas. This option automatically provides dispatchers with the caller's address and telephone number. Obtaining 911 service should be a top priority for all communities, and enhanced 911 is preferable.

The EMS Dispatch System. Rapid emergency medical dispatch has emerged as a vital part of the early access link.[44-48] Although the organization, structure, and protocols of EMS dispatchers may vary, most functions are similar.

EMS dispatchers should provide dispatcher-directed CPR. Dispatchers offer instructions to the caller on how to perform CPR until the EMS responders arrive. This method requires only 2 to 4 hours of additional dispatcher training and has been shown in controlled trials to be feasible and effective.[49,50] All EMS dispatch systems must be able to immediately answer all emergency medical calls, rapidly determine the nature of the call, identify the closest and most appropriate EMS responder unit(s), dispatch the unit(s) to the scene on average in less than 1 minute, provide critical information to EMS responders about the type of emergency, and offer telephone-assisted CPR instructions.

The EMS Responder System. The EMS responder system is usually composed of responders trained in both BLS and ACLS.[45] The system may be structured for either a one- or a multi-tier level of response.[51] Most one-tier systems use ACLS-trained (paramedic) responders, although some one-tier systems provide only BLS. Two-tier systems provide first-responder units staffed with EMTs or firefighters close to the scene,[45] followed by the second tier of ACLS responders. Two-tier systems in which the first responders are trained in early defibrillation are most effective in delivering rapid care.[37,52]

Once dispatched, EMS responders must quickly reach the site of the cardiac arrest, locate the patient, and arrive at the patient's side with all necessary equipment. Important considerations during this period are

- *EMS Travel Interval.* Communities have learned to shorten the EMS travel interval by placing response vehicles strategically and improving traffic paths. Multi-tiered systems appear to have the fastest response intervals because they have more first-responder units. Many communities report an EMS transit interval of approximately 5 minutes for first responders. This interval is too long when the goal is to provide CPR and defibrillation within 4 minutes of the call to 911. Providing rapid EMS response in rural areas, with smaller populations, remains a challenge.

- *Locating the Patient.* Few studies have noted the interval from the arrival of EMS responders at the scene to their arrival at the patient's side.[53] This interval, previously assumed to be negligible, is difficult to document because most systems have no means of recording this time.
- *Carrying the Correct Equipment.* The first EMS responders dispatched to a cardiac arrest must carry a defibrillator, oxygen, and airway management equipment.[32] They should arrive at the patient's side in less than 4 minutes from the call to 911.

The Second Link: Early CPR

CPR is most effective when started immediately after the victim's collapse. In almost all clinical studies, bystander CPR has been shown to have a significant positive effect on survival.[11,38,54-56] The one possible exception is when the call-to-defibrillation interval is extremely short.[57] Bystander CPR is the best treatment a cardiac arrest patient can receive until the arrival of a defibrillator and ACLS care.[58,59] Training in basic CPR also teaches citizens how to contact the EMS system efficiently, thus shortening the time to defibrillation. Bystander CPR rarely causes significant injury to victims, even when started inappropriately on people not in cardiac arrest.[31]

The 1992 National Conference on CPR and ECC recommended that communitywide CPR programs be developed wherever possible, including at schools, military bases, housing complexes, workplaces, and public buildings. Communities must remove any barriers that discourage citizens from learning and performing CPR. Rather, communities must proactively encourage training in the workplace and special focus on reaching the homes of those aged 50 years and over.

Although bystander CPR is unquestionably of value, it is only temporizing and loses its value if the next links (early defibrillation and early ACLS) do not rapidly follow. Communities must develop widespread CPR programs and target those groups most likely to observe cardiac arrest and thus have the opportunity to perform bystander CPR. They should also place a priority on activation of the EMS system. The dispatcher should be told "CPR is in progress." A single, unassisted rescuer with an adult victim should activate the EMS system after establishing unresponsiveness. In a pediatric arrest, the lone rescuer should activate the EMS system after initiating 1 minute of rescue support.

The Third Link: Early Defibrillation

Early defibrillation is the link in the chain of survival most likely to improve survival.[31,58-66] The placement of automated external defibrillators (AEDs) in the hands of large numbers of people trained in their use may be the key intervention for increasing the chances of survival for out-of-hospital cardiac arrest patients.[66] The AHA strongly endorses the position that every emergency vehicle that may transport cardiac arrest patients be equipped with a defibrillator and that the emergency personnel be equipped with, trained to use, and permitted to operate this device.[32] To achieve this goal, the International Association of Fire Chiefs has endorsed equipping every fire suppression unit in the United States with an AED.[67]

Several options exist for rapid defibrillation. Defibrillation can be performed with manual, automatic, or semiautomatic external defibrillators. Manual defibrillation requires interpretation of a monitor or rhythm strip. Even so, manual defibrillation by EMTs trained to recognize ventricular fibrillation improves survival.[60,61] Automatic, automatic advisory, or semiautomatic external defibrillators are also effective.[65] These devices analyze the rhythm and either automatically defibrillate or advise the operator to defibrillate. The widespread effectiveness and demonstrated safety of the AED have made it acceptable for nonprofessionals to effectively operate the device. Such persons must still be trained in CPR and the use of defibrillators. In the near future, more creative use of AEDs by nonprofessionals may result in improved survival.[31]

When EMS resources are limited, defibrillators should be given priority over many other medical devices, such as automatic transport ventilators or mobile 12-lead ECGs. The cost of defibrillators should steadily decline, permitting more to be purchased. Low-cost defibrillators for infrequent use are needed desperately. However, the price and cost of defibrillators is a product of sales volume and manufacturers' pricing. Government and the medical community must cooperate if we are to achieve healthcare cost containment, including low-cost defibrillators.

Participants in the national conference recommended that (1) AEDs be widely available for appropriately trained people, (2) all public safety units that perform CPR and first aid be equipped with and trained to operate AEDs, (3) AEDs be placed in gathering places of more than 10 000 people, and (4) legislation be enacted to allow all EMS personnel to perform early defibrillation. In addition, AEDs should be available to non–ACLS-qualified clinicians to ensure that defibrillation is available either immediately or within 1 to 2 minutes.

The Fourth Link: Early ACLS

Early ACLS provided by paramedics at the scene is the final critical link in the management of cardiac arrest. EMS systems should have sufficient staffing to provide a minimum of two rescuers trained in ACLS to respond to the emergency. However, because of the difficulties in treating cardiac arrest in the field, additional responders should be present. In systems that have attained survival rates higher than 20% for patients with ventricular fibrillation, the response teams have a minimum of two ACLS providers plus a minimum of two BLS personnel at the scene.[68] Most experts agree that four responders (at least two trained in ACLS and two trained in BLS) are the minimum required to provide ACLS to cardiac arrest victims. Although not every EMS system can attain this level of response, every system should actively pursue this goal.

The Advanced Cardiac Life Support Subcommittee and the Emergency Cardiac Care Committee of the American Heart Association recommend that all communities take the following actions to strengthen their chain of survival:

1. *Early Access*
   - All communities should implement an enhanced 911 system.
   - All communities should develop education and publicity programs that focus on cardiac emergencies and a proper response by citizens.

2. *Early CPR*
   - Communities should continue to vigorously implement and support communitywide CPR training programs.
   - Community CPR programs should emphasize early recognition, early telephone contact with the EMS system, and early defibrillation.
   - Community CPR programs should develop and use training methods that will increase the likelihood that citizens will actually initiate CPR.
   - Communities should adopt more widespread and effective targeted CPR programs.
   - Communities should implement programs to establish dispatcher-assisted CPR.

3. *Early Defibrillation*
   - All communities should adopt the principle of early defibrillation. This principle applies to all personnel who are expected, as part of their professional duties, to perform basic CPR: they must carry an automated external defibrillator and be trained to operate it.
   - Health professionals who have a duty to respond to a person in cardiac arrest should have a defibrillator available either immediately or within 1-2 minutes.
   - Responsible personnel should authorize and implement more widespread use of automated external defibrillation by community responders and allied health responders.

4. *Early Advanced Life Support*
   - Advanced life support units should be combined with first-responding units that provide early defibrillation.
   - Advanced life support units should develop well-coordinated protocols that combine rapid defibrillation by first-responding units with rapid intubation and intravenous medications by the advanced cardiac life support units.

Putting It All Together

The best way to evaluate the strength of the chain of survival is to assess the survival rates achieved by the system. The cost of data collection for a system may be considerable. However, it is only through evaluation that systems can improve their services. Therefore, participants in the national conference strongly endorsed the position that all ECC systems assess their performance through an ongoing evaluation process. For evaluation data to be meaningful, it is necessary to compare EMS systems. This, in turn, requires standardized definitions and terms of reference. Until recently, uniform terminology has not been available, producing a cardiac arrest Tower of Babel.[36] Reported survival rates in the literature range from 2% to 44%. It is not yet understood whether these profound variations are due to differences in population, treatment protocol, system organization, rescuer skills, response times, or reporting practices.

There is now international consensus on the importance of using standard terminology and methods to evaluate survival and the chain of survival.[43] Clear, unambiguous terminology has been created, a uniform method of reporting data has been established, and methods for cardiac arrest research have been improved.[36,42,43] Improving the ECC system, however, first requires an accurate measurement of the survival rate for each community. This can be achieved by implementing the following recommendations:

- Develop an evaluation process in every ECC system.
- Include an accurate assessment of survival rate using standardized nomenclature and reporting methods. This focus on quality improvement should identify practical goals given the structure and demographic characteristics of the local system; identify current performance, including the survival rate; identify gaps between goals and current performance; identify strategies to improve system performance; and evaluate whether performance improves with these modifications.
- Design the evaluation specifically to benefit the local community. As a secondary interest, information should be shared regionally and nationally to help other communities develop optimal systems.
- In assessments of survival, integrate into EMS systems evolving concepts of consensus terminology, data collection, system description, and CPR research methods.

Performing the Outcome Assessment: The Chain of Providers

The chain of survival model suggests an important dynamic to consider when performing an EMS system evaluation. It implies a chain of providers to treat victims of cardiac arrest. This chain of providers should also perform the system evaluation. The long-term goal is not merely to collect data but to improve the ECC system. All members of the chain of providers must be represented in the outcome assessment team because the assessment will naturally evolve into the improvement process.

The outcome assessment team should have representatives from health departments, EMS systems, police departments, hospitals, universities, industry, and organizations active in BLS and ACLS training. Often a nonpartisan organization like the AHA can facilitate the genesis of this diverse team and provide an umbrella over the work to be done. A representative team should assess the chain of survival, including all interested providers in the process, and identify (1) current performance, (2) community-specific goals, (3) gaps between current performance and goals, (4) ways to improve the ECC system, and (5) whether performance improves after modifications. This process of continuing quality improvement should be a long-term, ongoing effort in every community.

Design of Cardiac Arrest Studies

When developing a chain of survival assessment, the process of working together may be as important as scientific results. For example, EMS personnel may feel threatened by the review process. Paramedics may question why administrators wish to collect information on how long it takes to defibrillate, or dispatchers may think they are being singled out for scrutiny. Hospitals provide much of the outcome data, but they are also reluctant to undergo outside scrutiny. In reality local politics cannot be separated from the assessment. Most concerns, however, can be addressed, and the effort can move forward if the team represents all providers. Each community must develop its own assessment project to evaluate its chain of survival.

Summary

Cardiac arrest treatment continues to evolve. Adequate treatment of the individual patient requires that the whole ECC system function smoothly, consistently, and rapidly. To maximize communitywide survival rates, a careful evaluation of the entire chain of survival is required, using standard measurements of performance. The challenge for the next decade is to establish this infrastructure and to conduct multicenter, prospective, controlled clinical trials to better define the key factors that will improve survival of cardiac arrest in every community.

References

1. *Morbidity and Mortality Chartbook on Cardiovascular, Lung and Blood Diseases 1990*. Bethesda, Md: National Heart, Lung, and Blood Institute; 1990.
2. *1993 Heart and Stroke Facts Statistics*. Dallas, Tex: American Heart Association; 1992.
3. Kannel WB. Metabolic risk factors for coronary heart disease in women: perspective from the Framingham Study. *Am Heart J.* 1987;114:413-419.
4. Goldman L, Cook EF. The decline in ischemic heart disease mortality rates: an analysis of the comparative effects of medical interventions and changes in lifestyle. *Ann Intern Med.* 1984;101:825-836.
5. Bainton CR, Peterson DR. Deaths from coronary heart disease in persons 50 years of age and younger: a community-wide study. *N Engl J Med.* 1963;268:569-575.
6. Kuller L, Lilienfeld A, Fisher R. Sudden and unexpected deaths in young adults: an epidemiological study. *JAMA.* 1966;198:248-252.
7. Kuller L, Lilienfeld A, Fisher R. Epidemiological study of sudden and unexpected deaths due to arteriosclerotic heart disease. *Circulation.* 1966;34:1056-1068.
8. McNeilly RH, Pemberton J. Duration of last attack in 998 fatal cases of coronary artery disease and its relation to possible cardiac resuscitation. *Br Med J.* 1968;3:139-142.
9. Gordon T, Kannel WB. Premature mortality from coronary heart disease: the Framingham Study. *JAMA.* 1971;215:1617-1625.
10. Carveth SW. Eight-year experience with a stadium-based mobile coronary care unit. *Heart Lung.* 1974;3:770-774.
11. Cummins RO, Eisenberg MS. Prehospital cardiopulmonary resuscitation: is it effective? *JAMA.* 1985;253:2408-2412.
12. Shu CY. Mobile CCUs. *Hospitals.* 1971;45:14.
13. Kuller L, Cooper M, Perper J. Epidemiology of sudden death. *Arch Intern Med.* 1972;129:714-719.
14. Pantridge JF, Geddes JS. Cardiac arrest after myocardial infarction. *Lancet.* 1966;1:807-808.
15. Pantridge JF. The effect of early therapy on the hospital mortality from acute myocardial infarction. *Q J Med.* 1970;39:621-622.
16. Grace WJ, Chadbourn JA. The first hour in acute myocardial infarction. *Heart Lung.* 1974;3:736-741.
17. Division of Injury Control, Center for Environmental Health and Injury Control, Centers for Disease Control. Childhood injuries in the United States. *Am J Dis Child.* 1990;144:627-646.
18. Guyer B, Ellers B. Childhood injuries in the United States: mortality, morbidity, and cost. *Am J Dis Child.* 1990;144:649-652.
19. Rice DP, Mackenzie EJ, and Associates. *Cost of Injury in the United States: A Report to Congress.* San Francisco, Calif: Institute for Health and Aging, University of California and Injury Prevention Center, The Johns Hopkins University; 1989.
20. McIntyre KM. Cardiopulmonary resuscitation and the ultimate coronary care unit. *JAMA.* 1980;244:510-511.
21. Kannel WB, Doyle JT, Ostfeld AM, et al. Optimal resources for the primary prevention of atherosclerotic diseases: Atherosclerosis Study Group. *Circulation.* 1984;70:155A-205A.
22. Havlik RJ, Feinleib M, eds. *Proceedings of the Conference on the Decline in Coronary Heart Disease Mortality.* Washington, DC: National Heart, Lung, and Blood Institute; 1979. US Department of Health, Education, and Welfare publication 79-1610.
23. Higgins MW, Luepker RV, eds. *Trends in Coronary Heart Disease Mortality: The Influence of Medical Care.* New York, NY: Oxford University Press; 1988.
24. Stern MP. The recent decline in ischemic heart disease mortality. *Ann Intern Med.* 1979;91:630-640.
25. Thom TJ, Kannel WB. Downward trend in cardiovascular mortality. *Annu Rev Med.* 1981;32:427-434.
26. Kannel WB. Meaning of the downward trend in cardiovascular mortality. *JAMA.* 1982;247:877-880.
27. Hallstrom A, Eisenberg MS, Bergner L. Modeling the effectiveness and cost-effectiveness of an emergency service system. *Soc Sci Med.* 1981;15C:13-17.
28. Urban N, Bergner L, Eisenberg MS. The costs of a suburban paramedic program in reducing deaths due to cardiac arrest. *Med Care.* 1981;19:379-392.
29. Ornato JP, Craren EJ, Nelson N, Smith HD. The economic impact of cardiopulmonary resuscitation and emergency cardiac care programs. *Cardiovasc Rev Rep.* 1983;4:1083-1085.
30. Montgomery WH, ed. *Program Management Guidelines.* Dallas, Tex: American Heart Association; 1983.
31. Cummins RO, Ornato JP, Thies WH, Pepe PE. Improving survival from sudden cardiac arrest: the 'chain of survival' concept: a statement for health professionals from the Advanced Cardiac Life Support Subcommittee and the Emergency Cardiac Care Committee, American Heart Association. *Circulation.* 1991;83:1832-1847.

32. Kerber RE. Statement on early defibrillation from the Emergency Cardiac Care Committee, American Heart Association. *Circulation.* 1991;83:2233.

33. American College of Cardiology/American Heart Association Task Force on Assessment of Diagnostic and Therapeutic Cardiovascular Procedures. Guidelines for the early management of patients with acute myocardial infarction. *Circulation.* 1990;82:664-707.

34. Gunnar RM, Passamani ER, Bourdillon PD, et al. Guidelines for the early management of patients with acute myocardial infarction: a report of the American College of Cardiology/American Heart Association Task Force. *J Am Coll Cardiol.* 1990;16:249-292.

35. Weaver WD, Cobb LA, Hallstrom AP, et al. Considerations for improving survival from out-of-hospital cardiac arrest. *Ann Emerg Med.* 1986;15:1181-1186.

36. Eisenberg MS, Cummins RO, Damon S, Larsen MP, Hearne TR. Survival rates from out-of-hospital cardiac arrest: recommendations for uniform definitions and data to report. *Ann Emerg Med.* 1990; 19:1249-1259.

37. Eisenberg MS, Horwood BT, Cummins RO, Reynolds-Haertle R, Hearne TR. Cardiac arrest and resuscitation: a tale of 29 cities. *Ann Emerg Med.* 1990;19:179-186.

38. Becker LB, Ostrander MP, Barrett J, Kondos GT. Outcome of CPR in a large metropolitan area: where are the survivors? *Ann Emerg Med.* 1991;20:355-361.

39. Johnson JC. Quality assurance in EMS. In: Roush WR, Aranosian RD, Blair TMH, Handal KA, Kellow RC, Stewart RD, eds. *Principles of EMS Systems.* Dallas, Tex: American College of Emergency Physicians; 1989.

40. US Agency for Health Care Policy and Research. *Medical Treatment Effectiveness Research.* Rockville, Md: Agency for Health Care Policy and Research; March 1990.

41. Newman MM. The chain of survival concept takes hold. *J Emerg Med Serv.* 1989;14:11-13.

42. Jastremski MS. In-hospital cardiac arrest. *Ann Emerg Med.* 1993; 22:113-117.

43. Cummins RO, Chamberlain DA, Abramson NS, et al. Recommended guidelines for uniform reporting of data from out-of-hospital cardiac arrest: the Utstein Style. *Circulation.* 1991;84: 960-975.

44. Clawson JJ. Emergency medical dispatching. In: Roush WR, Aranosian RD, Blair TMH, Handal KA, Kellow RD, Stewart RD, eds. *Principles of EMS Systems: A Comprehensive Text for Physicians.* Dallas, Tex: American College of Emergency Physicians; 1989.

45. Pepe PE, Almaguer DR. Emergency medical services personnel and ground transport vehicles. *Probl Crit Care.* 1990;4:470-476.

46. Curka PA, Pepe PE, Ginger VF, Sherrard RC. Computer-aided EMS priority dispatch: ability of a computed triage system to safely spare paramedics from responses not requiring advanced life support. *Ann Emerg Med.* 1991;20:446. Abstract.

47. Clawson JJ. Emergency medical dispatch. In: Kuehl AE, ed. *EMS Medical Directors' Handbook.* St Louis, Mo: CV Mosby Co; 1989: 59-90.

48. National Association of EMS Physicians. Emergency medical dispatching. *Prehosp Disaster Med.* 1989;4:163-166. Position paper.

49. Eisenberg MS, Hallstrom AP, Carter WB, Cummins RO, Bergner L, Pierce J. Emergency CPR instruction via telephone. *Am J Public Health.* 1985;75:47-50.

50. Kellermann AL, Hackman BB, Somes G. Dispatcher-assisted cardiopulmonary resuscitation: validation of efficacy. *Circulation.* 1989; 80:1231-1239.

51. Braun O, McCallion R, Fazacherley J. Characteristics of midsized urban EMS systems. *Ann Emerg Med.* 1990;19:536-546.

52. Pepe PE, Bonnin MJ, Almaguer DR, et al. The effect of tiered system implementation on sudden death survival rates. *Prehospital Disaster Med.* 1989;4:71. Abstract.

53. Campbell JC, Gratton MC, Robinson WA. Meaningful response time interval: is it an elusive dream? *Ann Emerg Med.* 1991;20:433.

54. Bossaert L, Van Hoeyweghen. Bystander cardiopulmonary resuscitation (CPR) in out-of-hospital cardiac arrest: the Cerebral Resuscitation Study Group. *Resuscitation.* 1989;17(suppl):S55-S69.

55. Ritter G, Wolfe RA, Goldstein S, et al. The effect of bystander CPR on survival of out-of-hospital cardiac arrest victims. *Am Heart J.* 1985;110:932-937.

56. Cummins RO, Eisenberg MS, Hallstrom AP, Litwin PE. Survival of out-of-hospital cardiac arrest with early initiation of cardiopulmonary resuscitation. *Am J Emerg Med.* 1985;3:114-119.

57. Troiano P, Masaryk J, Stueven HA, Olson D, Barthell E, Waite EM. The effect of bystander CPR on neurologic outcome in survivors of prehospital cardiac arrests. *Resuscitation.* 1989;17:91-98.

58. Jaffe A, ed. *Textbook of Advanced Cardiac Life Support.* Dallas, Tex: American Heart Association; 1987.

59. Standards and guidelines for cardiopulmonary resuscitation (CPR) and emergency cardiac care (ECC), part VII: emergency cardiac care units (in EMS systems). *JAMA.* 1986;255:2974-2979.

60. Cummins RO. From concept to standard-of-care? review of the clinical experience with automated external defibrillators. *Ann Emerg Med.* 1989;18:1269-1275.

61. Stults KR, Brown DD, Kerber RE. Efficacy of an automated external defibrillator in the management of out-of-hospital cardiac arrest: validation of the diagnostic algorithm and initial clinical experience in a rural environment. *Circulation.* 1986;73:701-709.

62. Weaver WD, Hill D, Fahrenbruch CE, et al. Use of the automatic external defibrillator in the management of out-of-hospital cardiac arrest. *N Engl J Med.* 1988;319:661-666.

63. Wright D, James C, Marsden AK, Mackintosh AF. Defibrillation by ambulance staff who have had extended training. *Br Med J Clin Res.* 1989;299:96-97.

64. Paris PM. EMT-defibrillation: a recipe for saving lives. *Am J Emerg Med.* 1988;6:282-287.

65. Cummins RO, Thies W. Encouraging early defibrillation: the American Heart Association and automated external defibrillators. *Ann Emerg Med.* 1990;19:1245-1248.

66. Cobb LA, Eliastam M, Kerber RE, et al. Report of the American Heart Association Task Force on the Future of Cardiopulmonary Resuscitation: special report. *Circulation.* 1992;85:2346-2355.

67. Murphy DM. Rapid defibrillation: fire service to lead the way. *J Emerg Med Serv.* 1987;12:67-71.

68. Pepe P: Advanced cardiac life support: state of the art. In: Vincent JL, ed. *Emergency and Intensive Care.* New York, NY: Springer-Verlag NY Inc; 1990:565-585.

Index

Glucagon
  in β-adrenergic blocker overdose, 10.23
  in calcium channel blocker overdose, 10.23
Glucose
  administration in childhood, 1.64
  in cerebral resuscitation, 14.3
  hypoglycemia causing neurological disorders, 10.5
  serum levels in stroke, 10.6
Good Samaritan laws, 15.7
Guedel oropharyngeal airway, 2.2

Head
  injuries in childhood, 1.63-1.64
  positioning of
    for laryngoscopy, 2.4
    for venipuncture of subclavian and internal jugular veins,
      6.8
  stabilization in cervical spine injury, 1.6
Head tilt for airway control, 2.1
  chin lft with, 1.6, 2.1
  in severe trauma, 2.6
Heart block
  atrioventricular. See Atrioventricular block
  bundle branch
    electrocardiography in, 3.14, 3.15
    in myocardial infarction, 1.57, 9.5-9.6
Heart failure
  from β-adrenergic blockers, 8.12
  amrinone in, 8.7
  furosemide in, 8.13
  management of, 1.43-1.47
  in myocardial infarction, 9.6-9.8
  nitroglycerin in, 8.10
  nitroprusside in, 8.8-8.9
Heart rates in children, 1.62-1.63, 1.65, 1.66
Heimlich maneuver
  in airway obstruction, 2.1
  in near-drowning, 10.12
Hematoma
  from arterial puncture, 12.28
  from femoral artery cannulation, 12.6
Hemorrhage
  from arterial cannulation, 12.4
    in femoral artery, 12.6-12.7
  and bleeding caused by thrombolytic agents, 8.15, 9.10
  intracranial, 1.59
  pulmonary, in pulmonary artery catheterization, 12.25
  subarachnoid, 10.2
    therapeutic measures in, 10.9
Heparin
  contraindications for, 1.53
  interaction with nitroglycerin, 8.10
  in myocardial infarction, 1.49, 1.53, 9.10
  in stroke, 10.9
His bundle, 3.23
His bundle block, electrocardiography in, 3.14, 3.15
Hospitalized patients, resuscitation and life support decisions
  for, 15.5-15.7
Hyperglycemia in stroke, 10.6
Hyperkalemia, pulseless electrical activity in, 1.21
Hypertension
  from cocaine, 10.19

  in myocardial infarction, 1.58, 9.6
  nitroprusside in, 8.8-8.9
  in stroke, 10.4
    management of, 10.6, 10.8
Hyperventilation therapy
  cerebral perfusion in, 14.2
  in intracranial pressure increase, 10.9
Hypocalcemia in myocardial infarction, 1.58
Hypoglycemia
  in childhood, 1.64
  neurological signs in, 10.5
Hypokalemia
  in digitalis toxicity, 8.8
  in myocardial infarction, 1.58, 9.3-9.4
Hypomagnesemia in myocardial infarction, 1.58, 9.3-9.4
Hypotension
  in bradycardia, 1.29
  in cardiogenic shock, 9.7
  in childhood, 1.63, 1.65-1.66
  dobutamine in, 8.6
  dopamine in, 8.3
  in hypovolemic shock, 9.8
  morphine-induced, 7.16
  in myocardial infarction, 1.58, 9.6
    right ventricular, 1.32
  from nitroglycerin, 8.11
  norepinephrine in, 8.2
  in postresuscitation period, 1.26
  in pulmonary edema, 1.41
  from streptokinase, 8.15
  in tachycardia, 1.33
  treatment algorithm for, 1.41
  in tricyclic antidepressant overdose, 10.20
Hypothermia, 1.59, 10.9-10.12
  advanced cardiac life support in, 10.10-10.12
  basic life support in, 10.10
  cerebral metabolic activity in, 14.2-14.3
  in childhood, 1.64
  defibrillation in, 1.16, 4.11
  in near-drowning, 10.12, 10.13
  pulseless electrical activity in, 1.21
  treatment algorithm for, 10.11
Hypovolemia
  in cardiac tamponade, 13.1
  hypotension and shock in, 1.40, 9.8
  management of, 1.42
  pulseless electrical activity in, 1.21
Hypoxia, pulseless electrical activity in, 1.21

Immobilization in cerebral resuscitation, 14.3
Impedance, 4.3
  transthoracic, 4.4
    and current-based defibrillation, 4.7
    defibrillation shocks affecting, 4.6
Implantable cardioverter-defibrillators, defibrillation of patients
    with, 1.16, 4.7-4.8
  and use of automated external defibrillators, 4.13
Infants, defibrillation in. See Defibrillation, in pediatric patients
Infarction
  brain. See Stroke
  myocardial. See Myocardial infarction

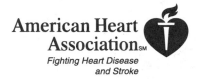

American Heart Association℠

Fighting Heart Disease and Stroke

National Center
7272 Greenville Avenue
Dallas, Texas 75231-4596
Tel 214 373 6300
Fax 214 706 1341

Keeping Up to Date in ACLS

Dear ACLS Provider:

Advances in cardiopulmonary resuscitation and emergency cardiac care are occurring so quickly that it is difficult for textbooks to remain current. The Committee on Emergency Cardiac Care of the American Heart Association is taking steps to help providers and instructors of advanced cardiac life support keep up to date.

- *Currents in Emergency Cardiac Care.* We think the most exciting and effective way to achieve this goal is through the official newsletter of the AHA and Citizens CPR Foundation, *Currents in Emergency Cardiac Care. Currents* was created to keep ECC providers up to date on advances in basic life support, pediatric advanced life support, and advanced cardiac life support. Reports on the biannual meetings of the ECC Committee and its subcommittees are published in *Currents.* Updated algorithms and treatment recommendations are published as well. *Currents in Emergency Cardiac Care* allows us to disseminate new knowledge and new ideas quickly.

  Subscribe to *Currents,* where, in addition to exciting new developments in CPR and ECC, you will find teaching tips, announcements of conferences and scientific meetings, abstracts from the world's literature, plus specific updates to the ECC Guidelines. Enclosed with this letter is an order form for *Currents.*

- *ACLS Handbook on Algorithms and Drugs for the ACLS and PALS Provider.* Already popular with ECC providers, the *ACLS Handbook* is a key tool for learning the algorithms and drugs used in emergency cardiac care. New editions of the *Handbook* will be published as additional new and useful information and changes in the guidelines become available.

We hope you will find *Currents* and the *Handbook* useful as you learn ACLS. Good luck!

Sincerely yours,

Richard O. Cummins, MD, MPH, MSc
Chairman, ACLS Subcommittee
Committee on Emergency Cardiac Care

Enclosure

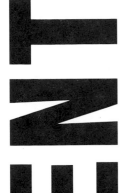

STAY CURRENT

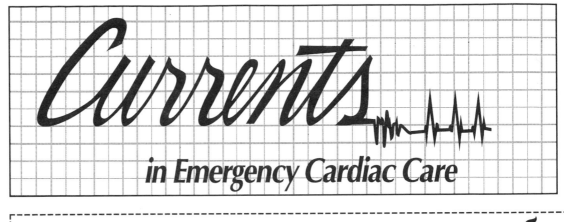

in Emergency Cardiac Care

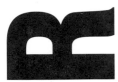 **Citizen CPR
Foundation, Inc.**

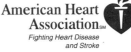 American Heart
Association℠
*Fighting Heart Disease
and Stroke*

Get to the heart of cardiac care
Make a critical decision to stay current

In this age of information overload, you need resources that keep you professionally current. CURRENTS IN EMERGENCY CARDIAC CARE saves you valuable time by getting to "the heart of the matter." It provides the most vital, up-to-date, authoritative data on CPR and ECC procedures, treatments, and guidelines in a style that's clear and concise. Each issue includes timely reports from the American Heart Association's Committee on Emergency Cardiac Care and its Basic, Advanced, and Pediatric Subcommittees as well as news on trends, developments, and innovations in emergency cardiac care from around the world.

The American Heart Association Council on Cardiopulmonary and Critical Care is an association for clinicians, scientists and emergency medical personnel interested in pulmonary circulation, lung/vascular interface and all aspects of critical care. Membership allows you to contribute your knowledge and expertise to the advancement of pulmonary, critical care and resuscitation science within the AHA as well as receive important information regarding research findings and patient education materials.

This offer expires 12/31/95

Fold here and tape at top - DO NOT STAPLE

_____YES, I want to subscribe to CURRENTS IN EMERGENCY CARDIAC CARE, the authoritative quarterly newsletter from the American Heart Association and the Citizen CPR Foundation, for only $12.00 (US) $16.00 (Non-US).

_____YES, I want to become a member of the Council on Cardiopulmonary and Critical Care for $25 per year.

_____YES, I want to become a member of the Council on Cardiopulmonary and Critical Care and receive CURRENTS IN EMERGENCY CARDIAC CARE for the special reduced price of $32 (US) or $36 (Non-US).

Please check all that apply:
- ❏ Physician
- ❏ Nurse
- ❏ EMS Personnel
- ❏ CPR/ACLS Instructors
- ❏ Pulmonary Circulation
- ❏ Anesthesiology
- ❏ Critical Care
- ❏ Cardiology
- ❏ Other _____

4ECC05/6

PRINT NAME _____ TITLE _____

ADDRESS _____

CITY _____ STATE _____ ZIP _____

COUNTRY _____ TELEPHONE _____

ADVANCE PAYMENT REQUIRED

❏ CHECK (in US currency, drawn on a US bank). If paying by check, enclose check and this card in envelope and mail to address on back.

❏ CHARGE MY: ❏ VISA   ❏ MasterCard   Exp. Date _____

Card # _____

Signature _____ Date _____

SCIENTIFIC PUBLISHING
AMERICAN HEART ASSOCIATION
PO BOX 843543
DALLAS TX 75284-3543